Liver Disease

Diagnosis and Management

Liver Disease

Diagnosis and Management

Bruce R. Bacon, M.D.

Professor of Internal Medicine
Director, Division of Gastroenterology and Hepatology
Saint Louis University School of Medicine
St. Louis, Missouri

Adrian M. Di Bisceglie, M.D.

Professor of Internal Medicine
Department of Internal Medicine
Saint Louis University School of Medicine
St. Louis, Missouri

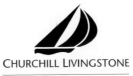

CHURCHILL LIVINGSTONE

A Division of Harcourt Brace & Company
New York   Edinburgh   London   Philadelphia   San Francisco

CHURCHILL LIVINGSTONE
A Division of Harcourt Brace & Company

The Curtis Center
Independence Square West
Philadelphia, Pennsylvania 19106

Library of Congress Cataloging-in-Publication Data

Liver disease: diagnosis & management / [edited by] Bruce R. Bacon,
Adrian M. Di Bisceglie.—1st ed.

p.   cm.

ISBN 0–443–05712–5

1. Liver—Diseases.   2. Biliary tract—Diseases.   I. Bacon, Bruce R.
II. Di Bisceglie, Adrian M. [DNLM: 1. Liver Diseases—diagnosis.
2. Liver Diseases—therapy.   3. Biliary Tract Diseases.
WI 700 L783265 2000]

RC845.L584 2000   616.3′62—dc21

DNLM/DLC   98–52043

LIVER DISEASE: DIAGNOSIS AND MANAGEMENT   ISBN 0–443–05712–5

Printed in the United States of America.

Last digit is the print number: 9   8   7   6   5   4   3   2   1

Preface

This is an exciting time for the discipline of hepatology. More and more liver diseases can now be identified and categorized and more and more treatments for liver disease have become available. For example, the use of liver biopsy has become routine, and it is now safely performed even in patients with decompensated liver disease. Sensitive and specific serologic tests for diagnosis of newly discovered viral agents have been introduced. The use of liver transplantation has provided a new lease on life for those with end-stage liver disease. The number of liver transplants done each year continues to expand rapidly. The use of interferon, ribavirin, and other nucleoside analogues has dramatically altered our management of patients with chronic viral hepatitis. As a consequence of all of these advancements and growth, the number of practitioners evaluating and caring for patients with liver disease has similarly expanded. The goal of our new textbook is to summarize these new developments and to provide an outline of the major clinical issues in hepatology for internists, gastroenterologists, and others involved in the care of these patients. We have attempted to create a "user-friendly" textbook that is easy to read with numerous illustrations and tables throughout. An international group of contributing authors takes advantage of expertise in hepatology from all corners of the globe. We hope you enjoy using *Liver Disease: Diagnosis and Management.*

Bruce R. Bacon, M.D.
Adrian M. Di Bisceglie, M.D.

This book is dedicated to our wives, Joan and Laureen, whose support and patience have allowed us to accomplish the things that we enjoy doing, including the completion of this new textbook.

Contributors

Vicente Arroyo, M.D.
Professor of Medicine, University of Barcelona Medical School; Director, Institute of Digestive Diseases, Hospital Clinic, Barcelona, Spain
Complications of Cirrhosis: Ascites, Hyponatremia, Hepatorenal Syndrome, and Spontaneous Bacterial Peritonitis

Bruce R. Bacon, M.D.
Professor of Internal Medicine; Director, Division of Gastroenterology and Hepatology, Saint Louis University School of Medicine, St. Louis, Missouri
Hereditary Hemochromatosis

John Baillie, M.B. Ch.B., F.R.C.P. (Glasgow)
Associate Professor of Medicine, Duke University Medical Center, Durham, North Carolina
Endoscopy in the Management of Biliary Tract Disorders

Alex S. Befeler, M.D.
Assistant Professor of Internal Medicine, Division of Gastroenterology and Hepatology, Saint Louis University School of Medicine, St. Louis, Missouri
Management of Bleeding Varices

Jean-Pierre Benhamou, M.D.
Professor Emeritus, Université Paris, Paris, France; Consultant, Hôpital Beaujon, Clichy, France
Disorders of the Hepatic Venous System, Peliosis, and Sinusoidal Dilatation

Henri Bismuth, M.D., F.A.C.S. (Hon.)
Professor of Surgery, Université Paris-Sud; Chairman, Centre Hépatobiliaire, Villejuif, France
Hepatobiliary Surgery

Andres T. Blei, M.D.
Professor of Medicine, Northwestern University Medical School; Attending Physician, Northwestern Memorial Hospital, Chicago, Illinois
Fulminant Hepatic Failure

Herbert L. Bonkovsky, M.D.
Professor of Medicine, Biochemistry, and Molecular Biology, University of Massachusetts Medical School; Director, Division of Digestive Disease and Nutrition; Director, The Liver, Biliary, Pancreatic Center, University of Massachusetts Memorial Health Care, Worcester, Massachusetts
The Porphyrias, α_1-Antitrypsin Deficiency, Cystic Fibrosis, and Other Metabolic Diseases of the Liver

Kyle E. Brown, M.D.
Assistant Professor of Internal Medicine, Saint Louis University School of Medicine; Staff Gastroenterologist, John Cochran Veterans Affairs Medical Center, St. Louis, Missouri
Liver Biopsy: Indications, Techniques, Complications, and Interpretation

Elizabeth M. Brunt, M.D.
Associate Clinical Professor of Pathology, Saint Louis University School of Medicine; Staff Pathologist, Saint Louis University Hospital, St. Louis, Missouri
Liver Biopsy: Indications, Techniques, Complications, and Interpretation

Robert L. Carithers, Jr., M.D.
Professor of Medicine, University of Washington School of
Medicine; Medical Director, Liver Transplantation Program; Director, Section of Hepatology, Division of Gastroenterology, University of Washington Medical Center, Seattle, Washington
Liver Transplantation: Long-Term Post-Transplant
Management

Connie L. Davis, M.D.
Associate Professor of Medicine, University of Washington
School of Medicine; Attending Staff, University of Washington Medical Center, Seattle, Washington
Liver Transplantation: Long-Term Post-Transplant
Management

Adrian M. Di Bisceglie, M.D.
Professor of Internal Medicine, Department of Internal
Medicine, Saint Louis University School of Medicine, St.
Louis, Missouri
Management of Chronic Viral Hepatitis

Charles S. Eby, M.D.
Assistant Professor of Pathology and Internal Medicine,
Saint Louis University School of Medicine; Associate Director, Saint Louis University Coagulation Consultants,
Saint Louis University Hospital, St. Louis, Missouri
Complications of Cirrhosis: Hemostatic Failure

Gregory T. Everson, M.D.
Professor of Medicine, University of Colorado School of
Medicine; Director of Hepatology, Medical Director of
Liver Transplantation, University Hospital, Denver, Colorado
Cystic Disorders of the Liver and Biliary Tree

Annie Fecteau, M.D.C.M., M.Sc., F.R.C.S.(C.)
Assistant Professor, University of Toronto; Staff Surgeon,
The Hospital for Sick Children, Toronto, Ontario, Canada
Hepatobiliary Surgery

Peter Ferenci, M.D.
Associate Professor of Medicine, University of Vienna, Vienna, Austria
Wilson's Disease

Jeff L. Fidler, M.D.
Assistant Professor of Radiology, University of Nebraska
Medical Center; Attending Staff, Nebraska Health System,
University Hospital and Veterans Affairs Medical Center,
Omaha, Nebraska
Imaging of the Liver

Lawrence S. Friedman, M.D.
Associate Professor of Medicine, Harvard Medical School;
Physician, Gastrointestinal Unit; Chief, Walter Bauer Firm
(Medical Services), Massachusetts General Hospital, Boston, Massachusetts
Evaluation of Surgical Risk in Patients with Liver Disease

Pere Ginès, M.D.
Faculty Member, Liver Unit, Institute of Digestive Diseases, Hospital Clinic, Barcelona, Spain
Complications of Cirrhosis: Ascites, Hyponatremia,
Hepatorenal Syndrome, and Spontaneous Bacterial Peritonitis

Stephanos Hadziyannis, M.D.
Professor of Medicine and Chairman, Department of Medicine, Athens University School of Medicine; Head of the
Academic Department of Medicine and the Center of Hepatology, Hippokration General Hospital, Athens, Greece
Viral Hepatitis: Clinical Features

Denise M. Harnois, D.O.
Senior Associate Consultant, Mayo Clinic Jacksonville,
Jacksonville, Florida
Primary Sclerosing Cholangitis

Mary F. Hebert, Pharm. D.
Associate Professor, Department of Pharmacy, University of
Washington School of Medicine, Seattle, Washington
Liver Transplantation: Long-Term Post-Transplant
Management

Lisa Higa, M.D.
Hepatology Fellow, Division of Digestive Diseases, University of California, Los Angeles, School of Medicine, Los
Angeles, California
Evaluation of Jaundice

Jay H. Hoofnagle, M.D.
Director, Division of Digestive Diseases and Nutrition, National Institute of Diabetes and Digestive and Kidney Diseases, National Institutes of Health, Bethesda, Maryland
Management of Chronic Viral Hepatitis

Christine G. Janney, M.D.
Professor of Pathology, Saint Louis University School of
Medicine; Director of Anatomic Pathology, Saint Louis
University Hospital, St. Louis, Missouri
Liver Biopsy: Indications, Technique, Complications, and
Interpretation

Philip J. Johnson, M.D., F.R.C.P.
Chairman, Department of Clinical Oncology, Chinese University of Hong Kong, Shatin, N.T.; Director of the Cancer
Centre, Chinese University of Hong Kong, Prince of Wales
Hospital, Shatin, N.T. Hong Kong, S.A.R.
Benign and Malignant Tumors of the Liver

J. Heinrich Joist, M.D., Ph.D.
Professor of Pathology and Internal Medicine, Saint Louis
University School of Medicine; Director, Saint Louis University Coagulation Consultants, Saint Louis University
Hospital; St. Louis, Missouri
Complications of Cirrhosis: Hemostatic Failure

Emmet B. Keeffe, M.D.
Professor of Medicine, Stanford University School of Medicine; Medical Director, Liver Transplant Program, Chief of Clinical Gastroenterology, Stanford University Medical Center, Stanford, California
Evaluation of Abnormal Liver Enzymes, Use of Liver Tests, and the Serology of Viral Hepatitis

Raymond S. Koff, M.D.
Professor of Medicine, University of Massachusetts Medical School, Worcester, Massachusetts; Chairman, Department of Medicine, MetroWest Medical Center, Framingham, Massachusetts
History and Physical Examination

Kris V. Kowdley, M.D.
Associate Professor of Medicine, University of Washington School of Medicine; Founder and Director, Iron Overload Clinic; Attending Physician, Gastroenterology/Hepatology, University of Washington Medical Center, Seattle, Washington
Liver Transplantation: Long-Term Post-Transplant Management

Stephan Krähenbühl, M.D., Pharm.D.
Associate Professor, University of Berne Medical School; Institute of Clinical Pharmacology, University of Berne, Berne, Switzerland
Drug Hepatotoxicity

Annette Kyprianou, M.D.
Clinical Instructor, Case Western Reserve University School of Medicine; MetroHealth Medical Center, Cleveland, Ohio
Portosystemic Encephalopathy

Nicholas F. LaRusso, M.D.
Professor of Medicine, Biochemistry, and Molecular Biology, Mayo School of Medicine; Chairman, Department of Internal Medicine; Consultant GI/Hepatology; Director, Center for Basic and Digestive Diseases; Consultant Biochemistry, Molecular Biology; Distinguished Investigator for Mayo Foundation, Mayo Clinic Rochester, Rochester, Minnesota
Primary Sclerosing Cholangitis

Ajit P. Limaye, M.D.
Assistant Professor of Medicine, University of Washington School of Medicine; Assistant Professor and Attending Physician, University of Washington Medical Center, Seattle, Washington
Liver Transplantation: Long-Term Post-Transplant Management

Michael R. Lucey, M.D., F.R.C.P. (I)
Associate Professor of Medicine, University of Pennsylvania School of Medicine; Associate Chief, Division of Gastroenterology; Director of Hepatology; Medical Director, Liver Transplant Program, University of Pennsylvania Hospital, Philadelphia, Pennsylvania
Liver Transplantation: Indications, Pretransplant Evaluation, and Short-Term Post-Transplant Management

Bruce A. Luxon, M.D., Ph.D.
Associate Professor of Internal Medicine, Division of Gastroenterology and Hepatology, Saint Louis University School of Medicine, St. Louis, Missouri
Anatomy and Physiology of the Liver and Biliary Tree

Michael P. Manns, M.D.
Professor of Medicine and Gastroenterology; Chairman and Director, Department of Gastroenterology of Hepatology, Medical School of Hannover, Hannover, Germany
Autoimmune Hepatitis

Paul Martin, M.D.
Associate Professor of Medicine, Division of Digestive Diseases, University of California, Los Angeles, School of Medicine; Director Hepatology, University of California Dumont Program, University of California, Los Angeles, Medical Center, Los Angeles, California
Evaluation of Jaundice

Arthur J. McCullough, M.D.
Professor of Medicine, Case Western Reserve University School of Medicine; Director of Gastroenterology, MetroHealth Medical Center, Cleveland, Ohio
Malnutrition in Cirrhosis

Klaus Mergener, M.D.
Associate in Medicine, Johannes-Gutenberg-Universität, Mainz, Germany
Endoscopy in the Management of Biliary Tract Disorders

Lisa A. Mueller, M.B., B.A.O., B.Ch.
Staff Gastroenterologist, Rhode Island Hospital, Providence, Rhode Island
Evaluation of Surgical Risk in Patients with Liver Disease

Kevin D. Mullen, M.B., F.R.C.P. (I)
Professor of Medicine, Case Western Reserve University School of Medicine; Director Hepatology Research, MetroHealth Medical Center and Cleveland Clinic Foundation, Cleveland, Ohio
Portosystemic Encephalopathy

Brent A. Neuschwander-Tetri, M.D.
Associate Professor of Internal Medicine, Division of Gastroenterology and Hepatology, Saint Louis University School of Medicine, St. Louis, Missouri
Fatty Liver, Nonalcoholic Steatohepatitis

Frederick A. Nunes, M.D.
Assistant Professor of Medicine, University of Pennsylvania School of Medicine, Philadelphia, Pennsylvania
Liver Transplantation: Indications, Pretransplant Evaluation, and Short-Term Post-Transplant Management

Kunio Okuda, M.D., Ph.D.
Professor Emeritus, Chiba University School of Medicine, Chiba, Japan
Noncirrhotic Portal Hypertension

Marco A. Olivera-Martínez, M.D.
Assistant Professor of Gastroenterology, Universidad La Salle, Mexico City, Mexico
Alcoholic Liver Disease

Kim M. Olthoff, M.D.
Assistant Professor of Surgery, University of Pennsylvania School of Medicine; Surgeon, Hospital of the University of Pennsylvania, Philadelphia, Pennsylvania
Liver Transplantation: Indications, Pretransplant Evaluation, and Short-Term Post-Transplant Management

Raoul Poupon, M.D.
Professor of Medicine, University Paris VI, Faculty of Medicine St. Antoine, Hôpital Saint-Antoine, Paris, France
Primary Biliary Cirrhosis

Renée Eugénie Poupon, Ph.D.
Directeur de Recherche, INSERM Unit 370, Faculté de Médecine Necker, Paris, France
Primary Biliary Cirrhosis

James H. Reicheld, M.D.
Instructor in Medicine, University of Massachusetts Medical School, Worcester, Massachusetts; Staff Physician, Lowell General Hospital, Lowell, Massachusetts
The Porphyrias, α_1-Antitrypsin Deficiency, Cystic Fibrosis, and Other Metabolic Diseases of the Liver

Jürg Reichen, M.D.
Professor and Chairman, Department of Clinical Pharmacology, University of Berne, Faculty of Medicine, Berne, Switzerland
Drug Hepatotoxicity

Juan Rodés, M.D.
Professor of Medicine, University of Barcelona Medical School; Director of Research, Hospital Clinic, Barcelona, Spain
Complications of Cirrhosis: Ascites, Hyponatremia, Hepatorenal Syndrome, and Spontaneous Bacterial Peritonitis

Hugo R. Rosen, M.D.
Assistant Professor of Medicine, Molecular Microbiology and Immunology, Oregon Health Sciences University; Staff Physician, Hepatology and Liver Transplant Program; Portland Veterans Affairs Medical Center and Oregon Health Sciences University, Portland, Oregon
Evaluation of Abnormal Liver Enzymes, Use of Liver Tests, and the Serology of Viral Hepatitis

Vinod K. Rustgi, M.D.
Clinical Professor of Medicine and Surgery; Medical Director, Liver Transplantation, Georgetown University Medical Center, Washington, D.C.
The Liver and Systemic Diseases

Zahid A. Saeed, M.D.
Professor of Internal Medicine, Division of Gastroenterology and Hepatology, Saint Louis University School of Medicine; Director of Endoscopy, Saint Louis University Hospital, St. Louis, Missouri
Management of Bleeding Varices

Arun J. Sanyal, M.B.B.S., M.D.
Associate Professor of Medicine, Medical College of Virginia Commonwealth University, Richmond, Virginia
Gastroesophageal Varices: Pathophysiology and Prevention of Bleeding

Steedman A. Sarbah, M.B.Ch.B.
Clinical Instructor, Case Western Reserve University School of Medicine; Gastroenterology Fellow, MetroHealth Medical Center, Cleveland, Ohio
Portosystemic Encephalopathy

Roshan Shrestha, M.D.
Associate Professor of Medicine, University of North Carolina School of Medicine; Medical Director of Liver Transplantation, University of North Carolina, Chapel Hill, North Carolina
Cystic Disorders of the Liver and Biliary Tree

David D. Stark, M.D.
Professor and Chairman, Department of Radiology, University of Nebraska Medical Center; Attending Staff, Nebraska Health Systems, University Hospital; Veterans Affairs Medical Center, Omaha, Nebraska
Imaging of the Liver

Rise Stribling, M.D.
Assistant Professor, Baylor College of Medicine; Medical Director of Liver Transplantation, The Methodist Hospital, Houston, Texas
Evaluation of Jaundice

Grace L. Su, M.D.
Assistant Professor of Medicine, University of Michigan School of Medicine; Staff Physician, University of Michigan Hospitals, Ann Arbor, Michigan
Liver Disease and Pregnancy

Dominique Valla, M.D.
Professor, Université Paris, Paris, France; Head, Hôpital Beaujon, Clichy, France
Disorders of the Hepatic Venous System, Peliosis, and Sinusoidal Dilatation

Rebecca Van Dyke, M.D.
Professor of Medicine, University of Michigan School of Medicine; Staff Physician, University of Michigan Hospitals; Ann Arbor Veterans Affairs Hospital, Ann Arbor, Michigan
Liver Disease and Pregnancy

Russell H. Wiesner, M.D.
Professor of Medicine, Mayo School of Medicine, and Medical Director of Liver Transplantation, Mayo Clinic Rochester, Rochester, Minnesota
Primary Sclerosing Cholangitis

Rowen K. Zetterman, M.D.
Professor, Department of Medicine, University of Nebraska Medical Center; Chief, Medicine Department, Veterans Affairs Medical Center, Omaha, Nebraska
Alcoholic Liver Disease

Contents

Normal Hepatic Function

Chapter

1

Anatomy and Physiology of the Liver and Biliary Tree

Bruce A. Luxon

OVERVIEW

The liver is a unique organ anatomically located to serve its dual role as a metabolic and biochemical transformation factory. The liver receives blood containing substances absorbed or secreted by the gastrointestinal organs including the pancreas, intestine, stomach, and spleen. The liver uses these substances as raw materials and modifies them or synthesizes completely new chemicals. These are then returned to the bloodstream or to bile for excretion.

On a cellular level, the liver allows maximal interaction between the blood and liver cells. In its unique design, liver cells are organized into cell plates, each plate being formed by one-cell-thick cords, which are surrounded by blood vessels (sinusoids). The perfusion of these sinusoids is unidirectional, proceeding from the portal tract to the hepatic venule. The specialized capillaries found in the sinusoids have large fenestrations, which allow free exchange between plasma and the extracellular space. Because blood flow proceeds sequentially down the length of the sinusoid, hepatocytes located in different positions along these cell plates contain differing amounts of enzymes and thus have distinct functional capabilities. As blood traverses the liver from its entry point at the portal inlet to its exit at the hepatic vein, the composition of sinusoidal blood is modified by removal and addition of compounds.

In this chapter, we describe the basic elements of the organization of the liver and emphasize how these elements determine its unique physiology. The anatomic organization of the liver is described first, concentrating on the gross anatomy of the liver, biliary system, and the blood vessels that supply both venous and arterial blood to the liver. The structure of the liver lobule is then described, and emphasis is placed on the concept of the liver cell plate. Included in this section is a description of the nonparenchymal cells:

endothelial cells, Kupffer cells, stellate cells, and pit cells. These nonparenchymal cells contribute to normal liver function in various important roles both in health and following hepatic injury. The remaining section deals with the functional organization of the cell plate, with emphasis on the uptake of compounds from plasma into hepatocytes, their metabolism and biotransformation.

ANATOMIC ORGANIZATION

The liver is the largest gland in the human body and accounts for approximately 2.5% of total body weight. In the adult, the liver weighs almost 1500 g. The liver is divided into four lobes. The left and right lobes are separated by the falciform ligament (Fig. 1–1). These lobes are supplied by the right and left branches of the portal vein and the hepatic artery. Bile is drained from the liver by the left and right hepatic ducts. The right lobe is further divided into two smaller lobes: the quadrate and the caudate. On occasion, the lower border of the right lobe may extend inferiorly to form a Riedel lobe.

The falciform ligament separates as it proceeds superiorly. There is, therefore, a segment on the superior surface of the liver that is devoid of this peritoneal covering. This is the so-called "bare area" (Fig. 1–2). Besides this peritoneal covering, the entire liver is covered by a thin connective tissue capsule (Glisson's capsule). This capsule completely surrounds the liver and consists of collagen fibers with accompanying small blood vessels. This capsule is thickest near the porta hepatis and the inferior vena cava. Strands of Glisson's capsule arborize to form a fine supporting network for the hepatic parenchyma. However, the only connective tissue within the liver lobule is the reticular network. These fibers presumably support the liver lobule and may

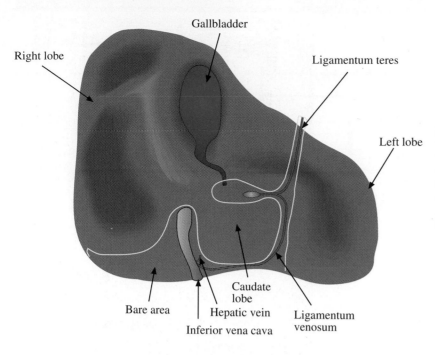

Figure 1–1
Diagram of the visceral surface of the liver. This view demonstrates the gallbladder in its position inferior to the liver. Also note the so-called "bare area" next to the inferior vena cava. An "H" pattern is formed by the ligamentum teres, ligamentum venosum, gallbladder, and inferior vena cava.

function to maintain sinusoidal blood flow. It is thought that these fibers are formed by hepatic stellate cells. After hepatic injury, these cells may produce increased amounts of collagen leading to the fibrosis seen in various disease states.

The blood supply to the liver is unique because it has a dual source. The portal vein carries the majority (75%) of the afferent blood volume to the liver. The remaining 25% is supplied by the oxygen-rich blood from the hepatic artery. These two vessels, along with their accompanying connective tissue, enter the liver through the porta hepatis. The porta hepatis is the area where the blood vessels enter and bile ducts leave the liver. It is contained in folds of the hepatoduodenal ligament. The vessels quickly arborize into smaller branches and ultimately form the blood channels of the liver (sinusoids).

The gallbladder serves as a reservoir for bile. It is located on the undersurface of the right lobe. In healthy humans, it may hold 30 to 50 mL of bile when fully distended. In its contracted state, it has numerous rugae, similar to those found in the stomach. Layers of smooth muscle form a muscularis that is fairly elastic. The serosal surface consists of numerous collagen fibers, blood vessels, and lymphatics as well as nerves from the autonomic nervous system.

Arterial blood reaches the gallbladder by the cystic artery. In almost three out of four humans, the cystic artery arises from the right hepatic artery. However, there is considerable anatomic variation in the origin of the cystic artery. The cystic artery can arise from the hepatic artery proper (6%), the left hepatic artery (3%), the gastroduodenal artery (3%), or from an accessory right hepatic artery (13%). Regardless of its origin, the artery divides into a su-

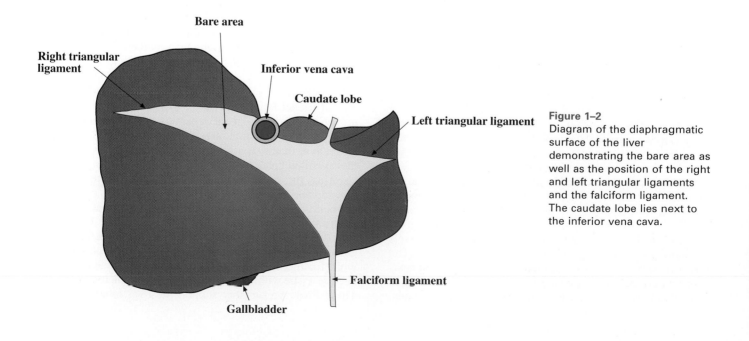

Figure 1–2
Diagram of the diaphragmatic surface of the liver demonstrating the bare area as well as the position of the right and left triangular ligaments and the falciform ligament. The caudate lobe lies next to the inferior vena cava.

perficial branch that supplies the serosal surface and a deep branch that supplies the interior layers of the gallbladder wall. The cystic vein drains the gallbladder and the cystic bile duct and ends in the right branch of the portal vein.

The neck of the gallbladder terminates in the cystic bile duct. This duct is approximately 4 cm long, and its walls contain numerous nerve cells. A series of folds form the "spiral valves." The cystic duct joins the common hepatic duct and forms the common bile duct. As the common bile duct passes through the duodenal wall, it is surrounded by the sphincter of Oddi. The components of the sphincter of Oddi regulate flow of bile and pancreatic enzymes into the duodenum.

LIVER LOBULE STRUCTURE

Liver Cell Plate

Histologic units within the liver parenchyma have been appreciated since the late 1600s. Most modern textbooks of histology provide detailed descriptions of two primary models of the organization of the liver lobule. These are the classic lobule and the liver acinus. These two models describe

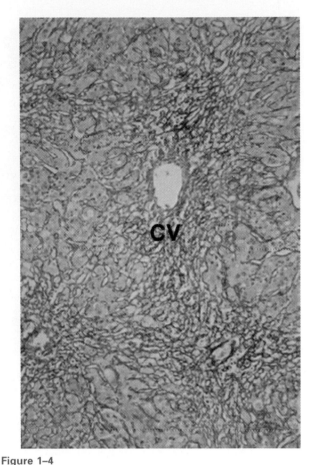

Figure 1–4
Photomicrograph of human liver demonstrating zone 3 hepatocyte damage due to acetaminophen. (CV, central vein.) (Photograph courtesy of E. Brunt, MD.)

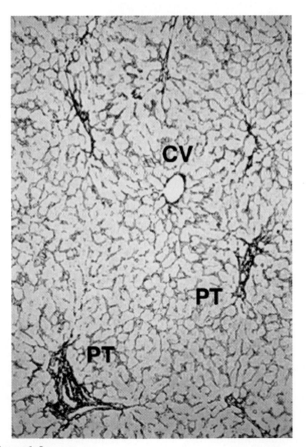

Figure 1–3
Photomicrograph of a normal human liver biopsy. The first 5 to 10 hepatocytes comprise the "periportal" region. Periportal sinusoids are interconnected and relatively narrow. The "perivenular" portion of the liver cell plate is the distal two thirds. Sinusoids in this region (zone 3) are wide and relatively straight as they drain into the hepatic vein. (CV, central vein; PT, portal triad.) (Photograph courtesy of E. Brunt, MD.)

the identical hepatic structure and are merely different interpretations of hepatic organization.

The classic lobule contains liver tissue with boundaries made by connective tissue. These are most prominent in nonhuman species such as the pig. The typical appearance is that of a hexagon with portal triads at the corners of the hexagon. In the center of the hexagon is the central vein. The liver cell plates radiate from the central vein to the portal triads, which are located at the circumference of the lobule. The lobulation in humans appears less well defined with no sharp demarcation between lobules owing to a paucity of connective tissue.

In the pioneering work of Rappaport, the organizational unit of the human liver was defined as an acinus. In this model, three concentric zones surround the portal triad (Fig. 1–3). Zone 1 cells are defined as those closest to the afferent blood vessels and are, therefore, the first in the sinusoid to receive blood. Cells in zones 2 and 3 are located at progressively greater distances from the afferent blood vessels, and thus these cells receive relatively oxygen-poor blood. These cells are the ones that are most likely to be damaged by ischemia (Fig. 1–4).

In both of the models, the key anatomic feature is the liver cell plate (Fig. 1–5), which consists of a group of 15 to 30 hepatocytes organized as a plate that is one cell thick. At one end of the plate, the afferent blood vessels are located in a portal tract. The other end consists of the central vein. Blood enters the liver sinusoid through the portal tract via

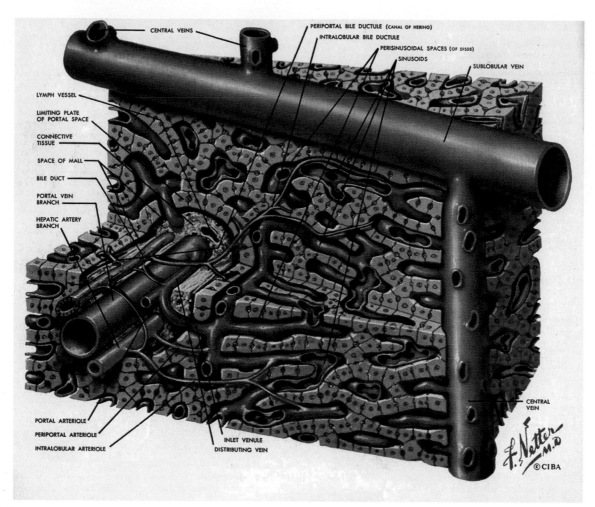

Figure 1–5
Classic view of the liver lobule. The central vein is on the right of the figure, draining the chords of hepatocytes. About the periphery of the lobule are portal areas consisting of branches of the portal vein, hepatic artery, and bile duct (From Netter F. In Oppenheimer, E [ed]: Digestive System: Liver, Biliary Tract and Pancreas, Vol 3, Part III. New York: CIBA Pharmaceutical Products, 1957, p 8. Copyright 1957. Novartis. Reprinted with permission from *The Netter Collection of Medical Illustrations, Vol. 3, Part 3,* illustrated by Frank H. Netter, M.D. All rights reserved.)

the portal vein and hepatic arteriole. Blood from these vessels empties into the hepatic sinusoids and flows unidirectionally along the liver cell plate. As it exits the cell plate, it empties into the central vein. Bile flows in the opposite direction to the blood, thus forming a countercurrent system similar to that in the kidney.

Nonparenchymal Liver Cells

The liver contains various different cells, each with distinct functions. Classically, liver cells are divided into parenchymal cells (hepatocytes) and nonparenchymal cells (Fig. 1–6). These latter cell types have only recently been extensively characterized and their various functions identified. This group of nonparenchymal cells includes endothelial cells, Kupffer cells, hepatic stellate cells, and pit cells. The nonparenchymal cells constitute only 6.3% of the liver volume but almost 35% of the total number of liver cells. Of the nonparenchymal cells, endothelial cells comprise 2.8% of the liver volume; 2.1% are Kupffer cells; 1.4% are hepatic stellate cells; and 0.2% are pit cells. Each type of cell has evolved special characteristics that allow the cells to

perform key roles both in normal liver function and liver injury. This section describes how endothelial cells, hepatic stellate cells, Kupffer cells, and pit cells contribute to normal hepatic function and what is emerging about their role in liver diseases.

Sinusoidal Endothelial Cells

In order for the liver to function as a major metabolic factory, there must be rapid and full exchange between the blood and liver cells. This requires special features within the sinusoidal endothelium to ensure such permeability (Fig. 1–7). In addition to allowing rapid exchange of both large and small molecules between sinusoidal plasma and the hepatocyte surface, sinusoidal endothelial cells have an important filtration role, selectively removing denatured and damaged proteins before they are presented to hepatocytes. The endothelial cells, when seen on electron microscopy, have a flattened profile. Rather than form a continuous boundary of the sinusoid, small gaps that are 1000 Å in diameter are found in the endothelial cell cytoplasm. These gaps, known as fenestrae, occur in patches and allow pro-

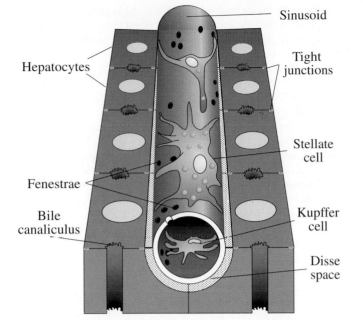

Figure 1–6
A schematic of a liver sinusoid. Hepatocytes surround the sinusoid forming thick plates that are 1 cell thick. Nonparenchymal cells are in close proximity to the sinusoid. Fenestrae allow solutes, including proteins, to permeate freely into the space of Disse. Bile canaliculi are located between pairs of hepatocytes. Tight junctions prohibit the passage of fluid and solutes from the space of Disse into the bile canaliculi. (Modified from Roll F, Friedman S: Role of sinusoidal endothelial cells, hepatic stellate cells, Kupffer cells, and pit cells. In Kaplowitz N [ed]: Liver and Biliary Diseases, 2nd ed. Baltimore: Williams & Wilkins, 1996, p 34.)

teins to move freely from the sinusoidal plasma into the space of Disse. The space of Disse varies in size and contains microvilli from hepatocytes that protrude into the sinusoidal lumen through the fenestrae. It is clear from scanning electron micrographs that the endothelial lining is not

a barrier between blood plasma and the space of Disse. It is also thought that hepatic lymph is formed in the extracellular space of Disse from excess water, solutes, and lipoproteins.

The fenestrae in the sinusoidal endothelial cells are responsible for the enhanced permeability seen in hepatic sinusoids. These pores occur in clusters called sieve plates. They do not have a diaphragm in contrast to the fenestrae found in other organs. They appear to be regulated by cytoskeletal filaments and respond to a variety of external signals both in the plasma and the extracellular matrix. It is unclear what tissue specific factors such as cytokines may be important in modulating the number and function of the fenestrae. Increased sinusoidal pressure and hypoxia cause the fenestrae to enlarge, whereas norepinephrine and serotonin cause acute contraction. Alcohol and other hepatotoxins cause a chronic decrease in the number of fenestrae.

Marked changes occur in the sinusoidal endothelial cells in response to liver injury (Fig. 1–8). All of these yield reduced endothelial permeability. The most striking feature is that the number of fenestrae is greatly decreased. In addition, a true continuous basement membrane forms beneath the endothelium. The space of Disse becomes filled with collagen bundles, thus further reducing the access of solutes to liver cells. This so-called "capillarization of sinusoids" has functional implications that have been documented using multiple indicator dilution curves in cirrhotic human and rat livers. This change in sinusoidal permeability leads to impaired liver clearance of solutes and appears to be irreversible.

Sinusoidal Endothelial Cell Filtration

Besides forming a permeable barrier for solutes, sinusoidal endothelial cells perform an important scavenger function. They bind a remarkable number of soluble compounds and remove specially designated proteins. The majority of the removal is controlled by receptor-mediated endocytosis. Pinocytosis and phagocytosis also remove larger particles,

Figure 1–7
Sinusoidal endothelial cells provide an important barrier to larger molecules such as chylomicrons. Fenestrae have a diameter of approximately 100 nm and exclude large chylomicrons. Smaller molecules permeate into the space of Disse and reach the microvilli of hepatocytes. (Modified from Roll F, Friedman S: Role of sinusoidal endothelial cells, hepatic stellate cells, Kupffer cells and pit cells. In Kaplowitz N [ed]: Liver and Biliary Diseases, 2nd ed. Baltimore: Williams & Wilkins, 1996, p 36.)

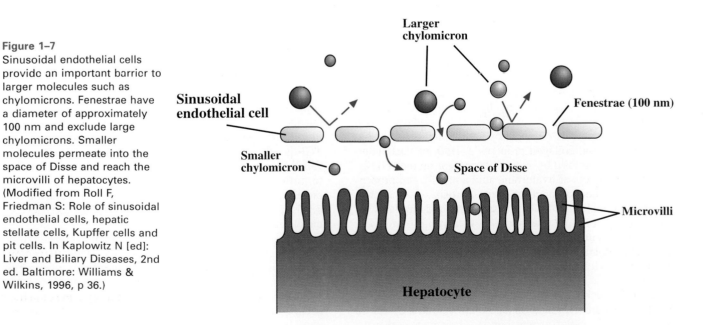

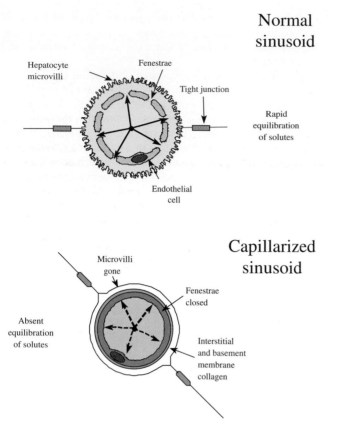

Normal sinusoid

Hepatocyte microvilli

Fenestrae

Tight junction

Rapid equilibration of solutes

Endothelial cell

Capillarized sinusoid

Microvilli gone

Fenestrae closed

Absent equilibration of solutes

Interstitial and basement membrane collagen

Figure 1–8

A normal sinusoid *(top)* has multiple fenestrae allowing rapid equilibration of solutes from the plasma into the space of Disse. Solutes reaching the space of Disse are exposed to hepatocyte microvilli. Normal sinusoids lack a basement membrane. A "capillarized" sinusoid *(bottom)* prohibits the rapid equilibration of solutes. A basement membrane formed of collagen is apparent and fenestrae are absent. Hepatocytes lose their microvilli, thus decreasing the surface area for absorption. (Modified from Roll F, Friedman SA: Role of sinusoidal endothelial cells, hepatic stellate cells, Kupffer cells, and pit cells. In Kaplowitz N [ed]: Liver and Biliary Diseases, 2nd ed. Baltimore: Williams & Wilkins, 1996, p 37.)

forming vesicles that eventually become degradative lysosomes.

The majority of receptor-mediated endocytosis is directed at the removal of waste compounds such as denatured collagens, glycosaminoglycans, aldehyde-modified proteins, and modified low-density lipoproteins. All of these compounds are destined for lysosomal degradation. Two important compounds removed by endothelial cells are hyaluronic acid and collagen propeptide. Both of these compounds are recognized by a specific receptor on the cell surface. Serum levels of hyaluronic acid and collagen propeptide are elevated in ongoing liver fibrosis. It is unclear whether the inability to clear these compounds initiates the fibrogenic process or whether it is merely an end result. Similarly, it is unclear if the cytotoxic products seen in liver inflammation lead to damaged endothelial cells.

Kupffer Cells

Kupffer cells are liver macrophages that were first described by Kupffer in 1876. Current thinking, however, is that the cell actually described by Kupffer is the hepatic stellate cell. Kupffer cells are currently described as cells that have phagocytic activity and are located along the lining of the sinusoid.

Kupffer cells are difficult to identify by light microscopy alone, and proper identification rests on using immunohistochemical techniques. Kupffer cells can most easily be recognized by their characteristic peroxidase reaction. This stains the endoplasmic reticulum, the perinuclear cisternae, and the lysosomes. Kupffer cells take up ^{99m}Tc sulfur colloid as demonstrated in liver spleen scans. Kupffer cells also can be identified by their phagocytic capacity. Research techniques involving phagocytosis of latex beads or formalin-fixed fluorescently labeled staphylococci have been used to identify Kupffer cells. Therefore, the cytoplasm of Kupffer cells often contains cellular debris intermixed with degradative lysosomes.

Kupffer cells account for 2.1% of the nonparenchymal cells on a volume basis. Electron scanning microscopy of liver sinusoids demonstrates a pronounced concentration gradient of Kupffer cells from zones 1 to 3. Besides the increased density in zone 1, Kupffer cells appear larger and have more phagocytic activity than do zone 3 cells. This acinar gradient positions the majority of Kupffer cells to efficiently remove unwanted organisms from the proximal part of the sinusoid.

The origin of Kupffer cells in the liver has remained controversial. Two current theories are that Kupffer cells are derived from circulating monocytes or by local self-perpetuation. Studies using human liver transplantation samples have demonstrated that the Kupffer cell population acquires the genotype of the recipient several months after transplantation. This observation would suggest that the Kupffer cells come from circulating monocytes. Other studies using mouse macrophages have demonstrated that Kupffer cells are generated from promonocyte-like precursors, under the control of macrophage colony-stimulating factor-1.

Whatever the source of Kupffer cells, it is clear that they are markedly decreased in cirrhosis. It has been speculated that cirrhosis causes portosystemic shunting of cytokines, decreasing the Kupffer cell population. The loss of Kupffer cells may lead to the increased susceptibility to infections in cirrhosis due to bacteria in the portal vein.

Kupffer cells, like hepatic stellate cells and macrophages in the other parts of the body, undergo activation. Under the influence of numerous biologic mediators, they become stimulated and continue their phagocytic role. When stimulated, they secrete numerous products, including cytokines, fibronectin, prostaglandins, platelet activating factor, and TGF-β. Kupffer cells are also subject to a phenomenon called "blockade." In blockade, Kupffer cells fail to respond to further stimulation and may even stop functioning completely. This is a reversible process and may contribute to sepsis with gut organisms that would otherwise be efficiently removed by Kupffer cells.

In normal conditions, portal vein blood is sterile. However, in bacteremia, the liver and spleen efficiently remove as much as 95% of the bacteria entering these organs. This is done primarily by Kupffer cells in the liver. In cirrhosis or in other conditions where shunting of blood around the liver occurs, there is impaired clearance of bacteria. In addition, those bacteria that are internalized by Kupffer cells may not be eradicated. Based on animal studies, the bactericidal capacity of the macrophages in cirrhosis is dramatically diminished. Thus, Kupffer cells may provide a sequestered site in which bacteria will temporarily elude host defenses, only to emerge later after the Kupffer cells die.

In addition to clearing bacteria from portal blood, Kupffer cells also function to remove viruses during viremia. During viral hepatitis in humans, Kupffer cells undergo hyperplasia. Each of the hepatitis viruses (A, B, and C) has been identified in Kupffer cells during chronic as well as acute infection. It is unclear whether the cleared viruses are actually destroyed. In some examples, Kupffer cells may serve as a reservoir for the virus, thus extending the period of viremia.

Finally, Kupffer cells are the primary site of endotoxin removal. Endotoxin circulates systemically during sepsis caused by gram-negative bacteria. Initial studies suggested that Kupffer cell uptake of endotoxin was beneficial. However, recent studies have suggested that endotoxin-mediated Kupffer cell release of tumor necrosis factor (TNF-α) may contribute to the lethal shock of sepsis. Studies on ameliorating the effect of TNF-α release caused by endotoxin are currently ongoing. Whether this effect can be blocked clinically remains to be determined. TNF-α release is also seen during ischemia-reperfusion injury. Kupffer cells appear to participate in the early phase of reperfusion injury.

Hepatic Stellate Cells

The biology of hepatic stellate cells has become the topic of intense investigation. However, the knowledge of the existence of the cells dates to 1876, when Kupffer identified these cells using a gold chloride histochemical technique. Confusion about their phagocytic capabilities continued to exist in the literature until 1951 when Ito suggested that hepatic stellate cells and Kupffer cells (as we now know them) were separate cell populations. Hepatic stellate cells are now known to represent a discrete population of nonparenchymal cells. Their most characteristic feature is that their cytoplasm contains large amounts of retinoids. They can be readily identified by the natural fluorescence of these vitamin A–like compounds.

Despite comprising only about a third of the nonparenchymal cells, hepatic stellate cells are recognized to play an important role in fibrogenesis in various liver diseases. The unique morphology and ultrastructure of hepatic stellate cells have allowed their identification and isolation. In a normal liver, they are located primarily in the periportal region of sinusoids, closely approximating the endothelial cells. Hepatic stellate cells have been shown to be contractile, and it has been proposed that they could regulate sinusoidal blood flow both in a normal or injured liver. As mentioned previously, hepatic stellate cells contain retinoid droplets. These are primarily perinuclear, especially in the "resting" hepatic stellate cell. Stellate cells contain prominent amounts of cytoskeletal elements. Desmin and α-smooth muscle actin are two proteins that have been used to characterize stellate cells.

Vitamin A and Stellate Cells

Hepatic stellate cells contain approximately 95% of the body's store of retinoids. The transport of retinoids from dietary sources to the liver has been well characterized. Dietary retinoids are absorbed from the intestine and transported in chylomicrons primarily in the ester form. These esters are subsequently taken up by receptor-mediated endocytosis into hepatocytes. Subsequently, retinol is formed by hydrolysis of the ester within endosomes. The retinol is transferred to hepatic stellate cells, and the retinol is re-esterified. The ester is then stored in cytoplasmic droplets as mentioned earlier. The mobilization of retinoids is essentially the reverse of the aforementioned process, using retinol-binding protein for secretion into the blood.

The control of retinoid transport is less well defined. Retinol-binding protein as well as the cellular retinol-binding proteins have both been shown to regulate the release of retinol esters. In addition, the amount of retinoid stored may control hepatic stellate function and modulate their response to cytokines from Kupffer cells or their response to changes in the extracellular matrix.

Fibrosis and Hepatic Stellate Cells

There is a growing body of literature that suggests that hepatic stellate cells, like other nonparenchymal cells, may undergo "activation" when the liver is injured. For hepatic stellate cells, this "activation" involves the transition from a resting cell to one that is predominantly a protein-secreting cell. During this activation, the hepatic stellate cell loses its vitamin A stores, develops receptors to various cytokines and proteins, and begins to secrete type I collagen. While they are activated, hepatic stellate cells express several smooth muscle markers.

Recent research has demonstrated that hepatic stellate cells are the major producers of the collagen found in cirrhosis. While the resting stellate cell produces small amounts of collagen types III and IV, the activated cell produces primarily collagen type I but also collagen III, IV, VI, fibronectin, hyaluronic acid, and other proteins. This matrix deposition by hepatic stellate cells seems to occur regardless of the type of liver injury and has been documented in human illnesses including viral and alcoholic hepatitis, hemochromatosis, and hypervitaminosis A.

In addition to vitamin A storage and matrix protein synthesis, hepatic stellate cells perform several other roles in humans. They express erythropoietin, hepatocyte growth factor, colony-stimulating factor, and epidermal growth factor. The role that hepatic stellate cells play in the biology of these compounds is an area of current research. Finally, recent studies have demonstrated that hepatic stellate cells may function in the regulation of blood flow to sinusoids. Hepatic stellate cells undergo contraction when stimulated by several mediators and may regulate blood flow to individual sinusoids as well as causing whole organ shunting in cirrhosis.

Pit Cells

Pit cells are the most recently recognized group of cells of the nonparenchymal cell types. They are also known as natural killer (NK) cells. They are generally found within the sinusoidal lumen and are fairly rare cells, being only about 20% as numerous as Kupffer cells. Their name is attributable to the first description by Wisse, when they were noted to have dense granules in their cytoplasm that resembled pits. In contrast to Kupffer cells, pit cells are nonphagocytic and do not have any endogenous peroxidase activity. Their identification relies on characteristic antigens that they express. All pit cells express OX-8 antigens just as NK cells do. However, unlike NK cells in the blood, pit cells do not express the T cell antigen OX-19.

The knowledge of the function of pit cells is rapidly emerging. Current evidence suggests that pit cells are part of the liver's antitumor defense. This is based on studies in which pit cells were observed to lyse lymphoma cells and cancer cells in culture. This is in the absence of other cells, such as Kupffer cells. There exists a large body of experimental evidence using both human and animal cell lines, which suggests that NK cells provide an important barrier in tumor defense. Recent evidence has also documented the accumulation of pit cells in viral hepatitis in humans. It is unclear whether pit cells are able to destroy virus-infected hepatocytes. Current thinking suggests that they may play a role both in the clearance of hepatotropic viruses as well as in tissue rejection after orthotopic liver transplantation.

HEPATOCYTE TRANSPORT

Electrolyte and Solute Transport

One of the principal functions of the liver is bile formation. There is a great deal of information regarding the mechanism by which individual hepatocytes extract electrolytes and solutes from the plasma, transport them across the plasma membrane, and excrete them into bile. Numerous transport mechanisms are associated with the sinusoidal plasma membrane. Specific transporters have been identified to facilitate the uptake of hydrophilic bile acids, amino acids, and organic anions such as sulfobromophthalein. All of these transporters rely on the potential difference maintained across the hepatocyte membrane (-35 mV) and the inward sodium concentration gradient (12 mM) (Fig. 1–9).

Amino acids are transported by at least eight different membrane proteins. These are traditionally grouped as follows: system A (neutral amino acids), system ASC (neutral amino acids containing -OH or -SH), system Z (dicarboxylic amino acids), system N (histidine, glutamine, and asparagine), and system gly (glycine). Each of these systems is affected by hormonal regulation, fasting, stereospecificity, and the electrogenic state of the hepatocyte.

Bile acids also enter hepatocytes by specific transporters located on the sinusoidal plasma membrane. Most studies have supported a sodium-coupled transporter for most of the bile acids found in humans. The hydrophobic unconjugated bile acids are transported more efficiently than are conjugated trihydroxy bile acids. This suggests that some bile acids may partition into the lipid bilayer, without the need for a specific energy dependent pump.

The liver transports a variety of organic anions other than bile acids. Historically, bilirubin and sulfobromophthalein have been studied the most extensively. These two compounds seem to compete for a common transporter. It is

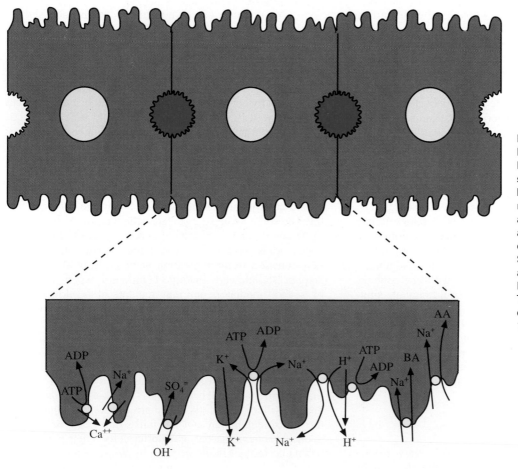

Figure 1–9
Multiple transport proteins have been identified in the sinusoidal plasma membrane. Each of these transporters relies on the sodium gradient and provides uptake of bile acids, amino acids, and organic anions. (Adapted from Scharschmidt B: Bile formation and cholestasis. In Zakim D, Boyer T [eds]: Hepatology: A Textbook of Liver Disease, 2nd ed. Philadelphia: WB Saunders, 1990, p 310.)

known that hydrophobic drugs share the transport system with bilirubin. This finding may explain the pronounced hyperbilirubinemia seen in clinical conditions, because the transporter is either overwhelmed by other organic anions or is displaced from the plasma membrane.

Bile Formation

The purpose of bile formation by the liver is two-fold: bile formation represents an important route of excretion for substances that have been extracted from plasma, metabolically altered by the liver, and excreted into bile. Bilirubin is a classic example. The second major function of bile is to aid in the absorption of lipids and fat-soluble substances. The bile acids are uniquely suited for this function.

The chemical composition of human hepatic bile varies relatively little. Human bile contains sodium (143 to 165 mEq/L), potassium (2.5 to 6 mEq/L), chloride (83 to 119 mEq/L), HCO_3^- (12 to 55 mEq/L), bile acids (3 to 45 mM), calcium (2.5 to 6.4 mg/dL), and protein (30 to 300 mg/dL). Bile is isosmotic with plasma having an osmolality of approximately 300 mOsm/kg.

Bile formation begins with hepatocytes actively secreting bile acids and electrolytes. Inorganic solutes, including bilirubin and various hydrophobic drugs, are also excreted into bile. Current evidence suggests that water follows by passive diffusion maintaining the isosmotic status with plasma. In the bile ducts, canalicular bile is further modified with secretion of water and electrolytes (especially sodium and bicarbonate). During storage in the gallbladder, water and electrolytes are reabsorbed (Fig. 1–10). The exact contribution of secretion and the absorption by the canalicular cells is unclear, owing to the technical difficulty of measuring the chemical composition of bile in the canaliculi.

FUNCTIONAL ORGANIZATION OF THE LIVER CELL PLATE

The organization of liver tissue centers around the individual liver cell plate. The cell plate is formed along a single sinusoid by a layer of hepatocytes, one cell thick, and comprises 15 to 30 hepatocytes. The plate extends from the portal space to the hepatic venule. Because each hepatocyte is approximately 30 μm across, the average length of a cell plate is approximately 500 μm. In addition to the hepatocytes, nonparenchymal cells also line the sinusoids.

In this section, liver function that is performed within the liver cell plate is discussed, concentrating on the design of the liver cell plate and how it affects hepatic function. Several features make this design unique. The unidirectional flow of plasma along the liver cell plate allows functional compartmentation to develop. Because of this, cells exposed to blood near the portal inlet are in contact with the highest concentration of incoming solutes, including oxygen. These cells are primarily responsible for the uptake of toxic compounds, whereas cells farther downstream are more active in the secretion of metabolic byproducts. Thus, as the plasma flows from its portal inlet to its hepatic outlet, its composition is modified. This leads to a dramatic difference in the microenvironment surrounding each hepatocyte and leads to a variety of injury patterns that are well documented in clinical practice.

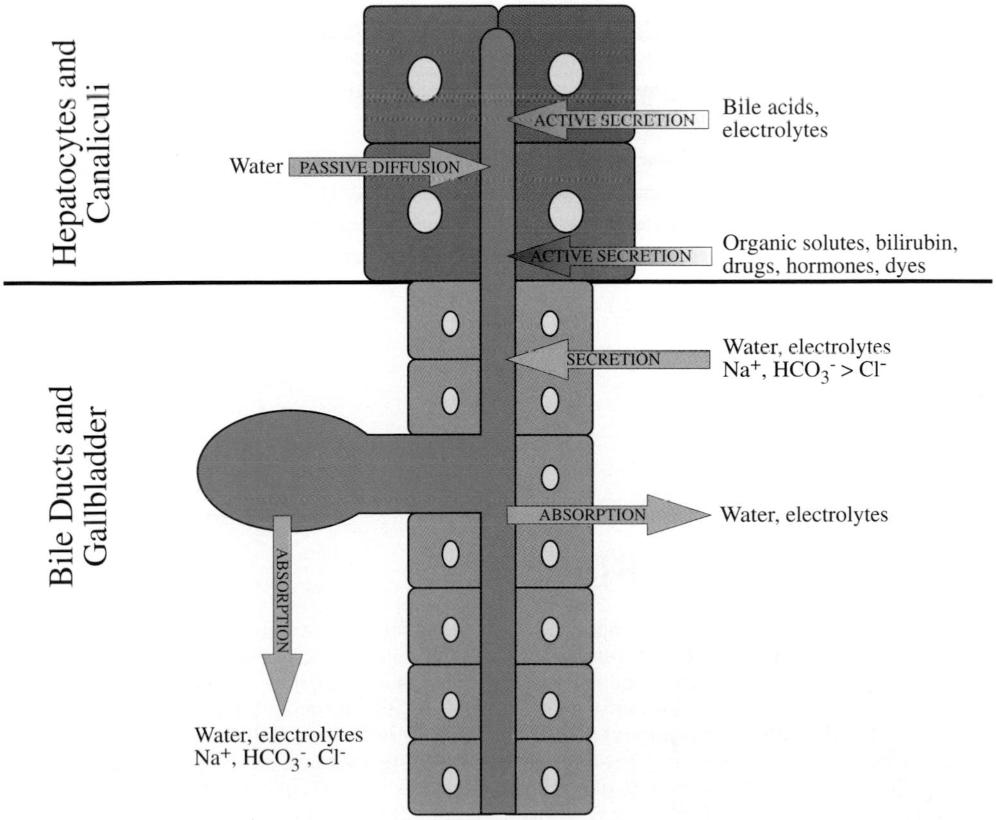

Figure 1–10
Bile formation involves the active transport of electrolytes, bile acids, and organic solutes such as bilirubin. Water follows passively into the canaliculi (top). Bile is modified in the bile ducts and gallbladder by secretion and subsequent absorption of electrolytes and water. (Modified from Scharschmidt B: Bile formation and cholestasis. In Zakim D, Boyer T [eds]: Hepatology: A Textbook of Liver Disease, 2nd ed. Philadelphia: WB Saunders, 1990, p 316.)

Limiting Plate

The limiting plate is defined as the row of hepatocytes that surrounds the portal space. It is from this location in the liver cell plate that bile leaves the hepatocytes that formed it. Bile moves along the liver cell plate in bile canaliculi and moves in a countercurrent direction compared with blood flow. Scanning electron microscopy has shown that bile canaliculi are approximately 1 μm in diameter. As they leave the liver cell plate, the bile canaliculi form bile ductules (canals of Hering). The bile ductules are formed by cuboidal cells, which form a duct that is 1 to 3 μm in diameter. As these canaliculi combine, they form an ampulla that is located at the junction of the limiting plate and the portal space. Bile flow along the bile ductule is enhanced by biliary cilia (7 to 15 μm), which run in the direction of bile flow. The bile ductules then form bile ducts as the bile leaves the limiting plate and proceeds into the biliary system.

Hepatocyte Heterogeneity Along the Liver Cell Plate

Along the liver cell plate, hepatocytes in general appear histologically uniform. However, when examined on a morphologic or histochemical basis, hepatocytes exhibit marked heterogeneity. This heterogeneity (also called zonation) is manifested by cells located in the periportal zone that differ from those downstream in the perivenous zone. Hepatocytes demonstrate zonation with respect to key enzymes, cell receptors, subcellular structures, and cell matrix interaction (Fig. 1–11). The heterogeneity is expressed by activation of the cellular genome in response to various inputs, including concentration gradients in hormones, oxygen, metabolic substrates, and neural input.

In the 1960s and 1970s, it became clear that there was a zonal organization for specific groups of enzymes and the concept of "metabolic zonation" became popular. In the original model of metabolic zonation, only two zones of equal size were defined. Later, as the concept of zonation became more prevalent, the periportal and perivenous compartments were subdivided into a proximal and distal part creating four zones.

Zonation of Specific Metabolic Pathways

Numerous experimental approaches using perfused livers, isolated hepatocytes, and hepatocyte cultures have been used to study differences in the metabolic specialization of hepatocytes. There are clear zonal differences in the metabolism of carbohydrates, amino acids and ammonia, and

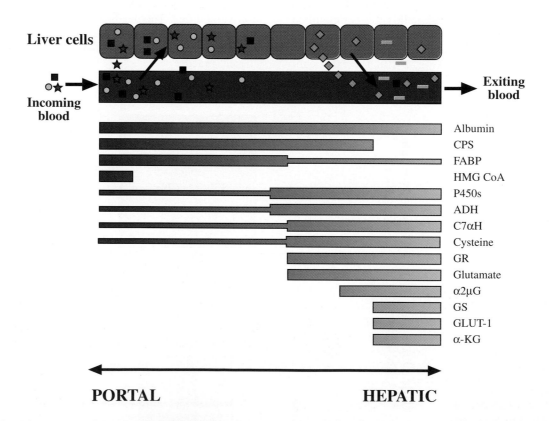

Figure 1–11

Sinusoidal blood flow composition changes as incoming solutes are removed by liver cells *(top)*. As solutes are taken up by hepatocytes, their concentration decreases. "Perivenular" plasma contains increased concentrations of material that have been secreted by zone 3 hepatocytes. Hepatic gene expression along the liver cell plate *(bottom)*. The 20 to 30 hepatocytes lining the liver sinusoid contain varying amounts of key enzymes. (CPS, carbamoyl phosphate synthetase; FABP, fatty acid–binding protein; HMG CoA, 3-hydroxy-3-methylglutaryl [HMG] coenzyme A reductase; P-450s, cytochromes of the P-450 family; ADH, alcohol dehydrogenase; C7αH, cholesterol 7 α-hydroxylase; Cysteine, cysteine transporter; GR, glucagon receptor; Glutamate, glutamate transporter; α2μG, α2μ-globulin; GS, glutamine synthetase; GLUT-1, glucose transporter; α-KG, α-ketoglutarate transporter.) (Modified from Gumucio J, Berkowitz C, Webster S, et al: Structural and functional organization of the liver. In Kaplowitz N: Liver and Biliary Diseases, 2nd ed. Baltimore: Williams & Wilkins, 1996, pp 9 and 11.)

Table 1–1   Heterogeneity of Hepatocyte Metabolism and Biotransformation

Periportal (Zone 1) Cells			Pericentral (Zone 3) Cells		
Physiologic Function	Metabolic Function	Enzyme Involved	Physiologic Function	Metabolic Function	Enzyme Involved
Oxidation		Succinate dehydrogenase			
Glucose formation	1. Gluconeogenesis 2. Glucose from glycogen 3. Glycogen from pyruvate	Glucose-6-phosphatase Phosphoenol-pyruvate carboxykinase	Glucose uptake	1. Glycolysis 2. Glycogen from glucose 3. Glycogen to pyruvate	Glucokinase
Urea formation	Urea from amino acid nitrogen and from NH_3	Carbamoyl phosphate synthetase	Glutamine formation		
Protective metabolism	1. Glutathione peroxidation 2. Glutathione conjugation	Glutathione peroxidase Glutathione level	Xenobiotic metabolism	1. Monooxygenation 2. Glucoronidation	Cytochrome P-450 UDP-glucuronosyltransferase
Plasma protein synthesis		Albumin α_2-Macroglobulin Fibrinogen	Plasma protein synthesis		α-Fetoprotein Angiotensinogen α_1-Antitrypsin
Cholesterol synthesis	Hydroxymethyl glutaryl-coenzyme A reductase				
Bile formation	Taurocholate uptake carrier Bile acid export carrier				

UDP, uridine diphosphate.

fatty acids. Bile formation as well as the metabolism of xenobiotics all demonstrate zonation. In the next sections, we present a brief overview of the current understanding of the zonation of each of these pathways (Table 1–1).

Carbohydrate Metabolism

Zonation of carbohydrate metabolism is divided into two phases: absorptive and postabsorptive phase. During the absorptive phase, glucose is primarily taken up by the perivenous cells. In these cells, it is used to synthesize glycogen. Following replacement of glycogen stores, glucose is converted to lactate and released into the hepatic veins. Lactic acid is then taken up by the periportal cells, where it is used as a substrate for gluconeogenesis. This concept is consistent with the observation that glycogen stores are refilled first in the perivenous hepatocytes whereas glycogen degradation starts periportally.

In the postabsorptive phase, glycogen is degraded to glucose in the periportal hepatocytes. As the glucose proceeds down the sinusoid, it is taken up by perivenous cells and degraded to lactate. Lactate is again released into the circulation, and, if unused by the peripheral circulation, it is used as a substrate for gluconeogenesis by periportal cells.

Fatty Acid Metabolism

The zonation of fatty acid metabolism is less pronounced than that described for carbohydrate metabolism. Perivenous cells appear to synthesize preferentially very low density lipoprotein, whereas periportal cells perform β-oxidation and ketogenesis. Fatty acid–binding protein, the chief intracellular transport protein for long chain fatty acids, is located predominantly in periportal cells. It is unclear whether the presence of this intracellular carrier promotes the preferential β-oxidation and ketogenesis seen in periportal cells. 3-Hydroxy-3-methylglutaryl coenzyme A (HMG-CoA) reductase is located almost exclusively in periportal cells.

Amino Acid and Ammonia Metabolism

Nutrient proteins in the form of amino acids are supplied to hepatocytes via the portal vein. Periportal cells preferentially convert the NH_3 to urea. If the quantity of ammonia presented to the periportal region is sufficient to escape ureagenesis, perivenous hepatocytes take up the NH_3 and convert it to glutamine. Glutamine is then released into the systemic circulation and returned to periportal cells, where again the NH_3 is preferentially formed into urea. The periportal and perivenous systems have different kinetics with the periportal system being a high-capacity, low-affinity pathway and the perivenous pathway having a high affinity but a low capacity. Work using perfused livers has demonstrated that the removal of ammonia in periportal cells (urea synthesis) is restricted to incoming ammonia concentrations higher than 50 μM and that glutamine synthesis in the perivenous cells occurs at concentrations of ammonia below 50 μM.

Zonation of Xenobiotic Metabolism

The cytochrome P-450 system is responsible for the metabolism of many xenobiotics. This process often involves monooxygenation followed by conjugation with either glucuronic or sulfuric acid. Sulfate formation predominates in periportal cells, whereas glucuronide formation is the major conjugation reaction in perivenous cells. The monooxygenation also occurs preferentially in the perivenous zone, leading to the formation of potentially toxic electrophiles. The perivenous zone, therefore, is predisposed to the toxicity of reactive oxygen intermediates. The combination of this predilection as well as the decreased ability of the cell to detoxify oxygen intermediates by glutathione leads to the perivenous necrosis caused by some hepatotoxins.

Regulation of Hepatocyte Heterogeneity

It is generally assumed that hepatocyte zonation develops as a consequence of the heterogeneity in the microenvironment of individual cells. This is controlled by various signals such as substrate concentration (including oxygen), hormones, neuromediators, nerves, and cell-to-biomatrix interactions. The differential expression patterns seen in the zonation may be attributed to different rates of mRNA transcription, mRNA degradation, mRNA translation, or end-protein degradation.

The expression of the genes for the enzymes of gluconeogenesis is regulated at the pretranslational level. Similarly, the amino acid metabolizing enzymes are regulated at the pretranslational level. Each of these alterations in gene expression occurs during a normal feeding rhythm. In contrast, glycolytic enzymes appear to be regulated mainly at the post-translational level during a normal feeding pattern. Each of these generalities regarding the regulation of zonal gene expression may change depending on the nutritional conditions.

Ammonia detoxification also appears to be regulated at the pretranslational level. Both the mRNA and the proteins of the key ureagenic enzymes are located exclusively in the periportal cells. In contrast, the mRNA and the protein for glutamine synthesis are located exclusively in parenchymal cells in the distal perivenous area. Neither these mRNA nor the enzyme levels themselves seem to vary with the nutritional state, suggesting that the organism needs to maintain tight control over ammonia despite external influences.

Physiologic Significance of Hepatocyte Heterogeneity

The pattern of organization described earlier indicates the complexity of the liver's ability to respond to a large variety

of input and output solute concentrations and the overall metabolic demands of the organism. Two control elements seem to dictate the degree of zonal responses: the sequential delivery of substrates and the zonal patterns of gene expression. Because of the unidirectional perfusion of the liver acinus, periportal cells are exposed to a high concentration of incoming solutes. Solutes using transport systems that have a great capacity for uptake (NH_3 and bile acids) are preferentially taken up by the first hepatocytes that they encounter. Refluxed material or substances escaping uptake by periportal cells are subsequently presented to "downstream" cells. The removal of ammonia, either as urea or by glutamine synthesis, is an example of this complexly controlled system. Each of these systems allow minute adjustments in the outflow concentration of substances of a splanchnic origin as well as new products formed by the synthetic machinery of the liver.

In summary, the zonation of hepatocytes allows the liver acinus to accomplish the regulation of substrate production and the metabolism of proteins and hormones in a dynamic fashion. Zonation appears to depend on the unidirectional perfusion of substrates as well as on basic gene expression by hepatocytes. Each of these control mechanisms is dynamic, responding to the overall needs of the organism.

SUGGESTED READINGS

Arias IM: The biology of hepatic endothelial cell fenestrae. Prog Liver Dis 9:11–26. 1990.

Blouin A, Bolender R, Weibel E: Distribution of organelle and membranes between hepatocytes and nonhepatocytes in the rat liver parenchyma. J Cell Biol 72:441–445, 1977.

Burt AD, LeBail B, Balabaud C, Bioulac-Sage P: Morphologic investigation of sinusoidal cells. Semin Liver Dis 13:21–38, 1993.

Erlinger S: Mechanisms of hepatic transport and bile secretion. Acta Gastroenterol Belg 59:159–162, 1996.

Fraser R, Dobbs BR, Rogers GW: Lipoproteins and the liver sieve: The role of the fenestrated sinusoidal endothelium in lipoprotein metabolism, atherosclerosis, and cirrhosis. Hepatology 21:863–874, 1995.

Hagenbuch B, Meier PJ: Sinusoidal (basolateral) bile salt uptake systems of hepatocytes. Semin Liver Dis 16:129–136, 1996.

Husztik E, Lazar G, Szilagyi S: Study on the mechanism of Kupffer cell phagocytosis blockade induced by gadolinium chloride. In Wisse E, Knook DL (eds): Kupffer Cells and Other Liver Sinusoidal Cells. Amsterdam: Elsevier/North Holland Biomedical, 1977, pp 387–395.

McCuskey RS, McCuskey PA: Fine structure and function of Kupffer cells. J Electron Microsc Tech 14:237–246, 1990.

Moseley RH: Hepatic amino acid transport. Semin Liver Dis 16:137–145, 1996.

Ramm GA, Britton RS, O'Neill R, et al: Vitamin A–poor lipocytes: A novel desmin-negative lipocyte subpopulation, which can be activated to myofibroblasts. Am J Physiol 269:G532–G541, 1995.

Rockey DC, Housset CN, Friedman SL: Activation-dependent contractility of rat hepatic lipocytes in culture and in vivo. J Clin Invest 92:1795–1804, 1993.

Rockey DC, Weisiger RA: Endothelin induced contractility of stellate cells from normal and cirrhotic rat liver: Implications for regulation of portal pressure and resistance. Hepatology 24:233–240, 1996.

Schaffner F, Popper H: Capillarization of hepatic sinusoids in man. Gastroenterology 44:239–242, 1963.

Smedsrod B, DeBleser P, Braet F, et al: Cell biology of liver endothelial and Kupffer cells. Gut 35:1509–1516, 1994.

Takezawa R, Watanabe Y, Akaike T: Direct evidence of macrophage differentiation from bone marrow cells in the liver: A possible origin of Kupffer cells. J Biochem 118:1175–1183, 1995.

Vanderkerken K, Bouwens L, Van Rooijen N, et al: The role of Kupffer cells in the differentiation process of hepatic natural killer cells. Hepatology 22:283–290, 1995.

Vujanovic NL, Polimeno L, Azzarone A, et al: Changes of liver-resident

NK cells during liver regeneration in rats. J Immunol 154:6324–6338, 1995.

Wang P, Ba ZF, Chaudry IH: Mechanism of hepatocellular dysfunction during early sepsis: Key role of increased gene expression and release of proinflammatory cytokines tumor necrosis factor and interleukin-6. Arch Surg 132:364–370, 1997.

Winnock M, Garcia Barcina M, Lukomska B, et al: Human liver-associated lymphocytes: An overview. J Gastroenterol Hepatol 10 (Suppl 1):S43–S46, 1995.

Wisse E, De Zanger R, Charels K, et al: The liver sieve: Considerations concerning the structure and function of endothelial fenestrae, the sinusoidal wall and the space of Disse. Hepatology 5:683–692, 1985.

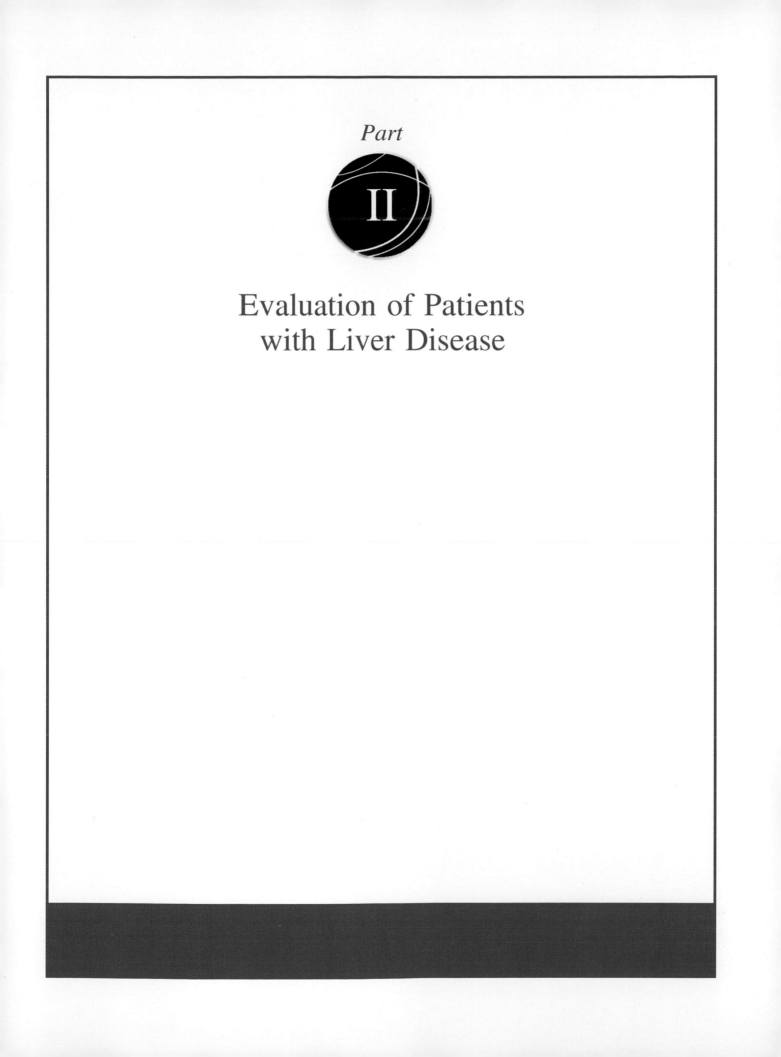

II

Evaluation of Patients
with Liver Disease

2

History and Physical Examination

Raymond S. Koff

As a consequence of an unusually rapid growth of knowledge, disorders of the liver are now recognized with increased frequency compared with just a few years ago. Their contribution to impaired wellness and premature death are becoming better known, and liver disease is increasingly appreciated as a common and costly health problem. As a result, the evaluation of patients for the presence of liver disease has become an important component of internal medicine and gastroenterology practices.

Accurate clinical diagnosis of liver disease remains one of the more challenging problems faced by the internist, primary care practitioner, and gastroenterologist. The wide availability of biochemical and serologic laboratory tests, high-technology imaging studies, and invasive procedures has clearly aided in the evaluation of the patient with suspected liver or biliary tract disease. Nonetheless, the essential evaluation tool that directs appropriate and timely further testing and diagnostic procedures continues to be the complete medical history and physical examination. Seasoned practitioners find that the history and physical examination provides an accurate diagnosis in more than three quarters of patients with liver disease. Furthermore, a focused repetition of the history on a separate occasion and sequential focused physical examinations may provide critical information and reduce diagnostic uncertainty. These "simple" tools are time consuming and intellectually demanding. Unfortunately, they are also often undervalued by the inexperienced practitioner. And if underutilized, costly, unnecessary testing and potentially risky procedures may result. Therefore, the complete history and physical examination constitute the most fundamental component of the evaluation. It is the foundation for the care of the patient with liver disease.

HOW PATIENTS COME TO ATTENTION

There are several possible ways by which an individual with suspected liver disease may come to the attention of the physician (Table 2–1). These patients are detected via a routine office evaluation during the course of an annual, biannual, or triannual check-up in which evidence of or a suspicion of liver disease may come to light through the interval history, review of systems, or physical examination. A more common occurrence today is the discovery of laboratory abnormalities identified from multiphasic health assessment screening tests (which include biochemical tests for liver dysfunction), as a result of laboratory testing required by life insurance underwriters or the routine laboratory screening of blood donors. Because these tests for liver disease are very widely used, internists and gastroenterologists are repeatedly confronted by apparently asymptomatic patients with laboratory findings of anicteric or early liver disease. The internist and gastroenterologist also see patients who may present with specific clinical features of acute or chronic liver disease (e.g., jaundice). However, the nonspecificity of many symptoms of liver disease requires that the physician maintain a high index of suspicion that liver disease may be present. Finally, some patients first come to the attention of physicians because of complications of previously unrecognized or undiagnosed liver diseases.

MEDICAL HISTORY

Approach to the History

The approach to the history varies from one patient to another and must remain flexible, depending on the circum-

Table 2–1 How Patients Come to Attention

- Routine office/clinic/insurance evaluation
- Discovery of unexpected laboratory abnormalities
- Symptoms of liver disease
- Symptoms of complications of liver disease

stances that have led to the encounter with the physician and with the patient profile. Key aspects, shown in Table 2–2, are reviewed here. For the patient with symptoms or for one in whom the evaluation is undertaken because of laboratory abnormalities that suggest hepatobiliary disease, the initial questions will be different but the same material will be covered. The symptoms and events of the presenting illness and its duration will be elicited in the first case by asking for an open-ended description of the illness and its influence on quality of life and lifestyle, best left uninterrupted by the physician except for questions of clarification. In the second case, the patient with laboratory abnormalities, it may be useful to review the patient's understanding of the abnormalities and their relationship to liver disease, before initiating questions concerning symptoms or changes in perception of quality of life.

The patient profile, defined simply as the age, gender, and occupational background of the individual, may provide general but nonspecific clues to the diagnosis. It may help to focus attention in the appropriate direction. For example, a 60-year-old man with known glucose intolerance is more likely to have iron overload disease than primary biliary cirrhosis; similarly, an 80-year-old person is unlikely to have Wilson's disease. Inherited disorders of bilirubin metabolism (e.g., Gilbert's syndrome) and acute viral hepatitis are the most common causes of jaundice in young patients. In contrast, extrahepatic biliary obstruction due to gallstones or malignancy is most common in middle-aged and elderly patients. Alcoholic liver disease might deserve important consideration in the bartender with unexplained liver disease; chronic viral hepatitis may be suspected in the patient with admitted injection substance abuse. Of course, alcoholic hepatitis and drug-induced liver disease have no specific age or sex predilections: they are suggested by other historical data. Exposure to potentially hepatotoxic chemicals in the workplace must also be queried and may lead to a presumptive etiologic diagnosis.

Dating the Disorder

One of the more useful aspects of the history is the establishment of some chronologic element to the story. Recog-

Table 2–2 Key Aspects of the Medical History

- The patient profile
- Events/symptoms of the presenting illness
- Dating the disorder
- Review of symptoms
- Family history
- Identification of risk factors

nized prior liver disease, a history of prior liver enlargement, or knowledge of previous liver biochemical abnormalities should be sought. Rejection as a blood donor or for life insurance because of abnormal laboratory testing may also help to date the onset or at least the first recognition of liver disease. A review of past medical records, laboratory data obtained earlier by other physicians or clinics, and previous hospitalizations may help to establish the duration of the disorder and to define whether the "illness" is acute or chronic. Critical information may be available in records of prior surgery, previous imaging studies and endoscopic reports, or previously undertaken liver biopsies. In symptomatic patients, the nature of the onset of illness may be helpful in the differential diagnosis. For example, an abrupt onset that can be dated to a specific day is characteristic of hepatitis A and may also be reported in gallstone-associated biliary tract obstruction. Other liver diseases tend to be more insidious in onset.

Symptom Review

Queries are directed at identifying symptoms that may be helpful in differential diagnosis. Jaundice, which is both a symptom and a sign, is a cardinal manifestation of liver disease but it must be recalled that its presence is simply a starting point for diagnostic evaluation. When jaundice is not accompanied by light-colored stools or dark urine, unconjugated hyperbilirubinemia should be suspected and Gilbert's syndrome and hemolysis should be considered in the adult patient. Unconjugated hyperbilirubinemia is also seen occasionally in patients with systemic diseases (e.g., congestive heart failure, sepsis, and malignancy) and as a consequence of some medications. In these cases the presence of mild jaundice is often overshadowed by clinical features of the principal disease, and extensive evaluation of jaundice is not usually warranted. In contrast, in most patients with jaundice as a consequence of hepatobiliary disease, the first change noted by the patient may be the passage of dark urine. Lightening of stool color may follow. Few patients identify their own scleral or mucosal icterus. It is usually a family member or a coworker who first draws the patient's attention to the presence of jaundiced sclerae or skin. Despite this, many jaundiced patients often delay in making an appointment with their physician until the pigmentation becomes cosmetically distressing or associated symptoms trigger the visit to the office or clinic. A full discussion of the importance of jaundice and its evaluation can be found in Chapter 4.

Although patients with acute liver disease may experience transient malaise, weakness, and fatigue, these symptoms may also be reported by patients with chronic liver disease and may reach disabling proportions, interfering with all activities of daily living. Abdominal pain may be a prominent feature of gallstone obstruction of the biliary tract and is frequent in biliary obstruction secondary to carcinoma of the pancreas. The abrupt development of abdominal pain is common in patients with choledocholithiasis, but the pain is usually steady and rarely waxes and wanes. It is not truly colicky. The presence of constant and deep boring pain is very frequent in pancreatic and bile duct carcinomas. Mild pain, which is usually described as abdominal discomfort or a heavy sensation rather than true pain, often localized to the right upper quadrant of the abdomen, is not unusual in acute viral hepatitis, alcoholic hepatitis, some cases of drug-induced hepatitis, and in passive congestion of the liver due to heart failure. The abdominal pain described in some patients with erythromycin-induced liver disease may simulate that of acute cholecystitis. Patients with chronic liver disease also occasionally mention right-sided discomfort over the liver when they are asked specifically.

Fever is a common accompaniment of the prodromal phase of hepatitis A and is often observed in alcoholic hepatitis and some cases of drug-induced hepatitis; however fever is infrequent in other forms of viral hepatitis. Fever may also reflect acute cholecystitis or the presence of cholangitis superimposed on biliary obstruction. Frank shaking chills are also found in patients with ascending cholangitis and in some patients with leptospirosis but are not usually present in patients with alcoholic, viral, or drug-induced hepatic inflammation. Arthralgias, arthritis, and skin rashes may precede the development of jaundice and other symptoms of hepatitis in acute hepatitis B; rashes may accompany some forms of drug-induced hepatitis.

Generalized pruritus without rash is occasionally the most salient feature of primary biliary cirrhosis, preceding the development of other symptoms (e.g., jaundice) by many years. Pruritus in a jaundiced patient is characteristic of the cholestatic syndromes—impaired bile flow caused by either intrahepatic or extrahepatic biliary tract obstruction or by parenchymal disease leading to a functional defect in bile formation or reduced bile excretion.

Patients with parenchymal, hepatocellular liver diseases may describe the nonspecific symptom of anorexia and accompanying weight loss. Significant weight loss that occurs over a period of months suggests the presence of a malignancy. On the other hand, a loss of 2 to 4 kg over a few weeks is commonly observed in some patients with severe acute viral or alcoholic hepatitis. Characteristically, in those in whom appetite is affected, breakfast is well tolerated but the desire for food wanes as the day goes on and caloric intake diminishes by the evening meal. Abnormalities in taste and smell have been noted in patients with liver disease, and in some diseases these changes have been correlated with symptoms of anorexia. In individuals who smoke cigarettes, intolerance for cigarette smoke and a transient aversion to tobacco may be prominent features of acute hepatitis. A few patients with acute viral hepatitis or alcoholic hepatitis mention diarrhea at the onset of their illness. Bloody diarrhea in a patient with liver disease might lead to the consideration of ulcerative colitis with its associated hepatobiliary disorders.

Current or past symptoms suggestive of portal hypertension or coagulopathy should be elicited. Increasing abdominal girth and ankle edema may be first recognized by the patient as tightness of clothing or slight difficulty in taking off the shoes at the end of the day. Fluid accumulation is often so insidious that the patient cannot identify when it began, and weight gain may not be noticed or is balanced by a loss of adipose tissue and muscle mass. In those few patients in whom the onset of ascites appears to be sudden, consideration of major hepatic vein occlusion or veno-occlusive disease seems appropriate. Symptoms of gastrointestinal bleeding resulting from gastroesophageal varices or nonvariceal lesions associated with portal hypertension include hematemesis, melena, and hematochezia. Easy bruising, unexplained ecchymoses, and the development of petechiae suggest a coagulopathy or thrombocytopenia—the former being a reflection of severe liver disease and the latter being a feature of hypersplenism.

Decreased libido in men and secondary amenorrhea in women may be spontaneously reported by some patients with advanced alcoholic or nonalcoholic chronic liver disease. In others, such information is not obtained unless the interviewer specifically questions the patient.

Patients with chronic liver disease and those with severe acute disease resulting in acute liver failure may describe reductions in mental concentrating ability, personality changes, or disruption of normal sleep patterns. In many cases, such changes are more likely to be noticed by a family member than by the patient. Hence, there may be considerable value in discussing current and past symptoms and behavior with a responsible family member.

Family History

Although the family history is routinely taken from the patient, verification of the patient's history and details of the family history sought from a family member may provide useful information, including insight into the family's understanding or lack of understanding of the patient's problems. Specific questions about familial liver disease, including alcoholic, autoimmune, and gallstone disease and confirmation of the patient's alcohol consumption, may provide rewarding information. A family history of alcoholism without recognition of alcoholic liver disease may also be vital information. A family history of jaundice in successive generations or first-degree relatives may be a clue to Gilbert's disease. Similarly, a history of Wilson's disease in a relative may be crucial in further evaluation of the index patient. Assessment of risk factors for liver disease may also be validated by involvement of the patient's spouse or family member.

Identifying Risk Factors for Liver Disease

In addition to exposure to occupational hepatotoxins and exposure to chemicals in the home, questions concerning the use of medications (including the use of injectable drugs) are essential. All prescribed drugs must be identified. Queries should include the enumeration of all nonprescription drugs, folk medicines, herbal remedies, and dietary supplements taken by the patient in the preceding months. Specific documentation of the dose and duration of oral contraceptive use in women may be important because of the association with hepatocellular adenomas; anabolic steroid ingestion in men is associated with various disorders, including hepatic adenoma, hepatic adenomatosis, hepatocellular carcinoma, and peliosis hepatis.

It may be helpful to have the patient or a family member bring in all drug containers for verification. It may also be helpful to ask whether the patient might have taken a drug used regularly or irregularly by another member of the household. In the case of the rare patient with unexplained acute liver failure, a history of ingestion of hepatotoxic mushrooms may resolve the etiologic mystery.

Detection of the problem alcohol drinker often depends

on establishing that the quantity of alcohol consumed is excessive, the presence of tolerance to alcohol intoxication, symptoms of physical dependence on withdrawal (e.g., tremulousness, sweating, anxiety), and interference with social relationships. Because some patients may grossly underestimate their alcohol consumption, minimize the importance of alcohol in their lives, or even deny using alcohol, discussion with a family member may be enlightening. Although most patients with alcoholic liver disease have ingested more than 160 g of absolute alcohol per day for more than 10 years, the threshold at which alcoholic liver injury occurs may be as low as 70 to 80 g in men and 35 to 40 g in women. As a consequence of cultural stereotyping, alcoholic liver disease may fail to be considered in the woman with unexplained liver disease, leading to errors or delays in diagnosis.

Risk factors for viral hepatitis should also be identified. These include recent exposure to a patient with known hepatitis or jaundice, living in a community currently experiencing an outbreak of hepatitis, recent travel, ingestion of uncooked or partially cooked bivalve mollusks, a history of injecting drug use, the transfusion of blood or blood products, tattoos, piercing of body parts, acupuncture, dental and medical exposures involving tissue penetrations, injections or venipunctures, and inapparent exposures that may be associated with the intranasal snorting of cocaine through a straw. Sexual orientation, numbers of sexual partners, and information on the use of safe sexual practices should be elicited.

PHYSICAL EXAMINATION

General Appearance

Key aspects of the directed physical examination are listed in Table 2–3. Many patients with liver disease look surprisingly healthy during the initial assessment. Patients with extrahepatic obstruction due to gallstones or those with acute viral hepatitis may appear healthy despite the presence of jaundice. Other patients, (e.g., those with severe or advanced parenchymal liver disease) may appear ill, with obvious weakness and decreased muscle mass and tone. The presence of cachexia with temporal wasting suggests advanced cirrhosis or malignancy. Exceptions are commonplace, however, and the initial assessment may be deceptive because advanced liver disease may be present even in the absence of any abnormalities on physical examination. Two such examples are the patient with chronic viral hepatitis or autoimmune hepatitis and the patient in an early phase of primary biliary cirrhosis. In the latter, the presence of multiple lacerations and repeated scratching during the interview may draw attention to that diagnosis.

Dermatomucosal Changes

Jaundice may be detected easily by examination of the sclerae or mucosa of the floor of the mouth when the tongue is elevated. Jaundice of the skin follows. The detection of pallor should suggest the anemia of chronic liver disease, blood loss due to gastrointestinal bleeding complicating portal hypertension, or neoplastic disease. The presence of

Table 2–3 Key Aspects of the Physical Examination

- General appearance
- Dermatomucosal changes
- Endocrine manifestations
- Abdominal examination
- Neurologic and ophthalmologic findings

petechiae or ecchymoses suggests thrombocytopenia or impaired hemostasis, which are both possible complications of hepatobiliary disease. The former may be a result of hypersplenism secondary to portal hypertension or a direct effect of alcohol on the bone marrow, whereas the latter may be associated with liver failure or vitamin K malabsorption due to extrahepatic bile duct obstruction. Cutaneous stigmata of chronic liver disease include spider angiomas and palmar erythema, neither of which is specific to chronic liver disease. Spider angiomas are seen in some normal individuals and also in pregnant women and may be present transiently in patients with acute liver disease. Palmar erythema is even more nonspecific, because it may be found in many normal individuals during pregnancy and in some patients with rheumatoid arthritis. Thickening of the palmar fascia, resulting in Dupuytren's contracture, is associated more closely with alcoholism than with liver disease but is also nonspecific. White, so-called *liver nails* are also nonspecific findings. In some patients with primary biliary cirrhosis or end-stage liver disease, clubbing of the fingers (and toes) may be detected.

The presence of xanthelasmas and xanthomas suggests primary biliary cirrhosis or long-standing cholestasis. Similarly, gray or brown pigmentation of the skin with sparing of a butterfly-shaped area of the back may be seen in primary biliary cirrhosis. The sparing may result from the inability of the patient to scratch the affected area. Slate-gray hyperpigmentation of the skin, which is often accentuated in exposed areas or in the axilla or groin, may suggest the presence of hemochromatosis.

Endocrine Manifestations

Unilateral or bilateral, occasionally painful, gynecomastia may occur in some male patients with chronic liver disease, perhaps related to abnormalities in sex hormone levels and metabolism, prolonged malnutrition, or after treatment of fluid accumulation with spironolactone. Testicular atrophy is particularly common in patients with alcoholism and alcoholic liver disease; along with feminization, testicular atrophy has been related to a direct toxic effect of alcohol on the testes and altered sex hormone levels.

Abdominal Examination

Dilated abdominal wall venous collaterals, a characteristic sign of portal hypertension or inferior vena cava obstruction, must be specifically identified. These vessels radiate from the umbilicus and carry blood centrifugally away from the umbilicus when identified in patients with portal hypertension. In inferior vena caval obstruction, flow below the umbilicus is also directed cephalad. Abdominal distention due to ascites suggests cirrhosis with portal hypertension or severe hepatitis, malignancy, or hepatic venous obstruction. Ascites may be detected by the demonstration of bulging flanks, shifting dullness, and a fluid wave. The presence of an umbilical hernia suggests that the ascites has been long-standing. Edema may be present in the lower limbs concomitantly with or developing after ascites becomes evident.

Hepatic enlargement is usually readily identified by measuring hepatic dullness on percussion in the right midclavicular line. Hepatomegaly may be defined by dullness greater than 11 cm in men and greater than 9 cm in women. The detection of an irregular, nodular, firm but not enlarged liver is compatible with the presence of cirrhosis. Similarly, a readily palpated left lobe of the liver is strongly consistent with cirrhosis. If the examination reveals the presence of rock-hard masses, hepatocellular carcinoma or metastatic involvement should be suspected. In acute hepatitis, in passive congestion of the liver due to heart failure and in the early phases of extrahepatic biliary tract obstruction, the liver may be mildly enlarged and slightly tender with a rounded edge, rather than the normally "sharp" edge. An exquisitely tender, enlarged liver might signal the presence of a pyogenic or amebic abscess. Neoplastic obstruction of the bile duct below the entry of the cystic duct may lead to enlargement of the gallbladder, which becomes palpable. Infrequently, an enlarged gallbladder may be detected in cystic duct obstruction because of a gallstone.

Although an enlarged spleen may be observed in some patients with acute liver disease, cirrhosis complicated by portal hypertension is more likely to be responsible, particularly if other manifestations of portal hypertension (e.g., ascites) are present. Infiltrative, granulomatous, and other space-occupying diseases of the liver (e.g., sarcoidosis) may result in hepatomegaly and may also be responsible for sple-

nomegaly. In the jaundiced patient with suspected carcinoma of the pancreas, the presence of an enlarged spleen suggests the development of splenic vein thrombosis.

Neurologic and Ophthalmologic Findings

Signs of hepatic encephalopathy (e.g., alterations of mental status, slowing of speech, constructional apraxia, the presence of asterixis, and fetor hepaticus) should be assessed in all patients with suspected liver disease. Simple bedside neuropsychologic tests, such as the trail-making test, may be useful in detecting subclinical encephalopathy. The golden-brown Kayser-Fleischer corneal rings of Wilson's disease may be visualized with the naked eye.

SUMMARY

The clinical evaluation of liver disease begins with the history and physical examination as outlined earlier. The synthesis of the information gathered into one or more hypotheses permits the physician to pursue the diagnosis quickly, efficiently, and effectively. Their importance cannot be overemphasized.

SUGGESTED READINGS

Gholson CF, Bacon BR: The history and physical examination in hepatologic practice. In Gholson CF, Bacon BR (eds): Essentials of Clinical Hepatology. St. Louis: Mosby-Year Book, 1993, pp 23–30.
Kirsch R, Robson S, Bass N: Clinical evaluation of liver disease. In Kirsch R, Robson S, Trey C (eds): Diagnosis and Management of Liver Disease. London: Chapman & Hall, 1995, pp 1–8.
Koff RS: Fundamentals of diagnosis. In Koff RS: Liver Disease in Primary Care Medicine. New York: Appleton-Century-Crofts, 1980, pp 1–20.
Schiff L: Jaundice: A clinical approach. In Schiff L, Schiff ER: Diseases of the Liver, 7th ed. Philadelphia: JB Lippincott, 1993, pp 334–342.

3

Evaluation of Abnormal Liver Enzymes, Use of Liver Tests, and the Serology of Viral Hepatitis

Hugo R. Rosen
Emmet B. Keeffe

A broad array of biochemical tests are used to provide indirect evidence of hepatobiliary disease. The term *liver function tests (LFTs)* is firmly entrenched in routine medical language, although its use has been criticized because the tests most commonly employed in the evaluation of liver disease (i.e., the serum aminotransferase and alkaline phosphatase levels) assess hepatocyte integrity rather than a known synthetic function. In fact, it might be argued that *liver injury tests* would be a more appropriate term. The asymptomatic individual who is found to have a mild elevation of one or more liver enzymes may represent a diagnostic challenge. Screening biochemical testing of healthy, asymptomatic populations has revealed that up to 6% have abnormal LFTs. However, the prevalence of liver disease in the general population is significantly lower (i.e., ~2%). Therefore, it is important to develop a rational and cost-effective approach to the assessment of asymptomatic patients with mild elevation of liver enzymes.

Limitations of the use of LFTs include problems with sensitivity (i.e., the likelihood of an abnormal test result in patients known to have liver disease). For example, cirrhotic patients may have minimally abnormal or even normal LFTs. Problems with specificity (i.e., the patient with elevated serum aminotransferase levels of cardiac or muscle origin) must also be considered. Even measures of specific hepatic functions, such as the serum albumin concentration, bilirubin concentration, and prothrombin time, can be affected by extrahepatic factors such as nutritional state, hemolysis, and use of antibiotics (Table 3–1).

In addition to describing the specific laboratory tests that reflect hepatobiliary injury and their efficient utilization, this chapter discusses the serologic and virologic tests used for the diagnosis and management of viral hepatitis.

TESTS THAT REFLECT HEPATOBILIARY INJURY

Aminotransferases

The aminotransferases are the most frequently utilized and specific indicators of hepatocellular necrosis. These enzymes—aspartate aminotransferase (AST, formerly serum glutamic oxaloacetic transaminase) and alanine aminotransferase (ALT, formerly serum glutamic pyruvic transaminase)—catalyze the transfer of the α-amino groups of aspartate and alanine, respectively, to the α-keto group of ketoglutaric acid. ALT is localized primarily to the liver, but AST is present in a wide variety of tissues, including the heart, skeletal muscle, kidney, brain, and liver. Whereas AST is present in both the mitochondria and cytosol of hepatocytes, ALT is localized to the cytosol. The evaluation of an asymptomatic individual with an isolated elevation of ALT is outlined in Figure 3–1.

Although no uniform definition of "mild," "moderate," or "severe" elevation of LFTs exists, a working definition has been outlined (Table 3–2). Diagnostic clues can often be garnered from the degree of elevation. Mild elevations of aminotransferases are typically found in patients with fatty liver, nonalcoholic steatohepatitis (NASH), and chronic viral hepatitis. The highest elevations occur in acute viral hepatitis, drug- or toxin-induced hepatic necrosis, and ischemic hepatitis related to circulatory shock or preservation injury following liver transplantation. The height of the elevation of aminotransferases does not appear to correlate with the extent of necrosis on liver biopsy specimens and therefore has no prognostic value. In fact, rapidly declining aminotransferase levels may be a reflection of decreased

Table 3–1   Nonhepatic Causes of Abnormal Liver Function Tests

Test	Nonhepatic Causes	Discriminating Tests
↓Albumin	Protein-losing enteropathy	Serum globulins, α_1-antitrypsin clearance
	Nephrotic syndrome	Urinalysis, 24-hour urinary protein
	Malnutrition	Clinical setting
	Congestive heart failure	Clinical setting
↑Alkaline phosphatase	Bone disease	GGT, SLAP, 5′-NT
	Pregnancy	GGT, 5′-NT
	Malignancy	Alkaline phosphatase electrophoresis
	Myocardial infarction	MB-CPK
	Muscle disorders	Creatine kinase
↑Bilirubin	Hemolysis	Reticulocyte count, peripheral smear, urine bilirubin
	Sepsis	Clinical setting, cultures
	Ineffective erythropoiesis	Peripheral smear, urine bilirubin, hemoglobin electrophoresis, bone marrow examination
	Shunt hyperbilirubinemia	Clinical setting
↑Prothrombin time	Antibiotic and anticoagulant use, steatorrhea, dietary deficiency of vitamin K (rare)	Response to vitamin K, clinical setting

GGT, γ-glutamyltranspeptidase; SLAP, serum leucine aminopeptidase; 5′-NT, 5′-nucleotidase.
Adapted from Moseley FH, Evaluation of abnormal liver function tests. Med Clin North Am 80:888, 1996.

numbers of viable hepatocytes and indicate a poor prognosis in fulminant hepatic failure. Moderately elevated aminotransferases (3- to 20-fold) are typical of acute or chronic hepatitis, including alcoholic hepatitis. A characteristic feature of chronic hepatitis C is an episodic, fluctuating pattern of serum ALT levels; periods of elevated enzyme activity alternate with periods of normal or near-normal ALT. In patients with extrahepatic biliary tract obstruction, serum levels of AST and ALT may increase to greater than 300 U/L but usually decline rapidly after peaking within the first 24 to 48 hours after obstruction. Although elevations in aminotransferases may be the first clue to liver disease and screening has proved useful for detecting subclinical liver disease in asymptomatic persons, patients with normal levels may have significant liver damage. For instance, recent studies have demonstrated that asymptomatic carriers of hepatitis C virus (HCV) may have evidence of chronic hepatitis or cirrhosis on liver biopsy despite repeatedly normal liver enzymes.

The ratio of AST to ALT may be helpful diagnostically, particularly in patients with alcoholic liver disease who characteristically have a ratio of more than two (Fig. 3–2). The reason for the elevation of the AST level out of proportion to the ALT level appears to be a differential reduction in hepatic ALT caused by a deficiency of the cofactor, pyridoxine-5-phosphate. In fact, oral administration of this cofactor to patients with alcoholic liver disease has been shown to result in an increase in serum ALT levels. Although an AST:ALT ratio of more than 2.0 strongly suggests the diagnosis of alcoholic liver disease, it does not preclude other diagnoses. Other biochemical clues to the presence of alcoholic liver disease include elevations of serum γ-glutamyltransferase (GGT), erythrocyte mean corpuscular volume, and desialyated transferrin. Conversely,

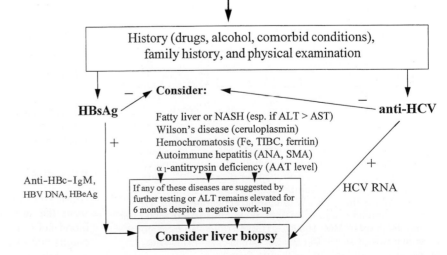

Elevated ALT in an asymptomatic person

Figure 3–1
Evaluation of an elevated serum alanine aminotransferase (ALT) in an asymptomatic person. Fe, iron; TIBC, total iron-binding capacity; ANA, antinuclear antibody; SMA, smooth muscle antibody; AAT, α_1-antitrypsin.

Table 3–2 Characteristics of Elevated Concentrations of Liver Enzymes

Test	Normal*	Mild†	Moderate†	Marked†
AST	11–32	<2–3	2–3 to 20	>20
ALT	3–30	<2–3	2–3 to 20	>20
ALP	35–105	<1.5–2	1.5–2 to 5	>5
GGT	2–65	<2–3	2–3 to 10	>10

*Units for normal are U/L; normal ranges vary with the assay used and should be obtained from the laboratory performing the test.
†Numbers in the table refer to multiples of the upper limits of normal.
ALT, alanine aminotransferase; AST, aspartate aminotransferase; ALP, alkaline phosphatase; GGT, γ-glutamyl transpeptidase.
From Keeffe ED: Diagnostic approach to mild elevation of liver enzyme levels. Gastrointestinal Dis Today 3:1–9, 1994.

NASH is typically associated with an ALT level greater than the AST level. In viral hepatitis, the ratio of AST to ALT is also usually less than 1.0 but may rise to values greater than 1.0 as cirrhosis develops.

It is important to note that certain clinical situations are associated with hypoaminotransferasemia. Yasuda and associates have shown that values higher than 20 U/L are definitely abnormal and possibly indicative of liver disease in patients undergoing dialysis, which suggests that the upper normal limits of AST and ALT in these patients should be

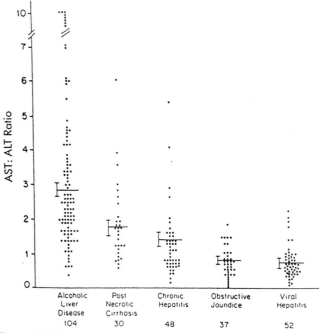

Figure 3–2

Ratios of serum aspartate aminotransferase (AST) to alanine aminotransferase (ALT) in patients with biopsy proven liver disease. Of patients with alcoholic liver disease, 70% had ratios greater than two, compared with 26% of patients with postnecrotic cirrhosis, 8% with chronic active hepatitis, 4% with viral hepatitis, and none with obstructive jaundice. (From Cohen JA, Kaplan MM: The SGOT/SGPT ratio—an indicator of alcoholic liver disease. Dig Dis Sci 24:835–838, 1979. With permission from Plenum Publishing Corp.)

reduced considerably. There is considerable evidence that hepatitis C viremia without biochemical evidence of hepatic dysfunction is common in patients with renal failure. Figure 3–3 outlines the evaluation of elevated LFTs in hemodialysis patients; as discussed in detail later in this chapter, the lack of sensitivity of antibody testing to HCV in this population warrants direct measurement of HCV RNA.

Alkaline Phosphatase and γ-Glutamyltranspeptidase

The usual markers to identify cholestasis are alkaline phosphatase (ALP) and GGT. Serum ALP is the name applied to a group of enzymes that catalyze the hydrolysis of phosphate esters at an alkaline pH. The enzymes are widely distributed and may originate from bone, liver, intestine, or placenta. In children and adolescents, in whom bone growth is active, the serum ALP may increase up to 3-fold. In patients with hepatobiliary disorders, elevated ALP levels result from increased hepatic production with leakage into the serum, rather than failure to clear or excrete circulating ALP. Markedly elevated levels of ALP suggest the possibility of disorders such as extrahepatic biliary obstruction, primary biliary cirrhosis (PBC), primary sclerosing cholangitis, or drug-induced cholestasis, but the degree of elevation does not differentiate extra- and intrahepatic cholestasis. Mild to moderate ALP abnormalities are seen in infiltrative processes such as amyloidosis, granulomatous disease, and neoplasms. Some patients with Hodgkin's disease and renal cell carcinoma may have elevated ALP without any direct involvement of bone or the hepatobiliary system. Depressed serum levels of ALP have been associated with congenital hypophosphatasia, hypothyroidism, pernicious anemia, and zinc deficiency. Moreover, fulminant Wilson's disease complicated by hemolysis is often manifested by undetectable levels of serum ALP, and whether this is due to replacement of the cofactor zinc by copper and subsequent inactivation of ALP remains unknown. Figure 3–4 shows the recommended algorithm for the evaluation of an isolated (or predominant) mild elevation of ALP.

GGT is useful to confirm whether an elevated ALP is secondary to hepatobiliary disease or is of extrahepatic origin. Unfortunately, because the enzyme is ubiquitous, an elevated GGT has poor specificity and may indeed be due to induction by alcohol, phenytoin (Fig. 3–5), or other drugs. 5'-Nucleotidase, on the other hand, is specific for liver disease, and its measurement is particularly helpful in diagnosing liver disease in children and pregnancy, clinical settings in which ALP is elevated physiologically but 5'-nucleotidase is not.

TESTS THAT MEASURE THE LIVER'S CAPACITY TO TRANSPORT ORGANIC ANIONS OR TO METABOLIZE DRUGS

Bilirubin

Bilirubin is an endogenous organic anion derived primarily from the degradation of hemoglobin released from red blood cells. Hyperbilirubinemia is classified as either unconjugated or conjugated (see Chapter 4). In patients with hyperbilirubinemia due to hepatocellular dysfunction or

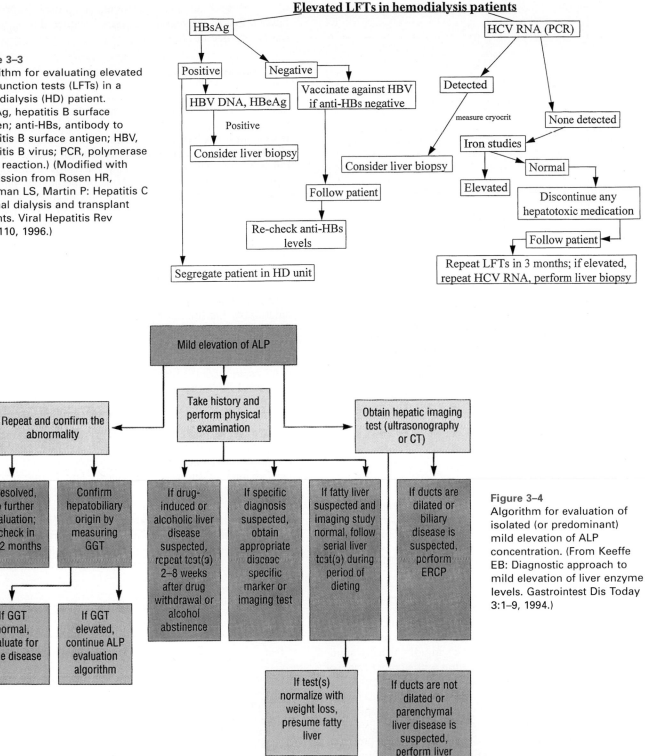

Figure 3–3
Algorithm for evaluating elevated liver function tests (LFTs) in a hemodialysis (HD) patient. (HBsAg, hepatitis B surface antigen; anti-HBs, antibody to hepatitis B surface antigen; HBV, hepatitis B virus; PCR, polymerase chain reaction.) (Modified with permission from Rosen HR, Friedman LS, Martin P: Hepatitis C in renal dialysis and transplant patients. Viral Hepatitis Rev 2:97–110, 1996.)

Figure 3–4
Algorithm for evaluation of isolated (or predominant) mild elevation of ALP concentration. (From Keeffe EB: Diagnostic approach to mild elevation of liver enzyme levels. Gastrointest Dis Today 3:1–9, 1994.)

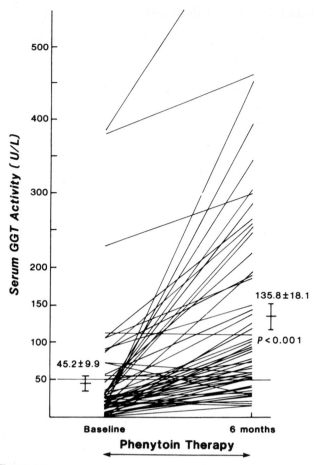

Figure 3–5

Individual and mean changes in serum γ-glutamyl-transpeptidase (GGT) activity from baseline to 6 months of phenytoin therapy in 58 patients. Of the total group, 52 patients demonstrated a rise and six patients a fall in GGT activity. (From Keeffe EB, Sunderland MC, Gabourel JD: Serum gamma-glutamyl transpeptidase activity in patients receiving chronic phenytoin therapy. Dig Dis Sci 31:1056–1061, 1986.)

of hyperbilirubinemia may provide prognostic information beyond that of the histologic score obtained during the initial recurrence of HCV.

Quantitative Liver Function Tests

Patients with essentially normal conventional LFTs may have significantly diminished hepatic function; conversely, hepatic function may be well preserved in some patients with abnormal LFTs. Although quantitation of functional reserve is not performed routinely in clinical practice, quantitative liver function tests (QLFTs) may provide useful data regarding the prognosis and effects of therapeutic interventions (Table 3–3). Because the Child-Pugh classification, initially designed to predict survival of cirrhotic patients following portosystemic shunting, does not differentiate patients with varying degrees of end-stage liver disease, it is possible that future QLFTs may quantitate differences in functional reserve in order to identify patients who have the greatest need of hepatic transplantation.

Indocyanine green (ICG) is a dye removed from the circulation by the liver after intravenous injection. Because it is taken up exclusively by hepatocytes, the clearance of low doses of ICG is used to measure liver blood flow. With administration of higher doses of ICG, the uptake process becomes saturated; the maximal removal of ICG can be calculated, and this reflects functional hepatic mass rather than blood flow in the liver.

The metabolism of aminopyrine is sensitive to alterations in the redox state, thyroid disease, infection, amino acid deficiency, and glutathione deficiency as well as folate and vitamin B_{12} deficiency. The aminopyrine breath test has been used to predict short-term prognosis and mortality in patients with alcoholic hepatitis, and in one study was a better predictor of outcome than standard LFTs. The caffeine breath test is comparable to the aminopyrine test, except without the need for radioisotope usage. Caffeine clearance appears to be impaired in advanced liver disease and has limited utility for screening mild or early liver disease.

cholestasis, the serum bilirubin is predominantly conjugated and hence water soluble, allowing easy renal excretion. Extreme hyperbilirubinemia (i.e., >25 mg/dL) usually signifies severe liver disease in association with another cause of unconjugated hyperbilirubinemia (i.e., hemolysis).

The level of serum bilirubin has been utilized to predict the natural history of specific liver diseases. Shapiro and others have reported that patients with PBC typically have a long and stable course followed by an accelerated preterminal phase of hyperbilirubinemia, with a mean survival of only 1.4 years in patients with a serum bilirubin greater than 10 mg/dL. Serum bilirubin is the most important variable, common to all prognostic survival models of PBC. The level of hyperbilirubinemia also has prognostic significance in patients with fulminant hepatic failure and acute alcoholic hepatitis, comprising the majority of the discriminant function scores derived by Maddrey and associates. Moreover, recent studies of liver transplant recipients have suggested that marked and transient hyperbilirubinemia is common after HCV reinfection of the allograft and that the level

Table 3–3 Quantitative Liver Function Tests

Test	Estimates
Galactose elimination capacity Maximal removal of indocyanine green	Metabolic capacity
Aminopyrine demethylation Caffeine clearance Antipyrine clearance	Microsomal enzyme function
Galactose clearance Sorbitol clearance Indocyanine green clearance Sulfobromophthalein clearance	Functional hepatic perfusion
Formation of monoethylglycinexylidide from lidocaine	Microsomal enzyme function and hepatic perfusion

From Hawker F: The Liver. London: WB Saunders, 1993.

The 14C-galactose breath test is a simple test that may provide good prognostic information in fulminant hepatic failure where the galactose elimination capacity (GEC) is reduced. In addition, serial measurements of the GEC were more accurate in predicting death in patients with PBC than the Mayo score. However, in multivariate analysis of survival in other patients with cirrhosis, determination of GEC appeared to provide little additional information compared with the Child-Pugh score. Unlike the ICG, the GEC is not suitable for assessment of hepatic reserve before hepatic resection for malignancy because some tumors may metabolize galactose.

Lidocaine is metabolized by oxidative *N*-demethylation to monoethylglycinexylidide (MEGX) by cytochrome P-450, and MEGX values above 30 ng/mL correlate with a lack of life-threatening complications of cirrhosis. MEGX has been shown to be a better predictor of primary nonfunction after liver transplantation than the ICG test or the GEC. Moreover, the MEGX test is essentially safe and is quick and easy to perform.

INDICATORS OF SYNTHETIC FUNCTION

Serum Albumin

Albumin is quantitatively the most important circulating protein synthesized by the liver, accounting for three quarters of the plasma colloid oncotic pressure. The liver is the only site of synthesis with approximately 12 to 15 g produced daily in the normal adult. Plasma albumin concentration is decreased in severe acute and chronic liver disease and is one of the criteria for the Child-Pugh classification widely used to grade severity of cirrhosis. In addition to liver disease, hypoalbuminemia may also result from gastrointestinal and renal losses, hormonal changes, increased catabolism, and hypergammaglobulinemia, which may lead to feedback inhibition of albumin synthesis. Prealbumin (or thyroid-binding prealbumin) appears to be a more sensitive

index of hepatic protein synthesis than albumin, particularly in acute liver failure because its half-life is shorter (1.9 days).

Prothrombin Time and Serum Coagulation Factor Levels

With the exception of factor VIII, all the clotting factors are synthesized in the liver. The clotting factors that determine prothrombin time (PT) are short-lived (hours), making the test suited for evaluating acute liver injury; indeed, PT is one of the key elements in prognostic scores for fulminant hepatic failure and acute alcoholic hepatitis. In general, a prolongation of 2 or more seconds greater than control is considered abnormal. Unfortunately, the PT is not a sensitive index of chronic liver disease, because it may be normal even in patients with cirrhosis; moreover, its specificity is low in the presence of malabsorption, because factors II, VII, and X are dependent on vitamin K. It is now generally accepted that the international normalized ratio (INR) should replace the PT, because the latter is based on different types of thromboplastin that have considerable variation in different countries.

SEROLOGY OF VIRAL HEPATITIS

Six major viruses (hepatitis A, B, C, D, E, and G) appear to be the etiologic agents responsible for clinical cases of viral hepatitis, and the patterns of development and presentation of antigens and antibodies are different in each (Table 3–4). The various hepatitides often cannot be distinguished from each other on clinical evaluation alone, and serologic assays are invaluable in the diagnosis and monitoring of therapy (see also Chapters 6 and 7). Immunoassays and molecular biologic diagnostic tests are important tools to test for viral antigen, viral antibody, or viral DNA or RNA in sera or secretions. Immunoassays may be an enzyme-linked immunoassay (ELISA or EIA) or solid-phase radioimmunoassay (RIA), depending on the type of indicator system uti-

Table 3–4   Types of Hepatitis Viruses

	Hepatitis A	Hepatitis B	Hepatitis C	Hepatitis D	Hepatitis E	Hepatitis G
Virus	HAV	HBV	HCV	HDV	HEV	HGV
Size	27 nm	42 nm	30–60 nm	35 nm	37 nm	30–60 nm
Genome	ssRNA	dsDNA	ssRNA	ssRNA	ssRNA	ssRNA
Antigens	HAAg*	HBsAg HBeAg HBcAg*	HCAg*	HDAg*	HEAg*	None available
Antibodies	IgM anti-HAV Anti-HAV	IgM anti-HBc Anti-HBc Anti-HBs Anti-HBe	Anti-HCV	IgM anti-HDV anti-HDV	anti-HEV	None available
Viral markers	HAV RNA*	HBV DNA DNA polymerase	HCV RNA†	HDV RNA	none	HGV RNA

*Research test.
†See the text for a discussion of HCV genotyping.
ss, single stranded.
Modified with permission from Lindsay KL, Hoofnagle JH: Serologic tests for viral hepatitis. In Kaplowitz N (ed): Liver and Biliary Diseases, 2nd ed. Baltimore: Williams & Wilkins, 1996, pp 221–234.

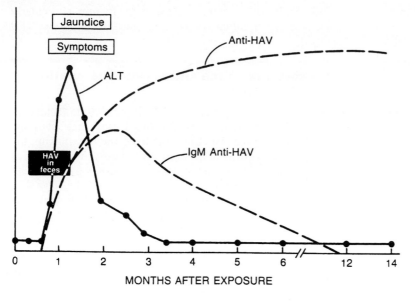

Figure 3–6
Typical course of acute icteric viral hepatitis, type A. (From Hoofnagle JH, Di Bisceglie AM: Serologic diagnosis of viral hepatitis. Semin Liver Dis 11:73–83, 1991.)

lized. Polymerase chain reaction(PCR) amplifies quantities of viral RNA or DNA that are often nondetectable by other methods.

Hepatitis A

Antibody to HAV (anti-HAV) appears in serum at the onset of illness or aminotransferase elevations. Tests for total anti-HAV detect both IgG and IgM and therefore are not helpful for detecting acute infection, unless IgM antibody is also measured. As IgM antibody wanes after a few months, IgG anti-HAV rises to high titers and probably lasts for life (Fig. 3–6). Rarely, patients may have low levels of detectable IgM anti-HAV for more than 1 year past the initial infection, and occasionally a patient may have a relapse of hepatitis A with reappearance of acute markers of infection. Used almost exclusively in the research setting, testing for HAV

RNA was demonstrated to be helpful in establishing contaminated factor VIII as the origin of an outbreak of hepatitis A.

Hepatitis B

The interpretation of tests for hepatitis B virus (HBV) markers is considerably more complex (Fig. 3–7). Like hepatitis A, viral replication appears during the incubation period (from 30 to 150 days), and the onset of disease with aminotransferase elevation is associated with a decrease in levels of replication. HBsAg arises first, rising to titers of 1 to 50 mg/mL. The markers of active viral replication—hepatitis B e antigen (HBeAg), HBV DNA, and HBV-associated DNA polymerase activity—become detectable shortly thereafter. In 90% to 95% of individuals, the infection resolves, and HBV DNA and HBeAg disappear first, usually at the peak

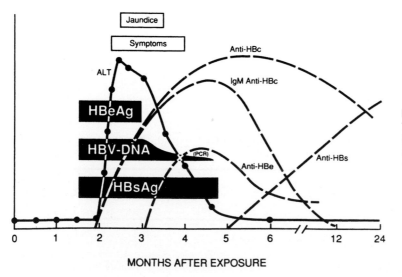

Figure 3–7
Typical course of acute icteric viral hepatitis, type B. (From Hoofnagle JH, Di Bisceglie AM: Serologic diagnosis of viral hepatitis. Semin Liver Dis 11:73–83, 1991.)

of clinical illness. HBV DNA can be detected by several molecular techniques with different sensitivities: slot blot or dot blot hybridization (10 to 500 pg/mL), liquid phase hybridization (1.6 pg/mL), and PCR (10 to 50 genome equivalents/mL). A transient, significant elevation of serum ALT often heralds seroconversion from HBeAg to anti-HBe, and the annual rate of seroconversion in chronically infected individuals is in the range of 2% to 20%. The disappearance of HBeAg signifies that replication has ceased or been reduced to the minimal levels and that the chronic HBV carrier has entered a *nonreplicative phase* of infection. However, anti–HBe-positive patients, particularly after treatment with chemotherapeutic agents, can develop reactivation of viral replication with reappearance of HBeAg, HBV DNA, and IgM anti-HBc. HBeAg and HBV DNA have historical significance as predictors of hepatitis B recurrence after liver transplantation, particularly before the availability of effective immunoprophylaxis (i.e., hepatitis B immunoglobulin) and antiviral agents (i.e., lamivudine). A subgroup of patients with precore gene mutants appear unable to synthesize the precore/core protein from which HBeAg is derived, leading to undetectable HBeAg and anti-HBe in serum despite detectable serum HBV DNA and elevated ALT. Initially described in patients with fulminant hepatic failure, precore mutants have also been isolated from patients with well-compensated chronic liver disease.

HBsAg persists for a long time and may last into convalescence, probably because of its long half-life. Persistent HBsAg without elevated serum ALT levels or evidence of liver disease denotes a *healthy carrier state,* which in one study was associated with no morbidity or mortality over a 10-year period. Antibodies to HBsAg (anti-HBs) arise during convalescence after clearance of HBsAg; however, in some cases, HBsAg and anti-HBs may coexist, representing low levels of a heterotypic anti-HBs (directed against different HBsAg subdeterminants) or an immunocomplex formation.

Although hepatitis B core antigen is not readily measurable in serum, antibody to HBcAg is detectable early during infection (initially of the IgM type) before the onset of symptoms and elevations in aminotransferases. Most infected individuals have total anti-HBc detectable throughout their lifetime. Anti-HBc was utilized as a "surrogate marker" for non-A, non-B hepatitis (NANB) before the availability of testing for HCV and is credited with reducing the incidence of post-transfusion NANB. Isolated anti-HBc in serum (without HBsAg or anti-HBs) may occur during the *window period* during which the HBsAg has disappeared but anti-HBs has not yet become detectable and can also be the only detectable antibody with recovery (i.e., no appearance or loss of anti-HBs). The administration of HBV vaccine to these latter individuals has been shown to evoke a prompt anamnestic appearance of anti-HBs. It should be noted that assays for anti-HBc can have false-positive reactions, particularly when a weak reactivity is obtained, and these individuals have an expected normal response to HBV vaccination rather than an amnestic response. In one study, 10 of 28 subjects known to have detectable anti-HBc without HBsAg or anti-HBs in serum for at least 6 months were found to harbor HBV DNA in serum or HBsAg and HbcAg in liver tissue. Moreover, the use of anti-HBc–positive do-

nors for liver transplantation has been associated with conversion to HBsAg positivity in the majority and allograft loss in a few recipients, prompting many centers to reject anti-HBc positive donors.

Hepatitis C

In 1989, HCV was identified as the major cause of parenterally transmitted and sporadic NANB hepatitis. HCV is a single-stranded RNA virus that is divided into a structural and nonstructural (NS) region. The structural region contains genes for the nucleocapsid protein and the envelope glycoproteins; the genes in the NS region encode various functional proteins. Whereas the 5′ "noncoding" or "untranslated" sequence of the genome is the most highly conserved region, the greatest heterogeneity occurs in the sequence encoding the envelope proteins. At least six major genotypes as well as numerous subtypes have been identified, and possible epidemiologic and clinicopathologic associations with specific genotypes and subtypes are currently under active investigation.

The currently available diagnostic armamentarium for HCV infection includes serologic assays for antibody to HCV and gene amplification techniques for detection of HCV RNA. Humoral responses to HCV are vigorous and directed to numerous antigenic sites. First-generation tests detected antibody to c100-3, a recombinant polypeptide expressed from the portion of the genome encoding NS proteins (Fig. 3–8). Because anti-c100-3 was not detectable in up to 20% of well-pedigreed cases of transfusion-associated hepatitis with detectable HCV RNA in serum and because of concerns regarding the nonspecificity of the first-generation tests, second-generation tests were developed. The second-generation enzyme immunoassay (EIA-2) detects antibodies to the core recombinant protein c22-3 and to a recombinant protein, c200, which represents a composite of the recombinant proteins c33c (in the NS3 region) and c100-3 (in the NS4 region). Compared with the first-generation assay, the EIA-2 detects anti-HCV in an additional 10% to 20% of patients with HCV infection. Moreover, the EIA-2 shortens the window period between the onset of clinical or biochemical illness and seroconversion by a mean of 8 weeks; in 70% to 80% of cases, EIA-2 can detect anti-HCV within 4 weeks of the onset of illness. In two US clinical trials, the detection rate of confirmed anti-HCV-positive blood donors was approximately 0.2% higher with EIA-2, and it has been estimated that substitution of EIA-2 for EIA-1 to screen blood donors for HCV has prevented an additional 50 transfusion-associated hepatitis cases per day. Recent reports underscore the limitations of even second-generation serologic testing for HCV in patients on chronic dialysis, implying that direct detection of HCV RNA may be required for diagnosing HCV infection in a substantial proportion of patients with chronic renal failure (see Fig. 3–3).

A strip immunoassay, the recombinant immunoblot assay (RIBA), uses recombinant proteins derived from HCV to confirm EIA anti-HCV results. In patients with liver disease, the confirmation rate is more than 90%; however, for blood donors the confirmation rate is below 50%. The second-generation RIBA (RIBA-2) consists of a nitrocellulose strip

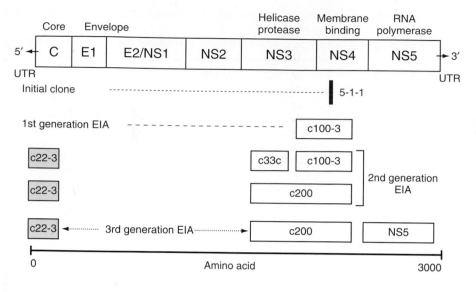

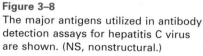

Figure 3–8
The major antigens utilized in antibody detection assays for hepatitis C virus are shown. (NS, nonstructural.)

to which recombinant HCV proteins 5.1.1. (from the NS4 region), c100-3 (from the NS4 region), c33c (from the NS3 region), and c22-3 (from the core region), have been blotted as discrete bands, along with two levels of human IgG and a superoxide dismutase (SOD) that serve as controls (Fig. 3–9). The result of the RIBA, which is performed by a technique similar to a Western blot test, is said to be positive when reactivity to two or more of the HCV antigens is demonstrated. More than 85% of patients with viremia (i.e., those who have HCV RNA in serum by PCR) demonstrate reactivity to two or more bands on RIBA-2.

The most widely used research method to detect HCV RNA in clinical specimens is PCR; HCV RNA has been detected in serum, plasma, whole blood, and fixed liver tissue. PCR primers are usually based on the highly conserved 5′ untranslated region (5′ UTR), which is less variable than other portions of the HCV genome. Several shortcomings may limit the usefulness of PCR as a diagnostic test; specifically, improper collection, handling, and storage of samples, including repeated thawing and freezing, may re-

sult in considerable variability in results among different laboratories. The branched DNA (bDNA) signal amplification system has been developed for detecting HCV RNA. Although less sensitive than PCR, bDNA testing is generally reliable and reproducible in detecting viremia and quantifying the viral load.

Table 3–5 outlines classification systems for HCV genotypes, including the generally accepted nomenclature. Methods for genotyping include genomic amplification of certain regions and nucleotide sequencing, PCR with genotype-specific primers, restriction fragment length polymorphism (RFLP) analysis of the PCR amplicons, differential hybridization, and serologic genotyping. Overall, there appears to be excellent concordance between the genotyping results obtained by these various systems utilizing different HCV genomic regions (5′UTR, NS4, and NS5). Only methods that include sequence analysis of specific gene regions of the HCV genome are completely reliable for genotyping. The line probe assay (LiPA) is based on the initial amplification of the 5′UTR and has excellent sensitivity and

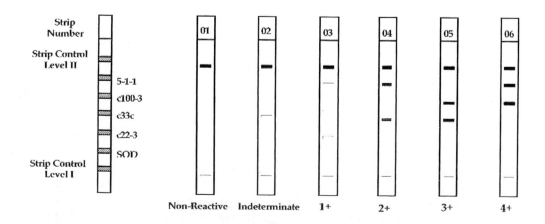

Figure 3–9
RIBA-II. Recombinant hepatitis C virus (HCV) antigens are absorbed on a nitrocellulose filter. When none of the HCV bands are observed, the test is read as nonreactive. If only one HCV band is visible, the test is read as indeterminate. The presence of two or more bands is interpreted as a positive test result. Gradation from 1+ to 4+ is done using the strip controls as reference. (From Sjogren MH: Serologic diagnosis of viral hepatitis. Gastroenterol Clin North Am 23:457, 1994.)

Table 3–5   Hepatitis C Genotype Classification

Standard System	Simmonds	Okamoto/Mori	Chayama	Houghton/Cha	Enomoto
1a	1a	I	I	I	PT
1b	1b	II	II	II	K1
1c					
2a	2a	III	III	III	K2a
2b	2b	IV	IV	III	k2b
2c				III	
3a	3	V		IV	
3b		VI	V	IV	
4a	4				
5a				V	
6a					

From Lau JYN, Mizokami M, Kolberg JA, et al: Application of six hepatitis C virus genotyping systems to sera from chronic hepatitis C patients in the United States. J Infect Dis 171:281–289, 1995.

specificity. Of note, direct nucleotide sequencing methods will detect a variant only if it represents more than 10% to 20% of the HCV genomes amplified. Therefore, genotyping of HCV may reveal only the predominant species in the patient's circulation at that point in time.

Hepatitis D

Hepatitis D (delta) virus (HDV) is a defective RNA virus that requires HBV to replicate. The commercially available assays for HDV markers are immunoassays for IgM and total anti-HDV. The diagnosis of acute HDV coinfection (both HBV and HDV) is suggested by the finding of anti-HDV in a patient with HBsAg or IgM anti-HBc. Whereas the majority of patients with acute HDV coinfection recover, most patients with superinfection (HDV infection in patients with pre-existing HBV infection) develop chronic HDV hepatitis manifested by persistent replication (Fig. 3–10). Titers of anti-HDV typically become nondetectable after acute self-limited coinfection but rise to high levels in patients with

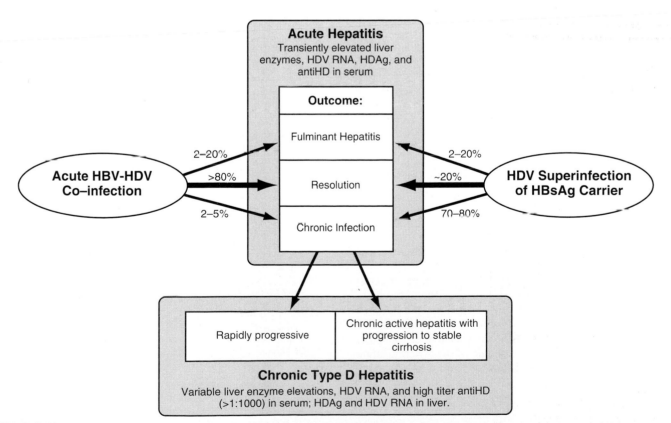

Figure 3–10
Patterns of hepatitis D virus (HDV) infection and disease. (HBV, hepatitis B virus; HDAg, hepatitis D antigen; HBsAg, hepatitis B surface antigen.) (From Casey JL: Hepatitis delta virus. Clin Lab Med 16:451–464, 1996.)

chronic superinfection. Because HDV infection exists only in the setting of concomitant HBV infection, persons immune to HBV are immune to HDV.

Hepatitis E

Hepatitis E virus (HEV) infection, previously called enterically transmitted or epidemic non-A, non-B hepatitis, has been recently cloned. The serologic profile resembles hepatitis A; HEV antigen can be found in the stool during the incubation period (which averages 40 days) and during the early symptomatic phase. The IgG anti-HEV appears to persist for at least 4 years.

Hepatitis G

Hepatitis G virus (HGV) is an identified RNA virus whose genomic organization is similar to HCV in that the genes encoding structural proteins required for viral assembly are located at the 5' end of the genome whereas the genes encoding nonstructural proteins required for viral replication are located at the 3' end. No antibody test to HGV is commercially available yet. A significant proportion of patients with liver disease, particularly those undergoing liver transplantation, have detectable HGV RNA by PCR, but a causative association with liver disease can only be inferred. In fact, preliminary reports suggest that HCV-positive patients coinfected with HGV are comparable to patients with HCV alone with regard to response to medical therapy and course after liver transplantation.

SUMMARY

The differential diagnosis of abnormal LFTs includes hepatic and extrahepatic conditions and is greatly narrowed by a comprehensive history and physical examination and by the recognition of classic patterns of liver injury. The limitations of these liver tests, including problems with specificity and sensitivity, must always be taken into account. Patients with essentially normal conventional LFTs may have significantly impaired hepatic function; conversely, hepatic function may be well preserved in some patients with abnormal LFTs. It is possible that in the future QLFTs (i.e., aminopyrine breath test, galactose elemination capacity) will gain wider clinical applicability. Furthermore, other indices of hepatic function, such as bilirubin and prothrombin time, are important prognostic indicators of the natural history of specific conditions such as PBC and alcoholic hepatitis.

Immunoassays and molecular biologic diagnostic tests are invaluable tools in the diagnosis and monitoring of therapy of the six etiologic agents responsible for viral hepatitis. Improved detection methods have resulted in improved prevention of transfusion-associated disease. Furthermore, an improved understanding of the different strains of viral hepatitis have provided insight into their epidemiology and pathogenesis.

SUGGESTED READINGS

Alter HJ: To C or not to C: These are the questions. Blood 85:1681–1695, 1995.

Bacon BR, Farahvash MJ, Janney CG, et al: Nonalcoholic steatohcpatitis: An expanded clinical entity. Gastroenterology 107:1103–1108, 1994.

Bukh J, Miller RH, Purcell RH: Genetic heterogeneity of hepatitis C virus: Quasispecies and genotypes. Semin Liver Dis 15:41–43, 1995.

Carithers RL Jr, Herlong HF, Diehl Am, et al: Methylprednisolone therapy in patients with severe alcoholic hepatitis. A randomized multicenter trial. Ann Intern Med 110:685–690, 1989.

Christensen E, Bremmelgaard A, Bahnsen M, et al: Prediction of fatality in fulminant hepatic failure. Scan J Gastroenterol 19:90, 1984.

Cohen JA, Kaplan MM: The SGOT/SGPT ratio—An indicator of alcoholic liver disease. Dig Dis Sci 24:835–838, 1979.

deFrancis R, Meucci G, Vecchi M, et al: The natural history of asymptomatic hepatitis B surface antigen carriers. Ann Intern Med 118:191–194, 1993.

Dickson RC, Everhart JE: Transmission of hepatitis B by transplantation of livers from donors positive for antibody to hepatitis B core antigen. Gastroenterology 110:A1182, 1996.

Dixit V, Quan S, Martin P, et al: Evaluation of a novel serotyping system for hepatitis C virus: Strong correlation with standard genotyping methodologies. J Clin Microbiol 33:2978–2983, 1995.

Estaban JI, Genesca J, Alter HJ: Hepatitis C: Molecular biology, pathogenesis, epidemiology, clinical features, and prevention. Prog Liver Dis 10:252–282, 1992.

Flora KD, Keeffe EB: Evaluation of mildly abnormal liver tests in asymptomatic patients. J Insur Med 22:264–267, 1990.

Friedman LS, Martin P, Munoz SJ: Liver function tests and the objective evaluation of the patient with liver disease. In Zakim D, Boyer TD (eds): Hepatology: A Textbook of Liver Disease. Philadelphia: WB Saunders, 1996, pp 791–833.

Hawker F: Liver function tests. In Hawker F: The Liver. London: WB Saunders, 1993, pp 41–70.

Hayashi PH, Beames MP, Kuhns MC, et al: Use of quantitative assays for hepatitis B e antigen and IgM antibody to hepatitis B core antigen to monitor therapy in chronic hepatitis B. Am J Gastroenterol 91:2323–2328, 1996.

Healey CJ, Chapman RWG, Fleming KA: Liver histology in hepatitis C infection: A comparison between patients with persistently normal or abnormal transaminases. Gut 37:274–278, 1995.

Huang Y-S, Lee S-D, Deng J-F, et al: Measuring lidocaine metabolism—monoethylglcinexylidide as a quantitative index of hepatic function in adults with chronic hepatitis and cirrhosis. J Hepatol 19:140–146, 1993.

Keeffe EBL: Diagnostic approach to mild elevation of liver enzyme levels. Gastrointest Dis Today 3:1–9, 1994.

Lau JYN, Davis GL, Prescott LE, et al: Distribution of hepatitis C virus genotypes determined by line probe assay in patients with chronic hepatitis C seen at tertiary referral centers in the United States. Ann Intern Med 124:868–876, 1996.

Lau JYN, Mizokami M, Kolberg JA, et al: Application of six hepatitis C virus genotyping systems to sera from chronic hepatitis C patients in the United States. J Infect Dis 171:281–289, 1995.

Linnen J, Wages J, Zhen-Yong Z-K, et al: Molecular cloning and disease association of hepatitis G virus: A transfusion-transmissible agent. Science 271:505–508, 1996.

Magarian GJ, Lucas LM, Kumar KL: Clinical significance in alcoholic patients of commonly encountered laboratory test results. West J Med 156:287–294, 1992.

Medrano FJ, Sanchez-Quijano A, Pineda J, et al: Isolated anti-HBc and hepatitis B virus occult infection. Vox Sang 61:140–144, 1991.

Mosely RH: Evaluation of abnormal liver function tests. Med Clin North Am 80:887–906, 1996.

Okamoto E, Kyo A, Yamanaka N, et al: Prediction of the safe limits of hepatectomy by volumetric and functional measurements of patients with impaired hepatic function. Surgery 95:586–591, 1984.

Pessoa MG, Wright TL: Hepatitis G: A virus in search of a disease. Hepatology 24:461–463, 1996.

Pietrangelo A, Panduro A, Chowdhury JR, Shafritz DA: Albumin gene expression is down-regulated by albumin or macromolecule infusion in the rat. J Clin Invest 89:1755–1760, 1992.

Roggendorf M, Lu M, Meisel H, et al: Rational use of diagnostic tools in hepatitis C. J Hepatol 24:26–34, 1996.

Rosen HR, Friedman LS, Martin P: Hepatitis C in renal dialysis and transplant patients. Viral Hepatitis Rev 2:91–110, 1996.

Rosen HR, Martin P, Goss J, et al: Significance of early aminotransferase elevation after liver transplantation. Transplantation 65:68–72, 1998.

Rothschild MA, Oratz M, Schreiber SS: Serum albumin. Hepatology 8:385–401, 1988.

Serfaty L, Chazouilleres O, Pawlotsky J-M, et al: Interferon alfa therapy in patients with chronic hepatitis C and persistently normal aminotransferase activity. Gastroenterology 110:291–295, 1996.

Shapiro JM, Smith H, Shaffner F: Serum bilirubin: A prognostic factor in primary biliary cirrhosis. Gut 20:137–140, 1979.

Sjogren MH: Serologic diagnosis of viral hepatitis. Med Clin North Am 80:929–956, 1996.

Wu J-C, Chen C-M, Chen T-Z, et al: Prevalence and type of precore hepatitis B virus mutants in hepatitis D virus superinfection and its clinical implication. J Infect Dis 173:457–459, 1996.

Yasuda K, Kunio O, Endo N, et al: Hypoaminotransferasemia in patients undergoing long-term hemodialysis: Clinical and biochemical appraisal. Gastroenterology 109:1295–1300, 1995.

4

Evaluation of Jaundice

Lisa Higa
Rise Stribling
Paul Martin

The presence of jaundice is a cardinal feature of liver disease, and its presence usually signifies a disturbance involving the hepatobiliary system. Jaundice is defined as a yellowish pigmentation of the sclerae, skin, and mucous membranes and occurs because of tissue deposition of excess serum bilirubin. Bilirubin pigment is most concentrated in tissues that contain a large amount of elastin (e.g., the sclerae and frenulum of the tongue), because bilirubin binds readily with this extracellular matrix protein. A patient becomes clinically icteric when serum bilirubin exceeds 2 to 3 mg/dL. True jaundice should be distinguished from yellow tinting of the skin, which can result from excessive intake of carotene- or lycopene-containing vegetables, drugs such as quinacrine, and associated conditions such as hypothyroidism and uremia. In these states, the serum bilirubin level is normal and there is no scleral icterus. Although an overlap exists, jaundice occurs in primarily four different disorders in bilirubin metabolism:

1. An increased bilirubin load delivered to the liver cell
2. An irregularity in the uptake or transport of bilirubin within the hepatocyte
3. A disturbance in bilirubin conjugation
4. Mechanical or functional obstruction of bile flow through the bile duct system

The initial step in evaluating the icteric patient is to determine if jaundice is caused by unconjugated (indirect) or conjugated (direct) hyperbilirubinemia. If indirect hyperbilirubinemia is present, there is either overproduction of bilirubin (e.g., in overt hemolysis) or a defect in hepatic uptake or conjugation. If direct hyperbilirubinemia is present, the differential diagnoses include hepatocellular, infiltrative, or cholestatic processes. If cholestasis is present, mechanical obstruction of the biliary tract needs to be excluded.

Because the wide differential diagnosis of jaundice ranges from benign to life-threatening diseases, a thorough clinical review of the patient is the cornerstone of efficient management. Within the past 20 years, various diagnostic studies have evolved to assess the liver and biliary tree. Because these methods have some risk and expense, tests should be chosen for their specific clinical usefulness and cost effectiveness.

BILIRUBIN METABOLISM

A brief review of bilirubin production, uptake and conjugation with the hepatocyte, transport, and excretion facilitates formulating an approach to jaundice (Fig. 4–1).

Bilirubin Production

Bilirubin is the end product of heme breakdown. Ninety percent of heme is derived from senescent erythrocytes that are phagocytized by reticuloendothelial cells in the spleen, liver (Kupffer cells), and bone marrow. The remaining 10% can come from cytochromes, ineffective erythropoiesis, and intravascular hemolysis as well as myoglobin breakdown. Under normal circumstances, ineffective erythropoiesis and intravascular hemolysis account for less than 5% of bilirubin production; however, this percentage can be greatly increased in certain pathologic processes. Whereas bilirubin is transported in the plasma bound primarily to albumin, hemoglobin and heme released into the serum as a result of hemolysis are bound to haptoglobin and to hemopexin, respectively, and each type of complex binds to specific hepatic receptors for hepatocyte uptake. Approximately 300 mg of bilirubin is formed daily. The level of serum bilirubin in 95% of healthy adults ranges from 0.2 to 0.9 mg/dL (1mg/dL of

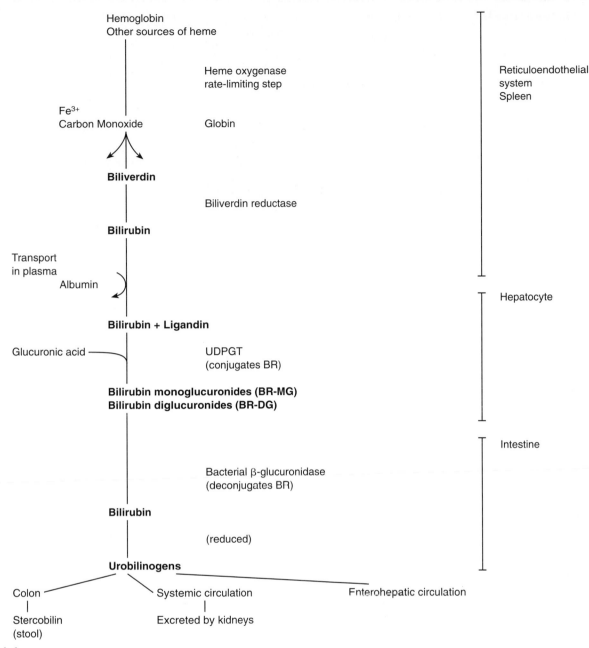

Figure 4–1
Bilirubin metabolism. (BR, bilirubin; UDPGT, uridine diphosphoglucuronyl transferase.)

bilirubin is ~17 mmol/L), and almost 95% of the total bilirubin present is in the unconjugated form. The concentration of unconjugated bilirubin in the serum is directly related to its rate of production and inversely proportional to its rate of hepatic and renal elimination from the body. Men have higher mean levels of bilirubin compared with women, usually because women have lower rates of bilirubin production and higher efficiency of bilirubin conjugation. Because up to 1500 mg of bilirubin can be broken down and excreted daily from heme, a massive increase in hemoglobin breakdown can occur without appreciable increase in serum bilirubin.

Within the reticuloendothelial system including the spleen, the first step in bilirubin synthesis is the rate-limiting oxidation of heme to biliverdin by the enzyme heme oxyge-

nase located on the endoplasmic reticulum. Iron and 1 molecule of carbon monoxide are also released in the reaction. Essentially all of the biliverdin is then reduced to bilirubin by the enzyme biliverdin reductase.

Bilirubin is a yellow tetrapyrrole compound that exists in two forms—unconjugated and conjugated. Unconjugated bilirubin is insoluble in water, because of intramolecular hydrogen binding that prevents ionization of the two external highly hydrophobic carboxylic acid groups. It is transported in the blood bound to serum proteins, primarily albumin. Thus, drugs that compete with bilirubin for binding sites on albumin (e.g., sulfonamides and anti-inflammatory drugs) will increase the free bilirubin concentration and increase the risk of kernicterus in infants.

Hepatic Uptake and Intracellular Binding

Upon arrival at the hepatocyte, the albumin-bilirubin complex freely crosses through the fenestrated endothelial cells that line the hepatic sinusoids and then dissociates, leaving albumin in the intravascular space and delivering the bilirubin to a carrier-mediated transport protein located on the basolateral membrane, which transports bilirubin into the cell. Within the hepatocyte, bilirubin binds to the ligandin glutathione acetyltransferase B, which traps it and prevents reflux of bilirubin back into the sinusoidal blood.

Bilirubin Conjugation and Secretion into Bile

Bilirubin conjugation facilitates bilirubin excretion from the hepatocyte into the bile canaliculi. Bilirubin is conjugated to glucuronic acid by the enzyme uridine diphosphoglucuronyl transferase (UDPGT) into water-soluble monoglucuronide (BR-MG) and diglucuronide (BR-DG). Of the conjugated bilirubin in bile, 80% is present as BR-DG. The conjugated bilirubin is then actively transported against a concentration gradient into bile via another carrier-mediated process into the bile canaliculi. Thus, in patients with hepatocellular dysfunction, bilirubin secretion is relatively more impaired than uptake and conjugation. The conjugated bilirubin accumulates intracellularly, is regurgitated back into the sinusoids, and returns ultimately to the systemic circulation.

Extrahepatic Transport, Metabolism, and Excretion

After biliary excretion, conjugated bilirubin passes throughout most of the small bowel without undergoing absorption or metabolism, because conjugation of bilirubin prevents its re-entry into the systemic circulation. In the distal ileum and colon, bacterial enzyme β-glucuronidase first deconjugates the bilirubin, which is then reduced to colorless urobilinogens. Urobilinogens are almost completely reabsorbed in the small intestine and predominantly enter the enterohepatic circulation. The remaining reabsorbed urobilinogens enter the systemic circulation and are excreted by the kidneys. Urinary urobilinogens may be increased, even before the onset of clinical jaundice, in patients with hemolysis (overproduction of bilirubin), gastrointestinal bleeding, or hepatocellular disease (impaired removal of urobilinogen from blood); conversely, in complete biliary obstruction with interruption of the enterohepatic circulation of bile pigments, urinary urobilinogens are absent. Thus, qualitative assessment of urinary urobilinogens can be helpful in the evaluation of jaundice. A false-positive urine dipstick test result for urobilinogens may be seen with increased urinary pH and certain drugs, including procaine, 5-hydroxyindoleacetic acid, and sulfonamides. The small number of urobilinogens that remain in the colonic lumen spontaneously oxidize to urobilins and several other compounds, which include stercobilin, the orange-brown pigment of stool. Bilirubin is not usually found in feces unless the intestinal flora is underdeveloped or altered by antibiotics.

Measurement of Serum Bilirubin

Measurement of serum bilirubin was first described by Van den Bergh in the early 1900s. The Van den Bergh or Diazo reaction involves multiple steps in which a bilirubin molecule combines with diazotized sulfinalol acid to form chromogenic pyrrolase moieties that can be quantitated spectrophotometrically. In general, total serum bilirubin represents all bilirubin that reacts within 30 minutes in the presence of alcohol, an accelerating agent. Direct (conjugated) serum bilirubin reacts quickly with the diazo reagent and is the fraction that reacts within 1 minute. Indirect serum bilirubin is determined by subtraction of the direct reacting fraction from the total bilirubin level. The Van den Bergh reaction is imprecise and often overestimates conjugated bilirubin; this is especially true in cases of mild hyperbilirubinemia with levels less than 5 mg/dL.

In patients with severe conjugated hyperbilirubinemia, up to 60% of the serum bilirubin may be bound covalently to serum proteins, usually albumin. Therefore, in these patients with significantly elevated serum albumin-bilirubin complexes (also known as delta bilirubin), the half-life of the serum bilirubin will approximate the half-life of albumin, which is approximately 14 to 21 days; this bilirubin will not be removed from the body until the albumin is degraded. This may account for the persistence of jaundice for days to weeks after the relief of a biliary obstruction, even after other parameters of liver function have improved or normalized. Because conjugated bilirubin is more soluble in water and can thus penetrate and become widely distributed in most body fluids and tissues, icteric patients with direct hyperbilirubinemia may appear more deeply jaundiced compared with those individuals with hemolytic anemia.

Urine Bilirubin

Conjugated bilirubin, but not unconjugated bilirubin, is excreted in the urine. Because the former is less hydrophobic than unconjugated bilirubin and as it is not highly protein-bound, it is excreted into the urine. In the kidney, the conjugated bilirubin is normally filtered at the glomerulus, and the majority is reabsorbed by the proximal tubules; only 1% to 2% is excreted in the urine. In contrast, unconjugated bilirubin is tightly bound to albumin. This large complex is not filtered at the glomerulus, and none will enter the urine. Therefore, bilirubinuria is an indication of conjugated hyperbilirubinemia and may be associated with consequent darkening of the urine even before the detection of overt jaundice. Conversely, however, delta bilirubin-albumin complexes in conjugated hyperbilirubinemia can result in persistent jaundice without elevated urinary bilirubin during the period of resolution of acute jaundice; in this setting, bilirubinuria is absent because the covalently protein-bound delta bilirubin is not filtered and thus does not exclude conjugated hyperbilirubinemia as the cause of jaundice.

CLASSIFICATION OF HYPERBILIRUBINEMIA

In general, hyperbilirubinemia is usually defined as a level greater than 1.5 mg/dL and is further characterized by the degree of excess conjugated or unconjugated hyperbilirubinemia. Hyperbilirubinemia is defined as unconjugated if more than 80% to 85% of the total bilirubin is unconjugated. Conjugated hyperbilirubinemia is present if more than 30% of the total bilirubin level is conjugated.

Unconjugated Hyperbilirubinemia

Hemolysis and Ineffective Erythropoiesis

Bilirubin overproduction most typically results from ineffective erythropoiesis or increased destruction from hemolysis of erythrocytes. Hemolysis can be induced by drugs (e.g., penicillin, ribavarin, and quinine) or primary erythrocyte disorders including thalassemia, sickle cell anemia, spherocytosis, glucose-6-phosphate deficiency, an ABO blood group incompatibility, and paroxysmal nocturnal hemoglobinuria. With normal hepatic function, a 50% reduction in erythrocyte survival leading to an increased load of bilirubin presented to the hepatocyte will not cause jaundice. In vivo studies demonstrate that the enzyme heme oxygenase can be stimulated up to 20-fold in the liver, kidney, or macrophages by the administration of heme or hemoglobin. Hence, the body has an effective adaptive mechanism for coping with increased heme breakdown. Bilirubin levels are rarely elevated above 5 mg/dL even in severe hemolysis in patients with normal hepatic function. However, even mild hepatic dysfunction can increase the degree of hyperbilirubinemia resulting from bilirubin overproduction. For instance, mixed direct and indirect hyperbilirubinemia can develop when hemolytic disorders are superimposed upon chronic liver disease from secondary iron overload or chronic hepatitis C as a result of a prior blood transfusion.

Hereditary Unconjugated Hyperbilirubinemia

Mild unconjugated hyperbilirubinemia is seen in approximately 5% of healthy blood donors. After hemolysis and ineffective erythropoiesis are excluded, the familial abnormalities of bilirubin metabolism, of which Gilbert's syndrome is the most common, should be considered. These disorders of bilirubin conjugation involve deficiencies in UDPGT activity. Patients are not pruritic because cholestasis is not present.

Gilbert's Syndrome: Gilbert's syndrome is benign, familial, mild unconjugated hyperbilirubinemia characterized by bilirubin levels usually less than 5 mg/dL and otherwise normal liver function tests and liver biopsy. There are no signs of portal hypertension on physical examination. Approximately 50% of patients may have an associated mild hemolytic anemia. Jaundice is noted to deepen during periods of fasting, stress, or intercurrent infection and may be associated with mild nausea, malaise, and abdominal discomfort. Otherwise, patients are clinically well and have an excellent prognosis with normal life expectancy. The diagnosis is often made after mild hyperbilirubinemia is detected on routine laboratory testing. Gilbert's syndrome is inherited in an autosomal dominant pattern and affects approximately 2% to 5% of the general population. The average age at presentation occurs in the late teens. Patients with Gilbert's syndrome are able to process most hepatically metabolized drugs, and no dose reduction is needed. No specific treatment other than reassurance is necessary.

The metabolic defect in Gilbert's syndrome is complex and is thought to involve several enzyme abnormalities including structural defects of the gene encoding for the conjugating enzyme UDPGT, leading to a reduction of UDPGT production, dyserythropoiesis, and alterations in membrane fluidity, thus impairing hepatocyte uptake of bilirubin.

The diagnosis of Gilbert's syndrome is easily made by clinical examination and history. Diagnostic challenging to see if hyperbilirubinemia increases after a period of fasting is not usually indicated. Older tests including the phenobarbital test (which induces UDPGT and thus causes a fall in bilirubinemia) and the intravenous nicotinic acid test (which increases the osmotic fragility of red blood cells causing them to lyse and increase the bilirubin load) are now obsolete.

Crigler-Najjar Syndrome: This rare form of jaundice is separated into two types (types I and II), both of which are associated with marked high serum unconjugated hyperbilirubinemia and deficiency of the conjugating enzyme UDPGT. Type I is inherited as autosomal recessive trait and is associated with a complete lack of conjugating enzyme and an absence of conjugated bilirubin in bile. Infants present with jaundice and high levels of unconjugated hyperbilirubinemia (as high as 30 mg/dL) by the first week of life. Patients usually die of kernicterus during the first 1 to 2 years of life. Conjugating enzyme levels are not induced by phenobarbital, because there is complete absence of UDPGT activity. Liver histology and tests of bilirubin uptake and storage are normal. Phlebotomy, plasmapheresis, and phototherapy are temporizing measures if kernicterus develops. Orthotopic liver transplantation in these patients is life saving. Type II, also known as Arias' disease, is an autosomal dominant disorder with very low levels of UDPGT activity (as low as 10% of normal), which is inducible by phenobarbital, although medical treatment is usually not necessary. Patients usually present with jaundice later in life than do patients with type I, ranging from 1 to 10 years of age. The degree of unconjugated hyperbilirubinemia can also be quite severe with bilirubin levels in the 20 mg/dL range; infants can also develop kernicterus.

Miscellaneous Causes (Impaired Hepatic Delivery or Uptake of Bilirubin): Drugs including penicillin, ribavirin, and quinine can also cause hemolysis and can lead to indirect hyperbilirubinemia. Other drugs such as probenecid and rifampin decrease hepatic uptake of bilirubin, which is reversible upon discontinuation of the drug. Sulfonamides, aspirin, and total parenteral nutrition (TPN) can displace bilirubin binding from albumin. Discontinuation or avoidance of these drugs will result in normalization of serum bilirubin concentration, generally within a few days. Postoperative patients, especially those following cardiac surgery, can frequently develop mild hyperbilirubinemia up to 5 mg/dL in the first few days after surgery. The etiology is multifactorial and may include multiple blood transfusions, resorption of a hematoma, mild hemolytic anemia, drug interactions, hypotension, and anesthesia. Pre-existing liver disease is a risk factor for developing postoperative jaundice, and cirrhotic patients must be monitored carefully after surgery for signs of hepatic decompensation including ascites, variceal bleeding, and hepatic encephalopathy.

Fasting can also cause reversible unconjugated hyperbilirubinemia. A diet consisting of less than 400 kcal/day for a normal adult can lead to an increase in the total bilirubin level by 0.4 mg/dL. Impaired delivery of bilirubin to the liver can occur in congestive heart failure or portosystemic shunting.

Conjugated Hyperbilirubinemias

Direct hyperbilirubinemia can be divided into hereditary and acquired causes. Acquired causes comprise the largest group of conjugated hyperbilirubinemia and include hepatocellular, infiltrative, and cholestatic, the latter being further separated into intrahepatic or extrahepatic etiologies. Patients with cholestasis may display pruritus, malabsorption, steatorrhea, and hypercholesterolemia. The degree of hyperbilirubinemia can range from mild to severe, and the degree of jaundice cannot distinguish the cause of hyperbilirubinemia.

Hereditary Conjugated Hyperbilirubinemia

Dubin-Johnson Syndrome: This form of jaundice is benign and intermittent and is associated with both conjugated and unconjugated hyperbilirubinemia along with bilirubinuria. The metabolic defect is impaired secretion of conjugated bilirubin. Total bilirubin levels are modestly elevated, typically below 5 mg/dL; other liver tests are normal. Most notably in this syndrome, the liver macroscopically appears greenish-black, although no bile or iron can be distinguished on liver biopsy. This is an autosomal recessive pattern and is most common in the Middle East. Patients typically present with nonpruritic jaundice during pregnancy or after taking oral contraceptives due to hormone-mediated decreased hepatic secretion of bilirubin. The prognosis is excellent. The diagnosis of Dubin-Johnson syndrome rests on the characteristic liver biopsy revealing dark pigment granules within hepatocytes and Kupffer cells. There is no correlation between the level of hyperbilirubinemia and the liver pigment. Previously, the Bromsulphalein (BSP) clearance test was used for a diagnostic tool. The characteristic finding is an initial immediate fall within 1 hour in BSP level to normal followed by a secondary increase in the level after 3 hours. Abnormal BSP testing reflects the hepatic secretory dysfunction in these patients.

Rotor's Syndrome: This syndrome is similiar to Dubin-Johnson syndrome; the main differences are a normal liver biopsy and no secondary increase on BSP testing. Rotor syndrome follows an autosomal recessive transmission pattern and results in mixed hyperbilirubinemia with usual elevation in serum bilirubin of less than 5 mg/dL. The exact metabolic defect is unclear. It has an excellent prognosis.

Acquired Forms of Conjugated Hyperbilirubinemia

Hepatocellular: Viral hepatitis and chronic liver diseases (including alcoholic liver disease and cirrhosis) are common etiologies of conjugated hyperbilirubinemia and usually present with elevated aminotransaminases. Cholestasis can also be seen with severe hepatocellular dysfunction or during the period of recovery from acute viral hepatitis.

Infiltrative and Intrahepatic Cholestasis: Drugs, infections, tumors, and chronic liver diseases are among the most common causes in this category. Drug hepatotoxicity is a common cause of jaundice. The diagnosis is often one of exclusion. Several mechanisms of drug hepatotoxicity can occur and may overlap. Drugs can produce a cholestatic reaction (e.g., cotrimazole, chlorpromazine) or hepatocellular damage (e.g., isoniazid). Drugs can also compete for binding sites on albumin and cause unconjugated hyperbilirubinemia.

Primary biliary cirrhosis and primary sclerosing cholangitis are the two main chronic cholestatic liver diseases. Patients with primary biliary cirrhosis typically present with pruritus and high alkaline phosphatase levels; serum bilirubin is usually normal early in the disease course due to the large adaptive mechanism of the liver for bile secretion. The onset of hyperbilirubinemia and jaundice is associated with an acceleration of the disease course of primary biliary cirrhosis. Primary sclerosing cholangitis is frequently associated with inflammatory bowel disease, typically ulcerative colitis. However, liver disease in these patients can antedate bowel symptoms.

By the time that primary hepatic tumors and metastatic carcinomas have infiltrated the liver massively enough to cause jaundice, the prognosis is poor. Lymphoma can cause an elevation of alkaline phosphatase, which is usually caused by diffuse hepatic infiltration. Amyloid, sarcoid, and tuberculosis are other examples of infiltrative hepatic diseases.

Infections that are bacterial, fungal, parasitic as well as related to acquired immunodeficiency syndrome can produce with jaundice by several mechanisms, including hyperbilirubinemia associated with intrahepatic cholestasis caused by sepsis, endotoxemia, or invasion of the hepatic parenchyma during fungemia. Liver biopsy findings may be diagnostic, especially when an elevated serum alkaline phosphatase level is present.

Extrahepatic Cholestasis: This is synonomous with obstruction of the bile duct by tumor, stones, stricture, blood, parasites, or external compression of the bile duct lumen. Extrahepatic obstruction should be considered early because these causes are potentially reversible and failure to recognize these cases may result in complications such as recurrent cholangitis or secondary biliary cirrhosis.

EVALUATION OF THE PATIENT WITH JAUNDICE (Table 4–1)

Clinical History

The clinical history may provide important clues to the diagnosis including the time course of jaundice, associated symptoms, and risk factors. The following points should be explored.

Demographics: With increasing age, the risk of malignancy is greater. In sexually active young adults, hepatitis B is a cause of acute jaundice. In Asian or African patients, hepatitis B may have been contracted in infancy or early childhood only to result in clinical liver disease in adulthood.

Onset of Jaundice: The insidious onset of icterus is a common complaint in patients with malignancy, whereas a prodromal viral syndrome is associated with viral hepatitis.

Table 4–1   Common Causes of Jaundice

Unconjugated Hyperbilirubinemia

OVERPRODUCTION	Hemolysis
	Blood extravasation (intra-abdominal bleed, resolution of hematoma)
	Ineffective erythropoiesis
	Multiple blood transfusions
HEREDITARY	Gilbert's disease
	Crigler-Najjar syndrome
MISCELLANEOUS	Drugs, neonatal disorders, fasting, thyroid disorders

Conjugated Hyperbilirubinemia

HEPATOCELLULAR	Acute/chronic viral hepatitis
	Alcoholic liver disease
	Hemochromatosis
	Toxins (Tylenol, *Amanita* mushrooms)
	Halothane anesthesia
	Hypotension
	Wilson's disease
INTRAHEPATIC CHOLESTASIS	Hepatitis
	Cirrhosis
	Infiltrative disorders (e.g., sarcoidosis)
	Drugs (e.g., anabolic steroids, chlorpromazine)
	Total parenteral nutrition
	Hypotension
	Congestive heart failure
EXTRAHEPATIC CHOLESTASIS	Choledocholithiasis
	Neoplasms (e.g., ampullary or bile duct CA, pancreatic CA, metastatic CA, extrinsic compression causing CBD obstruction and lymphoma)
	Oriental cholangiohepatitis (e.g., clonorchis)
	Choledochocele/choledochalcysts—Caroli's disease
	Iatrogenic (e.g., bile duct injury during surgery)
	Biliary strictures (malignant, benign, infectious)
	Cholangitis
HEREDITARY	Dubin-Johnson syndrome
	Rotor syndrome
FAMILIAL DISORDERS	Benign recurrent intrahepatic cholestasis
	Cholestasis of pregnancy
MISCELLANEOUS	Systemic disease
	Postoperative complications
	Renal disease
	Sepsis

Very High Bilirubin Levels

>30 mg/dL	Usually signifies hemolysis *plus* parenchymal liver disease or biliary obstruction
>60 mg/dL	Seen in patients with hemoglobinopathies (e.g., sickle cell anemia) or concomitant renal disease who develop obstructive jaundice or acute hepatitis

CA, carcinoma; CBD, common bile duct.

Abdominal Pain: The rapid onset of severe crampy right upper quadrant pain with posterior radiation and association with nausea and vomiting is suggestive of gallstone disease. Continuous dull epigastric discomfort may herald a malignant obstruction. In elderly patients, pain may be absent or atypical.

Systemic Symptoms: Fever is usually associated with cholangitis; hyperpyrexia can also be prominent in alcoholic hepatitis or granulomatous or malignant disease. Weight loss is associated with malignancy or advanced hepatic dys-

function. Fatigue and malaise are common complaints in viral hepatitis and cancer. Pruritus is often found in patients with cholestatic diseases such as primary biliary cirrhosis. It can also be present in advanced cirrhosis of any etiology. In severe hyperbilirubinemia, the ocular fluids are yellow, which may explain the symptom of xanthopsia (seeing yellow). Darkening of the urine may antedate the onset of jaundice in conjugated hyperbilirubinemia.

Associated Gastrointestinal Symptoms: Anorexia can be seen in both malignancy and viral hepatitis. Nausea or vomiting occurs with viral hepatitis or cholangitis. Aversion to smoking may be noted in smokers with acute viral hepatitis. Previous dyspepsia, fat intolerance, and biliary colic suggest choledocholithiasis.

Past Medical/Surgical History: Primary biliary cirrhosis may be associated with a history of other autoimmune disorders such as thyroiditis, sicca syndrome, Raynaud's phenomenon, or rheumatoid arthritis. A history of inflammatory bowel disease, in particular ulcerative colitis, may suggest primary sclerosing cholangitis. Bone pain and fractures, particularly vertebral collapse, can be seen in long-standing cholestatic diseases. Previous cholecystectomy raises the possibility of retained or recurrent choledocholithiasis. A thorough drug history to exclude hepatoxic medications is important; consumption of over-the-counter medications, vitamins, herbal supplements, and birth control pills must specifically be elicited. Pregnancy can be associated with a number of causes of jaundice that vary by trimester. Hospitalized patients with jaundice, especially in an intensive care unit, should have a careful review of the chart for episodes of hypotension or sepsis, use of TPN, surgical interventions, blood transfusions, gastrointestinal or other recent blood loss, and medication usage.

Risk Factors: A thorough review of social and personal history may elicit possible exposures for viral or chemical causes for jaundice. Accordingly, inquiry into previous blood transfusions, recreational drug use including intravenous drugs, sexual activity, and tattoos should be taken. A careful questioning for alcohol intake and previous complications of alcoholism is helpful in assessing the possibility of alcohol-related liver disease. Occupational and travel history as well as any known exposures to individuals with hepatitis should also be included.

Family History: Etiologies for chronic liver diseases such as the familial hyperbilirubinemias, chronic hepatitis B, primary biliary cirrhosis, or autoimmune hepatitis may be suggested by a positive family history.

Physical Examination

The physical examination may provide information regarding chronicity of disease, infection, and malignancy.

General: The overall nutritional state of the patient is important to note. Weight loss, muscle wasting, and cachexia may be present in chronic liver disease or malignancy. Mental status changes or asterixis may be elicited if hepatic encephalopathy is present. The degree of icterus should be assessed; mild jaundice usually accompanies hemolytic states, whereas deep jaundice signifies advanced cirrhosis or malignancy. Stigmata of chronic liver disease such as spider angiomata, palmar erythema, and Dupuytren's contractures should be noted; signs of feminization in male cirrhotic patients with gynecomastia, testicular atrophy, and hair loss are common. Scattered ecchymoses provide a clue to hepatic synthetic dysfunction. Excoriations suggest pruritus. Cutaneous xanthomas are present in approximately 10% of patients with primary biliary cirrhosis. Fetor hepaticus (the peculiar fruity odor of the breath characteristic of liver dis-

ease) is typically associated with decompensated cirrhosis. Careful inspection to detect evidence of extrahepatic primary malignant tumors is important and should include an examination of the lymph nodes, thyroid, breasts, abdomen, prostate, and rectum.

Cardiovascular System: Inspection for signs of right-sided heart failure including distended neck veins, hepatojugular reflux, and peripheral edema is necessary if passive congestion of the liver is suspected.

Abdomen: Note should be made of previous surgical scars consistent with cholecystectomy or other abdominal operations. The liver should be examined carefully for size, consistency, and tenderness; an enlarged firm liver is common in patients with primary or metastatic malignancies or infiltrative processes, whereas a tender large liver or painful right upper quadrant is seen in acute viral or alcoholic hepatitis, cholangitis, or congestive heart failure. A bruit may be audible if a hepatocellular carcinoma is present, whereas a rub suggests metastatic disease. A venous hum may be heard in the umbilical area if portal hypertension is present. Signs of portal hypertension, including splenomegaly, ascites, or caput medusae, should be sought. A palpable gallbladder (Courvoisier's sign) is associated with malignant distal bile duct obstruction. A positive Murphy sign (right upper quadrant pain on inspiration) suggests acute cholecystitis.

Laboratory Evaluation (Fig. 4–2)

A basic laboratory evaluation can distinguish between hemolysis and liver disease as the cause of jaundice. The first step is to determine whether the patient has unconjugated or conjugated hyperbilirubinemia. Patients with hemolytic disorders generally present with mild unconjugated hyperbilirubinemia. The hematologic work-up can reveal schistocytes or red blood cell fragments on the peripheral smear, an increased reticulocyte count in acute hemolysis, an increased red blood cell distribution width (RDW) on the cell count, and an increased serum lactate dehydrogenase (LDH) and aspartate transaminase (AST). ALT is generally normal. Gilbert's syndrome is suggested by mild unconjugated hyperbilirubinemia, if other liver function tests are normal and the hyperbilirubinemia is accentuated upon fasting or stress.

Conjugated hyperbilirubinemia is seen primarily in hepatobiliary diseases. The distinction between cholestatic and hepatocellular causes cannot always be based on the pattern of liver function test elevation. However, an increased serum alkaline phosphatase greater than two to three times normal (due to an accelerated hepatocyte synthesis of this enzyme during biliary obstruction) with mildly elevated AST and alanine transaminase (ALT) to levels usually less than 300 U/L suggests an obstructive process. A pattern of very rapid elevation followed by a rapid decline in transaminase levels (usually between 600 and 2000 U/L) can be the clue to acute intermittent biliary obstruction. Because serum alkaline phosphatase possesses a half-life of approximately 7 days, levels may remain elevated up to 1 week after relief from the obstruction and the return of serum bilirubin to normal. Because alkaline phosphatase is produced by bone, intestine, and placenta, thermostability fractionation can establish the hepatic origin of the alkaline phosphatase

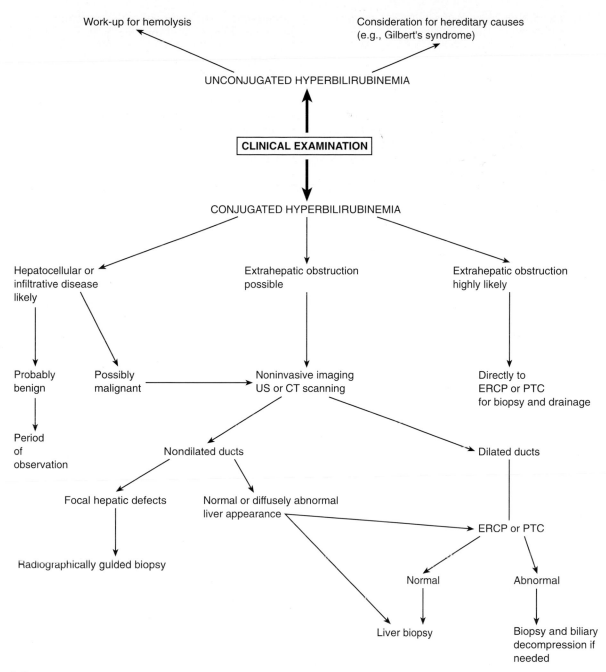

Figure 4–2
Algorithm for evaluation of jaundice and hyperbilirubinemia. (CT, computed tomography; ERCP, endoscopic retrograde cholangiopancreatography; PTC, percutaneous transhepatic cholangiography; US, ultrasound.

according to the aphorism "liver lives, bone burns"—thus, the heat stable fraction originates from the liver. An ancillary test is 5′ nucleotidase, which is another hepatic canalicular membrane enzyme physiologically similiar to alkaline phosphatase. A rise in both of these enzyme levels can also be used to confirm hepatic origin of the alkaline phosphatase. γ-Glutamyl transpeptidase (GGTP) is another hepatic microsomal enzyme that increases in both cholestatic and hepatocellular processes. However, it is overly sensitive and is useful mainly to confirm a hepatic origin for an isolated alkaline phosphatase elevation. GGTP has a long half-

life of 26 days and can be elevated after alcohol use; thus, it has been used as a marker of surreptitious alcohol consumption.

Hepatocellular causes of jaundice usually result from direct inflammation or injury of the hepatocyte. Laboratory findings include predominantly increased AST and ALT and are often the first biochemical abnormality detected in viral or drug-induced hepatitis. Degree of elevation may correlate with extent of hepatic injury but generally has no prognostic significance. Because ALT is synthesized only in hepatocyte whereas AST production is of a wider distribution, an elevated ALT is more specific for hepatocellular involvement. A notable exception occurs in alcoholic liver disease in which serum AST elevation to serum ALT evaluation is commonly 2 to 3:1; this may occur because of selective toxicity of alcohol on the hepatocyte with consequent depressed ALT production. Aminotransferase levels in alcoholic hepatitis are usually no greater than two to ten times above normal levels; higher values in these patients suggest an alternate etiology for hepatic dysfunction such as concomitant viral hepatitis or drug hepatotoxicity. Patients with end-stage renal failure and chronic viral hepatitis, for example, may display minimal aminotransferase elevations despite uremia and histologic abnormalities. Thus, normal or marginal elevation of aminotransferases does not preclude the presence of serious liver disease.

Further laboratory investigation depends on the specific clinical setting. If viral hepatitis is suspected, viral serologies may elucidate the cause of the patient's jaundice. Similarly, if autoimmune hepatitis or primary biliary cirrhosis are diagnostic possibilities, antinuclear antibody and antimitochondrial antibody testing are appropriate.

Imaging Modalities (Noninvasive Testing)

If the clinical examination and routine laboratory testing suggest that mechanical biliary obstruction is the likely cause, an imaging study is indicated. Prior studies have demonstrated that clinical examination is 80% to 90% sensitive in detecting the possibility of extrahepatic mechanical obstruction. The major limitation lies in the tendency to overdiagnose this cause of jaundice, as evidenced by a relatively low specificity of 76%. However, specificity improves to 98% if the results of history, physical examination, and routine laboratories are combined with ultrasound or computed tomography (CT) findings. Conversely, use of either of these imaging modalities alone without clinical examination yields a sensitivity that is less than that of the clinician's impression alone. Therefore, these studies should not be ordered indiscriminately. Initially, a noninvasive imaging study such as an ultrasound should be obtained. If biliary obstruction is then confirmed, then direct visualization by endoscopic retrograde cholangiopancreatography (ERCP) or percutaneous transhepatic cholangiography (PTC) is indicated to define and possibly treat the obstruction. If extrahepatic obstruction is highly likely, then evaluation by direct cholangiography should be done first.

Abdominal Films: In general, plain abdominal radiographs add little information in the diagnostic evaluation of jaundice. Occasionally, hepatic calcification can be detected and is caused by gallstones, deposits in the wall of echinococcal cysts, or an old granulomatous disease associated with tuberculosis or histoplasmosis. Tumors and vascular lesions can also become calcified. Other abnormalities that may be revealed on routine plain films include enlargement of the liver or spleen, elevation of the right hemidiaphragm due to cancer or abscess, pancreatic calcifications, and abnormal gas collections within the hepatobiliary system. Hence, these findings may be helpful to diagnose the jaundiced patient, but they probably do not justify routine ordering of plain abdominal films in the work-up of hyperbilirubinemia.

Ultrasound: High-resolution real-time ultrasound is usually the preferred initial imaging modality used for several reasons:

- Safety to the patient with no exposure to radiation
- Minimal need for preparation of the patient
- Relatively low cost
- More readily accessible in most centers
- Portable ultrasounds can be done at the bedside for very ill patients
- Diagnostic accuracy similar to an abdominal CT scan

Dilated intrahepatic bile ducts seen on ultrasound are a highly reliable sign of extrahepatic biliary obstruction, although the absence of biliary dilatation does not exclude this possibility. For example, false-negative ultrasound findings may be secondary to intermittent or incomplete obstruction, extraductular obstruction, or cirrhosis. It is estimated that approximately 25% to 40% of patients with documented choledocholithiasis will not have biliary dilatation on ultrasound. Although stones in the gallbladder are easily noted on ultrasound, detection of a common duct stone is not as reliable and may only be detected in a third of cases. Ultrasound is also very useful in detecting focal mass lesions within the liver, diffuse parenchymal abnormalities, spleen size, local lymphadenopathy, and the presence of ascites. Hepatic masses as small as 1 cm can be detected by ultrasound. Cystic lesions can be distinguished from solid masses. Clarity of image quality suffers, however, in patients who are obese or who have overlying bowel gas in the region of the distal common bile duct and pancreas; that is, increased tissue penetration is generally at the expense of decreased image resolution. Postcholecystectomy patients generally have mild common bile duct dilatation; the clinical significance of this finding is unclear. Sensitivities of 55% to 90% and specificities of 82% to 93% are reported for ultrasonographic determination of extrahepatic obstruction. Ultrasound is also helpful in facilitating percutaneous biopsy of solid masses, drainage of hepatic abscess, and paracentesis of loculated ascites. Combined with Doppler imaging, ultrasound can be utilized to assess the patency of hepatic and portal vasculature in liver transplant recipients with hepatic dysfunction.

CT Scan: Abdominal CT scanning is another excellent modality for determining the site of obstructive jaundice. Compared with ultrasound, CT scanning possesses slightly enhanced sensitivity and specificity for detecting biliary dilatation and hepatic mass lesions but has decreased precision in detection of choledocholithiasis. Because of its potential disadvantages of higher cost, radiation exposure, risk of intravenous contrast allergy, and the need for patient preparation with oral contrast, this study should be reserved for patients with equivocal ultrasound findings, need for superior definition of liver and surrounding structures, or possible film interpretation difficulties secondary to physical limitations. Potential advantages of CT scanning include:

- A small improvement in ability to define both the cause and the level of the obstruction
- If malignancy is suspected, examination for metastatic disease
- Improved imaging of obese patients

- No interference of overlying bowel gas in evaluating the distal bile duct and pancreas

Hepatobiliary Scintigraphy: Cholescintigraphy is a noninvasive study that evaluates biliary secretion and function rather than hepatobiliary anatomy. Hepatobiliary scintigraphy utilizing various ^{99m}Tc-labeled iminodiacetic acid (Tc-IDA) complexes is best at detecting common bile duct obstruction and acute cholecystitis with nonvisualization of the gallbladder. Sensitivities of 92% to 100% and specificities of 95% to 100% have been reported for the Tc-IDA scan in acute cholecystitis. False-positive results are often seen in patients who recently have passed a common bile duct stone, and false-negative results are common in patients with intermittent biliary colic. The second most common use of the Tc-IDA hepatobiliary scanning is for an evaluation of the biliary system after surgery. In these cases, ultrasound or CT interpretation may be quite difficult, because normal anatomic landmarks are altered. Furthermore, in patients with a biliary-enteric anastomosis, the anastomotic site may be remote from the duodenum and inaccessible by endoscope. Thus, in these postoperative patients, scintigraphy is helpful in checking for biliary leaks, strictures, and anastomosis patency. Hepatobiliary scintigraphy is also helpful in identifying an extrahepatic obstruction as characterized by the complete absence of ^{99m}Tc-IDA liver to bowel transit in a 24-hour period of monitoring. However, hepatocellular and intrahepatic causes of cholestasis demonstrate inconsistent results with decreased isotope uptake and transit times ranging from normal to absent. Another major disadvantage of hepatobiliary scintigraphy is its limited spatial resolution; for example, the etiology of biliary obstruction (including tumor, stones, or strictures) cannot be differentiated by nuclear scanning. Overall, the limitations encountered with nuclear medicine imaging technology in the differential diagnosis of jaundice weigh against its use as a primary screening tool.

Invasive Tests

Liver Biopsy: Acute jaundice rarely requires immediate liver biopsy. Liver biopsy is generally reserved for continued diagnostic difficulty after an appropriate noninvasive work-up. Liver biopsy is the definitive test to confirm a diagnosis of specific liver diseases (e.g., Wilson's disease), to assess the prognosis in many forms of parenchymal liver disease, or to evaluate allograft dysfunction in liver transplant recipients.

Direct Cholangiography: ERCP and PTC are invasive procedures that can directly image the bile ducts. These studies are indicated when initial imaging shows a biliary mechanical obstruction. These tests should also be considered for those patients in whom the possibility of extrahepatic obstruction remains great despite a negative or equivocal noninvasive imaging. Potential advantages include:

- Highly sensitive (99%) and specific (99%) in detecting ductal obstruction, its nature, location, and extent
- Opportunity for therapeutic intervention with relief of biliary obstruction
- Opportunity for tissue sampling with biopsy

The choice between the two modalities is determined by local availability and expertise. PTC can be effectively achieved in approximately 90% to 95% of patients with ductal dilatation; success rates of 70% are reported in the presence of nondilated ducts. PTC may be especially useful in patients with a tumor at the common bile duct bifurcation (Klatskin's tumors), because in these cases, separate ductal punctures may be required to fully opacify and evaluate the right and left intrahepatic systems. External biliary drainage, balloon dilatation, biopsy of bile duct strictures, and placement of biliary stents for drainage can be accomplished with PTC. Contraindications to PTC include massive ascites and uncorrectable coagulopathy. Possible complications include bile leaks, infection, and bleeding. Complication rates are reported in 4% to 10% of patients who undergo PTC. Pancreatograms are not easily achieved by PTC.

ERCP is a more technically demanding procedure than PTC but may offer more therapeutic options and diagnostic information with visualization of the papilla and an opportunity to perform a pancreatogram in addition to the cholangiogram. Success rates are higher than 90% in obtaining radiographic images by ERCP. ERCP also allows opportunity for therapeutic intervention such as nasobiliary drainage and endoscopic sphincterotomy with stone extraction. Hence, ERCP may be preferable to PTC in patients with suspected choledocholithiasis and in patients for whom an evaluation of the pancreatic duct or ampulla is desired. Contraindications to ERCP include an inability to tolerate intravenous sedation due to severe cardiac or pulmonary disease. ERCP in patients with a prior Billroth II procedure is more technically difficult. Complication rates with ERCP are approximately 7% and include pancreatitis, cholangitis, bleeding, perforation, and sedation reactions.

Laparoscopy: Laparoscopy is rarely used in the work-up of jaundice, because the other studies are less cumbersome and can successfully identify, define, and not infrequently treat the cause of biliary obstruction. At present, laparoscopy is reserved primarily for the following situations:

- To evaluate hepatic mass lesions or chronic parenchymal liver disease when ultrasound or CT-guided biopsy have failed to produce a definite diagnosis
- To search for an etiology of obscure abdominal or pelvic pain or mass

Contraindications to laparoscopy include an uncooperative patient, acute peritonitis, severe coagulopathy, diaphragmatic hernia, intestinal obstruction, and abdominal wall cellulitis. Relative contraindications are a history or prior abdominal surgery, marked obesity, tense ascites, and severe cardiopulmonary disease.

SUGGESTED READINGS

Berk PD, Noyer D: Bilirubin and hyperbilirubinemia. Semin Liver Dis 14:325–355, 1994.

Berk PD, Wolkoff AW, Berlin NI: Inborn errors of bilirubin metabolism. Med Clin North Am 59:803, 1975.

Borsch G, Wegener M, Wedmann B, et al: Clinical evaluation, ultrasound, cholescintigraphy, and endoscopic retrograde cholangiography in cholestasis: A prospective clinical study. J Clin Gastroenterol 10: 185, 1988.

Burnett DA: Rational uses of hepatic imaging modalities. Semin Liver Dis 9:1, 1989.

Chowdury JR, Wolkoff AW, Chowdury NR, et al: Hereditary jaundice and disorders of bilirubin metabolism. In Scriver CR, Beaudet AL, Sly WS (eds): The Metabolic Basis of Inherited Disease, 6th ed. New York: McGraw-Hill, 1995, p 2161.

Frank BB: Clinical evaluation of jaundice. JAMA 262:3031, 1989.

Hoofnagle JH, Di Bisceglie AM: The treatment of chronic viral hepatitis. N Engl J Med 336:347, 1997.

Ingidbashian VN, Jibin L, Goldberg BB: Hepatic ultrasound. Semin Liver Dis 9:16, 1989.

Kaplan MN: Primary biliary cirrhosis. N Engl J Med 316:521, 1987.

Larrey D, Pageaux GP: Hepatotoxicity of herbal remedies and mushrooms. Semin Liver Dis 15:183, 1995.

Lee WM: Drug-induced hepatotoxicity. N Engl J Med 333:1118, 1995.

Lee Y-M, Kaplan MM: Primary sclerosing cholangitis. N Engl J Med 332:924, 1995.

Lieber CS: Alcoholic liver disease. Semin Liver Dis 13:109, 1993.

Lindberg MC: Hepatobiliary complications of oral contraceptives. J Gen Intern Med 7:199, 1992.

Lyche KD, Brenner DA: A logical approach to the patient with jaundice. Cont Intern Med 5:43, 1992.

Moseley RH: Evaluation of the abnormal liver function test. Med Clin North Am 887:80, 1996.

Owens D, Sherlock S: The diagnosis of Gilbert's syndrome: Role of the reduced caloric intake test. Br J Med 2:559, 1973.

Pasanen PA, Pikkarainen P, Alhave E, et al: The value of clinical assessment in the diagnosis of icterus and cholestasis. Ital J Gastroenterol 24:313, 1992.

Pasha TM, Lindor KD: Diagnosis and therapy of cholestatic liver disease. Med Clin North Am 80:995, 1996.

Poupon RE, Poupon R, Balkau B, UDCA-PBC Study Group: Urosodiol for the long-term treatment of primary biliary cirrhosis. N Engl J Med 330:1342, 1994.

Radominska A, Treat S, Little J: Bile acid metabolism and the pathophysiology of cholestasis. Semin Liver Dis 13:219–234, 1993.

Richter JM, Silverstein MD, Schapiro R: Suspected obstructive jaundice: A decision analysis of diagnostic strategies. Ann Intern Med 99:46, 1983.

Roston AD, Carr-Locke DL: Nonsurgical treatment of biliary tract disease. In Zakim D, Boyer TD (eds): Hepatology, Vol 2, 3rd ed. Philadelphia: WB Saunders, 1996, p 1897.

Scharschmidt BF, Goldber HI, Schmid R: Approach to the patient with cholestatic jaundice. N Engl J Med 308(25):1515–1519, 1983.

Van Ness MM, Diehl AM: Is liver biopsy useful in the evaluation of patients with chronically elevated liver enzymes. Ann Intern Med 111:473, 1989.

Weiss JS, Gautam A, Lauff JJ, et al: The clinical importance of a protein-bound fraction of serum bilirubin in patients with hyperbilirubinemia. N Engl J Med 309:147, 1983.

Yasuda K, Okuda K, Endo N, et al: Hypoaminotransferasemia in patients undergoing long-term hemodialysis: Clinical and biochemical appraisal. Gastroenterology 109:1295, 1995.

Chapter

5

Liver Biopsy: Indications, Technique, Complications, and Interpretation

Kyle E. Brown
Christine G. Janney
Elizabeth M. Brunt

Needle biopsy of the liver plays an important role in the diagnosis, assessment of therapeutic response, and staging of many liver diseases. In addition, liver biopsy can sometimes be helpful in the diagnosis of conditions that are not primary diseases of the liver, such as metastatic cancer, sarcoidosis, amyloidosis, and fever of unknown origin. Information obtained from liver biopsy regarding the patient's response to treatment and the progression of disease is often an important factor in management decisions. Thus, liver biopsy is frequently utilized for both diagnostic and prognostic purposes.

Unless otherwise stated, the comments in this section pertain to the standard "blind" percutaneous liver biopsy (PLB). Focal liver lesions are often biopsied with the guidance of imaging modalities such as ultrasound or computed tomography (CT) or by direct visualization at laparoscopy. This approach maximizes the likelihood of obtaining diagnostic tissue while decreasing the need for multiple passes that are associated with an increased risk of hemorrhage in patients with malignancy. In patients with contraindications to PLB, such as coagulopathy or massive ascites, transjugular biopsy or percutaneous biopsy with embolization of the needle tract can be performed.

TECHNIQUE OF PERCUTANEOUS LIVER BIOPSY

Two types of needles can be used for PLB. The first category includes the cutting needles such as the Tru-Cut needle. Because this type of needle causes less fragmentation of fibrotic tissue, it may provide superior specimens in cases of cirrhosis. The second type of needle is the aspiration needle of which the Menghini and Jamshidi are examples. PLB done with an aspiration needle is simpler than with a cutting needle, and the intrahepatic phase of the biopsy is shorter, which may decrease the risks of the procedure. Although not a consistent finding, a higher rate of complications with the Tru-Cut needle than with aspiration needles has been reported in some series.

The aspiration biopsy is performed in the following manner. The patient is recumbent with the right arm extended. Liver dullness is identified by percussion. An area several centimeters caudad to the top of the liver dullness in the right midaxillary line is selected for the biopsy, usually in the eighth or ninth intercostal space. The site is infiltrated with local anesthetic, and care is taken to insert the needle along the superior margin of the rib in order to avoid the intercostal artery. A small skin incision is made so that the needle can be passed easily through the skin. The needle, which is attached to a syringe containing 2 to 3 mL of sterile saline solution, is inserted through the incision with its tip directed toward the xiphoid process. After the needle is passed through the subcutaneous tissue and intercostal muscle, 1 to 2 mL of the saline is expelled to flush the needle. The patient is then asked to hold his or her breath in expiration; with negative pressure exerted on the plunger of the syringe, the needle is quickly advanced into the liver substance and withdrawn. The specimen is transferred to an appropriate specimen container and inspected. If additional tissue is required, one to two additional passes can be made through the same entry site without significantly increased risk of complications. The patient is then asked to remain in the right lateral decubitus position for 1 hour and on bed rest for a further 2 to 3 hours while his or her vital signs are monitored every 15 minutes. In most cases, outpatients are observed for 6 to 8 hours after a liver biopsy, because most complications become evident within this period.

Contraindications and Complications

Although a liver biopsy is a safe procedure, the most common complication and the one that is most frequently fatal is bleeding. Approximately one quarter of patients undergoing ultrasound examination 1 day after liver biopsy were found to have intrahepatic or subcapsular hematomas. In general, these hematomas were not associated with significant hemodynamic changes and thus were clinically insignificant. Nonetheless, serious hemorrhagic complications occur in 0.06% to 0.35% of cases. Less common complications of liver biopsy include perforation of the gallbladder, bile peritonitis, puncture of the intestine or kidney, pneumothorax, hemobilia, hemothorax, arteriovenous fistula, and sepsis. Rates of these complications from several large series are summarized in Table 5-1.

Because of the risk of bleeding, coagulopathy is a contraindication to PLB. The adequacy of hemostatic mechanisms is commonly estimated using the platelet count and prothrombin time. Although acceptable levels are defined somewhat arbitrarily, a platelet count less 50,000/mm³ or a prothrombin time prolonged more than 3 seconds would be regarded as a contraindication to PLB in most cases. An attempt may be made to correct the deficiency by platelet transfusion or by administration of fresh frozen plasma; however, consideration of an alternative approach such as transjugular biopsy is often advisable in this situation. In addition to ensuring that the platelet count and prothrombin time are acceptable, the patient is counseled to avoid drugs such as aspirin and nonsteroidal anti-inflammatory agents that interfere with platelet function for 1 week before the biopsy. Hemorrhagic complications will occur occasionally despite these precautions. Direct observation of liver bleeding following laparoscopic biopsy has shown that the duration of bleeding from the biopsy site correlates poorly with indices such as the platelet count and prothrombin time. In addition to the possible inadvertent puncture of a large blood vessel, it has been speculated that the local concentration of clotting factors within the liver and mechanical compression of the needle tract by elastic tissue may be important determinants of excessive bleeding post biopsy. Other contraindications to PLB include massive ascites and the inability to cooperate.

Routine ultrasound examination prior to PLB has been advocated as a method of decreasing complications. One study in which ultrasound–guided PLB was utilized indicated a lower rate of complications than in a group of historical controls undergoing blind PLB. In a controlled study of ultrasound–guided versus blind PLB, the rate of hospitalization was significantly lower in the former group than in the latter. It should be noted, however, that the indication for admission in most cases was pain, and no difference was reported in the rate of complications requiring transfusion or surgery. Although ultrasound may often be helpful in avoiding puncture of adjacent organs, bowel perforation can occur despite sonographic guidance. In addition, it appears that prebiopsy ultrasound is less reliable in preventing hemorrhage. All three cases of fatal hemorrhage reported in a Swiss study had prebiopsy ultrasounds. Given the relatively low rate of serious complications associated with blind PLB, it is questionable whether the routine use of ultrasound guidance can be shown to be cost-effective. Nonetheless, if imaging studies are indicated on clinical grounds, it is reasonable that they should be obtained prior to PLB so that information regarding the size of the liver, the location of the gallbladder, and any anatomic abnormalities can be taken into account.

LIVER BIOPSY INTERPRETATION: PROCESSING, STAINS, AND GENERAL MORPHOLOGIC APPROACH

Processing

For interpretation of the morphologic processes encountered in most liver diseases, liver biopsies are best handled by immediate fixation in 10% neutral buffered formalin followed by paraffin embedding. It is not recommended that the liver biopsy be placed on a biopsy sponge, because the sponge results in artifacts in the cut sections caused by irregularly spaced holes and desiccation of tissue from the sponge. These artifacts result in triangular spaces with marked compression and distortion of parenchyma as well as artificial separation of hepatocytes from drying. In some clinical settings, such as acute fatty liver of pregnancy, special handling of the liver biopsy is necessary to perform the diagnostic evaluation (Table 5-2). In the rare circumstances when ultrastructural evaluation is desirable, a 1-mm² portion of the liver tissue may be fixed in 2.5% glutaraldehyde and further processed for plastic embedding.

Table 5–1 Complication and Fatality Rates from Liver Biopsy

Author, Date	Total Complications (%)	Hemorrhagic Complications (%)	Mortality (%)
Piccinino, 1986	0.22	0.06	0.009*
McGill, 1990	NR	0.35	0.11*
Froehlich, 1993	0.31	0.14	0.09*
Caturelli, 1996†	0.53‡	0.13	0

*All fatalities were caused by hemorrhage.
†All biopsies done under ultrasound guidance.
‡Included three vasovagal reactions.
NR, not reported.

Table 5–2 Tissue Processing for Specialized Analysis

Disease Process	Diagnostic Evaluation	Tissue Preparation
Hereditary hemochromatosis	Iron concentration; μg/g dry weight	Fresh tissue or paraffin block*
Wilson's disease	Copper concentration; μg/g dry weight	Fresh tissue or paraffin block*
Microvesicular steatosis	Microvesicular steatosis best seen with	Frozen sections of fresh or formalin-
Fatty liver of pregnancy	Oil Red O or Sudan Black stains	fixed tissue; cannot be done on
Reye's syndrome		paraffin-embedded tissue
Porphyria		
Porphyria cutanea tarda	Intracytoplasmic needle-shaped crystals	Unstained tissue sections examined under polarized light; ferric ferricyanide reduction test
Inborn errors of metabolism	Enzymatic assays	Fresh tissue obtained at biopsy*
Bacterial, viral, fungal, mycobacterial infections	Culture and identification	Fresh tissue supplied to the microbiology laboratory or PCR analysis on fresh or fixed tissue

*Submission of tissue to a reference laboratory is necessary.
PCR, polymerase chain reaction.

Stains

Routine histologic evaluation is done on multiple sections taken at various intervals through the paraffin block; predetermined sections are stained with a battery of stains to highlight morphologic features in order to add to the information obtained by the standard hematoxylin and eosin (H & E) stain. Connective tissue stains are part of the routine evaluation; trichrome stains are useful for demonstrating the presence and localization of increased collagen type I fibers; a silver stain for reticulin fibers delineates the type III collagen that invests hepatic plates, highlights the collapse of cords in areas of recent necrosis and widened cords in areas of regeneration, and helps in the evaluation of well-differentiated hepatocellular carcinoma in which tumor cords are abnormally thickened or from which reticulin fibers may be absent. An iron stain is more sensitive than H & E for confirming the presence of intracytoplasmic hemosiderin pigment. The diastase-pretreated periodic acid Schiff (PAS-d) stain is commonly used for evaluating three processes: PAS-d–reactive Kupffer cells, indicative of phagocytosis of necrotic hepatocytes; PAS-d positivity in intracellular globules in zone 1 hepatocytes, typical of the nonglycogen carbohydrate material seen in α_1-antitrypsin deficiency; and basement membrane that normally encircles interlobular bile ducts.

Table 5-3 lists additional histochemical and immunohistochemical stains available in most pathology laboratories, the disease processes for which they are useful, and reactivity in liver tissue. More sophisticated techniques such as in situ hybridization and polymerase chain reaction (PCR) are available in limited numbers of research facilities and, to date, are not available for diagnostic testing.

General Interpretation

The morphologic evaluation of a liver biopsy is a multistep process that incorporates architectural and cellular changes in the parenchyma (Table 5-4). The initial step is assessment of the architecture. Abnormal spacing between terminal hepatic venules and portal structures may be caused by necrosis with collapse or excessive scar tissue. Small, round fragments of parenchyma outlined by collagen and nodules of hepatocytes with no terminal hepatic venules are findings indicative of the remodeling of cirrhosis (Figs. 5–1 to 5–3). In addition to architectural assessment, the evaluation includes the portal tracts, the biliary and vascular components of the portal tracts, hepatocytes in the three zones of the acinus, and the location and structure of the terminal hepatic venules and the sinusoids. The types and location of inflammatory infiltrates are noted. Ultimately, the histologic findings are integrated with clinical information in an effort to establish the diagnosis.

HEPATITIS

Hepatitis may be broadly defined as inflammation of the liver accompanied by hepatocyte degeneration or necrosis. This pattern of liver injury is most commonly attributable to hepatotropic viruses or to drugs, but many other conditions including autoimmune disorders, nonviral and nonhepatotropic infections, and metabolic and biliary diseases can all

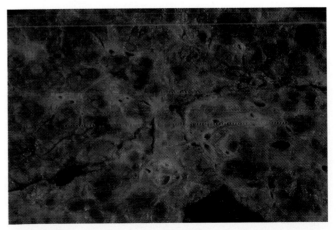

Figure 5–1
Cirrhosis. Scarring and nodularity of a cirrhotic liver are seen in this cross-section of an explanted liver (gross specimen).

Table 5–3 Histochemical and Immunohistochemical Stains

Histochemical Stains	Use in Diagnostic Liver Pathology	Pathologic Processes	Comments
Vierhoff Van Geison	Vessel wall connective tissue	VOD, Budd-Chiari syndrome	Helpful in the identification of obliterated vessels not readily seen by standard stains
Rhodanine	Copper in cytoplasm and lysosomes of hepatocytes	Wilson's disease	Most useful in late stages of Wilson's disease; uneven distribution in the liver so that a negative stain does not rule out the possibility of Wilson's disease
		Chronic cholestasis	Granular reactivity in zone 1 or periseptal hepatocytes
Orcein	Copper-associated protein	Wilson's disease, chronic cholestasis	Less sensitive than rhodanine for copper
	Elastic fibers	Recent necrosis, collapse	Passive septa: no elastic fibers detected
		Scar tissue formation	Active septa: elastic fibers present
	Hepatitis B virus (HBV) surface antigen	Eccentric cytoplasmic reactivity corresponds with the ground-glass change seen by hematoxylin and eosin; indicates the presence of viral components in hepatocytes	Less sensitive than immunohistochemical stain for HBV surface antigen
Oil Red O	Red globules correspond to fat droplets	Diseases in which microvesicular steatosis occurs in hepatocytes	Confirms the presence of microvesicular steatosis
Congo Red Crystal Violet Thioflavin-T	Confirmation of amyloid protein deposition in the space of Disse or hepatic arterioles	Amyloid infiltration	Immunohistochemical stains for protein A or immunoglobulin light chain will distinguish secondary (AA) from primary/plasma cell dyscrasia-related (AL) amyloidosis

Immunostains	Antigen	Reactivity in Liver Tissue	Diagnostic Utility
HBV surface antigen	HBsAg	Cytoplasmic reactivity: diffuse or inclusion; membrane reactivity	Confirmatory of the presence of HBV surface antigen in hepatocytes
HBV core antigen	HBcAg	Nuclear reactivity; may see cytoplasmic reactivity in occasional hepatocytes	Confirmatory of HBV core antigen in hepatocytes; indicates active replication of the virus
A_1AT	α_1-Antitrypsin protein	Immunoreactive globules or diffuse cytoplasmic blush	Reactivity with globules may be positive or negative with a positive rim; this is more specific for A_1AT in the secretory apparatus than diffuse cytoplasmic reactivity
Other viral antigens HSV	Herpes simplex, I and II	Immunoreactivity localizes to infected cells	Confirmatory of HSV in intranuclear inclusions
CMV	Cytomegalovirus	As above	Confirmatory of CMV in intranuclear and intracytoplasmic inclusions
Cytokeratins	CK 8,18	Hepatocyte cytokeratin	May be useful in confirming the hepatocellular origin of the tumor
	CK 8, 18, 7, 19	Biliary epithelium	Useful in delineating biliary differentiation in tumors; helpful in identifying bile duct epithelium in ductopenic conditions

Note: Immunohistochemical markers for other viral hepatitis markers, hepatitis delta agent, hepatitis C antigen, and hepatitis A antigen are available in research facilities.
VOD, veno-occlusive disease; A_1AT, α_1-antitrypsin deficiency; HSV, herpes simplex virus; CMV, cytomegalovirus.

Table 5–4 Evaluation of Morphologic Changes in Hepatic Parenchyma

Architecture

Terminal hepatic venules, portal tracts identified and in
  normal relationship
Abnormal vascular relationships
  Necrosis with collapse
  Fibrosis
Nodular architecture
  Without increased fibrosis
  With increased fibrosis; location of fibrosis: portal or central
Space-occupying lesion

Portal Tracts

Normal connective tissue, biliary and vascular structures
Increased fibrosis
  Periportal
  Bridging portal-portal
  Bridging portal-central
Cellular infiltrates
  Chronic inflammation; predominant cell types
  Acute inflammation
  Granulomatous inflammation
  Neoplastic infiltrate
Bile ducts
  Present in normal numbers, increased numbers; absent
  Inflammation, ductal infiltration/destruction
  Epithelial changes
  Bile ductular proliferation
Vascular structures
  Portal vein; changes suggestive of venopathy
  Hepatic artery; arteritis; arteriopathy

Vascular Structures of the Acinus

Terminal hepatic venules
  Location in the acinus, size
  Fibrosis; perivenular; intraluminal
Sinusoids
  Dilated
  Deposition of extraneous material: collagen, amyloid,* red
    blood cells
  Inflammation: chronic and acute
  Extramedullary hematopoiesis
Neoplastic infiltration

Hepatocytes

Normal cord and cellular architecture
Abnormal cords
  Hepatocellular unrest
  Single cell necrosis; apoptosis
  Zonal necrosis: submassive and massive
Cytologic features: ballooning or feathery degeneration; onco-
  cytic change
Inclusions
  Character of inclusions: fat, globules, pigment, hyaline,
    ground-glass
  Location of inclusions: intracytoplasmic, intercellular
  Zonal distribution of inclusions
Nuclear features
  Glycogenated
  Cytoplasmic pseudoinclusions
  N/C ratio: regenerative, large or small cell dysplastic change

*See Figures 5–4 and 5–5.

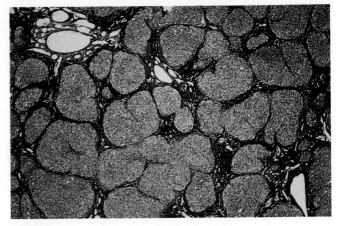

Figure 5–2
Cirrhosis. The distorted, remodelled hepatic architecture of cirrhosis is characterized by nodules of hepatocytes surrounded
by scar tissue. These features are well demonstrated by connective tissue stains (Masson's trichrome).

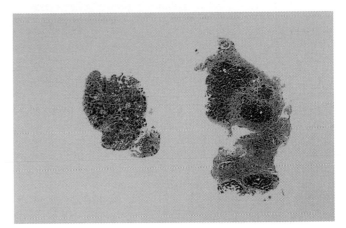

Figure 5–3
Cirrhosis. Fragmented hepatic parenchyma surrounded by
collagenous scars are typical findings in biopsies of cirrhosis
(Masson's trichrome).

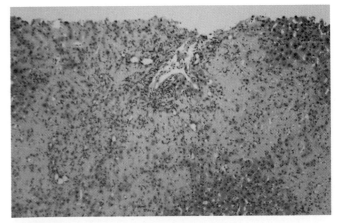

Figure 5–4
Amyloidosis. The hepatic parenchyma surrounding the portal
tract in the upper half is greatly distorted and nearly replaced
by amorphous, eosinophilic material. This pattern is
characteristic of amyloidosis involving the liver (H & E).

Table 5–5 Clues to Etiology of Acute and Chronic Hepatitis in Liver Biopsies

Histologic Features	Etiology
Zone 1 necrosis, predominantly plasma cell infiltrates, cholestasis, and iron-laden Kupffer cells	Hepatitis A
Cytoplasmic ground-glass change (demonstrates HBsAg by orcein or immunostain), sanded nuclei (demonstrate HBcAg by immunostain)	Hepatitis B (chronic)
Portal lymphoid follicles, bile duct injury, mild macrovesicular steatosis, scattered acidophil bodies. (Immunostains for HCV, PCR utilized in research)	Hepatitis C (chronic)
Severe hepatitis with massive or submassive necrosis, with HBsAg immunostaining	Hepatitis D (delta virus)
Predominantly plasma cell infiltrates, hepatocellular rosettes, giant cell transformation of hepatocytes, confluent acinar necrosis, collapse, or scar	Autoimmune hepatitis
Cholestasis, eosinophils, granulomas, steatosis	Drug-induced hepatitis
Acute hepatitis	e.g., isoniazid
Chronic hepatitis	e.g., α-methyldopa
Granulomatous hepatitis	e.g., aspirin, valium
Submassive or massive necrosis	e.g., acetaminophen, halothane
Atypical lymphocytes in portal areas and sinusoids*	Epstein-Barr virus
Focal granulomatous necrosis; microabscesses, nuclear and cytoplasmic viral inclusions in immunocompromised patients	Cytomegalovirus
Steatosis, glycogen nuclei, anisocytosis, copper demonstrated by rhodanine or orcein stains, Mallory's hyaline	Wilson's disease
Eosinophilic PAS-d-positive globules in zone 1 hepatocytes	α_1-Antitrypsin deficiency

*See Figure 5–10.

exhibit a hepatitic, inflammatory component in liver biopsy specimens. In many cases, the morphologic features will suggest a specific etiology (see Table 5-5), but definitive diagnosis usually requires correlation with viral serologies, liver enzymes, autoimmune markers, drug history, time course, and other clinical data. Liver biopsies are also useful in patients with hepatitis of known etiology to assess the degree of necroinflammatory activity and fibrosis as well as the response to therapy.

Acute Hepatitis

Hepatitis may be subdivided clinically and pathologically into acute and chronic disease. In acute hepatitis, common

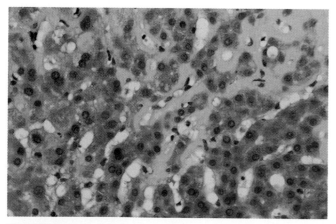

Figure 5–5
Amyloidosis. Examination of the same biopsy on higher power shows that the abnormal accumulation of protein is in the space of Disse with consequent compression of hepatocytes within the cords (H & E).

histologic changes include disarray of hepatic cords, acinar inflammation, ballooning degeneration of hepatocytes, acidophil (apoptotic) bodies, and Kupffer cell hypertrophy, with or without significant portal inflammation (Fig. 5–6). Cholestasis is usually mild or absent, with the exceptions of hepatitis A and drug-induced hepatitis, in which cholestasis may be quite prominent. Whereas the acute changes are panacinar, they are often most pronounced in zone 3. More severe injury is indicated by bridging necrosis, in which there is confluent hepatocyte necrosis connecting necrotic and collapsed zones of adjacent acini; a reticulin stain is helpful when confirming hepatocyte dropout and reticulin network condensation and collapse (Fig. 5–7). Submassive and massive necrosis are the terms used to indicate multiacinar, confluent necrosis and correlate with clinical subfulminant or fulminant liver failure. The acinar parenchyma is replaced by reticulin fibers, and chronic inflammation with macrophages. The histologic features of the recovery phase in survivors of acute hepatitis include regenerative changes such as hepatocyte mitoses and thickened hepatic plates. Pigmented, PAS-d-positive, and occasionally iron-laden, Kupffer cells become prominent (Fig. 5–8). Acute hepatitis can show complete clinical and histologic resolution, such as in hepatitis A and E viral infections, with disappearance of necroinflammatory activity and restoration of a normal reticulin architecture within months after the injury. However, confluent necrosis can result in scarring or postnecrotic cirrhosis, and smoldering disease can evolve into chronic hepatitis.

Chronic Hepatitis

Chronic hepatitis is characterized histologically by involvement and expansion of portal tracts by mononuclear, predominantly lymphocytic, inflammation. There is erosion of the limiting plate by inflammation, which is characterized

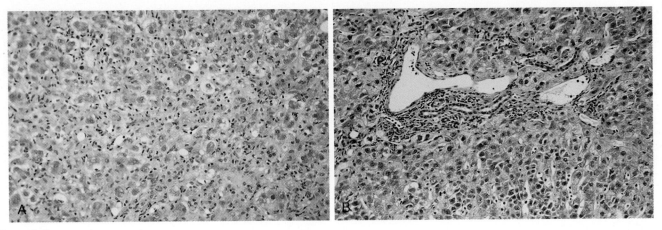

Figure 5–6
Acute hepatitis C virus. *A,* Hepatocellular swelling with panacinar disarray, sinusoidal inflammation, and ceroid-pigmented Kupffer cells are seen (H & E). *B,* The portal inflammation is relatively mild (H & E).

Figure 5–7
Reticulin collapse. A silver stain such as the reticulin stain highlights zonal collapse and appears as condensation of hepatic cords; this can be seen on either side of the centrally located group of regenerative hepatic cords (Sweet's reticulin).

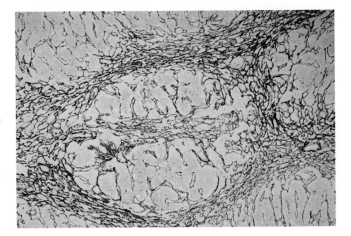

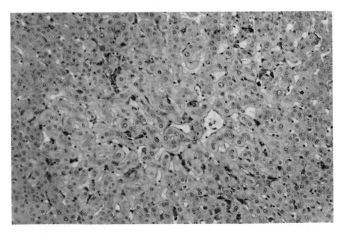

Figure 5–8
Intracellular pigment. The diastase-pretreated periodic acid–Schiff (PAS-d) stain highlights Kupffer cells in sinusoids that contain phagocytosed remnants of necrotic hepatocytes. These findings are indicative of a recent or resolving acute hepatitic process (PAS-d).

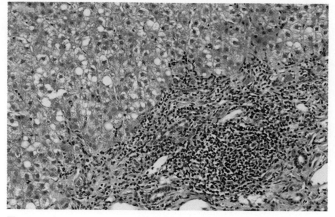

Figure 5–9
Chronic hepatitis C virus (HCV). Portal tract expansion by a lymphoid aggregate is one of the characteristic lesions of chronic hepatitis from HCV. Interface hepatitis is seen, characterized by loss of demarcation of the limiting plate due to inflammation and single hepatocyte necrosis. Mild bile duct injury and occasional hepatocytes with macrovesicular steatosis are also seen (H & E).

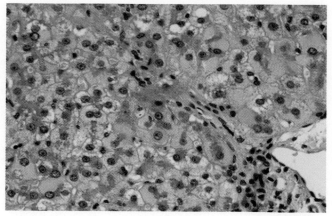

Figure 5–11
Chronic hepatitis B virus (HBV). One of the hallmarks of chronic hepatitis B infection is the presence of ground-glass cytoplasmic changes in hepatocytes. In this photomicrograph, several hepatocytes near the center and right of the frame contain ground-glass inclusions (H & E).

by spillover of inflammatory cells among the periportal hepatocytes, known as "piecemeal necrosis" or "interface hepatitis" (Fig. 5–9). Superimposed acinar activity of a variable degree is usually present, often with a pattern of spotty hepatocyte necrosis or confluent necrosis and inflammation. Fibrosis may or may not be present; with progression there is portal and periportal fibrosis, bridging fibrosis, and finally cirrhosis. The nomenclature for the diagnosis of chronic hepatitis has evolved; the classic terms chronic persistent hepatitis, chronic lobular hepatitis, and chronic active hepatitis have been replaced by diagnostic terminology that includes the etiology of the hepatitis (e.g., hepatitis B virus [HBV], hepatitis C virus [HCV], autoimmune diseases) as well as a statement about the extent of necroinflammatory activity (grade) and the stage of fibrosis (Figs. 5–11 to 5–14). Derived from the original Hepatic Activity Index

score by Knodell and associates, current grading and staging systems report separate scores for grade and stage.

GRANULOMAS

Granulomas, which are defined as more or less circumscribed aggregates of macrophages and lymphocytes, are a common finding in liver biopsies. Granulomas are usually present in small numbers; however, in some cases, extensive replacement of hepatic parenchyma may be seen. Etiologies include various infections, drugs, sarcoidosis and other systemic granulomatous diseases, Hodgkin's disease, primary biliary cirrhosis, and foreign material. Hepatic granulomas are of unknown etiology in 13% to 36% of cases. Although there are histologic clues that may suggest a certain cause (Table 5-6), most granulomas are of the nonspecific epithe-

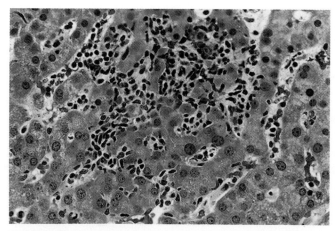

Figure 5–10
Epstein-Barr virus (EBV) hepatitis. In the setting of acute EBV infection, the histologic finding of atypical lymphocytes in the sinusoids is characteristic (H & E).

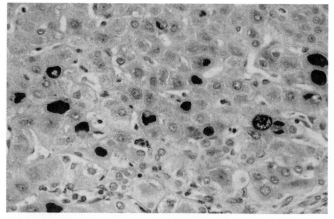

Figure 5–12
Chronic hepatitis B virus (HBV). This immunoperoxidase stain shows the intracytoplasmic inclusions of hepatitis B surface antigen. This finding corresponds with the ground-glass change described in the previous photomicrograph (alkaline phosphatase reaction).

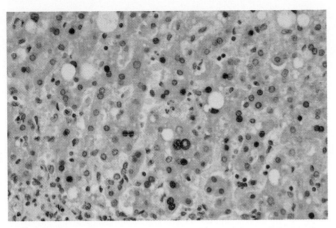

Figure 5–13
Chronic hepatitis B virus (HBV). The typical intranuclear reactivity of hepatitis B core antigen seen by immunohistochemical staining is illustrated in this photomicrograph (alkaline phosphatase reaction).

Table 5–6   Histologic Clues to Etiology of Hepatic Granulomas

Histology	Etiology
Necrotizing granulomas	Infections (e.g., tuberculosis, brucellosis, fungi)
Epithelioid granulomas with eosinophils	Drugs, parasitic infestations
Epithelioid granulomas "segmented" by fibrosis; Schaumann bodies	Sarcoidosis
Fibrin ring granulomas	Q fever, drugs (e.g., allopurinol)
Lipogranulomas	Steatohepatitis, exogenous lipids (e.g., mineral oil in processed foods)
Granulomas with polarizable talc crystals	Injection drug use

lioid type (Fig. 5–15). Specific diagnoses usually require correlation with clinical features, including drug and occupational history, special stains for organisms, microbiologic cultures, and serologic tests.

ACQUIRED IMMUNODEFICIENCY SYNDROME (AIDS)

Although there are no specific histologic features attributable solely to human immunodeficiency virus (HIV) infection of the liver, opportunistic infections, high-grade lymphoma, and Kaposi's sarcoma as well as granulomas, steatosis, peliosis, and Kupffer cell siderosis may be encountered in liver biopsies from these patients. Common infections include cytomegalovirus, *Mycobacterium avium intracellulare, Mycobacterium tuberculosis,* cryptococcosis, histoplasmosis, candidiasis, *Pneumocystis carinii,* and many others, in addition to hepatitis B and C. Infection of

the large bile ducts may lead to a sclerosing cholangitis-like syndrome (AIDS cholangiopathy), with biopsy changes of mechanical duct obstruction. Biopsies from patients with AIDS should be cultured routinely and stained with special histochemical stains for fungal and acid-fast organisms.

CHOLESTATIC LIVER DISEASE

Cholestatic liver disease may result from necroinflammatory lesions, congenital or metabolic processes, or external ductal compression. Two broad categories reflect the anatomic sites of abnormal bile retention: intrahepatic and extrahepatic (Table 5-7). This distinction is important for both diagnostic and therapeutic options: Extrahepatic biliary obstruction may respond to bile duct decompression procedures, whereas intrahepatic cholestatic processes will not.

The well-known morphologic changes of extrahepatic obstruction, which are categorized as acute cholestasis, do not discriminate the various etiologic possibilities. Histo-

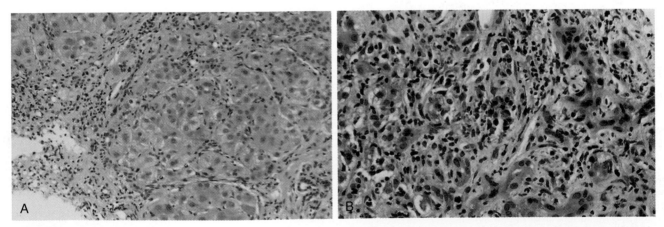

Figure 5–14
The low- *(A)* and high- *(B)* power views of this biopsy illustrate lesions seen from a patient with autoimmune hepatitis. Hepatitic rosettes and a prominent component of plasma cells in the inflammatory infiltrates, although not diagnostic of autoimmune hepatitis, are strongly suggestive of this disorder (H & E).

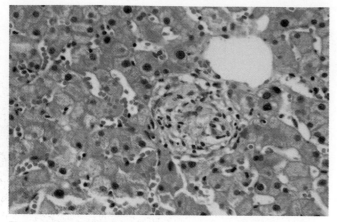

Figure 5–15
The well-formed epithelioid granuloma located near a terminal hepatic venule contains an occasional eosinophil. This raises the possibility of a drug-related etiology (H & E).

logic features in intrahepatic "chronic" cholestasis, however, may be characteristic of particular clinical syndromes. Acute and chronic cholestatic patterns of injury are described in Table 5-8. Different zones of the acinus are affected by cholestasis: The hepatocellular changes of acute cholestasis are present in the perivenular zone 3 hepatocytes, whereas zone 1, periportal or periseptal hepatocellu-

Table 5–7   Cholestatic Liver Disease

Intrahepatic Cholestasis

Primary Liver Disease	*Systemic Conditions*
Primary biliary cirrhosis	Cholestasis of pregnancy
Autoimmune cholangiopathies	Sepsis
Primary sclerosing cholangitis	Hodgkin's and
Paucity of intrahepatic bile ducts	non-Hodgkin's lymphoma
	Toxic shock syndrome
Idiopathic adulthood ductopenia	Congestive heart failure
	Sarcoidosis
	Cystic fibrosis
Metabolic Liver Disease	*Miscellaneous Liver Disease*
Byler's disease	Drug-induced hepatoxicity
α_1-Antitrypsin deficiency	Cholestatic viral hepatitis A and C
Wilson's disease	Alcoholic hepatitis
	Orthotopic liver transplant rejection
	Benign recurrent intrahepatic cholestasis

Extrahepatic Cholestasis

Choledocholithiasis
Benign and malignant strictures of extrahepatic bile ducts
Carcinoma of the bile ducts
Biliary atresia
Extrahepatic bile duct compression by tumors

Table 5–8   Histopathologic Features of Cholestasis

	Acute Cholestasis	Chronic Cholestasis
Zone 3 hepatocyte feathery degeneration	+	−
Canalicular bile plugs	+	±
Bile lakes/infarcts	+	−
Portal edema; cholangiolar proliferation; pmn infiltrates	+	−
Cholangiolar proliferation	+	+
Cholestatic liver cell rosettes	±	+
Periductal fibrosis	−	+
Ductopenia or loss of bile ducts	−	+
Xanthomatous transformation of hepatocytes	−	+
Periportal feathery degeneration; periseptal edema with loose fibrosis (cholate stasis)	−	+
Copper accumulation, periportal or periseptal hepatocytes	−	+
Mallory's hyaline, periportal or periseptal hepatocytes	−	+
Biliary fibrosis; cirrhosis	−	+

lar changes are characteristic of chronic cholestatic conditions.

Bile pigment may or may not be observed in histologic material. When present, the location of bile plugs is useful in suggesting pathogenesis. Canalicular bile plugs are seen most commonly in acute obstructive or necroinflammatory lesions (Figs. 5–16 and 5–17), but they may also be seen in the end stage of chronic cholestatic syndromes that are characterized by the loss of intrahepatic bile ducts. Bile plugs in zone 1 canals of Hering are characteristic of sepsis.

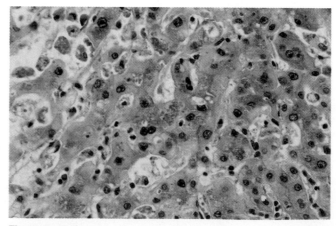

Figure 5–16
Acute cholestasis. The golden-brown pigment of bile can be seen in the intercellular canalicular spaces in hepatocytes and in enlarged, intrasinusoidal Kupffer cells. These changes, which are seen in acute bile flow obstruction, are predominantly in zone 3 (H & E).

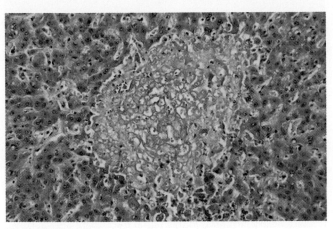

Figure 5–17
Acute cholestasis. Bile infarcts are usually associated with severe, acute cholestasis (H & E).

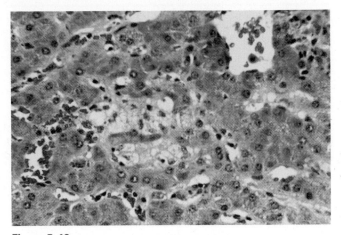

Figure 5–19
Chronic cholestasis. Xanthomatous cells are seen in clusters in sinusoids in chronic cholestasis (H & E).

CHRONIC CHOLESTATIC SYNDROMES

The clinical and histologic features of the major chronic cholestatic syndromes of adults are well described. Primary biliary cirrhosis (PBC), autoimmune cholangitis (AIC), primary sclerosing cholangitis (PSC), and idiopathic adulthood ductopenia (IAD) are clinically distinguished from one another by serologic assays for antimitochondrial antibodies (AMA), antinuclear antibodies (ANA), and cholangiographic findings. These processes share many of the histologic features of chronic cholestasis such as cholate stasis, copper reactivity, xanthomatous transformation of hepatocytes, and irregular "biliary" fibrosis (Figs. 5–18 to 5–20). In addition, in each process, there may be portal chronic inflammation with interface activity as well as sinusoidal chronic inflammation. Discriminating features are described in Table 5-9. The histologic stages for PBC and PSC reflect the progression of processes from bile duct–centered lesions to cirrhosis of the liver. Typically, these processes are inhomogeneous throughout the liver, and overlap of lesions among the four stages may be seen in an evaluation of a liver biopsy or resection specimen. The most advanced stage present in the biopsied material is reported (Figs. 5–21 to 5–25).

DRUG-INDUCED CHOLESTASIS

Drug-related cholestatic liver injury may result from a large number of commonly used drugs including antibiotics, anti-inflammatory agents, cardiac medications, and antineoplastic agents. A wide range of morphologic findings from "bland" cholestasis with subtle hepatocellular cytologic changes to the more common drug-related entity known as "cholestatic hepatitis," characterized by both hepatitic and cholestatic features, may be seen. Uncommonly, changes of chronic cholestasis may be induced by drugs, such as in the secondary sclerosing cholangitis seen after intra-arterial infusion of 5-fluoro-2′-deoxyuridine.

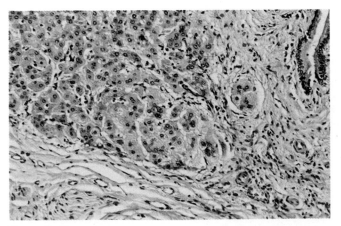

Figure 5–18
Chronic cholestasis. Chronic cholestasis results in copper accumulation in zone 1 or periseptal hepatocytes. The rhodanine stain reacts as red-brown granules with intracytoplasmic copper (Rhodanine).

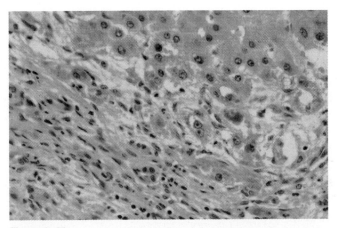

Figure 5–20
Chronic cholestasis. Mallory's hyaline, dense eosinophilic intracytoplasmic aggregates, can be seen in zone 1 or periseptal hepatocytes in chronic cholestasis (H & E).

Table 5–9 Chronic Cholestatic Syndromes

Morphology	PBC	AIC	PSC	IAD
Portal Tracts/Bile Ducts				
Ductopenia	+	+	+	+
With lymphoid aggregates	+	+	−	−
With residual fibrosis	−	−	+	−
Lymphoid aggregates	+	+	−	−
Granulomatous inflammation	+	+	−	−
Florid duct lesion	+	+	−	−
Concentric periductal fibrosis	−	−	+	−
Interface activity	+	+	+	±

PBC, primary biliary cirrhosis; AIC, autoimmune cholangiopathy; PSC, primary sclerosing cholangitis; IAD, idiopathic adulthood ductopenia.

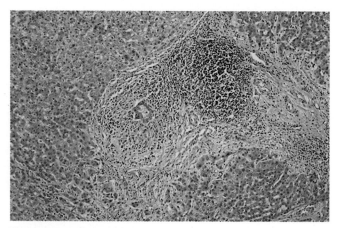

Figure 5–21
Primary biliary cirrhosis. There is both inflammatory and fibrous expansion in the illustrated portal tract. An epithelioid granuloma surrounds the bile duct and ductal epithelium is eosinophilic and shows regenerative nuclear irregularities (H & E).

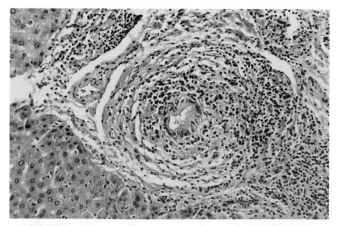

Figure 5–22
Primary biliary cirrhosis. The florid duct lesion is characterized by lymphocytic infiltration around and into the interlobular bile duct (H & E).

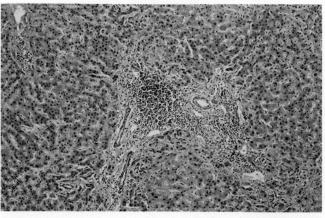

Figure 5–23
Primary biliary cirrhosis. In this portal tract, there are vascular structures and a large lymphoid aggregate, but the interlobular bile duct is not present (H & E).

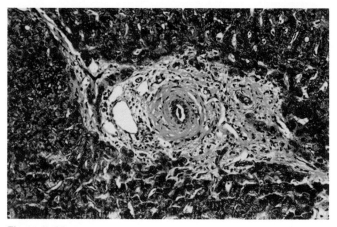

Figure 5–24
Primary sclerosing cholangitis. The interlobular bile duct in the center of the photomicrograph appears to be enlarged when compared with the hepatic artery branch nearby. This is due to the concentric, "onion-skin" fibrosis that surrounds it. This is a characteristic fibro-obliterative lesion of primary sclerosing cholangitis in the setting of cholangiographically demonstrated ductal changes (Masson's trichrome).

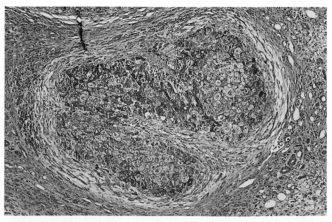

Figure 5–25
Primary sclerosing cholangitis. The cirrhotic nodule in biliary cirrhosis is irregular and surrounded not only by scar tissue but also by the loose, edematous stroma shown in this photomicrograph. This latter change is known as cholate stasis (Masson's trichrome).

CHOLESTASIS IN VIRAL HEPATITIS

Hepatocellular and canalicular cholestasis may be seen in hepatitis A and E infections; less commonly, cholestasis may also be a component of acute or chronic hepatitis C infections.

VASCULAR LESIONS

Primary vascular disorders of the liver are uncommon; more common is liver vascular involvement in a variety of hepatic and systemic diseases. For example, livers examined at autopsy often show sinusoidal dilatation, congestion, and fibrosis due to congestive heart failure; however, heart failure is usually clinically apparent, and raised liver enzymes in this setting do not usually result in a liver biopsy. Vascular lesions more commonly seen in liver biopsies, on the other hand, are perivenular and sinusoidal fibrosis of alcoholic liver disease or nonalcoholic steatohepatitis.

Two forms of hepatic vein lesions result in hepatic venous outflow obstruction: Budd-Chiari syndrome and veno-occlusive disease. Budd-Chiari syndrome refers to outflow obstruction at the level of the large hepatic veins or the inferior vena cava and may be attributed to various causes (Table 5-10). The large thrombosed veins are usually not sampled in a standard percutaneous liver biopsy, but the effects of the obstruction on the liver parenchyma have a characteristic histologic appearance. With acute obstruction, there is marked zone 3 sinusoidal dilatation, congestion, and hepatocyte dropout, with extravasation of red blood cells into the space of Disse and into the hepatic cords (the red blood cell trabecular lesion) (Fig. 5–26). With chronic obstruction, perivenular and sinusoidal fibrosis replaces the hepatic parenchyma; bridging fibrosis between adjacent acini produces a "reverse lobulation" pattern. In contrast, hepatic veno-occlusive disease results from fibrous obliterative occlusion of small intrahepatic outflow veins secondary to endothelial injury (see Table 5-10). The histology shows partial or complete fibrous obliteration of the lumen of terminal hepatic venules, along with the sinusoidal congestion, dilatation, and fibrosis (Fig. 5–27).

Table 5–10 Causes of Hepatic Venous Outflow Obstruction

Budd-Chiari Syndrome

Hematologic abnormalities, hypercoagulable states, myeloproliferative disorders, such as polycythemia vera
Membranous obstruction, often associated with hepatocellular carcinoma
Chemotherapy
Radiation therapy
Neoplasms, primary and metastatic
Oral contraceptives
Trauma
Pregnancy
Abscess

Hepatic Veno-Occlusive Disease

Chemotherapy, including thioguanine and 6-mercaptopurine
Azathioprine
Ingestion of toxic pyrrolizidine alkaloids (bush tea)
Radiation
After bone marrow transplantation

Decreased blood flow to the liver results in lesions of ischemic injury. Because of the dual portal vein-hepatic artery blood supply, even complete occlusion of major vascular branches does not necessarily cause infarction. Decreased blood flow secondary to systemic hypotension causes coagulative necrosis of zone 3 hepatocytes (Fig. 5–28). Obstruction of arterial branches due to causes such as thrombosis, polyarteritis nodosa, and inadvertent surgical ligation can result in infarcts as well as bile duct damage including strictures. Thrombosis of a branch of the portal vein leads to sharply demarcated, atrophic but viable "infarcts of Zahn" or to nodular regenerative hyperplasia rather than to true infarction.

Hepatoportal sclerosis may be seen with noncirrhotic portal hypertension and is characterized histologically by eccentric scarring and luminal narrowing of intrahepatic portal vein branches. These irregularly distributed venous lesions are associated with zones of hepatic cord atrophy,

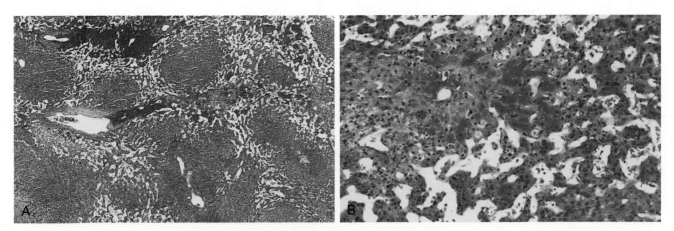

Figure 5–26
A and *B*, Budd-Chiari syndrome. The lesions of acute Budd-Chiari syndrome are characterized by the striking sinusoidal dilatation and red blood cell extravasation into hepatic cords seen in these photomicrographs (H & E).

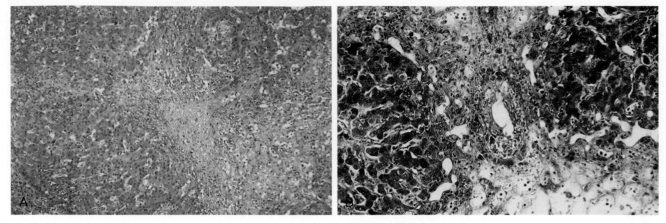

Figure 5–27
Veno-occlusive disease. *A,* The obliterative lesion of small, terminal hepatic venules characteristic of veno-occlusive disease is difficult to see in *A* but is well documented on a connective tissue stain such as the trichrome stain in *B* (H & E) (trichrome).

nodular hyperplasia, and portal or septal fibrosis. The gross appearance may be confused with cirrhosis. Although a biopsy sample often does not include the affected portal vein branches, hepatoportal sclerosis is one of the structural abnormalities to be considered in a biopsy performed for the evaluation of portal hypertension in the absence of cirrhosis (Fig. 5–29).

Nodular regenerative hyperplasia is a unique lesion characterized by nodularity of the parenchyma caused by hypertrophic cords surrounded not by scar tissue (e.g., in cirrhosis) but by atrophic hepatic plates (Figs. 5–30 and 5–31). This lesion may be associated with damage to portal tract structures (e.g., artery, vein, and bile duct) and is thought to be a result of an uneven blood supply to the affected acini.

METABOLIC LIVER DISEASE

Numerous primary metabolic disorders that affect the liver have been identified, but most are encountered only in pediatric populations. Common but nonspecific findings include fatty change, cholestasis, fibrosis, chronic hepatitis, and storage of abnormal metabolic products in hepatocytes or Kupffer cells. Histochemical stains, polarizing light, and electron microscopy are useful techniques in categorizing some disorders, but enzymatic or molecular analyses are usually required to confirm the specific metabolic defect. Among the more common metabolic disorders that are encountered in liver biopsies in the adult population are hereditary hemochromatosis, α_1-antitrypsin deficiency, Wilson's disease, and the porphyrias.

α_1-Antitrypsin deficiency is characterized histologically by round, 1- to 30-μm eosinophilic cytoplasmic inclusions within zone 1 or periseptal hepatocytes. These globules are strongly PAS-d positive and exhibit a halo-like peripheral staining pattern with an α_1-antitrypsin immunostain. In addition, features of chronic hepatitis may be seen (Figs. 5–32 and 5–33). When present, the cirrhosis is usually a mixed type in adults and a biliary type in children. In neonates, differentiation from viral hepatitis or biliary atresia may be

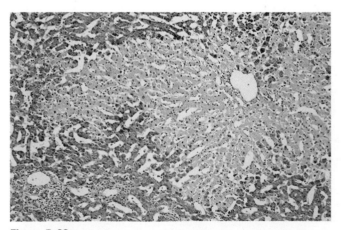

Figure 5–28
Ischemia. Zone 3 coagulative necrosis, as illustrated in this photomicrograph, is characteristic of ischemic liver disease and is usually associated with hypotension or shock (H & E).

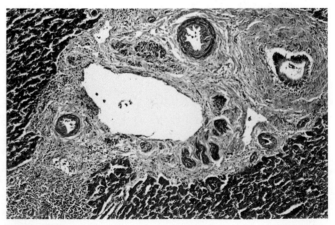

Figure 5–29
Hepatoportal sclerosis (HPS). The lesion of HPS is readily seen on a connective tissue stain as illustrated. The portal vein branch in this photomicrograph is very abnormal; numerous muscle bundles are absent (Masson's trichrome).

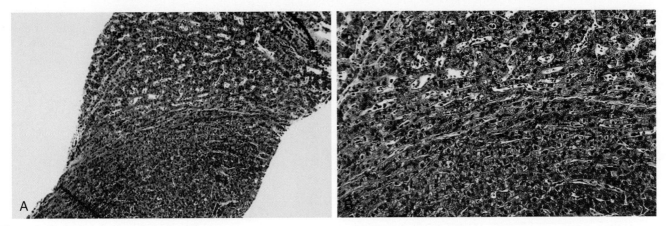

Figure 5–30
A and *B,* Nodular regenerative hyperplasia. The architecture of the hepatic parenchyma in this biopsy is very distorted by the bulging nodule seen in the upper portion of the photomicrograph. The nodule is not surrounded by scar tissue, as would be seen in cirrhosis; rather, compressed cords of hepatocytes form the edge of the nodule. This is a characteristic finding in nodular regenerative hyperplasia (Masson's trichrome).

Figure 5–31
Nodular regenerative hyperplasia. The reticulin stain from the same case as Figure 5–30 shows the typical findings of alternating groups of hypertrophic and atrophic hepatic cords (Sweet's reticulin).

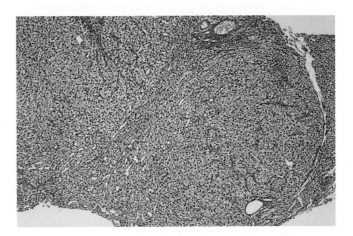

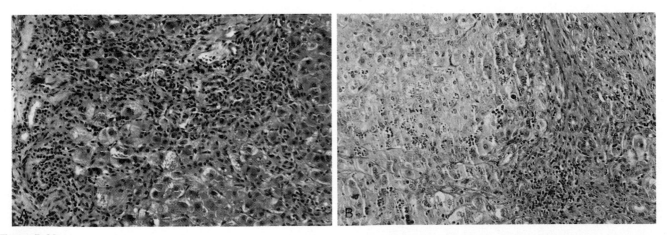

Figure 5–32
α_1-Antitrypsin deficiency. *A,* In the adult α_1AT may show changes similar to chronic hepatitis of other causes with cirrhosis and interface hepatitis as seen in the H & E. *B,* PAS-d stain, however, shows the characteristic intracytoplasmic globules of varying sizes located in hepatocytes adjacent to a fibrous septum (PAS-d).

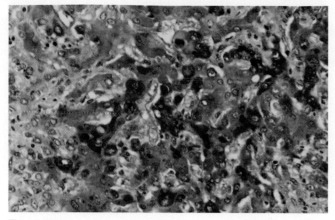

Figure 5–33
Immunohistochemical stain for α_1-antitrypsin protein demonstrates globules with either the positive solid red reactivity and globules with a negative center and a positive rim. In addition, regenerative hepatocytes may show a blush reactivity throughout the cytoplasm. This finding, however, is considered a "background" effect and is not considered to represent the inclusions of α_1AT deficiency (alkaline phosphatase reaction).

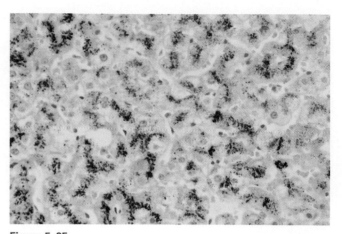

Figure 5–35
The high-power view of a Prussian blue stain highlights the typical pericanalicular localization of iron in affected hepatocytes (Prussian blue).

difficult because cytoplasmic inclusions are not usually apparent before 12 weeks of age. PAS-d-positive globules may be seen without associated liver disease in α_1-antitrypsin heterozygotes.

Hereditary hemochromatosis is associated with excess iron deposition and subsequent damage to the parenchyma of the liver as well as the pancreas, heart, joints, and other tissues. Liver biopsy is useful to confirm the diagnosis, assess the amount of fibrosis, and determine the hepatic iron concentration for calculation of the hepatic iron index. By routine H & E stains, iron is visible as a granular, slightly "chunky," golden-brown pigment (Fig. 5–34). Initially, the iron is seen only in zone 1 hepatocytes, with a distinct pericanalicular location within the cells (Fig. 5–35). As the ac-

cumulation continues, all hepatocytes acquire hemosiderin pigment, with a gradient decreasing in amount from zones 1 to 3. Eventually, iron pigment also accumulates in bile duct epithelium, Kupffer cells, portal macrophages, and vascular endothelium (Fig. 5–36). Using a Prussian blue stain to demonstrate the iron pigment, the amount of granular iron pigment observed is graded semiquantitatively; several grading systems exist, but the scale of 1+ (mild) to 4+ (massive) hepatocellular accumulation is relatively reproducible among pathologists and correlates with chemically determined amounts of iron present. The ultimate determination of the quantity of iron rests with chemical analysis of liver tissue (Table 5–2). Periportal fibrosis may progress to cirrhosis in the untreated patient. Occasionally, in a cirrhotic liver, small discrete regions devoid of hepatocellular iron are identified; the significance of these iron-free foci has been debated but may represent a preneoplastic change (Fig. 5–37). Hepatocellular carcinomas seen in cirrhotic livers in the setting of hereditary hemochromatosis do not contain iron. Iron reduction therapy can result in the complete removal of all stainable iron from the liver. Excess accumula-

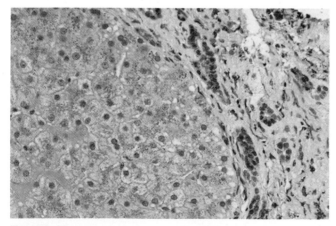

Figure 5–34
Hereditary hemochromatosis. Iron accumulation, when abundant, can be seen on H & E sections; in this example of a cirrhotic patient, the iron is granular and primarily located in periseptal hepatocytes as well as in bile duct and ductular epithelium (H & E).

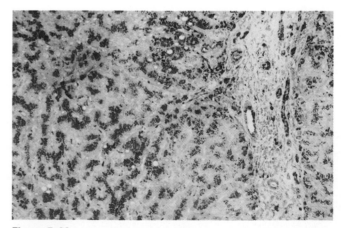

Figure 5–36
The Prussian blue stain also highlights the large clumps of iron in hepatocytes, Kuppfer cells, and ductular epithelium (Prussian blue).

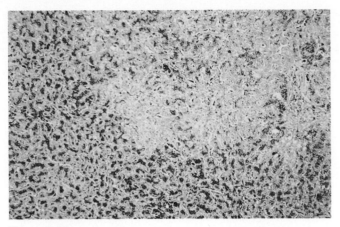

Figure 5–37

In this example, there are foci of nonreactive hepatocytes in an otherwise iron-loaded liver. This is an example of "iron-free foci." There was hepatocellular carcinoma elsewhere in the liver (Prussian blue).

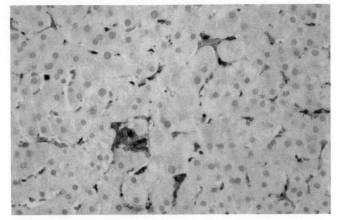

Figure 5–38

Iron overload, secondary to blood transfusion. This Prussian blue–stained liver biopsy shows the early lesions of secondary iron overload: Sinusoidal lining cell reactivity is highlighted by the stain. The hepatocytes are nonreactive (Prussian blue).

tion of iron in the liver can be seen in several clinical settings other than hereditary hemochromatosis; the distinction from hereditary hemochromatosis may be suggested based on both the quantity and the distribution of iron (Table 5-11 and Fig. 5–38), but the diagnosis rests with clinical evaluation and genetic testing.

The liver from a patient with Wilson's disease typically exhibits various nonspecific histologic findings, including nonzonal steatosis, glycogenic nuclei, anisonucleosis, and abundant "chunky" zone 1 lipofuscin granules (Fig. 5–39). Chronic hepatitis and massive or submassive necrosis can also be observed. In the cirrhosis of Wilson's disease, fat, cholestasis, and Mallory bodies are characteristic. Copper can be demonstrated in zone 1 hepatocytes (precirrhotic stage) or can be irregularly distributed throughout parenchymal nodules in cirrhosis. Copper accumulation may also be seen in zone 1 hepatocytes in chronic cholestatic liver diseases. It is important to recognize that a negative copper stain on a liver biopsy does not rule out the diagnosis of Wilson's disease, and in the appropriate clinical settings or when the diagnosis is considered by the pathologist, the serum ceruloplasmin, urinary copper excretion, and chemical hepatic copper determination should also be undertaken.

Electron microscopy can be helpful; the combination of intramitochondrial abnormalities, "fish-mouth" canaliculi, steatosis, glycogenic nuclei, lipofuscin, and "copperisomes" may be supportive of the diagnosis of Wilson's disease (Fig. 5–40).

Of the numerous porphyrias, only porphyria cutanea tarda is encountered with any frequency in adult populations. Liver biopsies in porphyria cutanea tarda may show macrovesicular steatosis, focal necrosis, and mild accumulation of hepatocellular and Kupffer cell iron or may include features of commonly associated alcoholic liver disease. Autofluorescence of uroporphyrin in hepatocytes may be detected in frozen sections; uroporphyrin crystals can sometimes be identified in paraffin sections with polarized light.

STEATOSIS AND STEATOHEPATITIS

Macrovesicular steatosis, or large droplet fat in which the hepatocyte nucleus is eccentrically located, is commonly encountered in varying amounts in liver biopsies. Frequently, this is a nonspecific finding but may be seen as a component of liver pathology in various settings including alcohol ingestion, obesity, diabetes mellitus, hepatitis C in-

Table 5–11   Distribution of Hepatic Iron* in Clinical Conditions with Iron Overload

Clinical Condition	Hepatocellular Iron	Kupffer Cell Iron	Bile Duct Iron
Hereditary hemochromatosis	1+–4+, zone 1 > zone 3	Large aggregates, only with 4+ hepatocellular iron	+
After portacaval shunt	1+–4+, zone 1 > zone 3	Only with 4+ hepatocellular iron	+
Alcoholic liver disease	1+–2+, nonzonal	+, panacinar	−
Porphyria cutanea tarda	1+–2+, nonzonal	+, panacinar	−
Transfusions, hemolytic anemias	1+–2+, up to 4+ with massive Kupffer iron	+, panacinar	±
Ineffective erythropoiesis (sideroblastic and chronic disease anemias, myelofibrosis)	1+–2+	+, panacinar	−

*The Prussian blue histochemical stain is necessary when evaluating increased iron deposition in liver parenchyma.

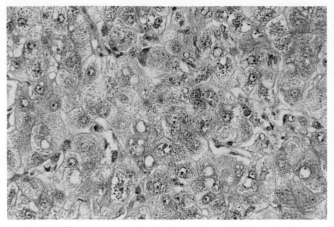

Figure 5–39
Wilson's disease. The H & E of a liver specimen from a patient with acute liver failure illustrates several of the lesions described in Wilson's disease, including the anisocytosis and anisonucleosis of hepatocytes, glycogenated nuclei, and golden-brown intracellular pigment. By special stains, some of the pigment can be shown to be bile; some is iron; and some is atypical lipofuschin (H & E).

fection, malnutrition, Wilson's disease, following jejuno-ileal bypass, and with certain drugs such as corticosteroids. Microvesicular fat is characterized histologically by numerous small cytoplasmic fat droplets; often this change is only suggested as delicate septa within hepatocytes but are well demonstrated by Oil Red O stain performed on frozen sections. The nucleus typically remains centrally located. This type of steatosis has a much more limited differential diagnosis but a significantly more ominous clinical prognosis. Included are Reye's syndrome, acute fatty liver of pregnancy, tetracycline, valproic acid and salicylate toxicity, alcoholic foamy degeneration, and some pediatric metabolic disorders.

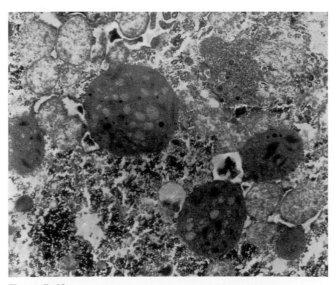

Figure 5–40
The ultrastructural photomicrograph highlights the abnormally enlarged mitochondria with intracristal widening and crystaloid inclusions (lead citrate and uranyl acetate).

Steatohepatitis refers to a characteristic combination of findings with hepatocellular damage and inflammation occurring in fatty liver; alcoholic liver disease is the prototype. There is predominantly macrovesicular steatosis with lobular disarray, ballooning degeneration of hepatocytes, acidophil bodies, lipogranulomas, and small lobular inflammatory infiltrates. The latter are unusual in that neutrophils are the primary cell type. Megamitochondria and Mallory's hyaline may be identified within ballooned hepatocytes. Fibrosis begins with deposition of collagen around terminal hepatic veins and in sinusoids and progresses with a "chickenwire" pattern of sinusoidal and pericellular fibrosis, eventuating in cirrhosis. Acute sclerosing hyaline necrosis is a particularly severe form of alcoholic liver disease with fibrous obliteration of terminal hepatic veins and extensive sinusoidal fibrosis, marked hydropic swelling of zone 3 hepatocytes, numerous Mallory bodies, and prominent neutrophilic infiltrates. This pattern carries a significantly worse clinical prognosis (Fig. 5–41).

Nonalcoholic steatohepatitis (NASH) is usually less severe clinically and pathologically than alcoholic steatohepatitis, but because of the overlap of histologic lesions may be distinguishable only with a complete and specific clinical history. Well-recognized associations include female gender, obesity, type II diabetes, jejunoileal bypass, and drugs such as amiodarone, but many patients lack these conditions. One histologic clue to a nonalcoholic etiology is the relative difficulty of finding Mallory's hyaline in NASH, and those that are present are often rather thin and poorly formed (Fig. 5–42). An exception is the steatohepatitis caused by amiodarone, in which Mallory bodies are prominent; however, the phospholipid-stuffed Kupffer cells are a clue to the use of amiodarone. Glycogenic nuclei are often notable in NASH and are not limited to patients with diabetes. Even though NASH is thought to be a milder disease than alcoholic steatohepatitis, a small percentage of biopsies will show cirrhosis.

SPACE-OCCUPYING LESIONS

The means by which the tissue is obtained for histologic evaluation of space-occupying lesions of the liver determines the assessment to be done: CT-guided liver aspirates with 22-gauge needles are best interpreted as a cytologic preparation, whereas intraoperative or CT-guided biopsies with larger-bore needles are more appropriately evaluated in the surgical pathology laboratory. Adequacy of sampled material is crucial for an accurate assessment of architectural as well as cytologic features of a clinically identified lesion in the liver.

As in evaluation of any liver biopsy, clinical history is necessary to adequately interpret the biopsy. It is important for the pathologist to be aware of predisposing clinical conditions such as underlying chronic liver disease and cirrhosis; use of medication and sex of the patient; size of the lesion and symptoms associated with it; and how the lesion was discovered are also useful to know. The differential diagnosis for an incidental nodule found in a young woman during cholecystectomy is quite different from a liver mass in a young woman taking oral contraceptives who presents to the emergency department with hemoperitoneum. The following is a descriptive list of the more common space-occupying lesions of the liver of adults and characteristic

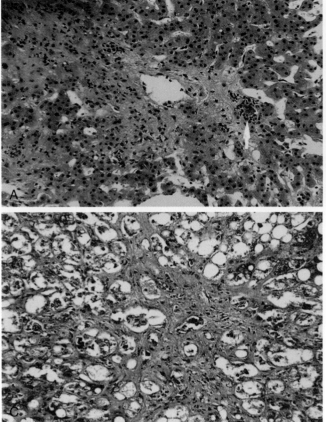

Figure 5–41
Alcoholic liver disease. *A,* Sclerosing hyaline necrosis is characterized by perivenular necrosis and fibrosis; the *arrow* points to a Mallory body surrounded by polymorphonuclear leukocytes (satellitosis) (H & E). *B,* In this case, there is hepatocellular ballooning, steatosis, Mallory's hyaline, and polymorphonuclear infiltrate (H & E). *C,* This trichrome stain highlights the dense sinusoidal fibrosis of steatohepatitis (Masson's trichrome).

histologic features of each. Some of these lesions are true neoplasms; others are of a reactive nature.

BENIGN PROLIFERATIVE LESIONS

Hepatocellular Adenoma: This consists of a tan or yellow tumor that may have hemorrhage or necrosis on the cut section; it consists of sheets of benign, uniform eosinophilic or clear hepatocytes separated by thin, sinusoidal-like vascular spaces with no cytologic atypia. No portal tracts or biliary structures are present within the tumor. Larger vascular structures are commonly seen at the periphery of the tumor and may show intimal lesions that are characteristic of oral contraceptive use (Fig. 5–43).

Focal Nodular Hyperplasia: This lesion is typically 2 to 3 cm in diameter and is frequently a pedunculated mass with

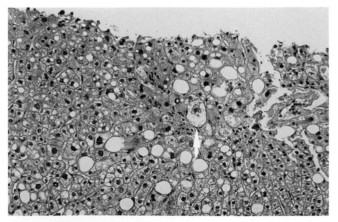

Figure 5–42
Nonalcoholic steatohepatitis (NASH). Compared with alcoholic steatohepatitis, in NASH the Mallory hyaline, when present, is less impressive. Steatosis and mild lobular inflammation are other features of NASH (H & E).

Figure 5–43
Hepatocellular adenoma. This benign tumor is characterized by sheets of cytologically bland hepatocytes. Although small vascular structures are present within the tumor, portal tracts are not (H & E).

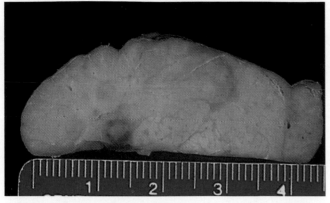

Figure 5–44
Focal nodular hyperplasia. The gross photograph shows the lesion is a nodular process with a large, centrally located scar attached to otherwise unremarkable liver (gross specimen).

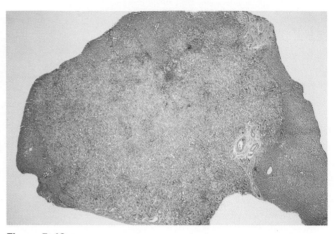

Figure 5–46
Bile duct adenoma. The subcapsular mass consists of benign ductular structures in a fibrous matrix (H & E).

a central scar containing abnormal vascular structures. The scar radiates into and separates groups of benign hepatocytes; ductular structures with mild inflammation are seen adjacent to the scar. Bile or copper reactivity may be present. Hepatocyte cytology is similar to the surrounding uninvolved liver (Figs. 5–44 and 5–45).

Dysplastic Hepatocellular Nodule: All or part of a cirrhotic nodule may bulge above the surface and appear bile stained or pale by gross examination; the nodule consists of a group of similar-appearing hepatocytes with nuclear or architectural features that are worrisome but not diagnostic of hepatocellular carcinoma. Cytologic changes include basophilia, eosinophilia, clear cell change, fatty change, Mallory's hyaline, increased bile or iron, and nuclear crowding.

Bile Duct Adenoma: A superficial subcapsular lesion is characterized histologically by a circumscribed proliferation

of benign glandular structures embedded in a fibrous matrix (Fig. 5–46).

Hemangioma: Thick-walled fibrous vascular spaces are lined by endothelium; calcifications and areas of myxoid degeneration are common (Figs. 5–47 and 5–48).

Angiomyolipoma: A large tumor includes vascular spaces, eosinophilic cells reactive with smooth muscle and HMB-45 immunohistochemical markers, and large droplet fat-containing cells (Fig. 5–49).

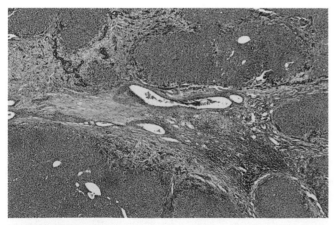

Figure 5–45
Focal nodular hyperplasia. The scar appears to radiate into nodules of hepatocytes and is demarcated from the hepatocytes by proliferated ductules and lymphocytic inflammation. Large, abnormal vascular structures are present in the center portions of the scar (H & E).

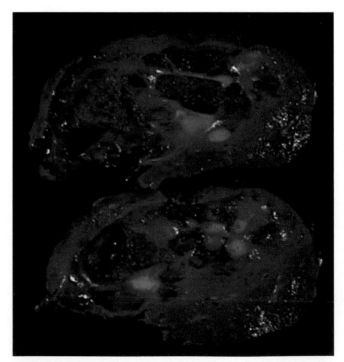

Figure 5–47
Hemangioma. A cross-section of a surgically removed hemangioma shows cystic spaces with foci of myxoid matrix (gross specimen).

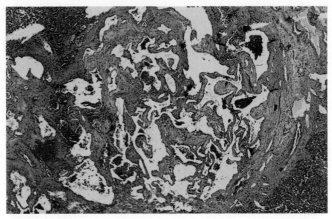

Figure 5–48
Hemangioma. The photomicrograph shows irregular
thick-walled vascular spaces, some of which contain blood
(H & E).

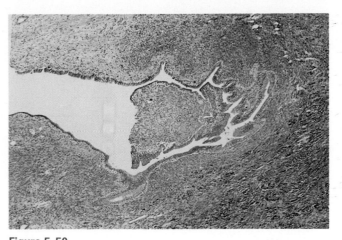

Figure 5–50
Biliary cystadenoma. The cystic space is lined by columnar
epithelium; the underlying stroma consists of spindled cells,
consistent with "mesenchymal" stroma (H & E).

Cystadenoma: A cystic tumor is present with a mucinous
epithelial lining on the basement membrane; dense, mesenchymal "ovarian" stroma are also present. The serous variant is uncommon, and mesenchymal stroma is not present
(Fig. 5–50).

Miscellaneous Benign Lesions

Focal Fatty Infiltration: Single or multifocal circumscribed areas of macrovesicular steatosis with no loss or replacement of acinar structures are present.

Peliosis Hepatis: Blood-filled lakes with or without an
endothelial lining are present (Fig. 5–51). A variant seen in
AIDS shows fibromyxoid stroma that contains Warthin-
Starry–positive rickettsial organisms.

Parasitic Cysts: An echinococcal cyst with parasitic con-
tents is usually identifiable.

Simple Cysts: A single cell lining of the basement membrane is present on the thin, fibrous wall.

Adult Polycystic Liver Disease: Cystic spaces of varying
size may occupy or replace large portions of the liver. Cysts
are lined by simple columnar epithelium; thick fibrous walls
frequently contain calcifications. Von Meyenburg complexes are commonly found in noncystic liver parenchyma
(Fig. 5–52).

Infections: In cases of pyogenic abscess, stains for bacteria and acid-fast organisms are indicated.

Amebic Abscess: With this destructive lesion, PAS-
positive trophozoites that contain ingested erythrocytes can
be seen.

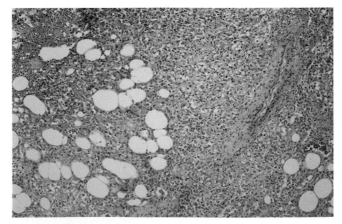

Figure 5–49
Angiomyolipoma. The three components of angiomyolipoma
are seen in this photomicrograph: a large arterial vascular
structure, the diffuse collection of eosinophilic cells with
abundant cytoplasm, and small nuclei and the foci of steatosis
(H & E).

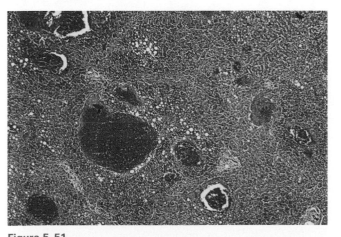

Figure 5–51
Peliosis hepatis. This unusual lesion of the liver is
characterized by blood-filled spaces scattered diffusely
throughout the parenchyma (H & E).

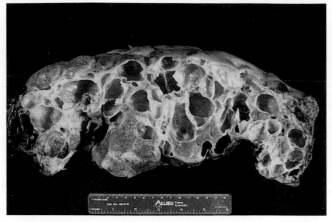

Figure 5–52
Adult polycystic liver disease. The gross photograph illustrates a cross-section of a liver nearly replaced by cystic spaces of varying sizes (gross specimen).

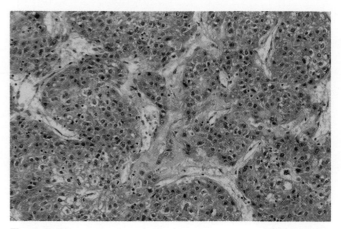

Figure 5–54
Hepatocellular carcinoma (HCC). This is the trabecular pattern of HCC. In this pattern, the tumor recapitulates hepatic parenchyma with liver cell cords invested by sinusoidal lining cells, but the trabeculae are significantly wider than normal. Cytologic features of malignancy are also present (H & E).

MALIGNANT LESIONS

Hepatocellular Carcinoma (HCC):   This variably sized, commonly encapsulated tumor may be stained with bile and bulging by gross examination; 60% of cases in North American are found in cirrhotic livers. Vascular invasion is apparent grossly or microscopically. World Health Organization (WHO) classifications describe the following architectural patterns: trabecular, pseudoglandular, compact, and scirrhous. Cytologic changes of HCC are variable and include an eosinophilic, clear cell change or steatosis and nuclear atypia. Mallory's hyaline or eosinophilic globules may be present in clusters of tumor cells. Intercellular bile is diagnostic when it is present. Nuclear features vary from an increased N/C ratio to hyperchromasia and abnormal mitoses. Positive or negative immunoreactivity is present with hepatocellular cytokeratins (Moll 8, 18) CAM 5.2, α-fetoprotein, α_1-antitrypsin, and canalicular immunoreac-

tivity with polyclonal carcinoembryonic antigen (CEA) (Figs. 5–53 to 5–57).

Fibrolamellar Hepatocellular Carcinoma: Large, eosinophilic granular tumor cells may contain intracytoplasmic pale inclusion bodies. Clusters of tumor cells are separated by broad bands of lamellar fibrosis (Fig. 5–58).

Cholangiocarcinoma (CCA):   Malignant glandular or ductular structures are embedded in desmoplastic stroma. Carcinoma-in-situ may be seen in the bile ducts; tumors may or may not be mucin-positive (Figs. 5–59 and 5–60).

Combined Cholangiohepatocellular Carcinoma: This entity may represent a "collision" tumor with distinct areas of HCC and CCA; other cases show a transition between areas of hepatocellular carcinoma and tumor cells with ductu-

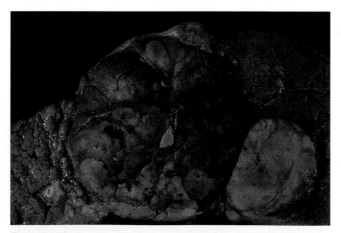

Figure 5–53
Hepatocellular carcinoma. The gross photograph shows two bulging nodules of hepatocellular carcinoma in a liver with underlying cirrhosis. The larger of the two nodules is stained with bile (gross specimen).

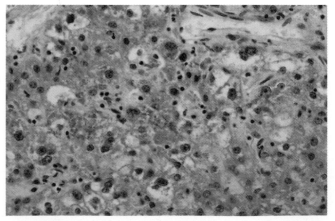

Figure 5–55
Hepatocellular carcinoma. In other areas of the same tumor (as illustrated in Fig. 5–54), clusters of tumor cells containing intracytoplasmic inclusions characteristic of Mallory's hyaline are seen (H & E).

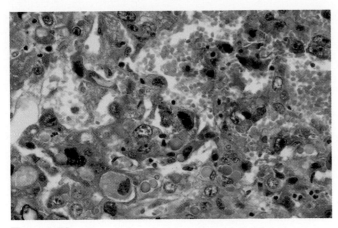

Figure 5–56
Hepatocellular carcinoma. Intracytoplasmic globules are quite
numerous in this area of malignant cells (H & E).

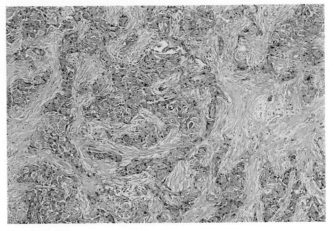

Figure 5–58
Fibrolamellar variant of hepatocellular carcinoma. The
lamellar pattern of fibrosis is apparent in this
photomicrograph. Clusters of fairly uniform, large eosinophilic
tumor cells are separated by the fibrosis (H & E).

lar or glandular architecture. Intercellular bile pigment is
present in the HCC component; mucin may be present in the
CCA component. The foci of CCA will react with biliary-
type cytokeratins Moll 7, 19.

Cystadenocarcinoma: Malignant nuclear and cytologic
features with a breach of the basement membrane by tumor
cells are typical. Mesenchymal stroma may or may not be
present.

Angiosarcoma: This multifocal destructive tumor is characterized by interdigitating vascular channels lined by atypical, large endothelial cells. The tumor may infiltrate along
the sinusoids and endothelial surfaces of the portal or central veins.

Epithelioid Hemangioendothelioma: Eosinophilic or
"dendritic" tumor cells are positive for factor VIII, Ulex endothelial cell markers by immunohistochemistry. Intracytoplasmic vacuoles, some of which contain RBCs, may be
seen in the tumor. The tumor infiltrates sinusoids and veins

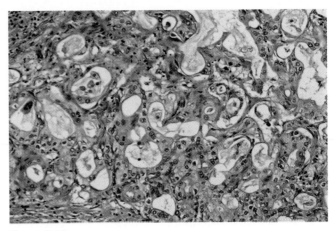

Figure 5–59
Cholangiocarcinoma. The tumor in this photomicrograph
contains haphazard glands with malignant cytologic features
(H & E).

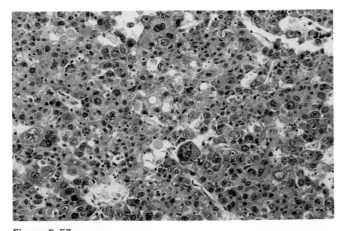

Figure 5–57
Hepatocellular carcinoma (HCC). This field illustrates poorly
differential HCC with tumor giant cells, marked nuclear
variability, and mitotic activity (H & E).

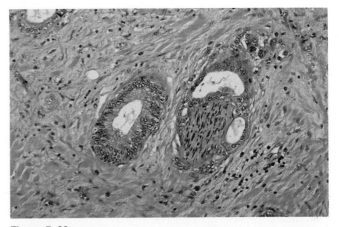

Figure 5–60
Cholangiocarcinoma. Perineural invasion is a frequent finding
(H & E).

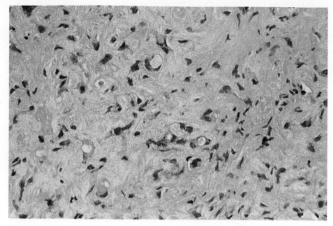

Figure 5–61
Epithelioid hemangioendothelioma. This unusual neoplasm consists of dendritic-type cells, some of which contain intracellular lumina. The tumor is embedded in a hyalinized stroma (H & E).

and may obliterate terminal hepatic venules. It may be present in fibrous or hyalinized stroma (Fig. 5–61).

Miscellaneous Sarcomas: These are usually metastatic but, rarely, primary sarcomas of the liver may occur.

Lymphoma: Lymphoma is rarely primary in the liver.

Extrahepatic Malignancy: Melanoma and carcinomas of renal, colonic, breast, and thyroid origin frequently metastasize to the liver; tumors may be seen as discrete nodules or may infiltrate into the hepatic cords. Immunohistochemistry may be necessary in some cases to distinguish metastases from HCCs. Hematopoietic malignancies may involve the liver as well; leukemic infiltrates typically involve the sinusoids, and lymphoid malignancies infiltrate portal tracts as well as sinusoids (Fig. 5–62). Hodgkin's disease may also

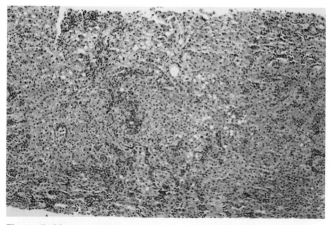

Figure 5–62
Leukemic infiltration of the liver. In this case of acute lymphoblastic leukemia, the tumor cells infiltrate and expand sinusoidal spaces (H & E).

involve the liver with cholestasis, neoplastic lymphoid cells, or a granulomatous infiltrate.

TRANSPLANT PATHOLOGY

Orthotopic Liver Transplantation

Biopsy of the donor liver before or during the transplant procedure may be indicated in two settings: pretransplant evaluation of the donor organ and for evaluation of post-transplant function. In the case of the former, the evaluation is most commonly a frozen section request for evaluation of possible pre-existing donor disease or steatosis. Necrotizing granulomas, malignancy, or evidence of chronic liver disease are criteria for exclusion in some centers; the presence of more than 30% steatosis has been correlated with subsequent dysfunction or nonfunction of the allograft. Because biochemical assays do not adequately discriminate immune-mediated, technical (biliary and vascular), or systemic complications that may cause allograft dysfunction, liver biopsy remains the "gold standard" in the diagnosis. Some centers have found post-transplant protocol biopsies done at predetermined intervals to be useful in detecting clinically inapparent graft injury.

Rejection remains a leading cause of allograft dysfunction; the terminology currently in use for rejection reflects both the pathogenesis and potential reversibility of the process. Acute rejection, a cell-mediated entity, is characterized by mixed portal infiltrates with lymphocytes and eosinophils, bile duct injury, and endothelial inflammation (endotheliitis) of terminal hepatic and portal veins (Fig. 5–63). Acute rejection is potentially responsive to increased immunosuppression. Ductopenic rejection, on the other hand, is caused by direct immune damage and secondary ischemia from immune injury of the vascular supply to the bile ducts. The portal tracts become devoid of bile ducts and inflammation. Features of chronic cholestasis may be seen in the lobules. Ductopenic rejection may be acute (of recent onset) or chronic (a manifestation of a progressive dysfunction of longer duration) and is generally irreversible (Figs. 5–64 and 5–65). Hyperacute rejection, a rare complication in liver transplantation, is caused by preformed antibodies usually in the ABO blood group system and is not responsive to medical intervention.

Table 5-12 shows the common causes of allograft dysfunction and their respective histologic lesions. In the early post-transplant period, acute rejection and preservation or surgically related processes are more common causes of dysfunction; in later time periods, although acute rejection may continue to be a problem, chronic ductopenic rejection, opportunistic infections of the graft (Figs. 5–66 and 5–67), recurrent disease, and post-transplant lymphoproliferative disorder (Fig. 5–68) are important considerations. At any time post-transplant, pathologic findings related to the transmission of clinically unknown donor disease, drug hepatotoxicity, and hepatic manifestations of sepsis may be seen. Finally, because the vascular supply to the biliary ductal system derives entirely from the hepatic artery, bile duct injury and related morphologic changes may be related to either the biliary anastomosis or to hepatic artery insufficiency from occlusion or immune-mediated injury (Fig.

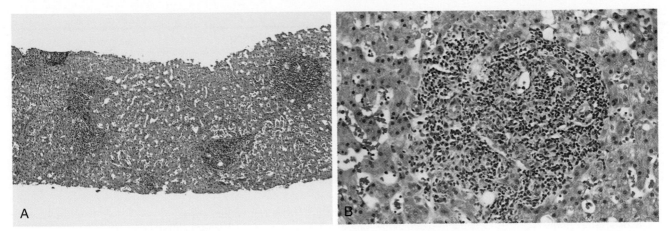

Figure 5–63
Acute rejection. *A,* Acute cellular rejection is characterized by inflammatory expansion of portal tracts with relative sparing of the acinar parenchyma (H & E). *B,* On higher power, the triad of acute rejection is seen: mixed chronic inflammation with eosinophils and occasional polymorphonuclear leukocytes, bile duct infiltration and damage, and subendothelial inflammation of the portal vein. The latter is known as endotheliitis (H & E).

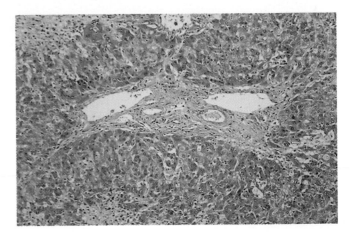

Figure 5–64
Chronic rejection. In ductopenic rejection, the portal tracts are nearly devoid of inflammation. Absence of the interlobular bile duct is apparent in this portal tract in which only the hepatic artery and portal vein branches are seen (H & E).

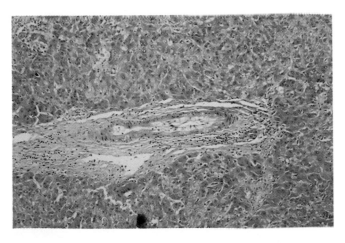

Figure 5–65
Chronic rejection. Foam cell arteriopathy is commonly found in chronic allograft rejection. The arteries involved are of medium to large caliber and are not typically represented in a percutaneous liver biopsy (H & E).

Table 5–12 Liver Transplant Pathology

Diagnostic Considerations	Morphologic Findings
Rejection	
Hyperacute	Hemorrhagic necrosis or polymorphonuclear infiltrates; IgM, complement in vessel walls
Acute	Triad: mixed chronic inflammation with eosinophils in portal tracts; bile duct infiltration, injury; portal or central endotheliitis; zone 3 necrosis, dropout in severe rejection
Acute vanishing bile duct syndrome	Paucity or loss of interlobular bile ducts with decreased portal inflammation; zone 3 cholestasis; foam cells in the sinusoids; zone 3 necrosis, dropout common
Chronic, irreversible rejection	Loss of interlobular bile ducts; zone 3 ballooning, cholestasis, or dropout; foam cells in the sinusoids; foam cell arteriopathy
Preservation-related changes	Zone 3 hepatocellular ballooning ± canalicular cholestasis; subcapsular necrosis
Vascular thrombosis	
Outflow compromise	Zone 3 congestion or red blood cell extravasation into cords
Venous or arterial inflow compromise	Zone 3 hepatocellular ballooning; less commonly, ischemic infarct
Arterial thrombosis	As above ± bile duct ischemic change or necrosis
Biliary obstruction	Acute cholestasis with portal edema, proliferating ductules, and polymorphonuclear leukocytes
Transmission of donor disease	Excess iron pigment (hemochromatosis); zone 1 PAS-d globules (α_1-antitrypsin globules); chronic hepatitis (HCV); malignancy
Recurrence of original disease	HBV surface and core antigens; HDV antigens may be demonstrated with immunohistochemistry with inflammatory changes associated with "hepatitis"; HBV and HCV recurrences may be seen as fibrosing cholestatic hepatitis Malignancy: hepatocellular carcinoma; cholangiocarcinoma Primary biliary cirrhosis Autoimmune hepatitis
Post-transplant lymphoproliferative disorder	Atypical lymphoid infiltrate, monoclonal B or T cell proliferation demonstrated by flow cytometry, DNA gene rearrangement studies on fresh tissue
Opportunistic Infections	
CMV	Microabscesses; intranuclear and intracytoplasmic inclusions in hepatocytes, biliary epithelium, or sinusoidal lining cells
HSV	Nonzonal "punched-out" necrosis; ground-glass viral inclusions at the periphery of the necrotic foci
EBV	Sinusoidal and portal atypical lymphocytic inflammation
Fungal	Hepatitis with organisms demonstrated by GMS or mucicarmine stains
Drug-induced hepatoxicity	As in nontransplant liver pathology

CMV, cytomegalovirus; EBV; Epstein-Barr virus; HBV, hepatitis B virus; HCV, hepatitis C virus; HDV, hepatitis D virus; HSV, herpes simplex virus; PAS-d, diastase-treated periodic acid–Schiff; GMS, Gomori methenamine silver.

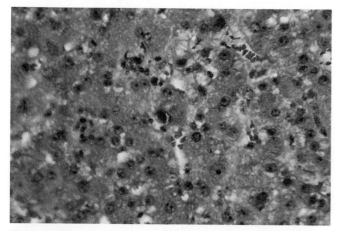

Figure 5–66
Post-transplant opportunistic infection. Cytomegalovirus infection, a common post-transplant opportunistic infection, may involve the allograft liver as well as other organs. The enlarged infected cells contain the characteristic intranuclear inclusion; frequently, a small cluster of acute inflammatory cells is present in adjacent parenchyma (H & E).

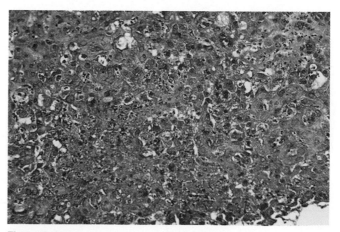

Figure 5–67
Post-transplant opportunistic infection. Herpes virus infection of the allograft liver shows similar histologic features as seen in the nonallograft liver: nonzonal "punched-out" necrosis of hepatic parenchyma. On the borders of these foci, hepatocytes with the ground-glass nuclear features of herpes simplex virus inclusions are present (H & E).

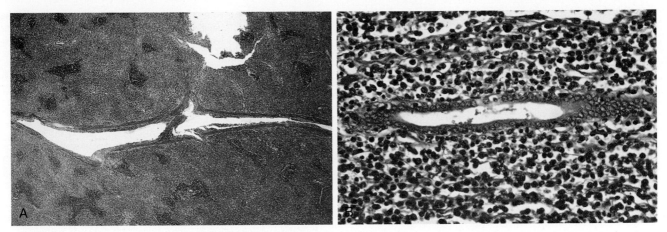

Figure 5–68
Post-transplant lymphoproliferative disorder. *A,* Post-transplant lymphoproliferative disorder is a process that may also lead to marked cellular expansion of portal tracts (H & E). *B,* High-power examination of the involved portal tracts shows that the infiltrate consists of atypical, monomorphic lymphoid cells. The bile duct is surrounded but not destroyed by the infiltrate. Further phenotypic and genotypic characterization of the infiltrate is necessary to determine the clonality of the process (H & E).

5–69). This change is more common in the later post-transplant period.

Recurrence of Viral Hepatitis

A major challenge occurs in distinguishing allograft injury caused by a recurrence of viral hepatitis B or hepatitis C infection from rejection. In some cases, there may be an overlap of findings, and more than one process may be present. Ground-glass change in hepatocytes and immunohistochemical stains for HBV antigens are helpful in documenting the presence of HBV. Bile duct injury and ductular proliferation may be seen in either acute rejection or infection with HCV; portal inflammation greater than acinar inflam-

mation and endotheliitis favors the former, whereas ballooning of hepatocytes, steatosis, acidophil bodies, and lymphoid aggregates are more indicative of the latter. Eosinophils may be seen in both processes. In some cases, serial biopsies are necessary for determining the causes of allograft dysfunction.

In addition, both recurrent HBV and HCV have been described in a unique process, fibrosing cholestatic hepatitis (FCH) characterized by clinical jaundice and graft deterioration. The histopathologic features include hepatocellular ballooning, marked ductular proliferation, periportal fibrosis, and cholestasis. Abundant intracytoplasmic viral antigens are readily demonstrated in HBV FCH (Fig. 5–70).

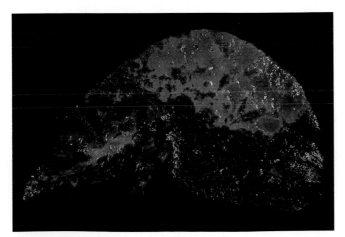

Figure 5–69
Hepatic artery thrombosis. The allograft liver shown on cut section in this photograph was removed for hepatic artery thrombosis. A large wedge infarct and several smaller foci of parenchymal necrosis are present. In addition, in the left lateral lobe, there is a large abscess that resulted from an ischemic, necrotic bile duct (gross specimen).

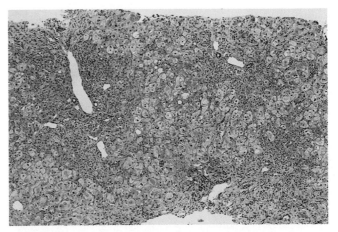

Figure 5–70
Recurrent hepatitis B. This biopsy is an example of a variant of recurrent hepatitis B infection known as fibrosing cholestatic hepatitis. There is panacinar hepatocyte ballooning; the portal tracts are expanded by chronic inflammation and ductular proliferation. In these cases, diffuse immunoreactivity with hepatitis B virus surface and core antigens will be present (H & E).

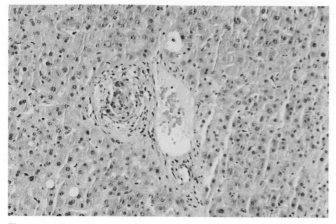

Figure 5–71

Graft-versus-host disease. Acute graft-versus-host disease may show significant damage to the interlobular bile ducts. As illustrated, the changes in the ductal epithelium include loss of nuclear polarity and cytoplasmic vacuolization. Inflammation is relatively mild (H & E).

LIVER PATHOLOGY FOLLOWING BONE MARROW TRANSPLANTATION

Liver dysfunction following bone marrow transplantation (BMT) may be attributed to processes that occur in the non-BMT setting, such as drug-induced hepatotoxicity or infections. Other causes of liver injury are unique to the post-BMT clinical setting. In a review of the changes that may be seen in post-BMT biopsies for liver dysfunction, the differential diagnoses for dysfunction should be considered in terms of post-transplant interval. In the initial 30 days after BMT, veno-occlusive disease and nodular regenerative hyperplasia from pretransplant cytoreductive therapies are more common considerations than graft-versus-host disease (GVHD). Between 30 and 100 days, acute GVHD is likely to occur; in more than 100 days, the differential diagnostic considerations include chronic GVHD as well as recurrent disease and viral hepatitis from transfusion.

Biopsies of the liver for acute GVHD may show single cell necrosis, ballooning, or lymphocytic infiltration and epithelial damage of the bile duct epithelium similar to that seen in allograft rejection; it is the latter that is the most characteristic finding in acute GVHD (Fig. 5–71). Chronic GVHD is characterized by mixed lymphoplasmacytic infiltration of bile ducts with minimal hepatocellular necrosis or ductopenia and cholestasis.

SUGGESTED READINGS

Caturelli E, Giacobbe A, Facciorusso D, et al: Percutaneous biopsy in diffuse liver disease: Increasing diagnostic yield and decreasing complication rate by routine ultrasound assessment of puncture site. Am J Gastroenterol 91:1318–1321, 1996.

Froehlich F, Lamy O, Fried M, Gonvers JJ: Practice and complications of liver biopsy: Results of a nationwide survey in Switzerland. Dig Dis Sci 38:1480–1484, 1993.

McGill DB, Rakela J, Zinsmeister AR, Ott BJ: A 21-year experience with major hemorrhage after percutaneous liver biopsy. Gastroenterology 99:1396–1400, 1990.

Minuk GY, Sutherland LR, Wiseman DA, et al: Prospective study of the incidence of ultrasound-detected intrahepatic and subcapsular hematomas in patients randomized to 6 or 24 hours of bed rest after percutaneous liver biopsy. Gastroenterology 92:290–293, 1987.

Piccinino F, Sagnelli E, Pasquale G, Giusti G: Complications following percutaneous liver biopsy: A multicentre retrospective study on 68,276 biopsies. J Hepatol 2:165–173, 1986.

Hepatitis

Desmet VJ, Gerber M, Hoofnagle JH, et al: Classification of chronic hepatitis: Diagnosis, grading and staging. Hepatology 19:1513–1520, 1994.

Ishak K: New developments in diagnostic liver pathology. In Farber E, Phillips MJ, Kaufman N (eds): Pathogenesis of Liver Diseases. Baltimore, MD: Williams & Wilkins 1987, pp 242–262.

Knodell RG, Ishak KG, Black WC, et al: Formulation and application of numerical scoring system for assessing histological activity in asymptomatic chronic active hepatitis. Hepatology 1:431–435, 1981.

Ludwig J: The nomenclature of chronic active hepatitis: An obituary. Gastroenterology 105:274–278, 1993.

Cholestatic Liver Disease

Ben Ari Z, Dhillon AP, Sherlock S: Autoimmune cholangiopathy: Part of the spectrum of autoimmune chronic active hepatitis. Hepatology 18:10–15, 1993.

Lefkowitch JH. Bile ductular cholestasis: An ominous histopathologic sign related to sepsis and "cholangitis lenta." Hum Pathol 13:19–24, 1982.

Ludwig J, Dickson ER, McDonald GS: Staging of chronic nonsuppurative destructive cholangitis (syndrome of primary biliary cirrhosis). Virchows Arch Pathol Anat 379:103–112, 1978.

Ludwig J, Kim CH, Weisner RH, Krom RA: Floxuridine-induced sclerosing cholangitis: An ischemic cholangiopathy? Hepatology 9:215–218, 1989.

Ludwig J, LaRusso NF, Weisner RH: Primary sclerosing cholangitis. In Peters RC, Craig JR (eds): Contemporary Issues in Surgical Pathology. Vol 8: Liver Pathology. New York: Churchill Livingstone, 1986, pp 193–213.

Ludwig J, Wiesner RH, LaRusso NF: Idiopathic adulthood ductopenia. J Hepatol 7:193–199, 1988.

Michieletti P, Wanless IR, Katz A, et al: Antimitochondrial antibody negative primary biliary cirrhosis: A distinct syndrome of autoimmune cholangitis. Gut 35:260–265, 1994.

Sciot R, Van Damme B, Desmet VJ: Cholestatic features in hepatitis A. J Hepatol 3:172–181, 1986.

Vascular Lesions

Lee RG: Vascular disorders. In Lee RG (ed): Diagnostic Liver Pathology. St. Louis, MO: CV Mosby, 1994, pp 324–333.

Wanless IR: Micronodular transformation (nodular regenerative hyperplasia) of the liver: A report of 64 cases among 2,500 autopsies and a new classification of benign hepatocellular nodules. Hepatology 11:787–797, 1990.

Metabolic Liver Disease

Bacon BR, Farahvash MJ, Janney CG, Nauschwander-Tetri BA: Nonalcoholic steatohepatitis: An expanded clinical entity. Gastroenterology 107:1103–1109, 1994.

Cortes JM, Oliva H, Paradines FJ, Hernandez-Guio C: The pathology of the liver in porphyria cutanea tarda. Histopathology 4:471–485, 1980.

Deugnier YM, Cheralambous P, LeQuillenc D, et al: Preneoplastic significance of hepatic iron free foci in genetic hemochromatosis: A study of 185 patients. Hepatology 18:1363–1369, 1993.

Nutritional and metabolic liver disease. In Sherlock S, Dooley J (eds): Diseases of the Liver and Biliary System. London: Blackwell Scientific, 1993, pp 410–411.

Olynyk JK, O'Neill R, Britton RS, Bacon BR: Determination of hepatic iron concentration in fresh and paraffin-embedded tissue: Diagnostic implications. Gastroenterology 106:674–677, 1994.

Searle J, Kerr JRF, Halliday JW, Powell LW: Iron storage disease. In Mac-Sween RNM, Anthony PP, Scheuer PJ, et al: Pathology of the Liver. London: Churchill Livingstone, 1994, p 224.

Stromeyer FW, Ishak KG: Histology of the liver in Wilson's disease: A study of 34 cases. Am J Clin Pathol 73:12–24, 1980.

Space-Occupying Lesions

International Working Party: Terminology of nodular hepatocellular lesions. Hepatology 22:983–993, 1995.

Ishak KG, Rabin L: Benign tumors of the liver. Med Clin North Am 59:995–1013, 1975.

Ishak KG, Sesterhenn IA, Goodman ZD, et al: Epithelioid hemangioendothelioma of the liver: A clinicopathologic and follow-up study of 32 cases. Hum Pathol 15:839–852, 1984.

Nzeako UC, Goodman ZD, Ishak KG: Hepatocellular carcinoma in cirrhotic and non-cirrhotic livers: A clinico-pathologic study of 804 North American patients. Am J Clin Pathol 105:65–75, 1996.

Transplant Pathology

Brunt EM, Peters MG, Flye MW, Hanto DW: Day five protocol liver allograft biopsies document early rejection episodes and are predictive of recurrent rejection. Surgery 14:511–517, 1992.

Davies SE, Portmann BC, O'Grady JG, et al: Hepatic histological findings after transplantation for chronic hepatitis B virus infection, including a unique pattern of fibrosing cholestatic hepatitis. Hepatology 13:150–157, 1989.

Ferrell LD, Wright TL, Roberts J, et al: Hepatitis C viral infection in liver transplant recipients. Hepatology 16:865–876, 1992.

Hubscher SG, Elias E, Buckel JAC, et al: Primary biliary cirrhosis. Histological evidence of disease recurrence after liver transplantation. J Hepatol 18:173–184, 1993.

International Working Party: Terminology for hepatic allograft rejection. Hepatology 22:648–654, 1995.

Markin RS, Wisecarver JL, Radio SJ: Hepatic allograft pathology. In Kolbeck P, Markin RS, McManus BM (eds): Transplant Pathology. Chicago: ASCP Press 1994, pp 241–265.

Neuberger J, Portmann B, Calne R, Williams R: Recurrence of autoimmune chronic active hepatitis following orthotopic liver grafting. Transplantation 31:363–365, 1984.

Schluger LK, Sheiner PA, Thung SN, et al: Severe recurrent cholestatic hepatitis C following orthotopic liver transplantation. Hepatology 23:971–976, 1996.

III

Diseases of the Liver
and Biliary Tree

6

Viral Hepatitis: Clinical Features

Stephanos J. Hadziyannis

Viral hepatitis can be defined as an infection in which necroinflammation of the liver is basically responsible for the majority of its clinical and laboratory features. It comprises a wide spectrum of clinical syndromes ranging from the most mild and subclinical to the most severe and rapidly progressive ones and is caused by at least five viral agents, the hepatitis viruses A, B, C, D, and E (HAV, HBV, HCV, HDV, and HEV), which are taxonomically diverse and belong to five different viral families.

Hepatitis caused by other viruses (e.g., the Epstein-Barr virus) will not be discussed in this chapter. Clinical manifestations in these infections are mainly caused by involvement of organs and tissues other than the liver.

In viral hepatitis, depending on its etiology, there is a variable incidence of clinically significant hepatic and extrahepatic manifestations, complications, and progression to chronicity. However, despite the fact that each virus has a gamut of clinical features, a distinction between the five virologic types of hepatitis is impossible on clinical grounds. On the other hand, the clinical diagnosis of viral hepatitis should also specify its etiology because of important implications in prognosis, management, epidemiology, and prevention. Thus, viral hepatitis will be discussed with and without distinguishing its five virologic types.

ETIOLOGY

At least five viruses belonging to different families have been implicated in the etiology of viral hepatitis. Four of the five viruses are RNA-containing agents, whereas the fifth, HBV, although a DNA-containing virus, utilizes an RNA transcript as its pregenome. Thus, none of the hepatitis viruses is a typical DNA virus. Three of the five viruses have envelopes, and all three viruses with envelopes are parenterally transmitted

and have the ability to cause not only acute but also chronic hepatitis. The main characteristics of the hepatitis viruses are summarized in Table 6–1. The viruses have been grouped according to modes of transmission and chronicity of infection, rather than by strict alphabetic order. The hepatitis A and E viruses comprise the orally transmitted group that cause only acute hepatitis, whereas viruses B, C, and D make up the parenterally transmitted group, causing both acute and chronic infection. Because HDV is dependent on HBV, it is listed immediately after HBV rather than after HCV. In addition to these five viruses, other agents called non–A-E viruses appear to be also involved in the etiology of viral hepatitis (see Table 6–1). However, claims on the identification of a new orally transmitted agent, prematurely designated as the hepatitis F virus, have not been substantiated. Another recently identified and well-characterized viral species, designated as "hepatitis" G virus and GB virus C, and a second transfusion-transmitted DNA virus, designated TTV, do not appear to be hepatotropic, causing little if any hepatitis. Consequently, they do not seem to belong to the hepatitis alphabet and will not be discussed in this chapter. The search for new hepatitis viruses continues.

SEROLOGY

All hepatitis viruses replicate in hepatocytes, and some of them also replicate in extrahepatic tissues. Detection of their specific nucleotide sequences and proteins and the antibodies produced by the host forms the basis of serologic diagnosis of acute and chronic infection with each hepatitis virus. This is summarized in Table 6–2. Mutations can modify the viral genes, change the antigenicity of the viral proteins, and cause difficulties in serologic diagnosis. Mutations are particularly common in chronic infection where mixtures of

Table 6–1 Characteristics of the Hepatitis Viruses, Modes of Transmission, Incubation Period, and Chronicity

Virus	Nucleic Acid and (n) of Nucleotides	Size of Virions (nm)	Envelope	Taxonomy a. Family b. Genus	Serotypes and Genotypes	Transmission	Incubation Period	Chronicity
HAV	ss RNA, positive polarity (7470)	27–28	No	a. Picornaviridae b. Hepatovirus, distinct from the enteroviruses	One with multiple genotypes	Fecal-oral: water, food, contact	4 weeks (2–7)	No
HEV	ss RNA, positive polarity (7500)	32 (27–34)	No	a. Caliciviridae b. Alpha-like super group of (+) RNA viruses	One with genetic heterogeneity	Fecal-oral: water, food, contact	6 weeks (2–9)	No
HBV	ds DNA (3200)	42	Yes	a. Hepadnaviridae b. Type I, orthohepadnavirus	Multiple	Parenteral (apparent or inapparent) including sexual contact	10 weeks (4 weeks to 6 months)	Yes
HDV	ss RNA, negative polarity (1768)	37 (36–38)	Yes provided by HBV	a. Deltaviridae (satellite viruses) b. Deltavirus	One with multiple genotypes	Parenteral similar to HBV	Similar to HBV (3 weeks to 5 months)	Yes
HCV	ss RNA, positive polarity (9400)	32	Yes	a. Flaviviridae but distantly related to flaviviruses and pestiviruses b. Hepacivirus	Six major genotypes and more than 80 subtypes	Parenteral and community	5 weeks (3–12)	Yes
Non–A-E	?	?	?	Flaviviridae? Other?	?	Parenteral and community	?	Yes

viral strains, referred to as quasi species, can be detected. Viral mutations bear important clinical implications not only in diagnosis but also in pathogenesis; severity and outcome of infection; evolution to chronicity and even response to treatment with antiviral agents; immunoglobulins; and interferons. Examples of clinically relevant viral mutations are represented by the precore HBV mutants that prevent formation and secretion of the hepatitis B e antigen (HBeAg), by the surface HBV mutants selected under immune pressure to the envelope epitopes of HBsAg, and by genotype III of HDV associated with a most severe form of liver necroinflammation.

The serologic diagnosis of viral hepatitis is further discussed together with the clinical features of acute and chronic infection caused by each of the five hepatitis viruses. The serologic profile of each virologic type in the course of the infection is shown schematically in Figures 6–1 to 6–6. In the case of HBV infection (see Table 6–2 and Fig. 6–3), the serologic profile seems complex because HBV components are rather numerous. These are shown schematically in Figure 6–7 in which their expression in the serum and liver is also summarized. Detection of these components in the liver by immunohistochemical and molecular biologic techniques can further facilitate diagnosis.

EPIDEMIOLOGY

Viral hepatitis is one of the most important infectious diseases worldwide. In the United States, it has ranked as the third most frequently reported infectious disease.

The five hepatitis viruses account for more than 95% of the acute viral hepatitis cases worldwide and for approxi-

Table 6–2   Serologic Diagnosis of Viral Hepatitis

Etiology	Serologic Marker	Term	Interpretation
HAV	Antibody to HAV class IgG	anti-HAV IgG	Current or past HAV infection; indicates immunity
	Antibody to HAV class IgM	anti-HAV IgM	Current, recent, or convalescent HAV infection
HBV	Hepatitis B surface antigen	HBsAg	Detectable in most patients with acute and chronic infection
	Hepatitis B e antigen	HBeAg	Transiently positive in acute or chronic wild type viral infection indicating high HBV replication and infectivity
	Antibody to HBeAg	anti-HBe	Becomes positive during convalescence and after HBeAg seroconversion
	Antibody to hepatitis core antigen	anti-HBc	Positive in chronic infection with negative or low level viremia. Positive in infection with precore HBV mutants regardless of HBV replicative level
	Class IgG	anti-HBc IgG	Positive in any HBV infection, acute, convalescence, past or chronic
	Class IgM	anti-HBc IgM	Reflects immune response to replicating virus. High levels in acute and fulminant hepatitis, in HBV reactivation, and in chronic hepatitis B with replicating virus (HBeAg minus or plus)
	Antibody to HBsAg	anti-HBs	Positive in convalescence of acute infection, in a previous infection and after HBV vaccination; protective
HCV	Antibody to hepatitis C virus (to structural and nonstructural cloned epitopes of HCV)	anti-HCV	Becomes positive 5–6 weeks after clinical onset, not protective. Most anti-HCV(+) patients are also positive for HCV-RNA
HDV	Antibody to hepatitis delta antigen	anti-HDV	Indicates current or past HDV infection. High titers of the IgG type and the detectable IgM type indicate active HDV replication
HEV	Antibody to hepatitis E antigen	anti-HEV	Indicates current or past HEV infection. Anti-HEV of IgM type indicates current or recent infection

Detection of viral nucleic acids indicates viremia.

mately 80% of the chronic hepatitis ones. Non–A-E agents are thought to be implicated in the etiology of the remainder as well as that of cryptogenic cirrhosis and probably hepatocellular carcinoma.

Prevalence and endemicity rates differ significantly among the five types of viral hepatitis, not only geographically but also by socioeconomic level, age, sex, and several other host and environmental factors.

Currently, approximately half (48%) of the cases of acute hepatitis in adults reported in the United States are caused by HAV, one third (34%) by HBV including HDV (2%), one sixth (15%) by HCV, and the remaining 3% to HEV and to unknown non–A-E viruses. These relative frequencies vary significantly geographically. Among children with viral hepatitis, different proportions of the five types are also encountered with hepatitis A being the most frequent. A significant decrease in HBV and HDV etiology has been observed in several countries, particularly in the Mediterranean area and in Japan. A decrease in the overall prevalence of hepatitis A has also been observed worldwide, mainly among industrialized and developing areas, resulting in its relative decrease among children and relative increase among adults because of lack of protective antibodies.

Hepatitis A: The frequency and endemicity level of hepatitis A ranges worldwide from low or very low to intermediate and high, depending on overall and age-related expo-

sure rates to HAV, which are reflected by seroprevalence rates of IgG anti-HAV. In general, disease patterns differ and correlate with prevailing sanitary conditions. In developing countries with low socioeconomic levels, the prevalence of anti-HAV of IgG class (previous infection) is approximately 100% already from the age of 5 years or soon thereafter. By contrast, in developed countries with high socioeconomic levels, the age-related anti-HAV seroprevalence rates increase slowly over the years and reach, at maximum, levels of 20% to 30% among the older age groups. In the United States, HAV endemicity is closer to the intermediate rather than the low endemicity pattern; foci of high endemicity and small outbreaks are observed occasionally throughout the country.

Improvement of socioeconomic and sanitary conditions and probably a decline in family size appear to account for the declining frequency of HAV infection worldwide. Longitudinal studies of anti-HAV seroprevalence in Greece and other Mediterranean countries have shown impressive changes in the HAV endemicity pattern moving from the high or intermediate to the low and very low ones. North Africa, South America, India, and China still represent areas of high HAV endemicity. Large epidemics of hepatitis A may occur when the number of susceptible individuals is high and wide exposure to contaminated water or food occurs, such as in Shanghai, where the ingestion of contaminated clams resulted in 300,000 affected individuals. Spo-

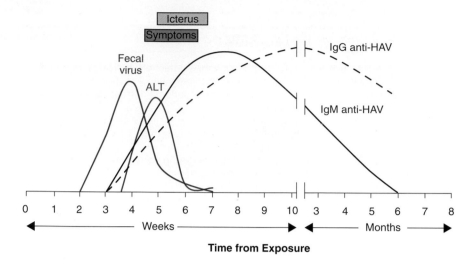

Figure 6–1
Sequence of events in acute hepatitis A. Fecal excretion of HAV occurs not only during the incubation period but also during the acute icteric phase. Transient viremia can also be detected.

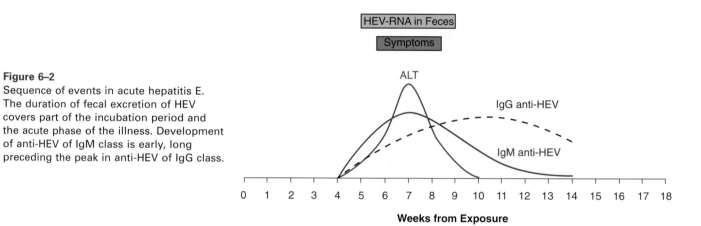

Figure 6–2
Sequence of events in acute hepatitis E. The duration of fecal excretion of HEV covers part of the incubation period and the acute phase of the illness. Development of anti-HEV of IgM class is early, long preceding the peak in anti-HEV of IgG class.

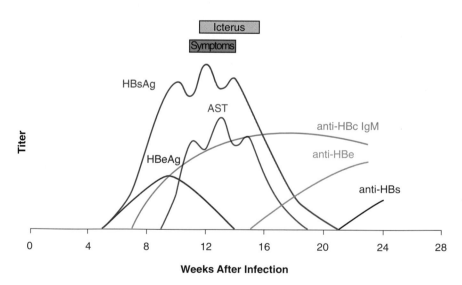

Figure 6–3
Sequence of events and course of hepatitis in acute HBV infection with complete recovery. The appearance of HBsAg precedes the development of anti-HBc. Viremia can be detected from the incubation period, lasts during the acute phase, and clears several weeks later. Anti-HBs usually develops after clearance of HBsAg.

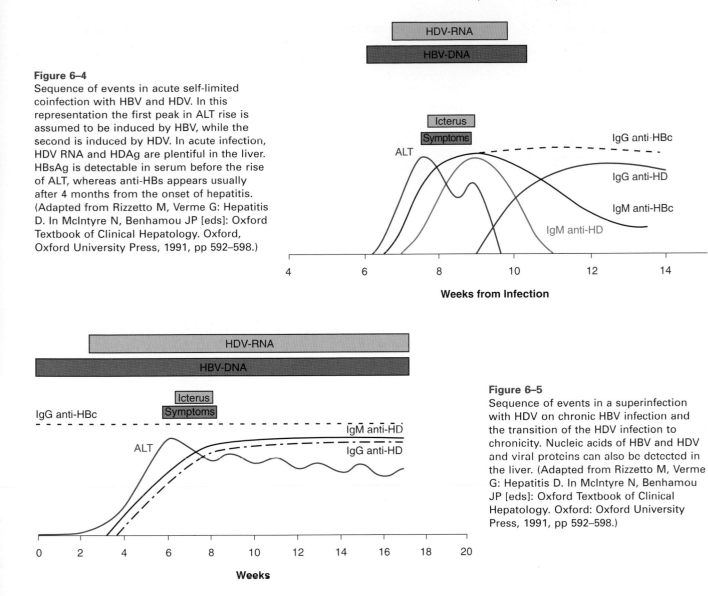

Figure 6–4
Sequence of events in acute self-limited coinfection with HBV and HDV. In this representation the first peak in ALT rise is assumed to be induced by HBV, while the second is induced by HDV. In acute infection, HDV RNA and HDAg are plentiful in the liver. HBsAg is detectable in serum before the rise of ALT, whereas anti-HBs appears usually after 4 months from the onset of hepatitis. (Adapted from Rizzetto M, Verme G: Hepatitis D. In McIntyre N, Benhamou JP [eds]: Oxford Textbook of Clinical Hepatology. Oxford, Oxford University Press, 1991, pp 592–598.)

Figure 6–5
Sequence of events in a superinfection with HDV on chronic HBV infection and the transition of the HDV infection to chronicity. Nucleic acids of HBV and HDV and viral proteins can also be detected in the liver. (Adapted from Rizzetto M, Verme G: Hepatitis D. In McIntyre N, Benhamou JP [eds]: Oxford Textbook of Clinical Hepatology. Oxford: Oxford University Press, 1991, pp 592–598.)

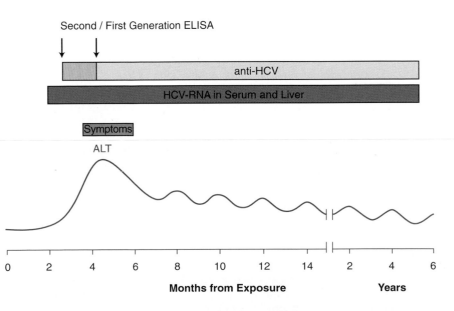

Figure 6–6
Sequence of events in acute HCV infection with a transition to chronicity. HCV RNA first appears in the liver and then in the serum, whereas antibodies to HCV proteins c22-3 and c33c can be detected by second-generation ELISA several weeks later. Antibodies to NS5 and c100-3, detectable by first-generation ELISA, appear much later on, sometimes after 3 or 4 months.

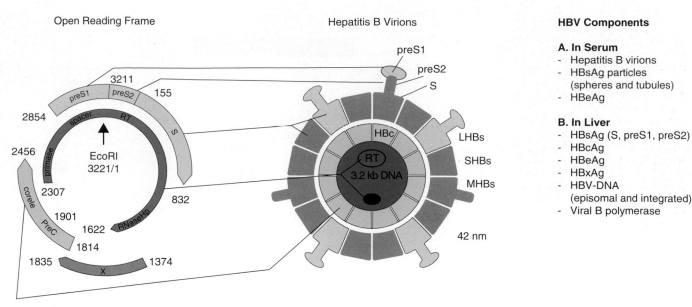

Figure 6–7
Schematic representation of the HBV gene products at the level of their open reading frames with configuration of their location within HBV particles. Circulating HBV components consist of hepatitis B virions and free HBsAg particles, which consist of pre-S1 and pre-S2 peptides, and secreted HBeAg, which contains precore/core sequences. HBV components in the liver comprise all HBV-encoded proteins as well as free and integrated HBV DNA.

radic cases of viral hepatitis A are usually attributable to the spread of HAV by direct person-to-person contact. An increased incidence of hepatitis has been observed among promiscuous homosexuals. Spread of HAV in day-care centers may involve not only children but also the staff and the families of affected children. Parenteral transmission of HAV may occur rarely and has been documented in transfusion-associated outbreaks in neonatal intensive care units (ICUs) and in hemophiliacs linked to the administration of factor VIII concentrates.

The reservoir of the HAV responsible for spread of the infection consists of clinically inapparent acute cases at the time of viral shedding. Fecal shedding occurs for 4 weeks or more. It starts from the last 2 weeks of the incubation period and ends later in the course of the disease, but not with the onset of the acute phase as was thought previously (see Fig. 6–1). A short-duration viremia also occurs during the same period and may account for the rare parenterally transmitted cases.

Hepatitis E: Hepatitis E occurs in epidemics in areas with very poor sanitary conditions such as refugee camps in developing countries (e.g., Sudan, Somalia, Libya, and Kenya). Large outbreaks have been reported in several parts of the world, including India, Pakistan, the former Soviet Union, China, southern Asia, Burma, Indonesia, Mexico, and many African countries. The disease is also endemic in certain areas where sporadic transmission occurs mainly among children (e.g., Egypt and Sudan). In the United States and Canada, all reported cases have been encountered among travelers to areas of HEV endemicity, and there has been no secondary transmission.

The virus is transmitted almost exclusively by the fecal-oral route. The source of infection is usually contaminated water, and epidemics are frequently observed after the rainy season. The secondary attack rate among exposed household contacts is low. In the described outbreaks, the highest attack rate was observed among individuals between 15 and 40 years of age and was probably caused by a loss of anti-HEV, permitting reinfection with a high fatality rate (20%) among infected pregnant women.

Hepatitis B: Infection with the hepatitis B virus occurs worldwide and is particularly common in heavily populated areas. HBV endemicity has been grouped on the basis of the frequency of chronic infection in the general population on three levels: below 2% (low); 2% to 7% (intermediate); and above 7% (high). In the high incidence areas, most of the population is seropositive for markers of HBV infection by the end of the first decade. Maternal-neonatal transmission and horizontal child-to-child transmission play the major role in the spread of HBV in these populations. In the intermediate prevalence areas, the peak of infection is observed much later with almost half of the population becoming seropositive by 25 to 30 years of age. Sexual contact seems to play a very important role in transmission in these areas. Finally, in the low HBV incidence areas, less than 10% of the general population becomes exposed to HBV by various mechanisms, usually related to high-risk behavior for parenteral viral transmission. It is estimated that worldwide billions of persons alive today have been infected with HBV and that approximately 350 million persons are chronic carriers of the virus. These chronically infected individuals represent the reservoir of HBV in nature, the source of new infection to others and the population at risk for development of severe chronic liver disease, including hepatocellular carcinoma. Hepatitis B is by far the most common type of acute viral hepatitis in adults in most parts of the world. In the

United States, the age groups that are predominantly affected are those between 15 and 40 years of age, indicating the importance of sexual transmission. The estimated annual number of new infections was higher than 200,000 up to the middle 1980s; the number of infections has decreased since then by approximately 50%. A significant decrease in the frequency of acute hepatitis B and the prevalence of chronic HBV infection has also been documented in Europe, particularly in the Mediterranean area as well as in Japan. The decreasing HBV prevalence has been attributed to improved socioeconomic level and hygiene conditions, to wide introduction of disposable needles and syringes, to behavioral changes among injection drug users and homosexual men, and in more recent years to hepatitis B vaccination.

The HBV is transmitted parenterally requiring either overt inoculation as in the case of blood transfusion and injection drug users or by inapparent modes of transdermal and transmucosal inoculation via intimate personal and sexual contact or through mother-infant transmission. HBV carriers with high levels of viremia, usually positive for HBeAg, are particularly contagious and readily transmit infection to others by such inapparent parenteral mechanisms. In horizontal and contact transmission, which are frequent in sub-Saharan Africa, a significant role may be played by eczematous, abrasive, and other skin lesions, scarification, and human or possibly even insect bites. The HBV infection has been found to be high in certain groups of individuals who are frequently exposed to procedures involving blood or blood products. These groups include health care workers, drug users who share needles and syringes, multiply transfused patients, hemophiliacs, hemodialysis patients, sexually promiscuous persons, and others. In a surveillance system operated by the Centers for Disease Control and Prevention (CDC) in four American counties, the most frequent risk factors were found to be heterosexual exposure to a contact with hepatitis (41%) or to multiple partners followed by injection drug use (15%) and homosexual activity (9%) (Fig. 6–8). In approximately one third of patients, no risk factor could be identified. These surveillance data do not include perinatal infection and hepatitis in young children, because acute infection among young children is usu-

ally asymptomatic. On the other hand, whereas the vast majority of HBV infection in adults is self-limited, HBV infection in early life often results in chronicity.

Hepatitis D: HDV infection occurs worldwide. High HDV prevalence areas with endemic hepatitis D have been identified in the Mediterranean basin, Eastern Europe, the Amazon territory, and parts of Africa. Epidemics may also follow the introduction of HDV in susceptible populations. A composite epidemiologic pattern has also been observed.

Although HDV is a virus satellite to HBV and modes of HDV transmission are similar to those of its helper virus, the frequency of hepatitis D does not parallel that of hepatitis B. Groups at high risk for HDV infection are injection drug abusers, sexual and other close contacts of individuals with HDV infection, and persons with chronic HBV infection who are exposed to parenteral procedures. The highest rates of HDV infection among HBsAg carriers have been detected in hemophiliacs and drug abusers (approximately 40%) and also in prisoners, dialysis patients, and homosexual men (18% to 20%).

HDV infection can be acquired either as a primary coinfection with HBV through inoculation of contagious blood or its products containing both viruses or as a superinfection by introduction of HDV into a person with a pre-existing chronic HBV infection. A third pattern has been observed in liver transplantation in which HDV infection and expression in the liver have been documented in the absence of detectable recurrence and expression of HBV.

Hepatitis C: Like the other hepatitis viruses, HCV is also distributed worldwide. In the early days of HCV testing, the prevalence of HCV infection was seriously underestimated being based mainly on data from volunteer blood donors who were not representative of the situation in the general population. Donors are highly selected groups that are screened for risk factors and serologic markers associated with a variety of infectious diseases. It is now appreciated that the frequency of HCV infection in the general population is several times higher than among blood donors. For example, although the prevalence of anti-HCV among blood donors in North America and Western Europe is approxi-

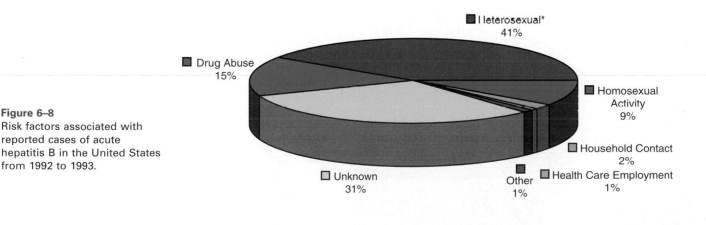

Figure 6–8
Risk factors associated with reported cases of acute hepatitis B in the United States from 1992 to 1993.

*Includes sexual contact with acute cases, carriers, and multiple partners
Source: Sentinel Counties, Centers for Disease Control and Prevention

mately 0.3%, its frequency in the general population of the United States has been found to be 1.8%, corresponding to a reservoir of about 4 million HCV-infected persons nationwide. Similar observations have been made in Europe. In selected populations from Africa, the Middle East, and the Mediterranean basin, prevalence rates of anti-HCV range from 4% to 12%, 4 to 10 times higher than among blood donors. In Greece, although the prevalence of anti-HCV among volunteer blood donors is 0.22%, ranging from 0.09% to 0.52%, its frequency in the general population ranges from 0.7% to 7.9% and is 3 to 30 times higher with a clear-cut age-dependent pattern of distribution.

HCV endemicity is generally higher in developing countries with low socioeconomic level compared with developed high, socioeconomic status communities as occurs with most other hepatitis viruses. The modes of HCV spread in the general population remain largely unknown. HCV is transmitted most efficiently by direct percutaneous exposure to blood and its products as by transfusion, transplantation of organs and tissues, and sharing of contaminated needles and syringes among injection drug users. Heavily transfused hemophiliacs and patients with thalassemia as well as injection drug users with many years of drug abuse have extremely high anti-HCV prevalence rates that may exceed 90%. In hemodialysis patients, the overall prevalence of anti-HCV is approximately 20%, ranging widely according to geographic location and the diagnostic methods used. However, the prevalence of HCV infection appears to decline in recent years.

Parenteral modes of viral inoculation prevailing among health care workers, sexual partners, and in mother-to-infant viral spread are not very efficient in HCV transmission, most probably because of rather low titers of HCV viremia. However, because of the large number of individuals with chronic HCV worldwide, such modes of HCV spread may be extremely important in the expansion of the viral pool in the community, with multiple possibilities for further transmission.

In the Sentinel Counties Study during 1990 to 1993, 36% of patients with acute hepatitis C had household contact with hepatitis or multiple sexual partners; 5% had a history of blood transfusion; 3% were health care workers; and 1%

were dialysis patients (Fig. 6–9). However, 40% to 50% of patients with hepatitis C have no identifiable parenteral risk factors. In these sporadic cases, the source of HCV infection and the modes of its transmission remain unknown, although low socioeconomic status is strongly associated. Arthropod-borne transmission has been hypothesized because HCV has structural similarities with the flaviviruses, but this is rather unlikely given the clustering of multiple viral subtypes within distinct age groups in similar geographic locations.

A recent event in the epidemiology of hepatitis C is the association of the infection with receipt of intravenous immune globulin. The Food and Drug Administration (FDA) of the United States now requires that all immune globulin products manufactured through a process that does not include a viral inactivation step be tested for HCV RNA.

Although infection with HCV is common worldwide, the frequency of transfusion associated hepatitis C is declining as a consequence of changing donor criteria connected with concerns about HIV contamination of the blood supply and the application of surrogate testing for ALT and anti-HBc and finally with the introduction of specific testing for anti-HCV. The risk has been reduced from 3.8% to 1.5% and with anti-HCV testing to 0.5% per patient or from 0.4% to 0.2% and then to 0.03% per unit of transfused blood. With second-generation anti-HCV assays, the risk has been further reduced. Thus, transfusion-associated transmission currently accounts for a negligible proportion of new HCV infections.

Hepatitis non–A-E: Approximately 4% of the acute hepatitis cases in the United States are negative for markers of any of the characterized hepatitis viruses. The prevalence of non–A-E agents seems to vary geographically, with socioeconomic factors and modes of viral transmission. In the post-transfusion setting, non–A-E agents appear to account currently for very few if any cases of hepatitis, whereas in community acquired hepatitis, non–A-E agents may be responsible for between 20% and 50% of cases. In fulminant hepatitis, non–A-E cases currently comprise the largest group worldwide. Finally, non–A-E agents may be implicated in the etiology of significant proportions of patients

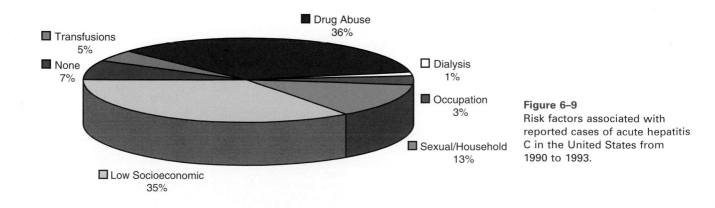

Figure 6–9
Risk factors associated with reported cases of acute hepatitis C in the United States from 1990 to 1993.

Source: Sentinel Counties, Centers for Disease Control and Prevention

with chronic hepatitis and cryptogenic liver disease. In recent studies of the possible role of the new flavivirus G/GBV-C, large series of patients with chronic liver disease of non–A-E etiology were reported from most parts of the world.

Table 6–3 summarizes the epidemiologic features and clinical aspects of the five established types of viral hepatitis and of the tentative non–A-E form.

PATHOPHYSIOLOGY

The process of initiating a hepatitis infection depends on the attachment of virus to hepatocytes, penetration through the cellular membrane into the cytoplasm, and uncoating. Attachment to hepatocytes depends on specific proteins of the virus, expressed on its surface, that bind to cellular receptors on the membrane of hepatocytes. The precise viral peptides that are involved in the binding of hepatitis viruses are not well defined, and cellular receptors are also largely unknown. Pre-S1 encoded polypeptides have been implicated in the binding of HBV to liver cells. Binding is ion and temperature dependent. Cells that lack viral receptors do not permit viral entrance but may be permissive to viral replication after transfection of viral nucleic acids.

After viral attachment, penetration occurs almost instantaneously via translocation across the plasma membranes or by endocytosis into cytoplasmic vacuoles. These mechanisms operate in the case of the nonenveloped viruses HAV and HEV, whereas a third mechanism of fusion is usually involved in enveloped viruses. In fusion, the viral envelope is retained within the plasma membrane and the nucleocapsid is transported into the cytoplasm. Virions in the cytoplasm become uncoated from their capsids, and their nucleic acids are expressed. In the case of HBV, the capsids traverse the cytoplasm to the nuclear membrane, and viral DNA is translocated into the nucleus. In the case of HAV, HBV and HDV viral assembly and maturation occur in the cytoplasm. For the exit of hepatitis viruses from hepatocytes, either cell lysis or secretion without cell destruction may occur; however, the exact molecular events and pathways in viral secretion are unknown. Extrusion of hepatitis viruses across the plasma membranes seems to be the preferred mode of release. However, insertion of the viral specific glycoproteins into the surface of hepatocytes provides an opportunity for easier cell destruction by host immune mechanisms.

In HBV, HDV and HCV infection transition to chronicity can be initiated and maintained through regulation of their lytic potential and evasion of the immunologic host surveillance to escape detection and elimination by the host. Downregulation of MHC expression, antibody-induced modulation of viral antigens on infected hepatocytes, nonneutralizing antibodies blocking the neutralizing ones, antigenic expression, and restricted expression of viral genes are among the possible mechanisms used by hepatitis viruses to evade immune clearance.

PATHOGENESIS

General Aspects: Infection with the hepatitis viruses is associated with inflammation and necrosis in the liver. However, none of the hepatitis viruses appears to be cytopathic to liver cells. The exact mechanisms involved in liver necroinflammation are not completely understood, but host immunologic reactions against the hepatitis viruses replicating in hepatocytes are thought to play a role in all forms of the disease.

In acute hepatitis, a multiclonal and multispecific host immune response involving several mechanisms is implicated and is responsible for viral clearance and liver cell injury. It involves rapid and nonspecific mechanisms such as interferon, antibody-dependent cell-mediated cytotoxicity (ADCC), natural killer (NK) cells, and complement lysis as well as virus-specific B and T cell responses that are relatively slow in their development. An extremely strong immune response probably related to viral factors and particularly to host genetic factors may result in rapid clearance of the infecting virus but also to massive hepatic necrosis causing fulminant hepatic failure. In general, the more active the host immune response, the greater will be the hepatic injury. On the other hand, a nonefficient immune response during the acute phase of the infection is associated both with mild or no hepatitis and, in the case of HBV and HCV infection, with frequent transition to chronicity.

In chronic viral hepatitis, immunologic responses are again pathogenetically responsible for the development of hepatic damage. They are linked to several host factors and are directed to viral components expressed in hepatocytes. They cause hepatic injury but rarely are multiclonal and multispecific to permit viral eradication with termination of chronic infection. In their absence, hepatocellular damage is either not existent or minor. However, cellular injury may eventually occur as a result of oncogenesis induced by oncogenes or inactivation of tumor suppression genes and from integration of the viral DNA into the host genome, such as in the case of HBV infection.

Hepatitis A: The HAV appears to be directly cytopathic to hepatocytes. The virus belongs to the Picornaviruses, a family known for its cytopathic properties. An asymptomatic viremic or fecal carrier state does not exist, and hepatitis appears to coincide to some extent with fecal shedding of the virus (see Fig. 6–1). Moreover, in experimental hepatitis in marmosets, the incubation period can be shortened by serial passages to only 7 days, which suggests direct hepatotoxicity. On the other hand, fecal shedding of HAV and transient viremia does occur before any evidence of liver necroinflammation; in cell cultures in which HAV has been propagated, no evidence of cytopathogenicity has been observed. Numerous observations further indicate that pathogenesis of liver damage is also related to immunologic mechanisms. Immune complexes containing antibodies to HAV of IgM and IgG class, viral A components and complement are detectable during the early phases of acute liver injury, and peripheral blood lymphocytes, which are activated against HAV, generate α-interferon and demonstrate HAV-specific cytotoxicity. Moreover, lymphocytes isolated from the liver are capable of destroying HAV-infected skin fibroblasts. The current view, therefore, is that in HAV infection, liver cell necrosis is mediated by HAV-specific, HLA-restricted cytotoxic T lymphocytes.

Hepatitis E: Information on immunopathogenesis of liver damage associated with this viral agent is still limited, but

Table 6–3 Prevalence, Transmission, and Clinical Features of the Five Established Types of Viral Hepatitis and of Possible Hepatitis Non–A-E

Type of Hepatitis	Prevalence	Perinatal Transmission	Sexual Transmission	Onset	Viremia	Massive Hepatic Necrosis	Chronic Infection	Risk for Cirrhosis, Hepatocellular Carcinoma
A	3 levels of endemicity; worldwide decrease; increased frequency in adults	No	No (rare)	Acute	Transient	Rare	No	No
E	Large outbreaks in developing countries; endemic in some areas; rare in USA, Canada, and Europe	No	No	Acute	Transient	Yes (pregnancy)	No	No
B	Worldwide occurrence; 3 levels of endemicity: more than 350 million chronically infected; decreasing prevalence	Yes (common in HBeAg+)	Yes (common)	Insidious and acute	Transient and chronic	Occasional	Yes (mainly in early life)	Yes
D	Worldwide decreasing prevalence; associated with HBV; foci of high endemicity and of severe hepatitis (South America)	Yes (infrequent)	Yes (rare)	Insidious and acute	Transient and chronic	Yes (coinfection)	Yes (mainly superinfection)	Yes
C	Worldwide; probably more than 300 million chronically infected; wide areas of high endemicity (Africa); in USA and Europe, more frequent than B	Yes (infrequent)	Yes (rare)	Insidious (mainly) and acute	Chronic and transient	Very rare	Yes (all ages)	Yes
Non–A-E	Sporadic; varying, probably worldwide	?	?	Insidious and acute	?	Yes	Yes	Yes

most observations are compatible with immunologically induced liver injury rather than with a direct HEV cytopathic
action. As in the case of hepatitis A, data on correlation between serum ALT levels and fecal viral shedding are conflicting. However, in recent studies in cynomolgus macaques and other primates, HEV particles and genomic
sequences of HEV were simultaneously present in stool and
serum before the ALT peak and were concordant with
HEVAg identification in the cytoplasm of hepatocytes. In
serial biopsies from HEV-infected nonhuman primates,
HEVAg was consistently identified prior to the ALT elevation. Small round cells are the predominant component of
the inflammatory infiltrates in the liver in hepatitis E. In areas of hepatocyte dropout, infiltration with lymphocytes and
activated Kupffer cells with direct contact between lymphocytes and hepatocytes was observed in infected cynomolgus
macaques. These observations are again indicative of immunologically mediated liver damage induced by the HEV.

Hepatitis B: HBV is not directly cytopathic to the liver in
humans, experimentally infected chimpanzees, or tissue culture systems. HBsAg-containing hepatocytes show no evidence of damage. When an efficient host immune response
is mounted against HBV, liver cell damage is caused by immune lysis of HBV-infected hepatocytes. The role of
soluble mediators of inflammation is important. Immune
complex–mediated responses are thought to play a pathogenetic role in some of the extrahepatic manifestations of
HBV infection but probably not for the liver changes of
hepatitis. Deposition of immune complexes has been demonstrated in skin, joints, and renal glomeruli, being responsible for the clinical features of urticaria and rashes, polyarthritis, and glomerulonephritis, respectively. When the
serum-sickness–like syndrome is present, then immune
complexes isolated from sera activate both the classic and
alternate complement pathways.

Cell-mediated immune mechanisms against viral B antigens are important for the development of acute hepatic injury and resolution of the infection. Hepatocytes expressing
HBV nucleocapsid antigens presented by HLA class I peptides are recognized by activated CTL (CD8), which are under the control of helper CD4+ lymphocytes (Fig. 6–10).
T helper cells are also important in the B cell immune response against HBV and in releasing cytokines that can sup-
press viral expression. Failure of these mechanisms is associated with tolerance of the virus, persistence of HBV
infection, and lack of eradication of HBV-infected hepatocytes. Chronic liver injury results from immunologic
responses to replicating HBV, regardless of whether it is a
wild type, precore, or core mutant. However, the strength of
the response is not enough to achieve viral clearance. It may
be continuous or intermittent and always follows periods of
HBV replication. Occasionally, a strong immune response is
mounted and HBV can be cleared. Clearance can also occur
subclinically without significant immune lysis of hepatocytes.

The importance of proinflammatory cytokines has been
studied in many ways both clinically and experimentally,
particularly with the transgenic mouse model. Their role in
the pathophysiology of liver cell necrosis and apoptosis and
in the suppression of HBV expression without immune lysis
of infected hepatocytes now seems to be central. A new pos-

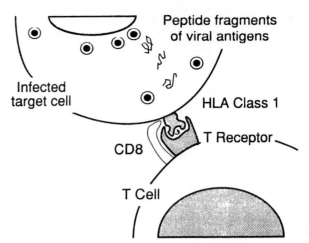

Figure 6–10
Interaction of cytotoxic T cell with hepatitis B viral protein and
HLA class I antigen on an infected hepatocyte. (From
Eddleston ALWF: Overview of HBV pathogenesis. In Hollinger
FB, Lemon SM, Margolis HS [eds]: Viral Hepatitis and Liver
Disease. Baltimore: Williams & Wilkins, 1991, pp 234–237.)

sibility has thus emerged that with appropriate inhibition of
excess cytokine production, survival with fulminant hepatitis B may improve. In chronic HBV infection, potentiation
of the cytokine effect may lead to eradication of the virus. In
this context, the role of individual viral epitopes has been
further elucidated, and the importance not only of core proteins but also of envelope proteins has been better understood.

Hepatitis D: Pathogenesis of hepatitis D is linked to that
of hepatitis B. However, the exact mechanisms of liver cell
injury remain elusive. A direct cytotoxic effect of HDV on
hepatocytes has been postulated on the basis of morphologic
and other observations and has been further supported by
the association of severe forms of hepatitis D with genotype
III in South America. However, several recent data argue
against HDV being intrinsically cytopathic. Liver grafts expressing only HDV without HBV are free of hepatocytic
damage. HDAg-expressing hepatocytes in woodchucks and
humans are rarely injured, and in transgenic mice, liver cells
expressing either the short or long form of HDAg are not
damaged. On the other hand, replication per se of the HDV
genome causes a moderate inhibition of cellular growth, and
it is possible that in acute hepatitis D an excess of the small
HDAg acting as a direct cytotoxic factor may play a major
pathogenetic role. By contrast, in chronic hepatitis D, host
immune reactions associated with the presence of HBV appear to be implicated pathogenetically. However, contrary to
HBV, CTL-mediated lysis of HDV-infected cells does not
seem to represent a major pathogenetic mechanism, but
CD4 helper lymphocytes are involved. The pathogenetic
mechanism in chronic hepatitis D has still to be linked with
the pathogenesis of hepatitis B. The presence of HBV, or at
least of its coat protein, seems to be a prerequisite for hepatocytic damage in chronic hepatitis D. As shown in the liver
transplant model, replicating HDV alone in the absence of
HBsAg is not associated with hepatocytic damage of the
graft, whereas a fully productive HBV infection is associ-

ated not only with enhanced HDV expression but also with a classical necroinflammatory picture of the liver.

Hepatitis C: Pathogenesis of hepatitis C remains poorly understood. There are reasonable analogies with HBV that suggest immune-mediated pathogenesis both in acute and chronic liver cell damage. An asymptomatic HCV carrier state with normal ALT seems to exist. The presence of lymphoid follicles on histopathologic examination of the liver and the occasional presence of cryoglobulins, circulating immune complexes, and autoantibodies argue for an immunologically induced pathogenesis. Cytotoxic T lymphocytes directed against more than one viral epitope have been shown in patients with acute and chronic HCV infection. Th1 reactions have been shown to occur in the liver; Th2 reactions predominate in peripheral blood mononuclear cells. In HCV persistence, antibody escape and CTL escape mutations have been implicated, probably resulting in hepatotropic and hematotropic HCV variants. In chimpanzees, the appearance of HCV RNA in hepatocytes paralleled the elevation of ALT, but no correlation could be demonstrated between hepatocellular necrosis and serum ALT. Furthermore, HCV RNA could not be detected in areas of liver cell necrosis, which clearly suggests that HCV replication and hepatocyte injury are not directly related. On the basis of these findings, it is currently assumed that mechanisms underlying liver cell injury in both acute and chronic HCV infection are probably similar to those in HBV infection. However, the immune response to HCV is usually milder than in HBV infection and rarely causes massive hepatic necrosis. Acute hepatitis C seems to be milder and more frequently asymptomatic than HBV, and transition to chronicity is much more frequent than in HBV.

Pathogenetic mechanisms of hepatocellular carcinoma in chronic HCV infection appear to be related to the development of cirrhosis and to continuous liver cell regeneration, which compensates the continuous loss of hepatocytes caused by the necroinflammatory process of chronic hepatitis C.

HISTOPATHOLOGY

Histopathologic features of viral hepatitis are described in detail in other chapters. In general, liver biopsy is not indicated in ordinary acute hepatitis; however, in difficult cases, liver histology may be helpful in establishing the diagnosis, in differentiating between acute and chronic disease, in obtaining clues to etiology, in determining the prognosis, and in therapeutic decision making.

Microscopic changes have been described extensively in the literature and can be grouped into: (1) cell death, (2) mesenchymal reactions, (3) cell regeneration, (4) inflammation, (5) changes in lobular architecture, and (6) fibrosis-cirrhosis. Apoptosis, which is frequently seen in viral hepatitis in the form of so-called acidophilic, councilman, and apoptotic bodies, has attracted renewed interest following the discovery of the mechanisms of programmed cell death involved in this form of cell necrosis. However, it is observed not only in acute but also in chronic viral hepatitis, and it is not restricted only to liver diseases of viral etiology. The type, location, and severity of hepatocellular necrosis and inflammation such as in-

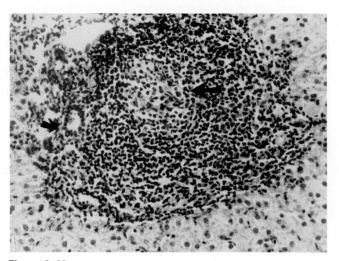

Figure 6–11
Hepatitis C with prominent portal changes. Heavy lymphoid infiltration of the portal tract, follicle formation with a germinal center *(big arrow)*, and bile duct damage *(curved arrow)*. Periportal necroinflammation is also obvious (H & E ×400).

tralobular, piecemeal, bridging has gained clinical importance particularly in terms of prognosis, and a histologic activity index (HAI) of necroinflammation is now widely applied in clinical studies, particularly of protracted acute and chronic viral hepatitis.

Histopathologic changes of bile ducts have also gained significance in the etiology and differential diagnosis of viral hepatitis, whereas liver immunohistochemistry can permit differentiation between acute and chronic hepatitis B and may be the only means to establish the diagnosis of HBV reactivation on the grounds of chronic HBV infection.

Figures 6–11 and 6–12 are examples of the diagnostic value of liver histology and immunohistochemistry in viral hepatitis C and B, respectively.

CLINICAL FEATURES OF ACUTE VIRAL HEPATITIS

Acute viral hepatitis produces a spectrum of clinical features and laboratory manifestations.

General Clinical Features

Acute viral hepatitis may be asymptomatic, marked only by increased aminotransferase levels, symptomatic but anicteric, icteric, subfulminant, or fulminant. Different types of illness (e.g., protracted, relapsing, cholestatic) and several extrahepatic manifestations are caused by the various hepatitis viruses.

Asymptomatic Hepatitis: This is also referred to as inapparent hepatitis, a term used to indicate that the infection with the hepatitis virus has not produced any symptoms. It is diagnosed by a rise in serum aminotransferase levels and the detection of serologic markers of acute viral infection, usually among individuals monitored because of viral exposure. Although such patients are also anicteric, the term an-

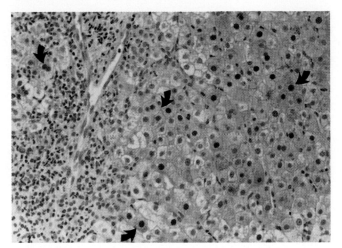

Figure 6–12
Immunohistochemical peroxidase staining of HBcAg in a case of viral hepatitis B. Liver necroinflammation is quite severe and associated with abundant cytoplasmic and nuclear expression of HBcAg *(arrows)* in numerous hepatocytes (×320).

icteric hepatitis should be reserved only for cases of symptomatic hepatitis without jaundice.

Acute infection with the hepatitis viruses may be not only asymptomatic but may also result in minimal biochemical changes and may only be detected by serologic evidence. This is probably the case of viral infection with HBV in neonates with complete tolerance of the virus and transition of the infection to chronicity.

It is a general rule that the younger the age of the patient, the milder will be the clinical form of hepatitis. Asymptomatic infections are usually more frequent than are symptomatic ones. For every icteric patient, 10 to 30 anicteric or completely asymptomatic cases may occur. Asymptomatic HBV infections have been detected in up to 90% of Eskimo children younger than 4 years of age but have only been found in two thirds of adults older than 30 years.

Symptomatic Hepatitis: Some clinical features are common to all types of acute viral hepatitis. The earliest symptoms are nonspecific (predominantly constitutional and gastrointestinal) and include malaise, fatigue, anorexia, nausea, vomiting, abdominal discomfort, and occasionally aching in the right upper abdomen or joint pains. To both patients and physicians, these symptoms may suggest influenza or an upper respiratory or gastrointestinal syndrome. The patient may also complain of loss of taste for coffee or the desire to smoke or drink alcohol. Low-grade fever is frequently present, but rigors are uncommon. In some patients, malaise is profound and increases in the evening. Occasionally, severe headache is also manifested. If the patient continues to remain anicteric, his condition usually also remains undiagnosed, unless there is a clear-cut history of exposure to hepatitis or recent transfusion of blood or its products.

The prodromal symptoms last for 3 or 4 days or even up to 2 to 3 weeks and may be followed by an icteric phase of varying severity, ranging from quick recovery in a few days or weeks to severe acute, subfulminant, and fatal fulminant

hepatitis. The earlier clinical manifestation is darkening of the urine, which is caused by bilirubinuria from rising concentrations of conjugated serum bilirubin. It is followed by stool discoloration and jaundice, which is first identified in the sclerae and then by yellow pigmentation of the skin. The person's temperature returns to normal, and he or she may have bradycardia. The person's appetite returns, and vomiting and abdominal discomfort abate.

Pruritus may appear transiently for a few days but may occasionally be protracted with cholestatic features that last for 8 to 29 weeks. This is particularly true for hepatitis A and poses several problems of differential diagnosis. On clinical examination, the liver is palpable with a smooth tender edge in more than two thirds of the patients, and slight splenomegaly occurs in about 10% to 15%. Most patients remain anicteric or develop very mild jaundice, this being particularly true for children especially with hepatitis A. Spider nevi may appear transiently, but their presence is more compatible with severe exacerbation of chronic hepatitis mimicking acute rather than with a frank episode of acute self-limited hepatitis.

The usual adult patient with acute viral hepatitis loses approximately 3 to 4 kg of body weight and makes an uneventful recovery. Fatigue may persist after apparent recovery for some weeks, and complete clinical and biochemical recovery usually occur within 6 months from the onset. Chronic hepatitis may follow acute hepatitis B, D particularly in infants and children, and hepatitis C in all ages. This unfavorable course is rare among nonimmunosuppressed adults with icteric hepatitis B.

A relapsing course has been observed in 2% to 15% of cases. This is characterized by duplication of the original attack, which is usually milder and may even be subclinical, identifiable only by a relapse in aminotransferase levels. Recovery may be complete as in hepatitis A, but relapses in hepatitis B and C also suggest a progression to chronicity.

In cases with a fulminant course, the patient is overwhelmed in less than 10 days from clinical onset. Jaundice becomes deep; fever may persist; there is repeated vomiting, confusion, drowsiness, fetor hepaticus with development of coma; and the full-blown picture of liver failure. The liver decreases in size, and clinical features of hemorrhagic diathesis develop. Currently, the major subset of fulminant viral hepatitis consists of non–A-E cases.

Extrahepatic Manifestations: Extrahepatic manifestations represent a clinically important aspect both of acute and chronic viral hepatitis. They include neurologic, hematologic, dermatologic, rheumatologic, genital tract, renal, pancreatic, gastrointestinal, and cardiopulmonary abnormalities. The serum sickness–like syndrome, which includes joint manifestations, skin rashes, polyarteritis nodosa, glomerulonephritis, mixed cryoglobulinemia, and papular acrodermatitis, are believed to be mediated by circulating immune complexes.

Neurologic Manifestations: Aseptic meningitis, meningoencephalomyelitis, or myelitis may occur rarely in viral hepatitis. However, a frequent headache may occasionally become severe and in children, it may be mistaken for meningitis when associated with neck stiffness.

The Guillain-Barré syndrome has been reported in association with viral hepatitis A, B, and C with recovery within 2 to 6 months from onset. Residual symptoms such as facial palsy, ataxia, or lack of reflexes have been described. Mononcuritis of various nerves, cranial and peripheral, has been observed in acute hepatitis but mainly in chronic viral hepatitis. It appears to be linked with polyarteritis and cryoglobulinemia related to HBV and HCV infections.

Hematologic Manifestations: A transient hematologic change, such as a decrease in hemoglobin and platelet count, is common in acute viral hepatitis. Cases of aplastic anemia have been reported in association with all types of acute viral hepatitis but mainly with hepatitis non–A-E. It is primarily a disorder of younger persons (median age of 18 years). Aplasia usually affects all three cell lineages, but pure red blood cell aplasia and agranulocytosis may also occur. The pathogenesis is unknown, and the mortality rate is high.

Immune thrombocytopenia has been seen in association with viral hepatitis, mainly hepatitis A, but is also included in the extrahepatic syndromes related to chronic viral hepatitis (mainly type C) (Table 6–4).

Dermatologic Manifestations: In addition to the described serum-sickness–like erythematosus and urticarial skin rashes, there are other rare dermatologic complications including Raynaud's phenomena, dermatomyositis-like syndrome, Henoch-Schonlein purpura, and papular acrodermatitis (Gianotti-Crosti syndrome) in children, mainly but not exclusively, with acute hepatitis B.

Other: They include proteinuria, membranous glomerulonephritis, and several cardiopulmonary and gastrointestinal disorders that may either represent manifestations of underlying vasculitis and cryoglobulinemia (e.g., glomerulonephritis and ischemic vasculitis) linked to viral hepatitis or complications of severe and fulminant forms of hepatitis (pancreatitis, cardiac arrhythmias, and pulmonary edema).

GENERAL LABORATORY FEATURES AND DIAGNOSIS

Biochemical changes provide evidence for the diagnosis of acute viral hepatitis, as well as for the assessment of its severity, but should be interpreted in conjunction with clinical and other laboratory findings.

Serum aspartate (AST) and alanine aminotransferase (ALT) levels increase prominently both in the icteric and anicteric patient already from the presymptomatic phase. By the time that acute hepatitis has become clinically manifest, peak AST and ALT have usually been reached and enzyme levels plateau or start to decline. Values above 1000 or 2000 U/L or even higher are usual. A higher than 10-fold ALT increase (>400 U/L) strongly suggests acute hepatitis. However, other hepatobiliary disorders such as shock liver, chronic active hepatitis, or occasionally acute biliary obstruction may also be associated with greatly increased aminotransferase levels. Consequently, the diagnosis of acute hepatitis should not be made only on the basis of AST and ALT values.

Bilirubin increases to a variable extent. Bilirubinuria appears before the serum bilirubin increases and may also be noted in the anicteric patient.

Serum alkaline phosphatase is only mildly elevated or normal, except in the cholestatic forms of viral hepatitis. Serum levels of albumin, prothrombin, and other proteins synthesized in the liver decrease significantly in the severe, subfulminant, and fulminant but not in the ordinary forms of the disease. Immunoglobulin changes are not diagnostic; serum complement levels may be low initially, and occasionally a patient can develop cryoglobulinemia. Specific immune responses to the infecting hepatitis viruses together with the detection of their viral proteins and nucleic acids form the current basis for the diagnosis and etiologic classification of acute and chronic viral hepatitis. These are summarized in Table 6–2 and shown schematically in Figures 6–1 to 6–6.

Hematologic changes are also frequent in acute viral hepatitis. The erythrocyte sedimentation rate is usually high in the presymptomatic phase but returns to normal with the appearance of jaundice. Hematopenia with atypical lymphocytes resembling those of infectious mononucleosis and with subsequent relative lymphocytosis is frequent. Red

Table 6–4 Nonhepatic Manifestations in Hepatitis C Virus Infection

Endocrine	Hyperthyroidism
	Hypothyroidism
	Hashimoto's disease
	Thyroid autoantibodies
	Diabetes mellitus
Salivary Gland and Eye	Sialadenitis†
	Mooren corneal ulcer
	Uveitis
Haematological and Lymphoid	Mixed cryoglobulinemia and vasculitis
	Aplastic anaemia
	Idiopathic thrombocytopenia
	Non-Hodgkin's B lymphomas*
Kidney, Neuromuscular and Joints	Glomerulonephritis*
	Muscle weakness*
	Latent muscular abnormalities
	Peripheral neuropathy*
	Arthritis/arthralgias*
	Rheumatoid arthritis*
Dermatological	Cutaneous necrotizing vasculitis* (Leukocytoplastic vasculitis)
	Porphyria cutanea tarda (PCT)
	Lichen planus (LP)
	Erythema multiforme*
	Erythema nodosum*
	Malacoplakia
	Urticaria*
	Pruritus
Autoimmune and Miscellaneous	Polyarteritis nodosa (PAN)
	Pulmonary fibrosis* and pulmonary vasculitis*
	Hypertrophic cardiomyopathy
	CREST syndrome
	Antiphospholipid syndrome
	Granulomas
	Autoimmune hepatitis Type 1 and 2
	Presence of autoantibodies

*From Hadziyannis SJ: The spectrum of extrahepatic manifestation in hepatitis C virus infection. J Viral Hepatitis 4:9–28, 1997.
†Frequently related to mixed cryoglobulinemia.

blood cell survival is reduced, and serum haptoglobin levels are low. Marked hemolysis occurs only rarely, mainly in patients with glucose-6-phosphate dehydrogenase (G6PD) deficiency. Thrombocytopenia and aplastic anemia are also associated with acute viral hepatitis.

Other laboratory changes include increased serum vitamin B_{12} levels and high ferritin and serum iron concentration. A transient increase in serum α-fetoprotein levels is also noted, particularly in the severe forms of hepatitis and usually when the ALT levels decrease; this is attributed to hepatocellular regeneration.

SPECIFIC CLINICAL AND LABORATORY FEATURES

Acute Hepatitis A

Serologic, virologic, and biochemical events in acute hepatitis A are schematically presented in Figure 6–1. Hepatitis A is generally considered as the mildest form of acute viral hepatitis. This is usually true but only for children. Most cases in childhood are clinically inapparent. In adults, the disease is more serious, more frequently symptomatic, and icteric and may be prolonged. Fulminant hepatitis A occurs rarely, usually among adults.

Cholestatic Hepatitis A: In adults, hepatitis A may have a protracted cholestatic course that lasts for 1 to 4 months or even longer. Itching is severe, but the final outcome and prognosis are excellent.

Relapsing Hepatitis A: A number of patients with hepatitis A (up to 4% to 20% of affected adults) have relapses 30 to 90 days after the onset of the icteric phase. The new episode resembles clinically and biochemically the original attack and is associated with continuing viremia and viral shedding in the feces. Pathogenesis probably involves an interaction between persistent infection and host immune responses to the continuing antigenic stimulation. Rarely, an association of the relapse with arthritis, vasculitis, and cryoglobulinemia is noted. More than one relapse may occur and return of serum aminotransferases to normal (usually within 3 months or less) may take up to 12 months. The final prognosis is excellent with complete recovery from hepatitis.

Acute Hepatitis E

The sequence of events in acute hepatitis E is shown schematically in Figure 6–2. Although the disease is usually mild and has a self-limited course, there is a high mortality (20%) rate in women in the last trimester of pregnancy. Like hepatitis A, hepatitis E can have a cholestatic course. Joint symptoms are frequently present. In all reported large epidemics of hepatitis E, jaundice was present in 100% of the cases; fever ranged from 23% to 97%; and anorexia ranged from 66% to 100%. Recovery has always been complete.

Acute Hepatitis B

The sequence of events in acute self-limited HBV infection is shown schematically in Figure 6–3. The course of acute hepatitis B is more variable and usually more prolonged than that of hepatitis A and E. Extrahepatic manifestations including a macular erythema, urticaria, other skin rashes and arthritis are not rare and are mediated by immune complexes consisting of HBsAg, anti-HBs, and complement components, whereas arthritic symptoms may be manifested in any type of viral hepatitis. Arthritis with redness, swelling, and effusion seems to occur only in hepatitis B. It may even be a presenting symptom that causes diagnostic confusion, particularly in the anicteric patient. Cutaneous involvement may also be the only manifestation of HBV infection.

Serum bilirubin levels tend to rise less steeply than in hepatitis A but reach higher levels and last longer particularly in older patients. The same is true for aminotransferase increases. The self-limited benign icteric disease usually lasts less than 4 months; jaundice rarely exceeds 4 weeks. Relapsing and cholestatic hepatitis are unusual but contrary to the orally transmitted hepatitis viruses, progression to chronic infection may occur. Chronicity is unlikely following florid acute hepatitis but is very frequent in asymptomatic infections common in childhood.

A fulminant course is much more frequent in hepatitis B (and D) than in other forms of viral hepatitis except perhaps for hepatitis E in pregnant women. Reactivation of HBV in individuals with chronic HBV infection occurring after cytotoxic therapy for leukemia and lymphomas, organ transplantation, or spontaneously, may mimic acute HBV infection and attain a severe clinical form of icteric hepatitis with nonfatal liver failure or death.

Diagnosis of HBV infection is based on the detection of HBV components in the serum and liver (see Figs. 6–3, 6–7, and 6–12) and of the immune responses elicited against them in the course of acute and chronic infection (see Table 6–2 and Fig. 6–3).

Acute hepatitis associated with HBsAg positivity is not synonymous with acute hepatitis B. Differential diagnosis includes several etiologic factors and superimposed conditions that can cause acute hepatitis with chronic HBV infection. The most important causes are exacerbations of hepatitis B at the time of HBeAg seroconversion to anti-HBe, HBV reactivation, superinfection by other hepatitis viruses (A, D, C, and E), infection by other viral and nonviral agents (e.g., Epstein-Barr virus, cytomegalovirus, leptospirosis, rickettsial infection) as well as development of acute liver cell injury from nonviral, noninfectious agents, such as alcohol, drugs, and ischemia. Figure 6–13 shows HBV reactivation in the setting of chronic B infection. In addition to lobular changes, numerous ground-glass hepatocytes are present indicating the existence of a chronic carrier state from integrated HBV sequences.

Acute Hepatitis D

Clinical features of acute hepatitis D differ between coinfection and superinfection on whether HDV is introduced in the host simultaneously with HBV or into a host with pre-existing chronic HBV infection. In coinfection of adults, an acute self-limited episode of hepatitis of varying severity is usually manifested which, as in the case of infection with HBV alone, depending on several virus-related and host factors, may range in severity from a completely asymptomatic hepatitis to a fulminant one. A fulminant course has been observed more frequently than in HDV superinfection and in infection with HBV alone. Worldwide HDV infection is the true or the major cause of 30% to 80% of fulminant cases that were formerly thought to be caused by HBV.

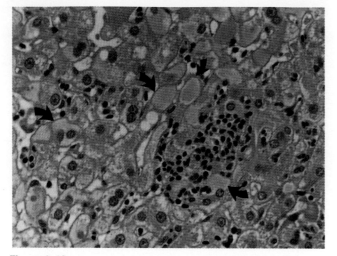

Figure 6–13
Spontaneous, severe HBV reactivation in chronic HBV infection, mimicking acute hepatitis B. The only clue to a correct diagnosis was the demonstration of numerous ground-glass hepatocytes *(arrows)* in the liver, harboring HBsAg from integrated HBV sequences. IgM anti-HBc was positive at high levels similar to those in acute hepatitis B.

A second episode of acute hepatitis may follow a few weeks from the first one, with each episode being pathogenetically distinct and attributable either to the D or B virus. This has clearly been noted in injection drug users. The distinction is clinically possible on the basis of virologic and serologic markers, particularly the timing and titers of anti-HD and anti-HBc of IgM and IgG class and has been well documented clinically and experimentally. The sequence of events in HBV/HDV coinfection is shown in Figure 6–4.

Transition to chronicity is rare in coinfected adults, but in children the situation seems to be different although information is limited. However, epidemiologic analysis of data in field studies suggest that coinfection in childhood may be associated more frequently with chronicity than with resolution of the infection.

In HDV superinfection, transition to chronicity seems to be the rule regardless of the patient's age (see Fig. 6–5). The acute episode is again of varying severity, ranging from subclinical to fulminant. Infection with genotype III of HDV has been associated with a very severe form of viral hepatitis found in the Amazon basin. This form is described as Labrea fever and Santa Marta hepatitis. The sequence of events in HDV superinfection is represented schematically in Figure 6–5.

Acute Hepatitis C

Acute hepatitis C in the adult is more frequently asymptomatic than acute hepatitis owing to the other hepatitis viruses. Only 25% of patients with post-transfusion hepatitis C develop clinical symptoms and jaundice, which are usually mild, whereas the risk for fulminant or subfulminant liver failure is rare. Despite its clinically silent features, HCV infection may be accompanied by various extrahepatic manifestations and systemic disorders, which are summarized in Table 6–4. However, most of the extrahepatic syndromes

listed in Table 6–4 have been recognized in association with chronic hepatitis C rather than with acute hepatitis C.

The most remarkable and alarming feature of acute HCV infection is its highly persistent rate and its ability to induce chronic liver disease, which can progress to cirrhosis and hepatocellular carcinoma. This unfavorable course appears to be unrelated to the age and sex of the patients and occurs in the majority of its cases. Follow-up studies have shown that, on average, more than two thirds of patients with acute infection have persistently increased ALT levels 6 months after the onset of the disease. Resolution of the acute infection is also possible but seems to be restricted to fewer than 25% of the acute infections.

The biochemical, serologic, and virologic profile of acute HCV infection with transition to chronicity is shown schematically in Figure 6–6. Serum HCV RNA is the earliest detectable marker of acute HCV infection. It precedes the appearance of anti-HCV by several weeks as well as the appearance of symptoms and the increase in ALT values. Antibodies to HCV proteins first become detectable in serum days or weeks after the onset of the disease with anti-C22-3 and anti-C33C being the first ones to appear. Anti-NS5 appears a little later, whereas anti-C100-3 is the last antibody to develop in acute self-limited infections. None of these antibodies are neutralizing or protective. In self-limited disease, serum enzymes return to normal; HCV RNA disappears; and antibodies to HCV decline in titer or disappear in 50% to 80% of the cases. However, in patients with transition to chronicity, not only anti-HCV but also HCV RNA positivity persist and serum aminotransferases remain elevated either in a persistent or intermittent pattern, reflecting waves of liver necroinflammation. Antibodies of the IgM class to HCV core proteins are a marker of persisting HCV replication. In a few patients ($\approx$10%) with chronic HCV infection, anti-HCV may decline or disappear spontaneously or after interferon treatment. Similar patterns in biochemical, virologic, and immunologic parameters have been observed in chimpanzees experimentally infected with inocula from patients with hepatitis C.

Clinical features and natural course of acute hepatitis C do not appear to be specifically related to modes of HCV transmission, HCV genotypes, age, sex, and other host- or virus-related factors, except perhaps for immunosuppression. A discussion follows on the natural course and severity of chronic HCV infection in the chronic sequelae of viral hepatitis.

Acute Hepatitis Non–A-E

Patients with acute viral hepatitis, either parenterally transmitted or sporadic, may be negative for markers of any of the established hepatitis viruses. Such patients are assumed to be affected by hepatitis of non–A-E etiology. Clinically and biochemically, they are indistinguishable from the other types of acute viral hepatitis. Their number is disproportionately high in the fulminant and subfulminant forms of the disease. A new flavivirus, the G/GBV-C, has been implicated in their etiology, but data are contradictory.

Infection with non–A-E hepatitis agents, particularly of the sporadic type, may also become chronic. Approximately 20% of patients with chronic viral hepatitis are assumed to be of non–A-E etiology.

CHRONIC SEQUELAE OF VIRAL HEPATITIS

Most patients with recognizable acute viral hepatitis recover completely either quickly or after a protracted or relapsing course. However, a proportion progresses to chronicity. It is restricted only to types B, C, and D. For hepatitis B, it is particularly high when infection occurs in the neonatal period or childhood, whereas hepatitis C seems to be similarly high in all ages.

Posthepatitic Syndromes

Patients with any type of self-limited acute hepatitis may exhibit some benign sequelae such as posthepatitic hyperbilirubinemia, persistence of nonspecific symptoms, and fatigue lasting for several months. These syndromes are collectively referred as the posthepatitic syndrome; they appear to be more frequent among doctors and nurses affected by hepatitis but they eventually subside.

The term chronic persistent hepatitis has also been applied in the past to patients with mild increases in ALT levels that persist for years after a presumable episode of acute viral hepatitis. Such patients are usually asymptomatic, and on liver histology they have portal inflammation but normal lobular architecture. They are now known to represent an etiologically heterogeneous group. Their prognosis has initially been reported to be excellent; however, subsequent studies have shown that the prognosis differs greatly and is dependent on the etiology. Most instances represent early cases of chronic viral hepatitis D and C; their histologic characterization as chronic persistent hepatitis is etiopathogenetically meaningless; and their inclusion in the benign posthepatitic syndrome can no longer be justified.

Chronic Viral Hepatitis

Nomenclature and Definitions

Chronic viral hepatitis is a term first introduced in the early 1970s for cases of chronic active liver disease, presumably of viral etiology, indicated by the chronic presence of HBsAg. This term is currently applied widely to all chronic infections with the hepatitis viruses with a specific denotation for the responsible agent (B, D, or C). It always implies the presence of some degree of liver damage (hepatitis). Patients with chronic viral infection, normal liver biochemistry, and completely normal liver histology are frequently referred to as chronic carriers of HBV or HCV. However, since the appearance, severity, and evolution of liver injury and inflammation fluctuate in the natural course of chronic infection with the hepatitis viruses, the broader term chronic viral hepatitis accompanied by its etiologic definition (B, D, or C) and by grading and staging of changes in the liver is currently recommended. Thus, an HBV carrier with normal enzymes and liver histology is defined as chronic viral hepatitis B, grade 0, stage 0; and an active late case of chronic hepatitis B will be considered as chronic viral hepatitis B, grade 4, stage 4. This classification combines clinical, etiologic, and histologic information and, in serial liver biopsies from the same patient, it can also evaluate if the disease is progressing or not.

General Clinical Features

Chronic infection with the hepatitis viruses covers a wide spectrum of clinical manifestations that range from a completely asymptomatic, subclinical state with minimal biochemical abnormalities to the fully developed picture of liver failure and decompensated cirrhosis.

In the asymptomatic states of chronic infection with the hepatitis viruses, signs of liver disease are minimal or completely absent; serum aminotransferase levels may be moderately increased whereas other liver chemistries are usually normal. Liver histology reveals liver necroinflammation and fibrosis ranging from none with a histologic activity index (HAI) of 0 to severe active cirrhosis with the maximum grades of necroinflammatory activity and stage of fibrosis. The most serious liver changes are encountered in approximately 20% of patients with increased ALT levels, whereas in those with normal ALT values such changes are detected in 1%. The old classification into chronic persistent, chronic active, and chronic lobular hepatitis has been abandoned, whereas the histologic grading and staging scores in association with etiology, pathogenesis, and natural course and response to interferon therapy are attaining greater clinical value.

The frequency and severity of liver changes, prevailing clinical features, laboratory abnormalities, and evolutionary patterns in each etiologic type of chronic infection with the hepatitis viruses are summarized below.

Specific Features

Chronic Hepatitis B: The early phases of chronic infection with HBV are usually completely asymptomatic. Despite high levels of HBV replication, liver cell damage is minimal or completely absent owing to immune tolerance of the virus (Fig. 6–14). In subsequent phases of the infection, an immune response to the replicating B virus is mounted and immune clearance of HBV infected hepatitis leads to varying degrees and duration of liver necroinflammation and fibrosis. Clearance of HBeAg and of replicating B virus is associated with quiescence of injury and inflammation, minimal residual liver changes, but persistence of HBsAg from viral sequence integrated into hepatocytes.

Precore HBV mutants that do not produce HBeAg become predominant during these phases and may keep replicating after HBeAg seroconversion has occurred, or they may reactivate, alone or in association with the wild type (wt) virus later in the course of chronic infection. However, although they do not express the HBeAg, they cannot escape host immune recognition. Whenever they resume replication at significant levels, liver necroinflammation develops through immune destruction of infected hepatocytes. Sometimes viral reactivation may be quite marked, and the immune response is strong enough to induce severe and even fulminant episodes of liver necroinflammation, which can be confused clinically with acute viral hepatitis B. The anti-HBc IgM levels reach very high values similar to those in acute or fulminant hepatitis B. If the patient manages to survive, then clearance of HBV may also occur. The natural course of the HBeAg-positive and HBeAg-negative phases of chronic HBV infection is shown schematically in Figure 6–14.

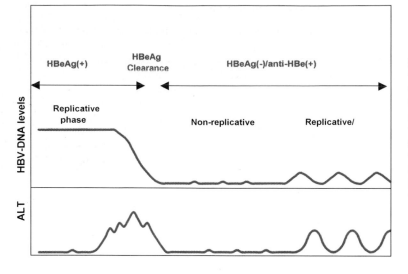

Figure 6–14
The natural course of a chronic HBV infection. The wild type (wt) HBV predominates during the HBeAg-positive phase. Emergence of precore HBV mutants occurs in the course of the infection before the phase of HBeAg clearance. These mutants are subsequently selected and become predominant in the HBeAg-negative phase of the disease. Residual HBV can be detected during the nonreplicative phase, but high HBV DNA levels are seen during periods of viral reactivation and disease activity (see text).

Chronic viral hepatitis B, acquired in early life, appears to last for decades. It may be complicated by superinfection with HDV and HCV, or it may result in compensated and decompensated cirrhosis and may be complicated by the development of hepatocellular carcinoma. The relative risk for development of HCC in chronic HBV infection acquired in early life is extremely high, and in some prospective studies the relative risk factor has been found to be higher than 200; in the case of concurrent chronic infections with HBV and HCV, it may attain even greater values.

Extrahepatic manifestations in chronic HBV infection are usually seen in patients with rather mild forms of liver disease. They include cryoglobulinemia, glomerulonephritis, polyarteritis nodosa, rare neurologic changes, hematologic abnormalities, and skin disorders.

Chronic Hepatitis D: The clinical syndrome of chronic hepatitis D also consists of a wide range of symptoms, none of which is sufficiently specific to provide a diagnosis. A history of acute hepatitis is reported more frequently than in chronic hepatitis owing to HBV alone. Splenomegaly is also more frequent and is sometimes out of proportion to the presence of portal hypertension, while in some patients with advanced disease cholestasis predominates with striking hyperbilirubinemia that is also out of proportion to other indices of liver failure.

In areas of HDV endemicity, numerous field studies sometimes even with normal serum aminotransferases have revealed that subclinical forms of chronic hepatitis D are quite common; in fact, these forms are two to four times more frequent than clinically overt cases.

In long-term studies, a bimodal evolution of the disease has been observed over the years with a rapidly progressive course to liver failure within 1 to 2 years in about 15% of cases; and a second very slowly progressive one during 1 or 2 decades in approximately 70% of patients. Remission, even with resolution of the infection, has been observed in 15% of patients on follow-up.

It is probable that evolution of cirrhosis in chronic HDV infection is not different from that with HBV alone. Serum aminotransferases return to normal or borderline values. Liver injury and inflammation diminish or disappear completely, and patients may enjoy a normal life for years. However, liver architecture has already been altered during the early phase of the infection, and a stable cirrhotic stage seems to be present in most of these patients.

Development of hepatocellular carcinoma has been thought to occur less frequently in chronic HDV than in HBV infection. However, it has now become apparent that if patients do not go quickly into liver failure, then the risk for development of HCC is quite high. In one study comprising a large number of patients who were monitored for many years, the development of HCC occurred in more than 40% with an annual rate of approximately 10%.

Chronic Hepatitis C: As already emphasized, a most important feature of viral hepatitis C is the high frequency with which acute disease progresses to chronicity. From follow-up studies it has been documented that at least two thirds of patients with acute hepatitis C have persistently increased ALT levels for more than 6 months after the onset of their illness. The majority of these patients are asymptomatic and run an indolent course for years up to the development of end-stage, decompensated cirrhosis or HCC. In fact, most patients with chronic hepatitis C are identified in screening or follow-up studies of transfused or other parenterally exposed groups. A dated onset of chronic hepatitis C with a history of symptomatic acute hepatitis is reported in less than 30% of these patients.

No specific factors have been documented to be associated with the transition to chronicity, except perhaps for certain HLA haplotypes. However, patients older than 50 years appear to manifest advanced chronic liver disease with histologically documented cirrhosis more frequently than do younger patients. This finding suggests a more rapid course. The mean time interval from exposure to HCV to cirrhosis and HCC has been estimated to be 21 and 29 years, respectively.

Biochemical changes in chronic hepatitis C (especially ALT elevations) are either persistent or intermittent ("sawtooth" pattern) with varying degrees of severity. Patterns of disease activity and severity fluctuate over time in relation to the stages of the disease.

Persistently normal ALT levels may be seen in some patients despite the presence of viremia, which suggests the existence, if not of a permanent healthy carrier state, at least of prolonged phases of HCV carriage in the absence of overt hepatitis. However, liver biopsy of such patients may bring into light significant changes of necroinflammation and fibrosis unexpected by the normal liver chemistries. Thus, liver histology in chronic HCV infection should be considered as a "clinical" procedure of diagnostic and prognostic value. Other laboratory abnormalities such as increased bilirubin and alkaline phosphatase, and low albumin concentration are unusual until late stages of liver disease have been reached; however, moderately and occasionally highly increased γ-globulin levels are not exceptional in earlier stages of chronic hepatitis C. Thrombocytopenia due to hypersplenism is related to the development of cirrhosis but may also occur in the absence of cirrhosis, being related to autoimmune mechanisms.

Despite its indolent course and the frequent lack of clinical features of liver involvement, chronic HCV infection may involve several organs and tissues outside the liver. The extrahepatic manifestations described in HCV infection are numerous, but the association with HCV has only been established in a few syndromes. These include essential mixed cryoglobulinemia, membranous glomerulonephritis, focal lymphocytic sialadenitis, lichen planus, thyroid dysfunction, autoantibodies and autoimmune hepatitis, and recently thrombocytopenia and the antiphospholipid syndrome (see Table 6–3).

The natural course of chronic HCV infection appears to be significantly accelerated in some patients with early termination to decompensated cirrhosis in less than 10 to 15 years. This appears to be particularly true in the liver transplantation setting.

Development of HCC on the grounds of chronic hepatitis C is usually associated with progression to cirrhosis, although cases not associated with cirrhosis have also been reported. In Japan, HCV-associated hepatocellular carcinoma is the most frequent form of HCC and greatly outnumbers the HBV-related cases of this tumor.

Chronic Hepatitis Non–A-E: Patients with chronic hepatitis of unknown etiology, which is clinically and biochemically indistinguishable from other forms of chronic viral hepatitis, are assumed to be affected by non–A-E hepatitis viruses. Evolution to cirrhosis and hepatocellular carcinoma has also been implicated on the basis of clinical and epidemiologic observations. Although this topic is still unresolved there is a general consensus that chronic viral liver disease of non–A-E etiology does really exist; it is worldwide and represents a causative factor of cirrhosis and probably of hepatocellular carcinoma.

SUGGESTED READINGS

Alter M: Epidemiology of hepatitis C in the West. Semin Liver Dis 15:5–14, 1995.

Alter MJ, Hadler SC: Delta hepatitis and infection in North America. In Hadziyannis S, Taylor JM, Bonino F (eds): Hepatitis Delta Virus: Molecular Biology, Pathogenesis, and Clinical Aspects, Vol 382. New York: Wiley-Liss, 1993, pp 243–250.

Alter HJ, Bradley DW: Non-A, non-B hepatitis unrelated to the hepatitis C virus (non-ABC). Semin Liver Dis 15:110–120, 1995.

Chisari FV, Ferrari C: Hepatitis B virus immunopathogenesis. Annu Rev Immunol 13:29–60, 1995.

Eddleston ALWF: Overview of HBV pathogenesis. In Hollinger FB, Lemon SM, Margolis HS (eds): Viral Hepatitis and Liver Disease. Baltimore: Williams & Wilkins, 1991, pp 234–237.

Esteban JI, Genesca J, Alter HJ: Hepatitis C: Molecular biology, pathogenesis, epidemiology, clinical features, and prevention. In Boyer JC, Ockner RK (eds): Progress in Liver Disease, Vol X. Philadelphia: WB Saunders, 1992, pp 253–282.

Green MS, Tsur S, Slepon R: Socioeconomic factors and the declining prevalence of anti-hepatitis A antibodies in young adults in Israel: Implication for the new hepatitis A vaccine. Intern J Epidemiol 21:136–141, 1992.

Hadziyannis SJ: Hepatitis delta: An overview. In Rizzetto M, Purcell RM, Serin JL, Verme G (eds): Viral Hepatitis and Liver Disease. Turin: Edjioni Minerva Medica, 1997, pp 283-289.

Hadziyannis SJ: Diagnostic flow chart in the hepatitis B carrier. In McIntyre N, Benhamou JP (eds): Oxford Textbook of Clinical Hepatology. Oxford: Oxford University Press, 1991, pp 599–605.

Hadziyannis SJ: HBe antigen negative chronic hepatitis B: From clinical recognition to pathogenesis and treatment. Viral Hepat Rev 1:7–36, 1995.

Hadziyannis SJ: Chronic viral hepatitis. Clin Gastroenterol 3:391–408, 1974.

Hadziyannis SJ: The spectrum of extrahepatic manifestation in hepatitis C virus infection. J Viral Hepat 4:9–28, 1997.

Hadziyannis S, Hess G: Epidemiology and natural course of G/GBV-C infection. In Zuckerman A, Thomas H (eds): Viral Hepatitis, 2nd ed. London: Churchill Livingstone, 1998, pp 427–436.

Hytiroglou P, Thung SN, Gerber MA: Histological classification and quantitation of the severity of chronic hepatitis: Keep it simple! Semin Liver Dis 15:414–421, 1995.

Koff RS: Viral hepatitis. In Schiff L, Schiff ER (eds): Diseases of the Liver, 7th ed. Philadelphia: JB Lippincott, 1993, pp 492–577.

Krawcynski K: Hepatitis E. Hepatology 17:932–941, 1993.

Lemon SM, Whetter LE, Chang KA, Brown ED: Recent advances in understanding the molecular virology of hepatoviruses: Contrasts and comparison with hepatitis C. In Nishioka K, Suzuki H, Mishiro S, Oda T (eds): Viral Hepatitis and Liver Disease. Tokyo: Springer-Verlag, 1994, pp 22–27.

Margolis HS, Alter MJ, Hadler SC: Hepatitis B: Evolving epidemiology and implications for control. Semin Liver Dis 11:84–92, 1991.

McIntyre N: Clinical presentation of acute viral hepatitis. Br Med Bull 46:533–547, 1990.

Ockner RK: Acute viral hepatitis. In Bennett JCB, Plum F (eds): Cecil Textbook of Medicine, 20th ed. Philadelphia: WB Saunders, 1996, pp 762–772.

Purcell RH: The discovery of the hepatitis viruses. Gastroenterology 104:955–963, 1993.

Reyes GR: Hepatitis E virus (HEV): Molecular biology and emerging epidemiology. In Boyer JL, Ockner RK (eds): Progress in Liver Disease, Vol XI. Philadelphia: WB Saunders, 1993, pp 203–218.

Rizzetto M, Hadziyannis S, Hansson BG, et al: Hepatitis delta virus infection in the world. Epidemiological patterns and clinical expression. Gastroenterology Intern 5:18–32, 1992.

Rizzetto M, Verme G: Hepatitis D. In McIntyre N, Benhamou JP (eds): Oxford Textbook of Clinical Hepatology. Oxford: Oxford University Press, 1991, pp 592–598.

Seeff LB: Diagnosis, therapy and prognosis of viral hepatitis. In Zakim D, Boyer TD: Hepatology: A Textbook of Liver Disease, 2nd ed. Philadelphia: WB Saunders, 1990, pp 958–10125.

Shapiro CN, Shaw FE, Mandel EJ, et al: Epidemiology of hepatitis A in the United States. In Hollinger FB, Lemon SM, Margolis HS (eds): Viral Hepatitis and Liver Disease. Baltimore: Williams & Wilkins, 1991, pp 71–76.

Sharara AI, Hunt CM, Hamilton JD: Hepatitis C. Ann Intern Med 125:658–668, 1996.

Sherlock S: Diseases of the Liver and Biliary System, 8th ed. London: Blackwell Scientific, 1997.

Toukan AU: An overview of hepatitis D virus infection in Africa and the Middle East. In Hadziyannis S, Taylor JM, Bonino F (eds): Hepatitis Delta Virus: Molecular Biology, Pathogenesis, and Clinical Aspects, Vol 382. New York: Wiley-Liss, 1993, pp 251–258.

7

Management of Chronic Viral Hepatitis

Adrian M. Di Bisceglie
Jay H. Hoofnagle

Chronic viral hepatitis is perhaps the major cause of chronic liver disease and cirrhosis worldwide, contributing significantly to morbidity and mortality from end-stage liver disease, liver failure, and hepatocellular carcinoma. Three viral agents are responsible for most cases: (1) hepatitis B virus (HBV), (2) hepatitis D virus (HDV) and (3) hepatitis C virus (HCV). The clinical symptoms, biochemical laboratory features, and histology of the three viral forms of chronic hepatitis are quite similar; they can be distinguished reliably only by virologic and serologic testing. Diagnostic tests are available for each form of chronic viral hepatitis. Methods of prevention and control of viral hepatitis are being developed, and the incidence of these diseases is declining. Therapies for chronic viral hepatitis are problematic and only partially effective but are the focus of considerable current research activity.

DIAGNOSIS

Chronic Viral Hepatitis. Chronic hepatitis is marked by persistent elevations in serum aminotransferases and chronic inflammation and hepatocellular injury on liver biopsy. This pattern of abnormalities, however, may not be present in all patients and may also occur with other conditions that must be distinguished from viral hepatitis (Table 7–1). The usual criterion for chronicity in viral hepatitis is the presence of abnormalities for 6 months. However, in many situations, chronicity can be assumed based on the pattern of aminotransferase abnormalities, the clinical symptomatology, and the history of exposure. The typical symptoms and clinical features of viral hepatitis are discussed in Chapter 6. In chronic viral hepatitis, symptoms are typically mild and nonspecific, being mainly chronic, and include intermittent fatigue and less frequently nausea, right upper quadrant discomfort, and muscle aches and pains. Even without symptoms, serum aminotransferase activities are typically 2- to 10-fold elevated, but they may be normal. Liver histology is usually diagnostic of chronic viral hepatitis but may be mimicked by other conditions and can be normal or almost normal in some patients with virologically documented chronic infection. Diagnostic features for each of the three types of chronic hepatitis have to be discussed separately.

Chronic Hepatitis B. Hepatitis B is diagnosed serologically by the finding of hepatitis B surface antigen (HBsAg) and hepatitis B e antigen (HBeAg) or HBV DNA in serum for 6 months or longer. In a proportion of patients, chronic hepatitis ultimately resolves into an "inactive" carrier state with persistence of HBsAg but absence of HBeAg and HBV DNA and normal serum aminotransferase. Persistence of HBV DNA in serum (as detected by hybridization or branched DNA assays) is characteristic of chronic hepatitis B and, with HBeAg, is the serologic marker used to evaluate the efficacy of therapy. Testing for antibody to hepatitis B core antigen (anti-HBc) is not helpful in the diagnosis of chronic hepatitis; this antibody is detected in almost all patients with acute and chronic hepatitis B as well as in patients who have recovered from infection. Tests for IgM-specific anti-HBc can be helpful to distinguish acute from chronic hepatitis B. This antibody is present in high levels during acute disease only. Antibody to HBsAg (anti-HBs) is also not helpful diagnostically; anti-HBs arises once hepatitis B has resolved but is detectable in some cases in low levels with HBsAg in patients with chronic hepatitis B.

Table 7–1 Differential Diagnosis of Chronic Hepatitis

Viral hepatitis
    Hepatitis B virus
    Hepatitis C virus
    Hepatitis D (delta) virus
Autoimmune hepatitis
    Type I
    Type II
    Overlap syndromes
Cryptogenic hepatitis
Metabolic diseases
    α_1-Antitrypsin deficiency
    Wilson's disease
Drug-induced hepatitis
    Isoniazid
    Oxyphenisatin
    α-Methyldopa
    Nitrofurantoin
Conditions which may mimic chronic hepatitis
    Hemochromatosis
    Fatty liver
    Primary sclerosing cholangitis

Chronic Hepatitis D. Chronic delta hepatitis is diagnosed by the finding of HBsAg and high titers of antibody to HDV (anti-HDV) in serum. HDV is a defective virus that requires HBsAg for replication and thus is found only in patients who also have hepatitis B. HDV RNA and HDAg are also usually present in the serum of patients with chronic HDV, but these assays are difficult to perform and are not routinely available. Acute HDV can occur either in a person who is a chronic HBsAg carrier (delta superinfection) or in one who has a concurrent acute hepatitis B (delta coinfection). These two possibilities can be differentiated by the presence of IgM anti-HBc, a characteristic feature of acute coinfection with HBV and HBV. There are no serologic assays that reliably separate acute from chronic HDV infection, and most cases are first detected after the disease has become chronic.

Chronic Hepatitis C. Chronic hepatitis C is diagnosed by the finding of antibody to HCV (anti-HCV) together with HCV RNA in serum. The current enzyme-linked immunoassays (EIAs) for anti-HCV are sensitive and detect this antibody in more than 95% of patients with chronic HCV. False-negative reactions for anti-HCV can occur in patients who are immunosuppressed or immunodeficient. Thus, in some cases, the diagnosis is made by the finding of HCV RNA without anti-HCV, and this pattern is more common among patients with agammaglobulinemia, renal failure, or solid organ transplant. Tests for anti-HCV can also yield false-positive results, these being most frequent when testing general populations or blood donors. For these reasons, confirmation of the anti-HCV reactivity is recommended, using supplementary tests such as immunoblot assays for anti-HCV or polymerase chain reaction (PCR) for HCV RNA. Detection of HCV RNA is particularly useful in acute HCV infection, in which it may take several months for anti-HCV to appear in serum. Detection of HCV RNA also provides evidence that infection is still ongoing. Unfortunately, tests for HCV RNA have not been rigorously standardized and can also have false-positive and false-negative reactions.

Cryptogenic and Other Forms of Viral Hepatitis. A proportion of patients with chronic hepatitis are negative for HBV and HCV markers yet seem to have viral hepatitis. This condition is variously referred to as non-A, non-B, non-C, non-D, non-E hepatitis, non–A-E hepatitis, hepatitis X, or more appropriately cryptogenic hepatitis. When viral markers are negative, a more careful search for other etiologies is warranted (see Table 7–1). The most important diagnoses to exclude are Wilson's disease, autoimmune hepatitis, sclerosing cholangitis, nonalcoholic steatohepatitis, and drug-induced liver disease. Only after careful exclusion of these diagnoses should the patient be considered to have cryptogenic hepatitis.

Hepatitis G virus (HGV) is a recently discovered blood-borne flavivirus related to HCV. It is diagnosed by the presence of HGV RNA in serum and is often found together with HCV infection. Between 1% and 2% of the general population have chronic infection with HGV, and higher rates are found in many of the same high-risk groups for hepatitis B and C, such as injection drug users, blood product recipients, and sexually promiscuous persons. It remains unclear whether HGV causes liver disease, or indeed whether HGV replicates in the liver. Most studies of cryptogenic hepatitis and cirrhosis indicate that HGV RNA is no more common in patients with this condition than in matched control patients. Thus, HGV does not seem to account for most cases of cryptogenic hepatitis or cirrhosis. Studies of patients treated with interferon alfa for hepatitis B or C have identified some who were coinfected with hepatitis G. Titers of HGV RNA fall during interferon therapy (but not during ribavirin therapy) but generally rise after interferon is stopped, whether or not HCV or HBV is cleared.

Another form of chronic hepatitis of unknown cause has been associated with syncytial giant cells, a variant found in adults that is associated with severe chronic hepatitis and cirrhosis. Some cases of this variant appear to be associated with paramyxovirus infection. Syncytial giant cells are found most commonly with autoimmune hepatitis, which responds well to corticosteroid therapy. Thus, this syndrome may be more related to autoimmune hepatitis than to cryptogenic hepatitis.

Liver biopsy confirmation of the diagnosis of chronic hepatitis is useful both in excluding other forms of liver disease (e.g., hemochromatosis, fatty liver, and α_1-antitrypsin deficiency) and in establishing the severity of liver injury and determining the presence and degree of fibrosis. Recently, the terminology for histopathologic descriptions of liver biopsies in chronic hepatitis has been revised. The terms "chronic persistent" and "chronic active" hepatitis have been replaced by a more complete description of the liver biopsy, which should include three elements: (1) the suspected *etiology* of the hepatitis (e.g., hepatitis B or C); (2) the *grade* of necrosis and inflammation (e.g., mild, moderate, or severe); and (3) the *stage* of fibrosis (e.g., none, minimal, portal expansion, bridging fibrosis, and cirrhosis).

Table 7–2 Diagnosis of Chronic Viral Hepatitis

Disease	Screening Tests	Supplementary Tests	Other
Hepatitis B	HBsAg	HBeAg HBV DNA	IgM anti-HBc
Hepatitis D	HBsAg	Anti-HDV	HDV RNA HDV Antigen
Hepatitis C	Anti-HCV	HCV RNA	Immunoblot for anti-HCV

In patients with suspected chronic hepatitis because of clinical history, persistent elevations in serum aminotransferases, or abnormal serologic tests from routine screening, testing should initially include hepatitis B surface antigen (HBsAg) and anti-hepatitis C virus (HCV) by enzyme immunoassay (EIA) (or radioimmunoassay [RIA]). If HBsAg is present, tests for hepatitis Be antigen (HBeAg), HBV DNA, and anti-HDV are appropriate and, if acute hepatitis is suspected, for IgM anti-HBc. If anti-HCV is present, testing for HCV RNA may be appropriate. In some cases seropositive for anti-HCV (if hepatitis C seems unlikely and if HCV RNA is negative), testing for anti-HCV by immunoblot is appropriate.

TREATMENT

Chronic Hepatitis B

The currently recommended regimen of therapy for chronic hepatitis B is a course of interferon alfa therapy given subcutaneously in doses of 5 million units (MU) daily or 10 MU three times weekly for 4 to 6 months. This regimen results in remission of disease in approximately one third of patients. Although the optimum dose and duration of therapy with interferon have not been completely determined for hepatitis B, few patients tolerate more than 10 MU of interferon three times weekly, and an extension of treatment for longer than 4 or 6 months seems to have little beneficial effect. The serologic tests used in diagnosing chronic hepatitis B are shown in Table 7–2.

The regimen should begin with careful documentation of the diagnosis as well as the grade and stage of disease, with an initial period of monitoring for serum aminotransferases, bilirubin, albumin, and prothrombin time followed by testing for HBeAg and HBV DNA and liver biopsy (Table 7–3). If the patient is a candidate for therapy, the expected results of treatment and side effects should be clearly defined for the patient. Acute side effects of fever, chills, malaise, nausea, headaches, and muscle aches typically occur with the first one or two injections and then resolve. Chronic side effects include fatigue, muscle aches and headaches, nausea, depression, irritability, and hair loss. More uncommon side effects involve the development of autoimmune disease, bacterial infections, severe depression, psychoses, suicidal ideation, and pulmonary, renal, or cardiac dysfunction.

The frequency of side effects and the nature of responses in hepatitis B make it important to monitor patients on therapy carefully, with visits at 1- to 4-week intervals. Patients should be interviewed regarding side effects and symptoms and tested for serum aminotransferases and complete blood counts. Tests for HBsAg, HBeAg, and HBV DNA should be repeated at the end of therapy and then approximately 6 months afterwards to document whether a beneficial virologic response has occurred. Testing for thyroid abnormalities, which are frequent with interferon therapy, is also appropriate before therapy and at the end of therapy.

A beneficial response to interferon alfa therapy in hepatitis B is defined by the loss of HBeAg and HBV DNA that persists for at least 6 months after therapy is discontinued. A transient exacerbation of disease with increases in serum aminotransferases occurs frequently during interferon alfa therapy for hepatitis B and occurs most commonly among patients with a sustained beneficial response. These flares of hepatitis during therapy are usually asymptomatic and transient and are rarely associated with changes in serum bilirubin or albumin. The dose of interferon may have to be adjusted or even discontinued if the exacerbation of disease is severe or if side effects are intolerable.

Table 7–3 Algorithm For Therapy of Hepatitis B

Initial Evaluation
Serial ALT levels
Presence of HBsAg, HBeAg, HBV DNA
Liver biopsy
Review side effects and expected results
Lack of contraindications

↓

Initiate Therapy
Alpha interferon given subcutaneously in a dose of 5 MU daily or 10 MU thrice weekly for 16 to 24 weeks

↓

Monitoring During Therapy
Every 2 to 4 weeks
  Symptoms and signs
  ALT, AST, bilirubin, albumin
  CBC and differential
At 2 and 4 months:
  HBeAg, HBsAg, prothrombin time, TSH

↓

Follow-up After Therapy
Every 2 to 3 months
  Symptoms and signs
  ALT, AST, bilirubin, albumin
  CBC
At 6 months:
  HBeAg, HBsAg, prothrombin time, TSH

ALT, alanine aminotransferase; AST, aspartate transaminase; HBV, hepatitis B virus; HBsAg, hepatitis B surface antigen; HBeAg, hepatitis Be surface antigen; TSH, thyroid-stimulating hormone; CBC, complete blood count.

Indications for interferon therapy in chronic hepatitis B are the presence of: (1) abnormal serum aminotransferases, (2) HBsAg and HBeAg or HBV DNA in serum, and (3) chronic hepatitis on liver biopsy. Patients with decompensated cirrhosis should be treated only with extreme caution because side effects are frequently severe and life threatening. Interferon alfa therapy is also not indicated in patients with normal serum aminotransferases, even when HBV DNA is present in serum, because these patients rarely respond to therapy. Finally, immunosuppressed patients should not be treated because therapy is ineffective and can be harmful in some cases (e.g., after solid organ transplant). When deciding which patients with chronic hepatitis B should be treated, it is important to distinguish the inactive or "healthy" carrier state from that involving chronic hepatitis B. Persons who are persistently HBsAg positive but have no evidence of ongoing hepatic injury or active viral replication (no HBeAg or HBV DNA in serum) are usually referred to as inactive or healthy carriers of HBsAg. Testing using sensitive PCR assays often demonstrates the presence of low levels of HBV DNA in these patients' liver and serum. However, the prognosis in these carriers appears to be excellent, and they are unlikely to benefit from antiviral therapy.

Ultimately, the goals of therapy in chronic hepatitis B are to cure the infection and to halt the progression of disease. These goals may not be achievable in most patients. More immediate and practical goals of treatment are the elimination of detectable viral replication as assessed by the loss of HBeAg or HBV DNA. The loss of HBeAg is usually accompanied by a fall of HBV DNA to undetectable levels (or levels detectable only by PCR) and is followed by improvement in serum aminotransferases and liver histology. These improvements may be somewhat delayed. Indeed, long-term follow-up indicates that the remissions of disease induced by interferon therapy are usually sustained and that many patients ultimately clear not only HBV DNA but also HBsAg and develop anti-HBs. If cirrhosis is not already present, prognosis in a patient who responds to treatment appears to be excellent.

Factors that correlate with a response to interferon alfa therapy include high serum aminotransferases and low levels of HBV DNA before therapy, active liver disease on biopsy, and short duration of hepatitis. However, the results of therapy in individual patients cannot be predicted reliably in advance. Low rates of response have been reported in patients with normal serum aminotransferases, immunosuppressed patients, and Asian patients who have acquired hepatitis B during childhood. Children have similar response rates to interferon alfa therapy and also tend to tolerate treatment better than adults. The dose of interferon for children is 6 MU/m^2 given subcutaneously three times weekly for 4 to 6 months.

Therapy with interferon alfa is beneficial in only one third of patients. Furthermore, interferon therapy is expensive, is often poorly tolerated, and is contraindicated in many patients. Obviously, other approaches to therapy for hepatitis B are needed. Therapeutic approaches that have been studied include use of other cytokines, nucleoside analogues, immunomodulatory agents, and gene therapies. The most promising other approach at present is the use of second-generation nucleoside analogues, several newly developed oral agents that have potent antiviral activity against HBV in vitro in cell culture systems and in vivo in animal models of hepatitis B. These drugs include lamivudine (3'-thiacytidine), famciclovir, lobucavir, and adefovir dipivoxil. Lamivudine has had the most extensive evaluation and was recently approved for use in chronic hepatitis B in the United States. Early dose finding studies showed a potent inhibitory effect of lamivudine against HBV at doses as low as 100 mg/day. These early data showed that although HBV DNA levels became undetectable in most treated patients, the rate of sustained clearance of HBV DNA and HBeAg was substantially lower than with interferon, typically less than 15%. For this reason, subsequent studies evaluated the use of lamivudine for as long as 12 months and this has now become the usual duration of therapy while 100 mg/day has become the standard dosage.

Results of prolonged treatment of chronic hepatitis B with lamivudine showed that over a period of 12 months, the 100-mg dose was associated with a 98% reduction in serum levels of HBV DNA compared with baseline, a 16% rate of HBeAg seroconversion (loss of HBeAg with development of antibody to HBeAg). Of significance though, treatment with lamivudine was also associated with significant improvement in liver disease activity as assessed by a decrease in serum aminotransferases and an improvement in liver histopathology. Thus, treatment was associated with a return to normal of serum ALT values in 72% of patients and a lessening in necroinflammatory activity noted on biopsy as well as a slowing of fibrosis progression compared with placebo-treated controls.

Thus, the use of lamivudine appears very attractive as a therapeutic option compared with interferon, even though it does not induce a very high rate of seroconversion. Furthermore, it is administered orally and is associated with very few significant side effects. One factor that may limit its use is the development of viral resistance to its antiviral actions. The mechanism of viral resistance appears to be a mutation that occurs in the gene coding for HBV DNA polymerase. Specifically, the amino acid motif YMDD is mutated to YIDD or YVDD. This genotypic resistance occurs with a typical clinical picture (phenotypic resistance) characterized by an initial beneficial response to therapy with clearance of HBV DNA from serum and a return to normal of serum aminotransferases with subsequent reappearance of HBV DNA in high titers. Resistance typically appears after at least 6 to 9 months of treatment and has been noted in as many as 15% of patients treated for at least 12 months. In cases of resistance where the lamivudine has been stopped, the viral mutant is promptly replaced by the wild type virus, which is often associated with an exacerbation of the hepatitis. The long-term significance of viral resistance is not known, and it is generally not recommended that lamivudine therapy be stopped when resistance develops.

On the surface the use of lamivudine in combination with interferon alfa appears to be a very attractive choice for the treatment of chronic hepatitis B, because both agents have independent effects and different mechanisms of action. To date, studies of combination therapy have not supported this presumption, and the addition of interferon does not seem to add substantially to the effect of lamivudine alone. This, therefore, raises the question of which of these two agents to choose in initiating therapy, and unfortunately there are no head-to-head comparisons of the therapies to help make this decision. The potential advantages of using interferon are that the duration of therapy is limited (no more than 6 months), and it seems to have a higher rate of HBeAg sero-conversion and sustained loss of HBV DNA. On the other hand, interferon has many side effects at the dosage used, some severe, and it must be given by subcutaneous injection. Lamivudine on the other hand is easy to take and has few side effects. It is also effective in immunosuppressed individuals whereas interferon is not. Its main limitations are the low rate of HBeAg seroconversion, a high relapse rate, and a high rate of viral resistance. Interferon might be a good first choice for patients with typical chronic hepatitis who are seropositive for HBeAg with elevated serum aminotransferases in the absence of decompensated liver disease, and if the patient does not respond to this treatment, then lamivudine could be tried. Lamivudine might be a good first choice in patients who have failed interferon therapy or don't fit into this typical pattern. For example, patients who are HBeAg negative but have HBV DNA in serum appear to have a better overall response to lamivudine than interferon and immunosuppressed patients (e. g., after organ transplantation or in chronic dialysis patients). Lamivudine has not been tested extensively in children and interferon is probably a better first choice in this group.

Chronic Hepatitis D

Therapy of chronic hepatitis D is difficult and not well standardized. Chronic hepatitis D is often severe, and natural history studies suggest that at least 70% of patients ultimately develop cirrhosis. Fortunately, chronic HDV is uncommon. The only therapy of benefit for HDV is interferon alfa therapy. The optimal regimen appears to be 10 MU subcutaneously three times weekly for at least 12 months. Between 30% and 50% of patients have a histologic and biochemical response to interferon alfa, and therapy can be stopped at 6 months if there has been no evidence of biochemical improvement. In patients who respond, serum HDV RNA falls to undetectable levels and HDV antigen in liver decreases. Unfortunately, many patients who respond later relapse when interferon therapy is stopped, and hepatitis activity and HDV RNA levels return to pretreatment levels. Longer courses of therapy have been tried with some success. Long-term remissions after interferon therapy have been reported, but remission occurs mainly among patients who become HBsAg negative during therapy—an outcome that occurs in only 10% to 20% of patients. Few other antiviral agents have been tried in cases of chronic delta hepatitis, and all agents have had little or no effect. Similarly, corticosteroid therapy has little or no benefit.

Indications for therapy in chronic delta hepatitis are the same as in hepatitis B, and general management, pretreatment evaluation, monitoring, and follow-up should follow the same regimen. In chronic delta hepatitis, therapy should not be continued for more than 6 months if there is no biochemical evidence of improvement. In patients who show a marked improvement on interferon and who are tolerating therapy well, long-term treatment should be considered. If HBsAg is lost during therapy, treatment with interferon can

be discontinued. Unfortunately, for most patients with chronic delta hepatitis, interferon therapy is not effective or is not well tolerated or practical.

Chronic Hepatitis C

Advances in therapy of hepatitis C have come rapidly since the first use of interferon alfa in the mid-1980s and the discovery of the hepatitis C virus (HCV) in 1989. The use of interferon alfa was codified at the NIH Consensus Conference held in 1997 in which interferon (3 MU three times weekly for at least 12 months) was recommended for most patients with chronic hepatitis C and raised serum aminotransferases. Unfortunately, this treatment regimen only achieved sustained response rates of about 20% to 25%. Since then, the use of interferon in combination with ribavirin, an oral nucleoside analogue, has become approved and currently appears to represent the best available initial therapy. The currently recommended therapy of chronic hepatitis C is a course of interferon alfa (3 MU subcutaneously three times a week) and ribavirin (1000 to 1200 mg/day orally, based on body weight) in combination for up to 48 weeks.

Ribavirin is a nucleoside analogue with a broad spectrum of antiviral activity, particularly against RNA viruses. Ribavirin can be taken orally and is generally well tolerated. Ribavirin monotherapy in patients with chronic hepatitis C results in significant decreases in serum aminotransferases and, after prolonged use, in improvement in liver histology. Interestingly, these improvements are not associated with the disappearance of or even a decrease in serum levels of HCV RNA, suggesting that ribavirin may act by mechanisms other than antiviral effects. The difficulty with monotherapy with ribavirin, however, is that the effects are only transient and almost all patients have a relapse when therapy is stopped.

In current studies of therapy for hepatitis C, a beneficial response to treatment is defined by serum biochemical, virologic, and histologic features and at set times, such as at 3 months (initial response), at 12 months (end-of-treatment response), and 6 to 12 months after therapy is discontinued (sustained response). Thus, a fall of serum aminotransferases into the normal range is referred to as a "biochemical" response, whereas the loss of HCV RNA from serum is referred to as a "virologic" response and an improvement in histologic score used to grade disease activity as a "histologic" response. In clinical practice, a combination of biochemical and virologic factors are suitable for defining a response. Thus, normal aminotransferases and lack of detectable HCV RNA in serum is evidence of a beneficial response. This response can be considered sustained if aminotransferases are normal and HCV RNA is not detectable 6 months or more after interferon therapy is discontinued. A follow-up liver biopsy is not needed.

McHuchinson and colleagues showed that sustained response rates as high as 38% could be achieved among patients treated with the combination of interferon and ribavirin for at least 12 months. Interestingly, this increase in response compared to interferon alone was noted even in some groups with low response rates (including those with cirrhosis) and high viral titers in serum and HCV genotype 1. The combination appears to substantially decrease the rate of relapse following therapy, which occurs frequently with interferon alone, and Davis and co-workers found a 10-fold increase in sustained response rate with the combination among patients who had previously relapsed when treated with interferon alone. An algorithm for evaluation, therapy, monitoring, and follow-up in chronic hepatitis C is given in Table 7–4.

The regimen should begin with documentation of the diagnosis and the grading and staging of the disease. Thus, there is an initial period of monitoring for serum aminotransferases, bilirubin, albumin, and prothrombin time followed by testing for HCV RNA in serum using the most sensitive assay available, which is currently PCR (Table 7–4). In some situations, testing for viral load (HCV RNA titer) and HCV genotype can be helpful when assessing the likelihood of a response to therapy. A liver biopsy should be done before therapy, if there are no contraindications, in order to assess the activity of the liver disease (grade) and the extent of hepatic fibrosis (stage). If the patient is a candidate for therapy, the expected results of treatment and side effects of interferon should be clearly defined for the patient.

Monitoring during therapy should include visits at 1- to 4-week intervals. Patients should be interviewed regarding side effects and symptoms and should be tested for serum aminotransferases and complete blood counts. Tests for HCV RNA should be repeated after 3 months, at the end of treatment, and approximately 6 months after stopping interferon therapy.

Table 7–4   Algorithm For Therapy of Hepatitis C

Initial Evaluation
Serial ALT levels
Presence of HCV RNA
Determination of HCV genotype (for combination therapy only)
Liver biopsy
Review side effects and expected results
Lack of contraindications
Ensure adequate and appropriate contraception

Initiate Therapy
Alpha interferon given subcutaneously in a dose of 3 MU thrice weekly with or without ribavirin 1000–1200 mg/day for 24–48 weeks

Monitoring During Therapy
Every 2 to 4 weeks
　　Symptoms and signs
　　ALT, AST, bilirubin, albumin
　　CBC and differential
At 3, 6, and 12 months
　　HCV RNA, TSH, prothrombin time
At 3–6 months:
　　If HCV RNA +ve <u>and</u> ALT abnormal
　　Stop therapy

Follow-up After therapy
Every 3 months
　　Symptoms and signs
　　ALT, AST, bilirubin, albumin
　　CBC
At 6 months after stopping therapy: HCV RNA

ALT, alanine aminotransferase; AST, aspartate transaminase; CBC, complete blood count; HCV, hepatitis C virus; TSH, thyroid-stimulating hormone.

Extreme caution should be exercised in the use of ribavirin in women of child-bearing age, who should be counselled to avoid pregnancy during and for at least 6 months after treatment with interferon. In fact, men are also advised to use contraceptives during and after a course of ribavirin. This agent should also be avoided in patients with pre-existing anemia and underlying coronary artery or other heart disease, which may be exacerbated by the development of anemia.

The side effects of interferon are similar to those described with therapy of hepatitis B (see Table 7–3). An important side effect that is somewhat specific to patients with hepatitis C is a paradoxic worsening of disease. Between 2% and 5% of patients have a flare of hepatitis during therapy that can be severe and even life threatening. This exacerbation may represent the induction of autoimmune hepatitis by the interferon therapy. For this reason, therapy should be stopped if alanine aminotransferase (ALT) levels double from baseline during the course of therapy, and patients should be followed carefully thereafter. This recommendation is very different in hepatitis B, in which a flare of hepatitis is common during therapy and often represents the first evidence of a beneficial response to therapy.

The main side effect of ribavirin is dose-dependent hemolysis whic may result in a drop in hemoglobin level of 3 to 4 g/dL during treatment. Although this drop in blood count is usually well tolerated, it may occasionally provoke episodes of ischemia among those with underlying coronary artery disease. Ribavirin is well known to be teratogenic in animals, although this has not been shown unequivocally in humans. Nonetheless, extreme caution is warranted, as described earlier.

Patients with hepatitis C who respond to interferon therapy generally demonstrate a rapid improvement in serum aminotransferases and disappearance of detectable HCV RNA within 1 to 2 months. In large clinical trials of interferon alone, patients who did not demonstrate evidence of a response by 3 months of therapy rarely responded later. For these reasons, it is recommended that serum be retested for HCV RNA by a sensitive PCR technique after 3 months of therapy. If ALT levels are not normal and HCV RNA is still present, a response is unlikely and therapy should be discontinued. This "3-month rule" for continuing or stopping therapy is a practical method of avoiding the expense and difficulty of a 12-month course of interferon in a patient who is obviously not responding to therapy. However, it is not always clear whether a response has occurred at 3 months. Thus, if the patient has normal ALT levels but is HCV RNA positive, or has abnormal ALT levels but is HCV RNA negative, the choice of whether to continue treatment or not is difficult. In general, it is prudent to continue therapy if either ALT levels are normal or HCV RNA is no longer detectable; therapy should be stopped only if both are abnormal.

Furthermore, these guidelines may not apply to patients treated with the combination of interferon and ribavirin. Thus, in the study reported by McHuchinson and colleagues, several patients who cleared HCV RNA beyond 12 weeks of therapy still went on to have a sustained response. Thus, for patients receiving this combination, HCV RNA and ALT should be assessed after 24 weeks of treatment in order to decide whether to complete the 48-week course of therapy.

Follow-up of patients who have received interferon alfa therapy with or without ribavirin for chronic hepatitis C demonstrates that the sustained loss of HCV RNA from serum is associated with sustained improvements in serum biochemical test results and also in liver histology studies. Most current evidence suggests that this sustained clearance of detectable HCV RNA represents a "cure" of hepatitis C. Patients with sustained clearance of HCV RNA generally have inactive liver disease and have been free of complications of chronic hepatitis C, such as development of cirrhosis, end-stage liver disease, hepatic failure, and hepatocellular carcinoma. A proportion of patients who have a biochemical response (normal ALT levels) have persistent detectable HCV RNA in serum. Histologic features also improve in these patients, but long-term follow-up studies show that most patients who remain HCV RNA positive ultimately have a relapse. Thus, persistence of HCV RNA with normal ALT levels after therapy should be considered a remission in, but not a cure of, chronic hepatitis C.

Sustained responses to interferon alfa therapy are not frequent but are clinically important. A major focus of therapy is therefore optimizing the possibility of achieving a sustained virologic response to a course of interferon alfa. Studies using higher doses and more prolonged courses of interferon have achieved only modestly better response rates, and these approaches are more expensive and are often poorly tolerated. Different forms of interferon alfa therapy (e.g., alfa-2a, alfa-2b, consensus alfa, and natural and lymphoblastoid interferon) may have slightly different potencies and side effects, but overall, one-on-one comparisons have found little difference in sustained responses with different formulations. Similarly, combination of interferon alfa with other nonspecific medications such as nonsteroidal anti-inflammatory drugs or ursodiol have not augmented the response rate to interferon alone.

An indirect method of increasing the response rate to interferon alfa is to select patients who are most likely to respond. Several factors have been identified that correlate with a high likelihood of a sustained response to interferon alone. These factors include: (1) low pretreatment levels of HCV RNA, (2) HCV genotypes 2 and 3 (as opposed to genotype 1), (3) lack of cirrhosis and lesser degrees of hepatic fibrosis, (4) short duration of disease, (5) young age, and (6) lack of other serious medical conditions such as renal failure, immunosuppression, or HIV infection. Thus, response rates to interferon in patients with HCV genotypes 2 and 3 have averaged 30% to 50%, whereas rates in patients with genotypes 1a or 1b have been as low as 5% to 15%. In like manner, response rates in patients with low levels of HCV RNA (<1 million genome equivalents per milliliter) have been 25% to 40%, whereas rates in those with high levels (>10 million) have been below 10%. Patients with cirrhosis also have low rates of response (usually less than 10%). It is important to point out that none of these features is completely reliable and that these factors are not really helpful in guiding management. Furthermore, most of these factors have been identified in studies using a 6-month course of interferon alfa therapy, a time frame that has been shown to be suboptimal.

The correlation of high rates of response with a short duration of illness, young age, and lack of fibrosis supports early therapy for hepatitis C in young persons with mild degrees of hepatic fibrosis. Unfortunately, age and degree of fibrosis, like most of the predictive factors for a response, are fixed and cannot be altered. A factor that correlates with a response that can be altered is the amount of hepatic iron. In several retrospective analyses, the amount of hepatic iron as assessed quantitatively on liver biopsy samples correlated inversely with the likelihood of a response. These findings have suggested that phlebotomy or chelation of iron before or during therapy with interferon may increase the rate of sustained response. This attractive hypothesis is currently being evaluated, but pilot studies to date suggest that phlebotomy does not increase the rate of sustained responses to interferon alfa.

Although the predictive factors described earlier hold true to some extent when patients are treated with interferon and ribavirin, this combination appears to offer hope of significant rates of sustained response even among patients in whom a poor response might be predicted (Table 7–5).

A recent National Institutes of Health (NIH) Consensus Development Conference on the Management of Hepatitis C provided fairly detailed guidance on indications for therapy and management. The Consensus Conference Panel recommended that therapy be offered to all patients between the ages of 18 and 60 years who have HCV RNA in serum, persistent elevations in serum aminotransferases, and liver biopsy histology demonstrating fibrosis or moderate degrees of inflammation and necrosis. For patients younger than 18 years of age or older than 60 years of age, patients with cirrhosis on biopsy, and patients with milder degrees of hepatitis, the relative benefits of current regimens of therapy are not clear. For these patients, therapy should be offered only after careful consideration of the potential benefits and risks of treatment. In these patients, monitoring on no therapy and reassessment at regular intervals is appropriate, especially as the field of therapy of hepatitis C is changing so rapidly and as current therapies have limited success rates despite

Table 7–5 Rates of Sustained Virologic Response According to Pretreatment Variables in Patients with Chronic Hepatitis C Treated with the Combination of Interferon and Ribavirin for a Period of 48 Weeks

Variable	Patients (No.)	Sustained Response (No.)	%
Genotype			
1	166	46	28
Other	61	41	66
Base-line serum HCV RNA level			
>2×10⁶ copies/mL	152	54	36
<2×10⁶ copies/mL	76	33	43
Degree of fibrosis at base line			
Cirrhosis or bridging fibrosis	55	21	38
Minimal or no fibrosis	159	62	39

*Adapted from McHuchinson JG, Gordon SC, Schiff ER, et al: Interferon alfa-2b alone or in combination with ribavirin as initial treatment for chronic hepatitis. N Engl J Med 339:1485-1492, 1998.

expensive and prolonged therapy. The Consensus Panel recommended that patients with normal aminotransferases not be treated, but be monitored with repeat serum aminotransferases at 6- to 12-month intervals or be enrolled in properly controlled trials of therapy. The Panel also recommended that patients with decompensated cirrhosis due to hepatitis C not be treated with interferon alfa but rather be referred for evaluation for liver transplantation. It was further recommended that treatment should be delayed in patients drinking significant amounts of alcohol or using illicit drugs until these habits have been stopped for at least 6 months. Relative contraindications to interferon include bone marrow compromise, active drug or alcohol abuse, severe psychiatric or neurologic problems, solid organ transplantation, and pregnancy, whereas relative contraindications to interferon with ribavirin include anemia, underlying heart disease, and the inability to practice appropriate contraception.

Patients who experience a relapse of hepatitis after treatment with interferon alone may be retreated with interferon alfa-con1 or the combination of interferon and ribavirin. (Heathcote et al; Davis et al). Options for those who are nonresponders to interferon include re-treatment with interferon alfa-con1, which is associated with a sustained response rate of 17%, expectant management, or some form of experimental therapy (Heathcote et al). Preliminary results from trials of combination therapy in interferon nonresponders show variable results, although as many as 25% have been reported to have a sustained response when retreated with interferon together with ribavirin. Some experimental options include use of high doses of interferon to initiate therapy ("induction therapy"), newer long-acting forms of interferon conjugated with polyethylene glycol (PEGylated interferons), and therapies aimed at suppressing liver disease activity rather than eliminating HCV infection (e.g., iron reduction by phlebotomy or long-term low-dose therapy with interferon alone).

A few patients with chronic hepatitis C have extrahepatic manifestations such as cryoglobulinemia and glomerulonephritis. In these patients, interferon therapy can be associated with a remission in the symptoms of cryoglobulinemia, a reduction in rheumatoid factor and cryoglobulins, and improvements in renal function. Unfortunately, a relapse of the disease and a return of serum HCV RNA occur in most patients when interferon therapy is stopped. In this group of patients, long-term, continuous therapy with interferon alfa may be appropriate. The combination of interferon and ribavirin has not been studied in this group.

Of course, the most likely method of increasing the response rate to therapy is by identification of more potent and effective antiviral agents, which might be used alone or in combination with interferon alfa. The lack of a reliable cell culture system and a convenient animal model for hepatitis C has made it difficult to identify new agents that might be effective against this disease. The complete characterization of the HCV genome and structural analysis of HCV proteins including the viral protease, helicase, and polymerase will clearly help to develop new antiviral agents.

Patients on immunosuppressive therapy or with untreated HIV infection do not seem to respond to interferon therapy as well as immunocompetent patients, possibly because interferon requires an intact immune effector system

to work. For hepatitis B patients, nucleoside analogues are probably more appropriate to use than interferon, although few studies have been conducted in this context. For hepatitis C, there are at present no suitable alternatives to interferon. Patients with early HIV infection (preserved CD4 counts), or who have been treated so as to reconstitute their immunity, may be treated with interferon either for hepatitis B or C.

LIVER TRANSPLANTATION FOR CHRONIC VIRAL HEPATITIS

Viral hepatitis is now the single most common indication for liver transplantation in adults and accounts for most cases. In some instances, transplantation may be done for hepatocellular carcinoma associated with chronic hepatitis B or C. Reinfection of the grafted liver occurs commonly with hepatitis B, particularly in patients who are seropositive for HBeAg and HBV DNA. The recurrent hepatitis B tends to be severe and rapidly progressive. As a consequence, the survival after liver transplantation for hepatitis B is poor (<50% at 2 years), and there is resistance to performing liver transplantation for this diagnosis. However, several recent publications have shown that prophylaxis with high doses of hepatitis B immunoglobulin (HBIG) started at the time of transplant and continued indefinitely, with repeated infusions aimed at keeping the titer of anti-HBs to above 500 IU/mL, is successful in preventing reinfection in more than 90% of patients and even in those with HBeAg and HBV DNA pretransplant. Survival in these patients has been excellent, above 90% at 2 years. Unfortunately, the HBIG must be continued indefinitely, and late recurrences have been reported even after years of successful use of HBIG. Furthermore, HBIG is expensive, difficult to administer, and in short supply, especially in the United States.

More recently, the second-generation nucleoside analogues have been used to treat and also prevent the recurrence of hepatitis B after transplantation. In preliminary studies, more than 80% of patients started on lamivudine before transplantation and continued on the agent afterwards have remained free of a recurrence of the disease up to 2 years post transplant. In this situation, some patients have developed viral resistance and breakthrough of infection. The ease of administration and lack of major side effects have made use of oral nucleoside analogues an attractive method of therapy and prevention of hepatitis B in the transplant situation. The efficacy and safety of these two approaches in preventing a recurrence of hepatitis B after liver transplantation have not been fully evaluated, but ultimately a combination of these two approaches may be optimal in making transplantation a reliable method of managing patients with end-stage liver disease due to HBV.

Liver transplantation for hepatitis C is almost always followed by reinfection of the grafted liver. However, the recurrent hepatitis C is usually mild and only rarely demonstrates a progressive course with redevelopment of cirrhosis. On the other hand, the long-term natural history of recurrent hepatitis C after liver transplantation is not well defined, and a recurrence of cirrhosis may develop years or perhaps decades after the transplant. For this reason, the development of safe and effective methods of prevention and therapy are greatly needed. Unfortunately, interferon alfa by itself has little effect on hepatitis C after transplantation and may be harmful, inducing acute or chronic rejection. Ribavirin and the combination of ribavirin with interferon are only now being evaluated but may provide a method of management for patients with severe progressive recurrent disease.

SUMMARY AND CONCLUSIONS

Therapy for patients with chronic hepatitis B, C, and D is appropriate for patients with active liver disease with accompanying detectable levels of viral replication. Therapy is generally not indicated for patients with minimal or mild disease or for those with normal serum aminotransferases. Therapy is not generally recommended for patients with decompensated liver disease or for patients who are immunocompromised. The goals of therapy are to eradicate viral replication or reduce it to low and nonpathogenic levels. Interferon alfa usually needs to be administered for prolonged periods (indefinitely for hepatitis D, 12 to 18 months for hepatitis C, and 4 to 6 months for hepatitis B) and appears to act by a combination of antiviral and antiproliferative actions. Unfortunately, only a few patients with chronic viral hepatitis have a sustained beneficial response to interferon therapy. The use of the second-generation nucleoside analogues offers considerable promise in the treatment of hepatitis B, and the combination therapy of ribavirin with interferon alfa shows promise as therapy for hepatitis C. New antiviral agents are badly needed for all forms of chronic viral hepatitis.

SUGGESTED READINGS

Belle SH, Beringer KC, Detre KM: Liver transplantation in the United States: Results from the National Pitt-UNOS liver transplant registry. United Network for Organ Sharing. In Teraska PI, Crecka JM (eds): Clinical Transplants 1994. Los Angeles: UCLA Press, 1994, pp 19–35.

Boyer N, Marcellin P, Degott C, et al: Recombinant interferon-a for chronic hepatitis C in patients positive for antibody to human immunodeficiency virus. J Infect Dis 165:723–726, 1992.

Brillanti S, Garson J, Foli M, et al: A pilot study of combination therapy with ribavirin plus interferon alfa for interferon alfa-resistant chronic hepatitis C. Gastroenterology 107:812–817, 1994.

Conjeevaram HS, Di Bisceglie AM: Management of chronic viral hepatitis in children. J Pediatr Gastroenterol Nutr 20:365–375, 1995.

Davis GL, Esteban-Mur R, Rustgi V, et al: Interferon alfa-2b alone or in combination with ribavirin for the treatment of relapse of chronic hepatitis C. N Engl J Med 339:1493–1499, 1998.

Desmet VJ, Gerber M, Hoofnagle JH, et al: Classification of chronic hepatitis: Diagnosis, grading and staging. Hepatology 19:1513–1520, 1994.

Di Bisceglie AM, Conjeevaram HS, Fried MW, et al: Ribavirin as therapy for chronic hepatitis C: A randomized, double-blind, placebo-controlled trial. Ann Intern Med 123:897–903, 1995.

Dienstag JL, Perrillo RP, Schiff ER, et al: A preliminary trial of lamivudine for chronic hepatitis B infection. N Engl J Med 333:1657–1661, 1995.

Dienstag JL, Schiff ER, Mitchell M, et al: Extended lamivudine retreatment for chronic hepatitis B (Abstract). Hepatology 24:188A, 1996.

Farci P, Mandas A, Coiana A, et al: Treatment of chronic hepatitis D with interferon alfa-2a. N Engl J Med 330:88–94, 1994.

Heathcote EJL, Keeffe EB, Lee SS, et al: Re-treatment of chronic hepatitis C with consensus interferon. Hepatology 27:1136–1143, 1998.

Hoofnagle JH: Type D (delta) hepatitis. JAMA 261:1321–1325, 1989.

Hoofnagle JH, Di Bisceglie AM: Serologic diagnosis of acute and chronic viral hepatitis. Semin Liver Dis 11:73–83, 1991.

Hoofnagle JH, Di Bisceglie AM: The treatment of chronic viral hepatitis. N Engl J Med 336:347–356, 1997.

Kim JL, Morgernstern KA, Lin C, et al: Crystal structure of the hepatitis C virus NS3 protease domain complexed with a synthetic NS4A cofactor peptide. Cell 87:343–355, 1996.

Lau JYN, Mizokami M, Ohno T, et al: Discrepancy between biochemical and virological responses to interferon-a in chronic hepatitis C. Lancet 342:1208–1209, 1993.

Ling R, Mutimer D, Ahmed M, et al: Selection of mutations in the hepatitis B virus polymerase during therapy of transplant recipients with lamivudine. Hepatology 24:711–715, 1996.

Linnen J, Wages J, Zhang-Keck Z-Y, et al: Molecular cloning and disease association of hepatitis G virus: A transfusion-transmissible agent. Science 271:505–508, 1996.

Lunel F, Musset L: Hepatitis C virus infection and cryoglobulinemia. Viral Hep Rev 2:111–124, 1996.

Marcellin P, Boyer N, De Gott C, et al: Long-term histologic and viral changes in patients with chronic hepatitis C who responded to alpha interferon. Liver 14:302–307, 1994.

Martinot-Peignoux M, Marcellin P, Pouteau M, et al: Pretreatment serum hepatitis C virus RNA levels and hepatitis C virus genotype are the main and independent prognostic factors of sustained response to interferon alfa therapy in chronic hepatitis C. Hepatology 22:1050–1056, 1995.

McDonnell WM, Lok ASF: Testing for hepatitis C virus RNA in serum: When and how? Viral Hep Rev 2:81–84, 1996.

McHuchinson JG, Gordon SC, Schiff ER, et al: Interferon alfa-2b alone or in combination with ribavirin as initial treatment for chronic hepatitis C. N Engl J Med 339:1485–1492, 1998.

National Institutes of Health Consensus Development Conference Panel Statement: Management of hepatitis C. Hepatology 26:2S–10S, 1997.

Niederau C, Heintges T, Lange S, et al: Long-term follow-up of HBeAg-positive patients treated with interferon alfa for chronic hepatitis B. N Engl J Med 334:1422–1427, 1996.

Olynyk JK, Reddy KR, Di Bisceglie AM, et al: Hepatic iron concentration as a predictor of response to interferon alfa therapy in chronic hepatitis C. Gastroenterology 108:1104–1109, 1995.

Phillips MJ, Blendis LM, Poucell S, et al: Syncytial giant cell hepatitis. Sporadic hepatitis with distinctive pathological features, a severe clinical course, and paramyxoviral features. N Engl J Med 324:455–460, 1991.

Polito AJ, DiNello RK, Quan S, et al: New generation RIBA hepatitis C strip immunoblot assays. Ann Biol Clin 50:329–336, 1992.

Reichard O, Norkrans G, Fryder A, et al: Randomised, double-blind, placebo-controlled trial of interferon alpha-2b with and without ribavirin for chronic hepatitis C. Lancet 351:83–87, 1998.

Renault PF, Hoofnagle JH: Side effects of alpha interferon. Semin Liver Dis 9:273–278, 1989.

Rosina F, Pintus C, Meschievitz C, Rizzetto M: A randomized controlled trial of a 12-month course of recombinant human interferon-a in chronic delta (type D) hepatitis: A multicenter Italian study. Hepatology 13:1052–1056, 1991.

Samuel D, Muller R, Alexander G, et al: Liver transplantation in European patients with the hepatitis B surface antigen. N Engl J Med 329:1842–1847, 1993.

Tanaka E, Alter HJ, Nakatsuji Y, et al: Effect of hepatitis G virus infection on chronic hepatitis C. Ann Intern Med 125:740–743, 1996.

Wong DKH, Cheung AM, O'Rourke K, et al: Effect of alpha-interferon treatment in patients with hepatitis B e antigen-positive chronic hepatitis B: A meta-analysis. Ann Intern Med 119:312–323, 1993.

Chapter

8

Autoimmune Hepatitis

Michael P. Manns

The existence of autoimmune hepatitis (AIH) has been a challenging concept since its first description in young women by Waldenström. Shortly thereafter, the syndrome was described in the United States. Owing to the association of AIH with antinuclear antibodies (ANAs), Mackay proposed the term *lupoid hepatitis*. The International Autoimmune Hepatitis Group has defined diagnostic criteria for AIH. At the time of diagnosis, the disease has usually been present for 6 months or longer, and patients show high levels of serum aminotransferases. Histology reveals periportal or periseptal hepatitis (piecemeal necrosis). The disease progresses further to bridging necrosis, panlobular and multilobular necrosis, and active cirrhosis. Without treatment, AIH is associated with a high mortality rate (up to 50% of patients with severe AIH die in approximately 5 years) and a low rate of spontaneous remission. The diagnosis of AIH is based on particular features that are typical for AIH and on exclusion of other causes of chronic hepatitis (Tables 8–1 and 8–2). Excluded are patients with ongoing infections with hepatitis viruses or significant alcohol intake. Features characteristic for autoimmune hepatitis are female sex (female-to-male ratio of 4:1), hypergammaglobulinemia, circulating autoantibodies, benefit from immunosuppression, extrahepatic clinical autoimmune syndromes, and over-representation of human leukocyte antigen (HLA) alleles DR3 or DR4. These features are summarized in a provisional scoring system for the diagnosis of AIH (see Table 8–1). According to the autoantibodies found in AIH, it was proposed to classify AIH into subtypes 1 to 3 (see Table 8–2). AIH type 1 is characterized by antinuclear or antismooth muscle autoantibodies; AIH type 2 by antibodies specific for liver and kidney microsomes (LKMs), and AIH type 3 by autoantibodies against cytosolic liver antigens or antibodies to the liver-pancreas antigen (anti-LP). Further autoantibodies associated with AIH are directed against the asialoglycoprotein receptor (ASGPR) and the liver cytosol 1 antigen (anti-LC1).

EPIDEMIOLOGY

Compared with other liver diseases, AIH is a rare disorder. The prevalence is estimated to be between 50 and 200 cases per 1 million for Northern European and North American white populations. This is comparable with the prevalence of other autoimmune diseases, such as primary biliary cirrhosis, systemic lupus erythematosus, and myasthenia gravis. In Northern European and North American white populations, AIH occurs in up to 20% of all patients with chronic hepatitis. Owing to the overwhelming prevalence of viral hepatitis, the relative frequency of AIH is rather low in countries endemic for viral hepatitis such as Africa and Asia. In Japan, AIH does occur, however, at a lower frequency and is usually associated with HLA DR4 and a higher age at onset. Most data used today are from the period before the discovery of the hepatitis C virus. It is necessary, therefore, to obtain current epidemiologic data based on our present knowledge of the etiology of the heterogeneous syndrome of chronic hepatitis, in particular based on modern technology to discover hepatitis C virus (HCV) infection and to diagnose AIH.

ETIOLOGY AND PATHOPHYSIOLOGY

Several agents have been considered as triggers for the self-perpetuating autoimmune process in AIH (e.g., viruses, bacteria, chemicals, drugs, genetics), and recent attention has focused on viruses. All the major hepatotropic viruses have

Table 8–1 Scoring System for Diagnosis of Autoimmune Hepatitis: Minimum Required Parameters

Parameter	Score
Gender	
Female	+2
Male	0
Serum biochemistry	
Ratio of elevation of serum alkaline phosphatase versus aminotransferase, ALT	
>3.0	−2
<3.0	+2
Total serum globulin, γ-globulin, or IgG	
Times upper normal limit	
>2.0	+3
1.5–2.0	+2
1.0–1.5	+1
<1.0	0
Autoantibodies (titers by immunofluorescence on rodent tissues)	
Adults	
ANA, SMA, or LKM-1	
>1:80	+3
1:80	+2
1:40	+1
<1:40	0
Children	
ANA or LKM-1	
>1:20	+3
1:10 or 1:20	+2
<1:10	0
or SMA	
>1:20	+3
1:20	+2
<1:20	0
Antimitochondrial antibody	
Positive	−2
Negative	0
Viral markers	
IgM anti-HAV, HBsAg or IgM anti-HBc–positive	−3
Anti-HCV positive by ELISA or RIBA	−2
HCV positive by PCR for HCV RNA	−3
Positive test result indicating active infection with any other virus	−3
Seronegative for all of the above	+3
Other etiologic factors	
History of recent hepatotoxic drug usage or parenteral exposure to blood products	
Yes	−2
No	+1
Alcohol (average consumption)	
Male <35 g/day; female <25 g/day	+2
Male 35–50 g/day; female 25–40 g/day	0
Male 50–80 g/day; female 40–60 g/day	−1
Male >80 g/day; female >60 g/day	−2
Genetic factors: HLA DR3 or DR4	+1
Other autoimmune diseases in patients or first-degree relatives	+1

Interpretation of aggregate scores: definite AIH, greater than 15 before treatment and greater than 17 after treatment; probable AIH 10 to 15 before treatment and 12 to 17 after treatment. (According to Johnson PJ, McFarlane IG, Meeting report of the International Autoimmune Hepatitis Group. Hepatology 18:998-1005, 1993).

been suggested to cause AIH, such as measles viruses, hepatitis A virus (HAV), hepatitis B virus (HBV), HCV, hepatitis D virus (HDV), herpes simplex virus type 1 (HSV-1), and Epstein-Barr virus (EBV).

There are several observations that AIH can develop after acute HAV infection. This observation has also been made regarding hepatitis B infection. In the early 1990s, there was a lively discussion on the relationship of HCV to the induction of AIH. Hepatitis C does not induce AIH, but HCV infection is associated with autoimmune markers that are also seen in AIH (Table 8–3). Hepatitis D is also associated with several autoimmune reactions, in particular with several autoantibodies. However, there is no proof that HDV can cause AIH. Recent interest has concentrated on hepatitis G (GBV-C). This recently discovered group of viruses is also not the major cause of AIH. The prevalence of GBV-C RNA in AIH is between 9% and 15%, depending on the serologic subgroup. This is about the range seen for cryptogenic chronic hepatitis and is below the prevalence of GBV-C in other liver diseases (e.g., chronic viral hepatitis).

The major B cell epitope of antibodies against cytochrome P-450 2D6, the major LKM-1 antigen, shares sequence homology with the immediate early protein IE 175 of herpes simplex virus type 1 (Fig. 8–1). Although there are some observations that AIH may develop after herpes virus infection, this does not seem to be a major cause of AIH. Furthermore, another peptide of cytochrome P-450 2D6 (epitope E2) shares sequence homology with the 21 hydroxylase of the adrenal gland and the carboxypeptidase H of the pancreas. Therefore, an exogenous agent sharing a sequence with these enzymes of different organs may trigger autoimmunity, leading to an autoimmune process that attacks various tissues. The clinical presentation, however, could depend on additional factors, including the genetic background of the patient.

The earlier observation that measles virus infection was found to be associated with AIH could not be confirmed. AIH has been associated with EBV infection. It is unknown whether certain drugs or chemicals can cause AIH. The mechanisms for immune-mediated drug-induced hepatitis may serve as models. Drugs may be a trigger of AIH. However, no particular drug has been identified as a true etiologic agent for AIH. It is interesting that drug-metabolizing enzymes of phase I and phase II (i.e., cytochromes P-450 and UDP glucuronosyltransferase proteins) are targets of virus-induced and drug-induced autoimmunity as well as of AIH. It seems that different etiologic agents may trigger autoimmunity against the same molecular target. For example, P-450 2D6 is the target for autoantibodies in AIH and hepatitis C. P-450 1A2 is the target in AIH as part of the autoimmune polyendocrine syndrome type 1 (APS-1) and in dihydralazine-induced hepatitis. In any case, a specific immunogenetic background seems to be an important prerequisite for AIH. Most likely, the manifestation of AIH is a result of multiple factors. One could think of a necessary specific genetic background and a specific agent triggering the autoimmune process (Fig. 8–2). This can be a virus or a chemical. Other cofactors may be necessary; for example, female hormones and environmental reagents that upregulate or downregulate mediators or components of the immune system, or even autoantigens. One could think of environmental reagents such as nicotine, alcohol, and nutrients

Table 8–2 Classification of Chronic Hepatitis on the Basis of Etiology

Hepatitis Type	HBsAg	HBV DNA	HDV Antibody (HDV RNA)	HCV Antibody (HCV RNA)	Autoantibodies
B	+	±	–	–	—
D	+	±	+	–	10–20% anti-LKM-3
C	–	–	–	+	2–10% anti-LKM-1
Autoimmune					
Type 1	–	–	–	–	ANA, SMA
Type 2	–	–	–	–	LKM-1
Type 3	–	–	–	–	SLA/LP
Drug-induced	–	–	–	–	Some: ANA, LKM, LM
Cryptogenic	–	–	–	–	—

HBV, hepatitis B virus; HDV, hepatitis D virus; SLA, soluble liver antigen antibody; LP, liver-pancreas antigen antibody; LM, liver microsomal antibody; ANA, antinuclear antibody; LKM-1, liver and kidney microsomes.
Modified from Desmet V, Gerber MA, Hoofnagle JH, et al: Classification of chronic hepatitis: Diagnosis, grading and staging. Hepatology 9:1513–1520, 1994.

Table 8–3 Comparison of Clinical Features of Autoimmune Hepatitis Type 2 and HCV-Associated Autoimmunity (LKM)

	Autoimmune Hepatitis Type 2	Chronic Hepatitis C Associated with LKM-1 Autoantibodies
Age	Young	Older
Sex	90% Female	No prevalence
ALT	↑↑↑	↑
LKM-1 titer	↑↑↑	↑
LKM-1 antigen	P-450 2D6	P-450 2D6, 59 kD, 70 kD
Conformational autoepitopes	+	+++
Immunosuppression effective	+++	–
Interferon effective	–	(+) Possibly side effects increased
HLA DR3	++	+
C4A-Q0	+	+
Anti-HCV/HCV RNA	–	+

HCV, hepatitis C virus; LKM-1, liver and kidney microsome type 1.

that up- or downregulate drug-metabolizing enzymes, which then become autoantigens.

A loss of tolerance against the patient's own liver is regarded as the primary pathogenetic mechanism (see Fig. 8–2). A genetic predisposition is an absolute prerequisite. It is unclear whether the autoimmune disease process develops spontaneously or whether specific environmental agents trigger the process in genetically susceptible individuals. Autoantibodies to liver tissue are hallmarks of such an autoimmune process (Table 8–4). Typical for AIH type 1 are significant titers of ANAs and smooth muscle antibodies (SMAs). The most frequent method of detection of ANA is indirect immunofluorescence on Hep-2 cells. Depending on the autoantigens detected, different patterns of fluorescence

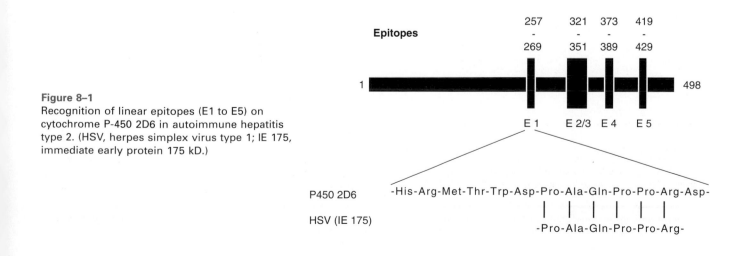

Figure 8–1
Recognition of linear epitopes (E1 to E5) on cytochrome P-450 2D6 in autoimmune hepatitis type 2. (HSV, herpes simplex virus type 1; IE 175, immediate early protein 175 kD.)

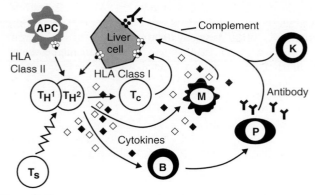

Figure 8–2
Pathogenesis of autoimmune hepatitis. (Modified from Vergani D, Mieli-Vergani G: Autoimmune hepatitis: Cellular immune reactions. In Meyer zum Büschenfelde KH, Hoofnagle J, Manns M [eds]: Immunology and Liver. Boston: Kluwer, 1993, pp 233–239.)

are found: homogeneous-nuclear (58%), speckled (21%), homogeneous-speckled (10%), centromere (9%), or homogeneous-perinuclear (6%). Each pattern is associated with the recognition of several nuclear antigens with a wide range of molecular weights. Among ANAs are autoantibodies directed against ss-DNA, ds-DNA, sn-RNPs, t-RNA, lamin A, and lamin C. Recently, cyclin A was discovered as another species of antigens of antinuclear antibodies. To date, neither a liver-specific nuclear antigen nor a liver disease–specific ANA has been identified. No convincing data are available to prove that some or all of these ANA specificities contribute to tissue destruction.

SMAs are directed against structures of the cytoskeleton. SMAs are measured by indirect immunofluorescence on smooth muscle cells that have a well-developed cytoskeleton, owing to their contractile function. Antibodies to actin represent a subset of SMA antibodies that are found at particular frequency in AIH type 1. In AIH, SMA are predominantly directed against F-actin. Antiactin antibodies in AIH have been further analyzed. Actin antibody–positive patients were younger, were more commonly HLA DR 3–positive, and death and transplantation occurred more frequently in these patients than in actin antibody–negative patients with ANA. Again, the diagnostic relevance of SMA goes far beyond their possible involvement in pathophysiology.

AIH type 2 is characterized by the presence of LKM-1 autoantibodies. Their characteristic feature is the exclusive staining of liver tissue and of the P3 portion of the proximal renal tubules. Western blots with hepatic microsomes reveal a protein band at 50 kD. In addition to the 50-kD protein, a 55-kD protein and a 64-kD protein were detected at a lower frequency. In up to 67% of patients with AIH type 2, antibodies to liver cytosol type 1 (anti-LC-1) are detected. The significance of anti-LC-1 autoantibodies in AIH type 2, however, is not clear. Cytochrome P-450 2D6 is the major antigen for LKM-1 autoantibodies. In vitro, the enzymatic activity of cytochrome P-450 2D6 is inhibited by LKM-1 autoantibodies. Cytochrome P-450 2D6 in humans shows a significant polymorphism. The absence of functional cytochrome P-450 2D6 results in a low metabolizer phenotype for debrisoquine or sparteine, which are both substrates for cytochrome P-450 2D6. Studies with sparteine as a test substrate permitted measurement of P-450 2D6 activity in vivo. To date, all patients with LKM-1 antibodies are extensive metabolizers of sparteine and express functionally intact cytochrome P-450 2D6 protein. LKM-1 autoantibodies inhibit P-450 2D6 activity in vitro, but not in vivo. An adequate ex-

Table 8–4 Major Autoantibodies in Liver Diseases

	Antigen	Disease Association
ANAs	Very heterogeneous	Autoimmune hepatitis
		Minor: PBC, PSC, viral hepatitis, drug-induced hepatitis
LKM antibodies		
LKM-1	Cytochrome P-450 2D6	Autoimmune hepatitis type 2, hepatitis C
LKM-2	Cytochrome P-450 2C9	Ticrynafen-hepatitis
LKM-3	UDP-glucuronosyltransferases	Hepatitis D, autoimmune hepatitis type 2
LM	Cytochrome P-450 1A2	Dihydralazine-hepatitis, hepatitis in the APS-1 syndrome
Anti-SMA	F-actin	Autoimmune hepatitis, chronic viral hepatitis C
Antibodies to cytosolic antigens		
SLA	Cytokeratins	Autoimmune hepatitis type 3
LP	?	Autoimmune hepatitis type 3
Anti-LC1	?	Autoimmune hepatitis type 2
Anti-LC2	?	Autoimmune hepatitis type 2
Autoantibodies to hepatocellular membrane antigens	Asialoglycoprotein receptor (ASGPR)	Autoimmune liver diseases, namely autoimmune hepatitis
AMAs	Acyltransferases, in particular PDH-E2	PBC
ANCAs		PSC (minor) autoimmune hepatitis

LKM, liver-kidney-microsomal; SMA, smooth muscle antibodies; AMA, antimitochondrial antibodies; ANCA, antineutrophilic cytoplasmic antibodies; ANAs, antinuclear antibodies; PBC, primary biliary cirrhosis; PSC, primary sclerosing cholangitis.

pression of P-450 2D6 seems to be a prerequisite for the development of LKM-1 autoantibodies directed against P-450 2D6.

The epitopes recognized by LKM-1 autoantibodies have been characterized. AIH sera recognize at least four different linear epitopes as well as additional conformational epitopes on cytochrome P-450 2D6. Linear epitope No. 1 consists of a short linear sequence of eight amino acids that span amino acids 257 to 269 DPAQPPRD (see Fig. 8–1). The inhibitory activity of LKM-1 antibody is caused by the presence of autoantibodies to conformational epitopes. This hypothesis has been confirmed. As multiple epitopes are recognized by most of the patients' sera, the original immune response may be polyclonal; later on an oligoclonal response is attributed to epitope spreading or affinity maturation. The immunodominant sites are believed to be caused by the structural and sequential characteristics of the protein and also by the genetic background of the patient. LKM-1 autoantibodies are widely used as diagnostic markers for AIH type 2 or related to autoimmunity associated with hepatitis C. However, the role of these autoantibodies in liver cell injury is unknown. One possible mechanism of liver cell injury mediated by these autoantibodies could be by direct binding of LKM autoantibodies to hepatocytes, resulting in lysis of hepatocytes either by complement or by antibody-directed cell-mediated cytotoxicity (ADCC). A prerequisite for the activation of both mechanisms would be the expression of P-450 2D6 on the surface of the hepatocyte of patients with AIH-2. The surface expression of cytochrome P-450, however, has been controversial for many years, but recent publications demonstrate the surface expression of different cytochromes of family 2. Robin and associates even succeeded in describing the route of transport to the surface membrane. Using fluorescence-activated cell sorter (FACS) analysis and electron microscopy, the authors demonstrated the surface expression of cytochrome

P-450 2B and showed that cytochrome P-450 2B follows a vesicular route from the endoplasmic reticulum to the Golgi apparatus. Interestingly, the authors found that cytochrome P-450 2B, expressed on the cytoplasmatic surface of the endoplasmic reticulum, was located at the outer surface of the plasma membrane. A location of cytochrome P-450 on the outer surface might suggest a pathogenic role of autoantibodies and their antigens in AIH.

LKM-2 autoantibodies have only been observed to date in patients with drug-induced hepatitis caused by tienilic acid and have not been found with AIH. These autoantibodies are directed against cytochrome P-450 2C9. LKM-3 autoantibodies may be found in approximately 10% of patients with AIH type 2. These autoantibodies are directed against family UDP-glucuronosyltransferases (Table 8–5). LKM-3 antibodies were first described in 10% to 20% of patients with chronic hepatitis D. Epitope mapping of UDP-glucuronosyltransferases in AIH revealed a large minimal epitope from amino acids 264 to 373, indicating that the autoantibody binds to conformation-dependent epitopes. Anti-microsomal antibodies that react only with liver tissue and recognize P-450 1A2 are called LM antibodies. LM antibodies are found in drug-induced hepatitis caused by dihydralazine and in AIH as part of the APS-1. There does not seem to be a serologic overlap between LKM-1 antibodies in AIH type 2 and LM antibodies in APS-1. The pathogenetic mechanisms in dihydralazine-induced immune-mediated hepatitis seem clear. Cytochrome P-450 1A2 metabolizes dihydralazine, which then binds with its reactive metabolite to the cytochrome P-450 1A2 protein. After covalent binding of the reactive metabolite to P-450 1A2, this enzyme becomes immunogenic. The autoantibodies, however, react with the native enzyme. In hepatitis as part of the APS-1, the pathogenetic mechanisms are less clear. If the patient develops adrenal insufficiency, autoantibodies become detectable in the patient's serum, which reacts with

Table 8–5   Heterogeneity of Cytochrome P-450s and UDP Glucuronosyltransferases as Human Autoantigens

Antibody	kD	Target Antigen	Disease Association
LKM-1	50	Cytochrome P-450 2D6	Autoimmune hepatitis Hepatitis C
LKM-2	50	Cytochrome P-450 2C9	Tienilic acid–induced hepatitis
LKM-3	55	Family 1 UGT Family 2 UGT	Hepatitis D, autoimmune hepatitis
LM	52	Cytochrome P-450 1A2	Dihydralazine-induced hepatitis Autoimmune polyendocrine syndrome type 1
	54	Cytochrome P-450 2E1	Halothane hepatitis, alcohol-induced liver disease
	57	Disulfide isomerase	Halothane hepatitis
	59	Carboxylesterase	Halothane hepatitis
	59	?	Chronic hepatitis C
	64	?	Autoimmune hepatitis
	70	?	Chronic hepatitis C
	50	Cytochrome P-450 c21	Adrenal and ovarian failure
	50	Cytochrome P-450 scc	
	50	Cytochrome P-450 C17a	
	53	Cytochrome P-450 3A1	Anticonvulsant hypersensitivity
	53	Cytochrome P-450 2C11	Phenobarbital, phenytoin, carbamazepine

LKM, liver-kidney-microsomal; LM, liver-microsomal.

cytochrome P-450 enzymes that are specifically expressed in the adrenal gland. These adrenal P-450 antigens, which are targets for disease-associated autoantibodies, are involved in the synthesis of corticosteroid hormones, the deficiency of which leads to the clinical features. If the liver is involved as part of the multiorgan autoimmune process, liver cytochrome P-450 enzymes are recognized by autoantibodies. They differ from those found in AIH type 2. Although cytochrome P-450 2A6 is the most prevalent cytochrome P-450 autoantigen in APS-1, only anti-P450 1A2 antibodies are associated specifically with liver disease in this syndrome. Therefore, a pathogenetic relevance of immune reactions toward this antigen seems possible. Precise mechanisms, however, must be elaborated.

Autoantibodies against the ASGPR, a liver-specific membrane receptor, are found at high frequency in autoimmune liver diseases, particularly in AIH. They may also be detected in primary biliary cirrhosis, viral hepatitis, and other liver diseases, although at a lower frequency. Anti-ASGPR antibodies correlate with disease activity, and anti-ASGPR antibodies against human-specific epitopes seem to be closely associated with AIH. T lymphocytes directed against the ASGPR were isolated from liver tissue of patients with AIH type 1. Tissue expression of the ASGPR is most evident in the periportal areas, where piecemeal necrosis is found as a marker of severe inflammatory activity.

Histologically, the liver in AIH shows dense mononuclear infiltrates, which consist mainly of T cells. Several years ago, studies on cellular immunity had concentrated on the characterization of suppressor cell defects. Aminotransferase levels often fluctuate in patients before the initiation of immunosuppressive therapy, indicating that the disease process is regulated rather than being caused by a single upregulated autoreactive T cell clone. Therefore, the concept was developed that an aberrant autoimmune response is present in AIH and that attempts by the immune system to downregulate this autoimmune process cause spontaneous immunosuppression. Patients with AIH show significant T cell reactivity to autologous liver antigens, whereas very low, if any, reactivity could be detected in patients with HCV and HBV infection. While in remission with immunosuppressive treatment, T cell reactivity to liver antigens become undetectable. Active immunosuppression can be detected in the in vitro T cell response of such patients. Patients with AIH in remission show a lack of T cell proliferative response to tetanus toxoid, whereas healthy subjects and patients with chronic hepatitis B and C have strong reactions. Therefore, active immunosuppression is involved in the immunoregulation of AIH. The role of autoreactive T cells with antigen specificity for liver antigens is still in question. Furthermore, there is still a question regarding whether the pathogenetically relevant T cell response is directed against antigens that are targets of disease-associated autoantibodies, such as antibodies to cytochrome P-450 or the ASGPR. A first step toward the elucidation of this question was the isolation of T cell clones from liver tissue of patients with AIH and specificity for such autoantigens.

It is generally accepted that an immunogenetic background is a prerequisite for the manifestation of AIH and also presumably its severity. In white populations, AIH type 1 is associated with the HLA B8-DR3 haplotype. HLA B8 is in linkage disequilibrium with HLA DR3, resulting in a close association between AIH type 1 and B8. A subsequent association was found with HLA DR4. Patients with the HLA DR3 allele have a lower age at onset and a more active form of the disease compared with patients with other HLA alleles. These patients are less likely to enter remission and have more frequent relapses during corticosteroid therapy and after treatment is withdrawn. Consequently, liver transplantation is needed more often in HLA DR3–positive patients. It seems that patients with DR4 are more likely to develop concurrent extrahepatic diseases. The situation is different in Japan, where AIH type 1 is rare and no association with HLA DR3 is found, whereas there is an association with HLA-DR4. There is also a highly significant association with HLA B54. The HLA class III region was studied in AIH with particular emphasis on the complement genes C2, C4A, C4B, and factor B (Bf). Studies on complement polymorphism revealed low complement C4 levels for AIH type 1. This is associated with C4A-Q0 alleles due to gene deletions. Because C4 is involved in clearance of immune complexes and viruses, low levels might indicate the involvement of a viral agent in the pathogenesis of the disease.

Only limited data are available on the genetic background of AIH type 2, but an association of AIH type 2 with HLA DR3 is reported. Further preliminary findings indicate an association with HLA B14, HLA DQ2, and C4A-Q0.

Progress on the immunogenetic background in AIH has resulted from recent advances in molecular biology, particularly from x-ray crystallography of the purified antigens A2 and DR1 and the development of PCR-based HLA genotyping techniques. Patients with AIH type 1 have a very high frequency of the HLA DRB1*0301-DRB3*0101-DQA1*0501-DQB1*0201 haplotype, and there is a strong secondary association with one of the DR4 alleles DRB1*0401. DRB genes are more strongly associated with the disease than DQA or DQB. There is a strong association of a single amino acid residue, lysine, at position 71 of the HLA DRβ-polypeptide. Lysine DRβ71 is encoded by DRB1*0301 and DRB1*0401 as well as by all of the DRB3 alleles (Fig. 8–3). The implication of DRβ71 is supported by studies on patients from North America but not by data from Asia or Argentina. Studies on Japanese patients indicate that basic amino acids at position 13 of the HLA DR β polypetide (DRβ13) are responsible for the second HLA DR4 association found in Japanese patients with late onset AIH type 1. Our knowledge of the immunogenetic susceptibility to liver disease is still incomplete. However, future work will help to define better the genetic background at the amino acid level (i.e., identify particular amino acids at the bottom of the groove of the HLA class II molecule as risk factors for the various serologic, clinical, genetic, and racial subgroups of AIH). These studies should help to identify patients at risk and those likely to develop a severe course of the disease or concurrent extrahepatic syndromes. Hopefully, we will better understand the pathogenetic mechanisms of tissue destruction by T lymphocytes, so that new therapeutic strategies can emerge.

Several animal models for experimental autoimmune hepatitis (EAH) have been developed in order to increase our understanding of the pathophysiology of AIH. Most experiments have been done in mice, but experiments performed in the rat or rabbit are also reported. In a recent

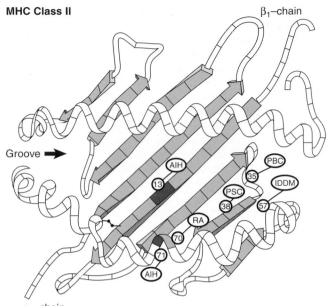

MHC Class II

β₁–chain

Groove ➤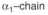

α₁–chain

Figure 8–3
Risk amino acids in the groove of the HLA class II molecule. Lysine at position 71 of the DRβ chain is a risk factor for DRB1*0301, DRB1*0401, and all DRB3 alleles. A basic amino acid at position 13 of the HLA DRβ polypeptide is a risk factor for Japanese patients. Other particular amino acids are risk factors for other autoimmune diseases and are located at position 35 (PBC), position 38 (PSC), position 57 (IDDM, insulin-dependent diabetes mellitus), and position 70 (RA, rheumatoid arthritis).

mouse model, EAH was induced by intraperitoneal immunization with the 100,000-g supernatant of syngeneic liver homogenate (S100) in complete Freund's adjuvant (CFA). The most susceptible inbred mouse strain was C57B1/6, and less susceptible strains were Balb/c or C3II mice. EAII could not be induced in Lewis rats. A single injection of S100 in CFA led to biochemical and histologic signs of hepatitis. At week 2 alanine aminotransferase (ALT) values were elevated, and perivascular inflammatory infiltrates and moderate liver damage were visible histologically. The peak of disease occurred at week 4, followed by biochemical and histologic recovery. Aminotransferase values were normal at 8 weeks, and histologic recovery took up to 6 months. In EAH, characteristic autoantibodies directed against only a few target proteins appeared several weeks after induction of disease, and titers rose continuously, even after biochemical and histologic parameters had regressed. However, targets differed from those in human AIH. In contrast, T cell reactivity was critical for the development of EAH, because it could be induced by the transfer of T cells from diseased animals to naive animals. However, the adoptively transferred form of the disease was milder than the antigen-induced active disease. In the course of EAH, T cell reactivity to liver antigens precedes histologic disease. At the peak of the disease, the T cell response is already suppressed. The suppression of T cell response is active and antigen-specific. The effect is even more pronounced in in vivo studies with tetanus toxoid at the peak of the disease, when more than 90% inhibition is found in animals with EAH. These results

demonstrate in vitro and in vivo immunosuppression, which is associated with recovery from EAH, and stress the involvement of immunoregulatory circuits in AIH. This finding indicates that in human AIH, active immunosuppression may facilitate recovery from AIH.

CLINICAL FEATURES

AIH may present at any age in either sex, although it occurs most frequently in women between the ages of 10 and 30 years or it occurs also in late middle age. In approximately 30% of cases, the presentation is acute and may mimic acute viral hepatitis. Therefore, this disease should nowadays be named AIH and not autoimmune chronic active hepatitis. In the remainder, the onset is insidious and the disease may not be recognized until damage to the liver is at an advanced stage. The frequency of the various clinical manifestations have been similar in the major reported series. A significant number of patients will be jaundiced at presentation. Anorexia, fatigue, and amenorrhea (in women) are common. Abdominal pain, which is often related to hepatic tenderness, occurs in 10% to 40% and up to 20% may have a fever at presentation. Most patients will have palpable hepatomegaly and 50% will have a palpable spleen. Patients frequently have spider nevi, which may reflect changes in the activity of the disease. Between 30% and 80% of patients will already have progressed to cirrhosis by the time of presentation, and 10% to 20% may already have evidence of decompensated cirrhosis with ascites and less commonly encephalopathy. Approximately 20% of patients will have evidence of esophageal varices.

Extrahepatic manifestations occur frequently. In a study of 108 patients with chronic hepatitis of various etiologies, 63% had evidence of disease in at least one organ other than the liver. Arthropathy and periarticular swelling occur in 6% to 36% and affect both large and small joints. The swelling is usually transient and reflects disease activity; however, occasionally, an erosive arthritis may occur. Skin rashes occur in approximately 20% of cases and may take the form of a pleomorphic maculopapular or an acneiform rash. Allergic capillaritis, lichen planus, and leg ulcers occur commonly. Occasionally, the patient may appear cushingoid and have abdominal striae before the start of any therapy. There are associations with other diseases, particularly ulcerative colitis, in which there appears to be an overlap syndrome with primary sclerosing cholangitis. Particularly in children, primary sclerosing cholangitis may present initially as chronic hepatitis. There is also an increased incidence of various autoimmune diseases and other diseases, including autoimmune thyroiditis, Sjögren's syndrome, renal tubular acidosis, fibrosing alveolitis, peripheral neuropathy, and glomerulonephritis.

DIAGNOSIS

As in many other autoimmune diseases, the diagnosis of AIH is based on several clinical and laboratory parameters. The International Autoimmune Hepatitis Group has defined the diagnostic criteria and has given them specific scores (see Table 8–1): hypergammaglobulinemia, female sex, genetic markers, absence of markers of viral hepatitis, and last but not least, autoantibodies. Several autoantibodies are relevant for the diagnosis of AIH (see Table 8–4). Most are listed as diagnostic criteria for AIH by the International Autoimmune Hepatitis Group (see Table 8–1). ANAs, the most important and earliest defined markers of AIH, have diagnostic relevance when they are detected by immunofluorescence at a titer of more than 1:40. ANAs are determined by indirect immunofluorescence on rodent liver and kidney tissue. Tissue cultures with Hep G-2 cells are currently preferred in many laboratories. For routine purposes, the detection by immunofluorescence is sufficient and subtyping of antinuclear antibodies has not shown any diagnostic relevance for routine clinical practice.

Cytoskeleton antibodies are also of diagnostic relevance. Smooth muscle antibodies (SMAs) are detected by indirect immunofluorescence on rodent liver and kidney (owing to staining of vessel walls) and stomach (owing to staining of the muscle layer). SMAs in liver diseases, in particular AIH, are directed against F-actin. A titer of more than 1:80 is regarded as diagnostically significant. SMAs can be the only marker of AIH. If at high titer, this is particularly relevant in children. Low SMA titers are frequently observed in chronic viral hepatitis but usually lack F-actin specificity.

Liver-kidney microsomal (LKM) antibodies are also determined primarily by indirect immunofluorescence. Owing to their staining of the cytoplasm of liver cells and proximal renal tubules, they can be distinguished from antimitochondrial antibodies (AMAs) in primary biliary cirrhosis (PBC), which stain proximal and distal renal tubules (see Fig. 8–2). LKM-1 antibodies are heterogeneous themselves (see Table 8–5). LKM-1 antibodies are markers of AIH type 2. Their main target antigen is human cytochrome P-450 2D6. LKM-1 antibodies occur in some cases of chronic hepatitis C in which they react with either cytochrome P-450 2D6 or with other microsomal proteins at 59 kD and 70 kD. Antibodies to cytochrome P-450 2D6 in AIH type 2 react with a major B cell epitope of eight amino acids (E1 epitope) (see Fig. 8–1). In chronic hepatitis C, LKM-1 antibodies are more heterogeneous because, in addition to the 59-kD and 70-kD antigens, they react with conformational epitopes and with additional linear epitopes on cytochrome P-450 2D6. LKM-2 antibodies react with cytochrome P-450 2C9 and are associated with drug-induced hepatitis caused by tienilic acid. LKM-2 antibodies were never found in AIH. LKM-3 antibodies react with UDP-glucuronosyltransferase family 1 proteins at approximately 55 kD, and a few sera also recognize family 2 UGT proteins. In 10% of patients with AIH type 2, LKM-3 antibodies against UGT proteins can be detected and may be the only marker of autoimmune liver disease (see Table 8–5). LM antibodies are microsomal antibodies that react with a liver-specific antigen. LM antibodies reacting with cytochrome P-450 1A2 occur either in drug-induced hepatitis due to dihydralazine or in AIH as part of the APS-1 (see Table 8–5).

Antibodies to cytosolic antigens can be detected by immunofluorescence as anti-LC-1 and anti-LC-2 antibodies, or they are only detectable by ELISA or radioimmunoassay techniques. This also holds true for antibodies to soluble liver antigen (anti-SLA), or liver-pancreas antigen (anti-LP). Although anti-LC-1 and anti-LC-2 antibodies usually occur together with LKM-1 antibodies and seem to characterize AIH type 2, anti-SLA and anti-LP seem to characterize a third subgroup of AIH. Although the International Au-

toimmune Hepatitis Group regarded it as preliminary to define subgroups of AIH, anti-SLA and anti-LP antibodies may be the only markers of AIH in patients who are ANA, SMA, and LKM-1–antibody negative.

Further autoantibodies are directed against antigens of the liver cell membrane, notably the ASGPR. The ASGPR is specific to the liver and is membrane-associated. This antigen is interesting for pathogenetic studies. Anti-ASGPR antibodies occur at high frequency in AIH type 1; in addition, they occur in PBC and in some patients with chronic viral hepatitis. Anti-ASGPR against specific human epitopes were reported to be closely associated with AIH. Anti-ASGPR antibodies may be diagnostically helpful in those cases in which ANA, SMA, anti-LKM-1, and anti-SLA/LP are negative and AIH is suspected.

AMAs are determined by indirect immunofluorescence and are markers of PBC. They should be negative in AIH and, therefore, received a negative score by the International Autoimmune Hepatitis Group as a diagnostic criterion of AIH. There are several PBC specific subtypes of AMA. AMAs against the E2 subunit of pyruvate dehydrogenase (PDH-E2) occur in more than 90% of patients with PBC and are, therefore, of particular diagnostic relevance for PBC.

Other autoantibodies as well as other immunologic markers apart from circulating autoantibodies are of minor diagnostic relevance. Determination of HLA phenotypes or even HLA alleles at the DNA level are not usually necessary for daily clinical practice. Certainly, there are a few cases of AIH that respond to corticosteroids but are negative for all marker autoantibodies; in these cases, HLA DR3 and HLA DR4 would support a diagnosis of AIH. Possibly more sophisticated and more specific genetic markers of the MHC locus determined by molecular technology at the DNA level may be even more helpful in the future.

The determination of immunoglobulins may be helpful because AIH is characterized by hypergammaglobulinemia even when cirrhosis is absent. In AIH hypergammaglobulinemia is mainly due to polyclonal IgG elevation, whereas PBC is associated more with elevated IgM levels and IgA is increased in alcoholic liver disease. Monoclonal gammopathy is sometimes associated with AIH.

Liver biopsy is important to determine activity (grading) and fibrosis (staging) of chronic hepatitis. However, histology is less effective for defining the etiology of liver diseases, particularly AIH. Some decades ago, plasma cells as part of the inflammatory infiltrate were regarded as a diagnostic hallmark for AIH, but several standard textbooks on liver pathology lack specific histologic comments on AIH. Definitely, the syndrome of AIH has become more precise due to internationally proposed criteria as well as improvements of autoantibody testing. Early studies had indicated the importance of plasma cells as significant components of the inflammatory infiltrate. In more recent studies, plasma cells are not a hallmark of AIH, at least compared with hepatitis B and hepatitis C. There is no specific histologic pattern of AIH; furthermore, no specific features are associated with either of the three subtypes of AIH defined by patterns of autoantibodies. However, broad hypocellular areas of collapse extending from the portal tracts into the parenchyma and encompassing groups of hepatocytes with microacinar transformation were found to be characteristic as was hydropic swelling of hepatocytes. In contrast, the eosinophilic cell damage with acidophilic bodies frequently seen in non-A, non-B hepatitis (hepatitis C) were not specific nor a characteristic finding in AIH.

SUBTYPES OF AUTOIMMUNE HEPATITIS: A CONTROVERSIAL ISSUE

There is a debate regarding whether AIH may be further differentiated into several serologically distinct subgroups. There are two possibilities for distinct subgroups of AIH. The most widely used is based on autoantibody profiles. AIH type 1 is characterized by ANA with or without SMA and represents by far the most common subgroup of AIH. Despite the fact that recent research focused on AIH type 2 in many centers with its anti P-450 and anti-UGT autoimmunity, it should be noted that AIH type 1 is by far the most common form. AIH type 2 characterized by LKM-1 antibodies against P-450 2D6 is rarely seen in the United States, Australia, and Japan. Furthermore, most of our knowledge on the genetic background, on the treatment response as well as on long-term results after liver transplantation, is based on AIH type 1.

On the other hand, there are several arguments that support the distinction of AIH type 1 from types 2 and 3. AIH type 2 has a more specific autoantibody profile compared with the heterogeneous ANA response (see Table 8–4). Furthermore, these patients seem to suffer more frequently from fulminant hepatic failure and extrahepatic syndromes; low IgA levels are also more common. AIH type 2 is particularly frequent in the pediatric patient population, and the geographic difference observed for the prevalence of autoimmune hepatitis type 2 argues for a different etiology. The case of AIH type 3 is more difficult. Certainly there are cases of AIH that are negative for the usual autoantibody markers (ANA, SMA, LKM-1), and anti-SLA/LP antibodies and anti-ASGPR may identify such patients. However, these patients with AIH type 3 share the clinical and genetic characteristics of AIH type 1.

Another subgrouping is based on the genetic background. Patients with HLA DR 3 are younger at onset, have a more rapid disease progress, and more frequently experience a relapse after treatment. HLA DR3-positive patients are overrepresented in AIH patients being candidates for liver transplantation. A second subgroup is associated with HLA DR 4. These patients have a later age at onset, a slower disease process, and usually respond better to immunosuppressive treatment. In Japan, AIH is restricted to the HLA DR4–positive group. A further development of the DNA-based technology to identify HLA alleles and even particular amino acids as risk factors will further help to clarify the issue of AIH subgroups.

DIFFERENTIAL DIAGNOSIS

Liver Disease in the Autoimmune Polyendocrine Syndrome Type 1

The APS-1 is a rare autosomal recessive disorder characterized by a variable combination of disease components. The first clinical manifestation of APS-1 usually occurs in childhood, and progressively new components may appear throughout life, with the majority (63%) of the patients suffering from three to five of them. The most frequent are chronic mucocutaneous candidiasis, hypoparathyroidism, adrenocortical failure, and gonadal failure in females, with AIH as a serious but less frequent component. Compared with other autoimmune diseases, female predominance and linkage to HLA-DR do not exist. The APS-1 locus has been assigned to the long arm of chromosome 21. Lymphocytic infiltration of the affected organs and the presence of organ-specific autoantibodies are typical features of APS-1. The major hepatic autoantigen in AIH related to APS-1 is cytochrome P-450 1A2, whereas microsomal autoantibodies in APS-1 do not react with the LKM-1 antigen cytochrome P-450 2D6.

Autoimmunity Associated with Viral Hepatitis

Chronic infection with HCV is known to induce autoimmune reactions. Hepatitis C is associated with an array of extrahepatic manifestations, including mixed cryoglobulinemia, membranoproliferative glomerulonephritis, polyarthritis, porphyria cutanea tarda, Sjögren's syndrome, and autoimmune thyroid disease. Not surprisingly, numerous autoantibodies are found to be associated with chronic hepatitis C. As for AIH, antitissue antibodies including ANA, SMA, LKM, and antithyroid antibodies are found at high frequency. Anti-GOR is a disease-specific autoantibody that is present in at least 80% of sera from patients with hepatitis C. The epitope recognized by anti-GOR, GRRGQKAK-SNPNRPL, is located on a nuclear protein that is overexpressed in hepatocellular carcinoma. Interestingly, anti-GOR is not associated with AIH but is specific for hepatitis induced by HCV. Depending on the geographic origin, a variable proportion of patients with anti-LKM-1–associated liver disease are infected with HCV. The prevalence of HCV infection among LKM-1–positive patients is approximately 90% in Italy, about 50% in France and Germany, and less than 10% in England. Overall less than 10% of patients with chronic hepatitis C are positive for LKM-1 antibodies. Interferon seems to be effective; however, liver disease may worsen in some of these patients. LKM-1 antibodies in chronic hepatitis C react with linear, and in particular, conformational epitopes of cytochrome P-450 2D6. Fifty percent of sera do not react by Western blot. HCV-induced LKM-1 antibodies may react with other microsomal protein in addition to cytochrome P-450 2D6 (see Table 8–3).

Chronic Hepatitis D

Ten percent of patients with chronic hepatitis D express serum antibodies against microsomes of liver and proximal renal tubules. Because these antibodies differed from LKM-1 and LKM-2 antibodies, they were called LKM-3. The molecular target of the LKM-3 autoantibody was identified by screening a cDNA library, which revealed UDP-glucuronosyltransferase 1.6 (UGT 1.6) as the reactant. Western blotting with recombinant rabbit UGT 1.6 was used to characterize the clinical associations of LKM-3 autoantibodies. These were detected only in hepatitis D and AIH and not in hepatitis B, hepatitis C, PBC, primary sclerosing cholangitis, or systemic lupus erythematosus.

Immune-Mediated Drug-Induced Hepatitis

Because of its central role in xenobiotic metabolism, the liver is an important target for adverse drug reactions. In the course of the normal metabolism of drugs, many may form unstable metabolites that bind to cellular proteins or DNA; this direct toxic effect may lead to cell death or cancer. However, if the protein adducts formed in this process are presented to the immune system as neoantigens, eventually an immune response may be induced, including the production of autoantibodies, inflammation of the liver, and necrosis. This type of immunoallergic reaction represents drug-induced hepatitis. Hepatitis induced by tienilic acid and dihydralazine has been investigated intensively and provides a hypothesis for the induction of autoantibodies and T cell responses possibly also relevant to idiopathic AIH.

Tienilic Acid–Induced Hepatitis

Tienilic acid was a uricosuric agent used in hypertension, but it was withdrawn from the market because of rare cases of drug-induced severe hepatitis. This type of hepatitis was dose independent and always occurred with a delay ranging from 14 to 240 days of drug treatment. Women and men were equally affected. After discontinuation of drug treatment the liver damage resolved, but rechallenge resulted in symptoms after a shorter period than before. These patients produced a new specific antibody directed against unmodified liver and kidney microsomal proteins (LKM-2), which was later identified as cytochrome P-450 2C9, the major tienilic acid–metabolizing enzyme in the liver.

Dihydralazine-Induced Hepatitis

Long-term treatment with the hypertensive drug dihydralazine has led to many reports of hepatitis. This type of drug-induced hepatitis affects more women than men, the ratio being 7:2. Most patients are of the slow acetylator phenotype. The onset of hepatitis is usually delayed, with a latent period of several months, and it resolves after the drug is discontinued. Rechallenge with the drug results in a recurrence of hepatitis. Inflammatory infiltrates include mononuclear cells, neutrophils, and eosinophils. In several patients, a positive lymphocyte transformation was reported. Dihydralazine hepatitis is associated with liver microsomal (LM) antibodies that do not stain kidney sections. The target protein was identified as cytochrome P-450 1A2 (see Table 8–5). LM autoantibodies are very specific. Despite a high sequence homology between cytochromes P-450 1A1 and P-450 1A2, no cross-reaction with cloned human P-450 1A1 is observed. LM antibodies against P-450 1A2 may also indicate AIH as part of APS-1.

Cryptogenic Hepatitis

Approximately 10% to 20% of patients with chronic hepatitis are classified as cryptogenic, because no specific cause can be identified. These cases may be due to either unknown viruses or mutants of known viruses, or they may be of autoimmune type but negative for characteristic autoantibodies. One still has to think of other yet unidentified nonviral, nonautoimmune, and nondrug–related etiologies for cryptogenic hepatitis. The prevalence of GBV-C/HGV RNA in cryptogenic hepatitis is only between 10% and 20%. Therefore, this virus is not a major cause of cryptogenic hepatitis.

Overlap Syndromes

PBC is not usually a diagnostic problem due to the detection of AMAs against acyltransferases, in particular antibodies to the E2 subunit of pyruvate dehydrogenase. Several groups have observed patients with clinical and morphologic characteristics of PBC being negative for AMAs but positive for ANAs. Such studies do not include enough patients to draw final conclusions. These cases are called autoimmune cholangitis and seem to respond to immunosuppressive treatment. The condition of another group of patients became known as the CAH/PBC overlap syndrome. These patients share the characteristics of both AIH as well as PBC. Histologically, these patients present with piecemeal necrosis and periductular infiltration of the portal tracts with bile duct destruction. They are seropositive for AMA and ANA and seem to benefit from immunosuppressive treatment. A specific AMA does not seem to be associated with this syndrome as had been presumed. Although the overlap syndrome between PBC and AIH was described in the adult population, overlap between primary sclerosing cholangitis and AIH was described in the pediatric population. These patients show typical bile duct strictures and dilatations on endoscopic retrograde cholangiography (ERCP) while typical histologic lesions for chronic hepatitis are evident on liver biopsy. Again, high-titer ANAs are serologic hallmarks.

TREATMENT AND PROGNOSIS

The treatment of choice for AIH is immunosuppression. Standard treatment is either prednisolone alone or a combination of prednisolone and azathioprine (Table 8–6). Both prednisolone monotherapy or combination treatment are effective in inducing remission. We prefer prednisolone monotherapy in children and young females, and in adults we prefer combination therapy if there are no contraindications to the use of azathioprine, such as leukopenia or drug-induced cholestasis. Either prednisolone or prednisone can be used; prednisone is the prodrug that is converted to prednisolone in the liver. Prednisone metabolism into prednisolone is not affected in patients with liver cirrhosis. The standard treatment regimes have been used worldwide for many years. Immunosuppression was shown to improve survival of patients with severe AIH (Fig. 8–4). It is suggested that cases with mild-to-moderate inflammatory activity need not be treated. Clinical remission is followed by biochemical and then histologic remission. Approximately 65% of patients experience complete clinical, biochemical, and histologic remission. Treatment should be continued for at least 2 years. If complete remission is not achieved within 24 months, there should be no further continuation of treatment. Up to 80% of treatment responders may experience a relapse after the end of the 2-year treatment period; if so, a long-term low-dose immunosuppressive treatment should be introduced for the maintenance of remission. There are two alternatives—either low-dose prednisolone with a dose between 5 and 15 mg/day or azathioprine monotherapy, 2

Table 8–6 Treatment of Autoimmune Hepatitis

	Single Drug Regimen	Combination Regimen
Prednisolone	50 mg for 10 days; maintenance 20 mg or lower as required	50 mg for 10 days; taper 5 mg q 10 days; maintenance 10 mg or lower as required
Azathioprine	None	100 mg for 3 wk; 50 mg
Upon remission (treatment 24 mo)		
Prednisolone	Taper 2.5 mg q/wk	Taper 2.5 mg q/wk
Azathioprine	None	Taper 25 mg q 3wk
Follow-up		

Test	Before Therapy	During Therapy (q 4 wk)	Remission	After Therapy (q 3 wk × 4)	After Therapy (q 3 mo)
Physical examination	+	+	+	+	+
Liver biopsy	+	−	+	−	−
Blood count	+	+	+	+	+
Aminotransferases	+	+	+	+	+
Bilirubin	+	+	+	+	+
Coagulation	+	+	+	+	+
Autoantibodies	+	±	+	±	±
Thyroid function	+	±	+	±	±

mg/kg body weight. Although azathioprine alone does not induce remission this drug as monotherapy can maintain remission for a long time (Fig. 8–5).

Recent data on the long-term use of azathioprine in the transplant population have shown that this confers less oncogenic risk and teratogenic complications than was previously suspected from animal experiments. There seems to be a difference in the response to standard treatment concerning the genetic background. Patients with HLA DR3 experience a full remission less frequently, and relapse rates are higher than for the HLA DR3–negative patients. Consequently, HLA DR3 is more prevalent among the transplanted population of patients with AIH from Europe and North America. If standard treatment with prednisolone alone or in combination with azathioprine fails to induce re-

mission, other immunosuppressive drugs including cyclosporin A, FK 506, mycophenolate-mofetil, and cyclophosphamide may be tried. However, a sufficient response is shown only for a minor proportion of such patients in single case reports.

Liver transplantation was shown to be very effective in the end stage of AIH with cirrhosis; cirrhosis may develop despite complete biochemical remission under long-term immunosuppressive treatment. AIH is among the best indications for liver transplantation, with long-term survival rates of more than 90% after 5 years. Although a recurrence of AIH after liver transplantation has been reported in some cases, this is uncommon and does not prejudice the long-term outcome. Furthermore, immunosuppressive treatment started immediately after liver transplantation not only prevents rejection but may also treat or prevent recurrent AIH. Furthermore, donor and recipient MHC complex are differ-

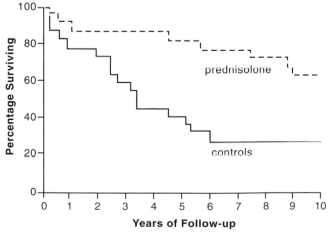

Figure 8–4

Effect of corticosteroids on patients with autoimmune hepatitis compared with the placebo group. The life table survival curves of control (——) and prednisolone-treated (-----) patients are shown.

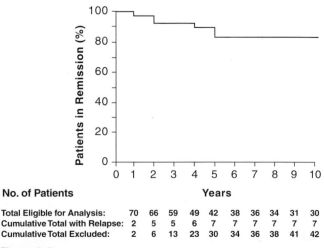

No. of Patients										
Total Eligible for Analysis:	70	66	59	49	42	38	36	34	31	30
Cumulative Total with Relapse:	2	5	5	6	7	7	7	7	7	7
Cumulative Total Excluded:	2	6	13	23	30	34	36	38	41	42

Figure 8–5

Cumulative probability of sustained remission during 2 mg of azathioprine/kg/day in patients with autoimmune hepatitis.

ent, which may have an impact on the autoimmune response after transplantation.

Topical steroids like budesonide are under clinical investigation for AIH. Budesonide has a 90% first-pass effect in the liver. The idea is that the drug reaches pathogenetically relevant lymphocytes within the liver before being metabolized. Hepatic metabolism then prevents severe systemic side effects, such as bone disease. A Swedish group has shown that budesonide therapy does reduce elevated aminotransferase levels to normal in AIH. Studies in a limited number of patients have confirmed that budesonide is effective in reducing levels of liver enzymes, and cortisol levels in the peripheral blood are hardly changed if the patient has not yet developed cirrhosis with portosystemic shunts. In particular, in middle-aged women with AIH, immunosuppressive treatment should be applied in combination with vitamin D and calcium (1000 mg/day orally) treatment to prevent or treat bone disease such as osteoporosis.

SUGGESTED READINGS

Ahonen P, Myllrniemi S, Sipil I, Perheentupa J: Clinical variation of autoimmune polyendocrinopathy-candidiasis-ectodermal dystrophy (APECED) in a series of 68 patients. N Engl J Med 322:1829–1836, 1990.

Czaja AJ: Autoimmune hepatitis: Current therapeutic concepts. Clin Immunother 6:413–429, 1994.

Czaja AJ, Cassani F, Cataleta M, et al: Frequency and significance of antibodies to actin in type 1 autoimmune hepatitis. Hepatology 24:1068–1073, 1996.

Czaja AJ, Manns MP: The validity and importance of subtypes in autoimmune hepatitis: A point of view. Am J Gastroenterol 90:1206–1211, 1995.

Danielson A, Prytz H: Oral budesonide for treatment of autoimmune chronic active hepatitis. Alim Pharm Ther 8:585–590, 1994.

Desmet V, Gerber MA, Hoofnagle JH, et al: Classification of chronic hepatitis: Diagnosis, grading and staging. Hepatology 9:1513–1520, 1994.

Homberg JC, Abuaf N, Bernard O, et al: Chronic active hepatitis associated with anti-liver/kidney microsome antibody type I: A second type of "autoimmune hepatitis." Hepatology 197:1333–1339, 1987.

Johnson PJ, McFarlane IG: Meeting report of the International Autoimmune Hepatitis Group. Hepatology 18:998–1005, 1993.

Johnson PJ, McFarlane IG, Williams R: Azathioprine for long-term maintenance of remission in autoimmune hepatitis. N Engl J Med 333:958–963, 1995.

Krawitt EL: Autoimmune hepatitis. N Engl J Med 334:897–903, 1996.

Lohse W, Kögel M, Meyer zum Büschenfelde K-H: Evidence for spontaneous immunosuppression in autoimmune hepatitis. Hepatology 22:381–388, 1995.

Mackay IR, Taft CO, Cowling DS: Lupoid hepatitis. Lancet 2:1323–1226, 1956.

Manns M, Gerken G, Kyriatsoulis A, et al: Characterization of a new subgroup of autoimmune chronic active hepatitis by autoantibodies against soluble liver antigen. Lancet 1:292–294, 1987.

Manns M, Griffin KJ, Sullivan KF, Johnson EF: LKM-1 autoantibodies recognize a short linear sequence in P450 II D6, a cytochrome P450 monooxygenase. J Clin Invest 88:1370–1378, 1991.

Robin MA, Maratrat M, Loeper J, et al: Cytochrome P450 2B follows a vesicular route to the plasma membrane in cultured rat hepatocytes. Gastroenterology 108:1110–1123, 1995.

Stechemesser E, Klein R, Berg PA: Characterization and clinical relevance of liver-pancreas antibodies in autoimmune hepatitis. Hepatology 18:1–9, 1993.

Strassburg CP, Manns MP: Viral hepatitis and autoimmunity: Chicken or egg? Viral Hepatitis Rev 1:97–102, 1995.

Yamamoto AM, Cresteil D, Boniface O, et al: Identification and analysis of cytochrome P450IID6 antigenic sites recognized by anti-liver-kidney microsome type-1 antibodies (LKM1). Eur J Immunol 23:1105–1111, 1993.

Chapter

9

Alcoholic Liver Disease

Marco A. Olivera-Martínez
Rowen K. Zetterman

The association of excessive ethanol intake with the development of chronic liver disease has been known for centuries. However, despite this knowledge, consumption of ethanol continues to be a public health problem in Western countries and remains the most abused drug worldwide. In the United States, it is estimated that there are at least 10 million alcoholics, representing approximately 6% to 7% of the adult population. Although the direct medical cost associated with alcoholism may approach $12 billion annually, this number may actually represent only 10% of total societal costs from alcoholism. Most medical costs can be attributed to the development of cirrhosis and its attendant complications. Although cirrhosis of the liver ranks as the 11th most common cause of death overall in the United States, it is the 6th to 8th most common cause in 15- to 74-year-old men due to ethanol consumption and accounts for a large number of cases.

EPIDEMIOLOGY

The reason why only some humans develop alcoholism remains a mystery. From studies to date, it would appear that genetic, social, and psychological factors may all have a potential role. In studies of adoptees, a history of alcoholism in the biologic parents is more predictive of alcohol abuse in the child than the presence of alcoholism in the adoptive parents. Male gender and antisocial behavior have also been associated with alcohol abuse.

It is equally unclear why only 10% to 15% of chronic alcoholics develop alcoholic cirrhosis and up to one third lack clinically apparent liver injury. There does seem to be some relationship to total consumption of ethanol. For men, those who develop advanced liver injury have typically ingested the equivalent of 80 g/day or more of pure ethanol for 10 years or more. This is approximately equivalent to 8 bottles of beer or 6 oz of 80 proof distilled spirits daily. For women, the threshold seems to be less or approximately 40 g or more equivalent daily. Women may also present clinically with alcoholic liver disease (ALD) at an earlier age compared with men. What makes women more susceptible is unclear. Differences in body composition, a smaller body habitus, a greater propensity for women to develop autoimmune diseases, and gender-related differences in the metabolism of ethanol have all been implicated. Some have suggested that a reduction of alcohol dehydrogenase (ADH) content in the gastric mucosa of women could increase delivery of unmetabolized ethanol to the liver and thus increase levels of its proximate metabolite, acetaldehyde, within the hepatocyte. However, there is little evidence to support this concept.

The "safe" quantity of daily ethanol consumption is difficult to determine. Some have suggested that daily consumption of less than the equivalent of 80 g of pure ethanol for men and of 40 g for women is best. Others have been more restrictive. The group at the King's College, London, suggests that if 10 g of alcohol is equal to 1 U, then alcohol intake should not exceed 21 U/wk for men or 14 U/wk for women.

PATHOPHYSIOLOGY

The pathophysiology of alcoholic liver disease is unknown, and the lack of a suitable animal model continues to hinder our understanding. Potential mechanisms for liver injury include associated malnutrition, direct ethanol/acetaldehyde toxicity, development of a hypermetabolic state, and immune reactivity.

Malnutrition: Malnutrition is one of the oldest suggested mechanisms for development of liver injury in the alcoholic. The frequent association of cirrhosis with the malnourished "Skid Row" alcoholic popularized this theory. In some studies, up to 82% of patients with advanced alcoholic liver disease have concurrent protein-calorie malnutrition. However, alcoholic cirrhosis can develop in the absence of malnutrition, and alcoholics with minimal liver disease may have significant malnutrition. Ethanol is a substantial source of energy at 7.1 kcal/g. However, long-term ethanol intake may not be followed by an increase of body weight due to associated negative nitrogen balance and nutrient displacement. Ethanol also increases the daily requirements of choline, thiamine, folate, and other nutrients such as pyridoxal-5'-phosphate. Vitamin A deficiency has also been implicated in alcohol-related liver injury.

Direct Ethanol/Acetaldehyde Toxicity: Ethanol is mainly absorbed by the small intestine, and a lesser amount is absorbed through the stomach mucosa. Gastric mucosa contains ADH, and it has been proposed that the metabolism of ethanol begins there. Because women have less gastric mucosal ADH, the reduction of ethanol metabolism in the stomach would cause more ethanol to reach the liver cell and result in greater exposure of the hepatocyte to acetaldehyde, the proximate metabolite of ethanol. However, the gastric mucosal metabolism of ethanol appears to have little significance in the overall metabolism of ethanol.

Three enzyme systems account for hepatic metabolism of ethanol: (1) cytosolic ADH; (2) the microsomal ethanol-oxidizing system (MEOS); and (3) peroxisomal catalase. There appears to be a minimal role for catalase in ethanol-oxidation. Hepatic ADH is a cytosolic zinc metalloenzyme and the rate-limiting step of ethanol oxidation. The majority of ethanol oxidation occurs via ADH to form acetaldehyde. Once formed, acetaldehyde is a highly reactive molecule that may have multiple in vivo effects (Table 9–1) and is subsequently metabolized to acetate by aldehyde dehydrogenase (ALDH). Both ADH and ALDH enzyme reactions reduce nicotinamide-adenine dinucleotide (NAD) to NADH with the production of excess reducing equivalents that can diminish fatty acid oxidation, increase triacylglycerol formation, and favor the development of a fatty liver.

Polymorphism of both ADH and ALDH occurs. ADH has multiple molecular forms coded in five different gene loci on chromosome 4. ALDH also exists as varying isoenzymes coded by genes on four different chromosomes. Acetaldehyde is principally metabolized by ALDH-1 and ALDH-2. It has been proposed that enzyme polymorphism could enhance liver injury due to increased acetaldehyde formation or reduced acetaldehyde clearance. ADH-2 is associated with more rapid formation of acetaldehyde and ALDH-2 with reduced acetaldehyde oxidation. However,

Table 9–1 Metabolic Effects of Acetaldehyde

Hyperlactacidemia
Hyperuricemia
Hyperlipidemia
Lipid perioxidation

the data presently available do not support a role for altered enzyme activity as a cause of alcoholic liver injury.

The MEOS system has a greater role in those with sustained ethanol consumption and high blood alcohol levels. MEOS, in the presence of oxygen and nicotinamide-adenine dinucleotide phosphate (NADPH), oxidizes ethanol to acetaldehyde and water. MEOS refers to the specific cytochrome P-4502E1 (CYP 2E1), an inducible enzyme system with a high Km for ethanol at 8 to 10 mmol/L, compared with 0.2 to 2 mmol/L for ADH. Cytochrome P-4502E1 is contained within hepatocyte smooth endoplasmic reticulum (SER), especially centrilobular hepatocytes. It has been suggested that its centrilobular preponderance may be the reason why alcoholic liver injury first occurs in this region. MEOS can also oxidize acetaldehyde and higher aliphatic alcohols. MEOS and other hepatocellular enzymes can be induced by ethanol and enhance conversion of other substances to intermediates that may be toxic. For example, therapeutic quantities of acetaminophen can result in hepatic injury in chronic alcoholics due to enhanced formation of the toxic intermediate of acetaminophen. Enzyme induction has also been implicated in the enhanced susceptibility of alcoholics to cancer formation through carcinogen or co-carcinogen activation.

The possible mechanisms by which ethanol could induce liver injury are complex. Intake of ethanol will increase the intracellular accumulation of triacylglycerol by increasing fatty acid uptake while reducing fatty acid oxidation and lipoprotein secretion. Protein synthesis, glycosylation, and secretion are also impaired. Accumulation of both triglycerides and proteins within the hepatocyte can contribute to both fatty liver and hepatomegaly. Lipid peroxidation of the hepatocyte membrane lipid bilayer due to the formation of a reactive oxygen species during ethanol metabolism has also been proposed as an initiating step in hepatocyte injury. The proximate metabolite of ethanol, acetaldehyde, is a highly reactive molecule that can bind to essential lysine moieties of proteins to form protein-acetaldehyde adducts. These adducts form rapidly following ethanol ingestion and could be a marker of underlying alcohol consumption. Adducts form with various proteins and may interfere with specific enzyme activities, intracellular processes, or integrity of the hepatocyte membrane. For example, the formation of acetaldehyde-tubulin adducts may alter tubulin polymerization and microtubule formation and decrease hepatic protein trafficking. This may be the explanation for hepatocyte protein accumulation, which, in conjunction with fat and osmotically retained water, results in hepatocyte and ultimately in hepatic enlargement of alcoholics. Similarly, alteration of protein synthesis and trafficking may alter hepatocyte membrane integrity and lead to cell injury.

Hypermetabolic State: Chronic ethanol intake causes enhanced oxygen consumption by the liver because of an increased rate of ethanol metabolism. This hypermetabolic state may result in relative or absolute hypoxia due to a diminished oxygen gradient along hepatic sinusoids. As the centrilobular region (zone 3) where ethanol is principally metabolized is relatively hypoxic compared with periportal areas, a further decline in oxygen availability might cause zone 3 liver injury in the alcoholic. Because propylthiouracil (PTU) reduces oxygen consumption by the liver, it has been proposed as a protective agent against alcohol-mediated liver damage.

Immune-Mediated Injury: Immune mechanisms for alcoholic liver injury have been proposed because of the initial progression of liver injury despite cessation of ethanol intake, the occurrence of a chronic hepatitis-like histology, the association of hypergammaglobulinemia, circulating immune complexes, anti-DNA, nonorgan–specific autoantibodies, and an almost anamnestic recurrence of liver injury when ethanol consumption is resumed. However, cell-mediated immunity seems more likely than humoral mechanisms to account for alcoholic liver injury. Peripheral blood lymphocyte reactivity to autologous liver, alcoholic hyalin, membrane epitopes, and the presence of circulating interleukins in those with alcoholic hepatitis support this contention.

Whether immune mechanisms initiate injury to the liver in the alcoholic or develop as a result of the initial injury to the liver is unclear. However, they may play a role in the manifestations and sequelae of alcoholic hepatitis and cirrhosis. Chemoattractants for polymorphonuclear neutrophils (PMNs) such as metabolites of leukotriene B_4 and chemotactic factor may increase PMN infiltration of centrilobular regions. Secretion of interleukin-6 (IL-6) may increase γ-globulin production. Tumor necrosis factor (TNF-α) may cause fever; and a reduction of the secretion of IL-2 may impair cell-mediated immunity in the alcoholic cirrhotic.

Role of Viral Infections: Hepatitis C virus (HCV) is frequently associated with alcoholic liver disease, and 10% to 18% of those with advanced alcoholic liver disease have concurrent infection. In addition, chronic hepatitis in the alcoholic may be a result of coexisting HCV, because these patients have more portal and lobular inflammation. False-positive test results for anti-HCV antibodies can occur in the alcoholic owing to hypergammaglobulinemia. However, this is less likely with second-generation enzyme-linked immunosorbent assay (ELISA) testing. The cause of increased prevalence of HCV in those with alcoholic liver disease is unclear. With concurrent HCV and ethanol, there is a greater risk of the development of advanced liver disease. The frequent association of hepatocellular carcinoma (HCC) and alcoholic cirrhosis could also be caused by concurrent infection with HCV.

Hepatitis B virus (HBV) infection of the alcoholic may also be more common as indicated by the higher prevalence of HBV serum markers in alcoholics compared with the general population and in those with both alcoholic liver disease and HCC, including the identification of HBV DNA in HCC cells of those with alcoholic cirrhosis.

HISTOPATHOLOGY

General: A liver biopsy is essential in the diagnosis of alcoholic liver disease, because alcohol consumption potentially alters the enzyme pattern of any liver injury to that of the typical alcoholic.

The pathologic spectrum of alcoholic liver disease classically includes hepatocellular steatosis (fatty liver), alcoholic hepatitis (alcoholic steatonecrosis), and cirrhosis. In addition, lipogranulomas, perivenular fibrosis, cholestasis,

hepatocellular foamy degeneration, chronic hepatitis, veno-occlusive disease, and hepatocellular carcinoma can be associated with ALD.

In some alcoholics, significant liver disease does not develop clinically. The liver may appear normal by light microscopy, although hepatocytes may be enlarged due to induction of SER and retention of fat, protein, and water. Whereas sinusoidal lining cells are typically fenestrated in normal persons, fenestration is reduced in the alcoholic. There is also deposition of IgA continuously along sinusoidal lining cells of both pericentral and periportal regions in the alcoholic. Pericellular IgA deposition has been related to more advanced disease. Collagenization of the space of Disse may also be observed. Lipogranulomas form when hepatocytes rupture and release intracellular fat and macrophages and mononuclear cells accumulate at the site. Focal fibrosis of a lipogranuloma can develop.

Fatty Metamorphosis: The most common pathologic change with excessive ethanol consumption is the macrovesicular accumulation of fat, usually within liver cells. Alcoholic fatty liver can develop within days of ethanol intake. Fatty change typically involves cells in acinar zones 2 and 3, although diffuse fatty change can be seen (Fig. 9–1). Hepatocytes are enlarged by the fat vacuoles, and the nuclei are displaced. Fatty change can also be observed in nonalcoholic diseases such as obesity, malnutrition, or diabetes mellitus. Microvesicular fatty change of hepatocytes (alcoholic foamy degeneration) is typically centrilobular (perivenular) and is associated with cholestasis and perivenular fibrosis. It can coexist with macrovesicular steatosis. Fatty change from alcohol is reversible with abstinence.

Alcoholic Hepatitis: Alcoholic hepatitis develops in 15% to 20% of chronic alcoholics and is thought to be the most common precursor lesion for the development of alcoholic cirrhosis. It is characterized by hepatocyte necrosis, PMN inflammation, and frequently alcoholic hyalin (Mallory's bodies) in acinar zone 3 (centrilobular) (Fig. 9–2). Other pathologic features may include hepatocyte enlargement,

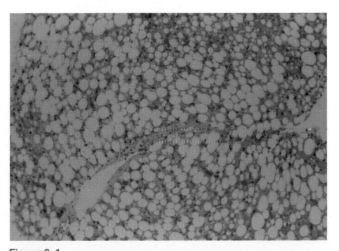

Figure 9–1
Fatty change manifested as mixed macrovesicular and microvesicular fatty metamorphosis of hepatocytes.

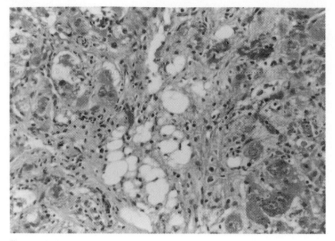

Figure 9–2
Fatty metamorphosis of hepatocytes, eosinophilic alcoholic hyalin, and focal hepatocellular necrosis typical of acute alcoholic hepatitis.

apoptotic bodies, oncocytes (hepatocytes densely packed with mitochondria), perivenular and pericellular fibrosis, Kupffer cell proliferation, portal inflammation with increased mononuclear cells, and megamitochondria. Megamitochondria may be confused at light microscopy with intracellular crystalloid bodies. Portal inflammation can be prominent. Ductular proliferation, cholestasis, and polymorphonuclear leukocyte inflammation of proliferating periportal ducts (cholangiolitis) may occur. Centrilobular cholestasis may also be prominent. Although Mallory's hyalin is often present (Fig. 9–3), it is observed in other liver diseases including sclerosing cholangitis, Wilson's disease, autoimmune hepatitis, primary biliary cirrhosis, and hepatocellular carcinoma. There are three ultrastructural types of Mallory's hyalin: type I formed by intermediate fibril bundles of 5- to 20-nm-thick fibrils in parallel array; type II formed by ran-

domly oriented fibrils; and type III with an amorphous or granular appearance. Type II Mallory's hyalin is most commonly observed. Perivenular fibrosis and terminal hepatic venule occlusion may accompany alcoholic hepatitis and produce portal hypertension in the absence of cirrhosis (acute sclerosing hyalin necrosis). Pericellular fibrosis also develops with the transformation of the quiescent stellate cell (Ito cell, lipocyte) to a collagen-producing myofibroblast. Approximately 50% of patients with alcoholic hepatitis will have cirrhosis at clinical presentation.

Veno-Occlusive Disease: Although alcoholic hepatitis may be the precursor of alcoholic cirrhosis for most alcoholics who develop cirrhosis, veno-occlusive disease may be an alternate pathway to cirrhosis for some. Some patients with alcoholic cirrhosis do not have a history or changes of alcoholic hepatitis.

Alcoholic Cirrhosis: Alcoholic cirrhosis develops in approximately 20% of those with chronic alcoholism. It is characterized by the progression of fibrous septa from perivenular to periportal areas and from periportal to periportal areas with a regenerative process that results in small nodules of hepatocytes surrounded by fibrous tissue (Fig. 9–4). This micronodular cirrhosis typically has nodules that are 1 to 3 mm in diameter. With ethanol abstinence, macronodules can develop and produce a mixed nodular or eventually frankly macronodular cirrhosis. Continued ingestion of ethanol impairs regeneration and may also result in persistent inflammation and fatty change of hepatocytes. Hepatocyte copper and iron accumulation, and α_1-antitrypsin globules may be noted. With excessive accumulation of iron, differentiation from hereditary hemochromatosis may be difficult and tissue iron levels as well as genetic testing should be obtained. Coexisting HCV infection may also be associated with iron accumulation.

Hepatocellular Carcinoma: Hepatocellular carcinoma develops in at least 5% to 10% of abstinent patients with al-

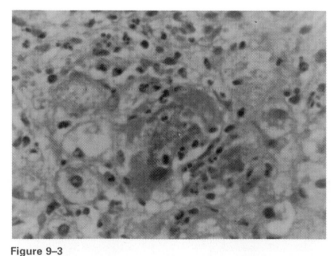

Figure 9–3
A hepatocyte containing alcoholic hyalin with an accumulation of polymorphonuclear leukocytes at its periphery (sometimes called satellitosis).

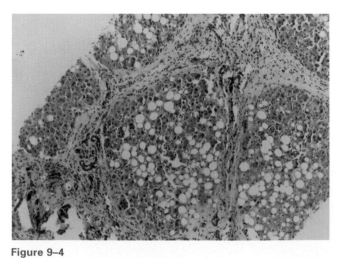

Figure 9–4
Micronodular cirrhosis. The nodules are encircled by fibrosis. Some hepatocytes contain fat.

coholic cirrhosis. It seems to correlate with the transformation from micronodular to macronodular cirrhosis and develops at a median of 4.5 years after the diagnosis of cirrhosis.

CLINICAL FEATURES

The diagnosis of ALD is based in part on a history of significant ethanol consumption, and it is incumbent on the examiner to ask appropriate questions about drinking. A number of screening tools have been developed. One of the simplest is the CAGE questionnaire (Table 9–2). Suspicion should also be high in patients with social or family disruption, depression, or abnormal behavior.

Patients with alcoholic liver disease typically present with nonspecific symptoms including right upper quadrant abdominal pain, fever, nausea, vomiting, diarrhea, anorexia, and malaise or with more specific symptoms caused by complications of portal hypertension such as abdominal swelling, peripheral edema, confusion, and gastrointestinal hemorrhage.

Fatty Liver: Although patients may not have symptoms with fatty liver, hepatomegaly is often present. In rare cases, microvesicular steatosis (alcoholic foamy degeneration) can develop and present with hepatic encephalopathy, cholestasis, jaundice, and portal hypertension. In uncomplicated fatty liver, cessation of ethanol intake should allow the liver to return to normal. Fatty liver can rarely be associated with sudden death, apparently as a consequence of fat embolism to the lungs, hypoglycemia, or alcohol withdrawal.

Alcoholic Hepatitis: Patients with acute alcoholic hepatitis typically present with jaundice, right upper quadrant abdominal pain, fever, and hepatic failure, although patients may even be asymptomatic. Those with abdominal pain, fever, and jaundice can be confused with acute cholecystitis. It is imperative to differentiate between the two because of the high perioperative mortality of patients with alcoholic hepatitis. A tender enlarged liver, jaundice, and an arterial bruit over the liver can also be observed. Protein-calorie malnutrition, parotid gland enlargement, spider angiomata, and testicular atrophy may also be present. Fevers associated with alcoholic hepatitis are typically low grade, although spiking remittent fevers can occur.

Up to 50% of patients with alcoholic hepatitis will have coexisting cirrhosis at clinical presentation, and approximately 50% of the remainder develop cirrhosis despite continued abstinence. Signs of portal hypertension can be present even in the absence of cirrhosis owing to perivenular inflammation and fibrosis or veno-occlusive disease of terminal hepatic venules.

Table 9–2   CAGE Questionnaire

Felt like you should **C**ut down your drinking?
Are you **A**nnoyed by questions about your drinking?
Have you ever felt **G**uilty about your drinking?
Do you need an **E**ye opener in the morning to get started?

Table 9–3   Maddrey's Discriminant Function

- DF-(4.6 × Prothrombin time in seconds − control) + serum bilirubin mg/dL
- If DF greater than 32, then there is a 50% increase in hospital mortality
- If DF greater than 32, consider corticosteroid therapy unless contraindicated

DF, discriminant function.

The prognosis of alcoholic hepatitis depends partly on the severity of the underlying clinical disease and can be estimated utilizing the discriminant function (DF) or Maddrey index (Table 9–3). Patients with a DF greater than 32 have a 50% chance of dying during their current hospitalization.

Alcoholic Cirrhosis: Patients with alcoholic cirrhosis can be well compensated or have symptoms and signs of portal hypertension including ascites, peripheral edema, increasing icterus, confusion, and variceal hemorrhage. Physical signs may include hepatosplenomegaly, ascites, edema, dermovascular findings of palmar erythema, spider angiomata over the upper torso, loss of nail lunulae, proximal muscle wasting, parotid enlargement, gynecomastia, testicular atrophy, periumbilical collateral vessels (caput medusa), and Dupuytren's contractures.

White nails related to hypoalbuminemia may be present. Loss of hair on the axilla and chest and alteration of the distribution of pubic hair to a female pattern can also occur. A hyperdynamic cardiovascular state with increased cardiac output can be observed. Cyanosis is rarely present owing to right-to-left shunting of blood mainly within the pulmonary vascular bed. This so-called hepatopulmonary syndrome may be associated with reduced oxygen saturation and dyspnea that improves when the patient is supine. Pulmonary hypertension and clubbing may also develop.

The clinical presentation of hepatic encephalopathy can be as subtle as minor personality changes and day-night sleep reversal or as severe as deep coma (Table 9–4). The classic physical finding of hepatic encephalopathy is asterixis (although it can be seen in other metabolic encephalopathies such as uremia, heart failure, or hypercarbia). At electroencephalography, hepatic encephalopathy is characterized by a slowing of the normal alpha rhythm to a delta rhythm. The pathophysiology of encephalopathy is still unclear, although a relationship with ammonia has long been suspected. Increased levels of circulating γ-aminobutyric acid (GABA), a neuroinhibitory peptide, have also been described.

Table 9–4   Classification of Encephalopathy

Grade	Symptoms
Grade I	Behavioral changes, sleep rhythm reversal
Grade II	Asterixis, drowsy, confusion, arousable
Grade III	Stupor, poorly arousable, asterixis
Grade IV	Flaccid, unresponsive

The most immediately life-threatening complication of portal hypertension is variceal hemorrhage. Varices are typically esophageal or gastric in location, and mortality from initial hemorrhage can be as high as 50%. Portal hypertensive gastropathy may also be observed and can result in bleeding.

Hepatorenal failure is a functional renal failure that develops in otherwise normal kidneys associated with liver failure. It rarely recovers spontaneously, although resolution with orthotopic liver transplantation or after spontaneous improvement in liver function may occur.

Protein-calorie malnutrition is commonly associated with advanced ALD as the calories from excessive ethanol intake displace normal nutrients from the diet. Inadequate dietary consumption also leads to reduction in folate and C and B vitamins; scurvy, pellagra, Wernicke's encephalopathy, and anemia may coexist.

LABORATORY FINDINGS

As ethanol metabolism enhances lactate production, hyperuricemia may be present as lactate interferes with uric acid excretion by the kidney.

Alcohol Screening: Chronic alcohol consumption can result in red blood cell enlargement and be observed as an increased mean corpuscular volume (MCV) on a complete blood count (CBC). Chronic alcoholics may also have an elevation of serum γ-glutamyltranspeptidase (GGT) due to hepatocyte enzyme induction. Although GGT and MCV have been suggested as potential screening tests for alcoholism, both are weak indicators. However, a decline in serum GGT level during a forced abstinence such as hospitalization may be more indicative. Isolated elevation of serum GGT in healthy people also occurs. Carbohydrate-deficient (desialylated) transferrin may also be indicative of alcohol intake.

Hematology: Coexistent anemia may be a consequence of iron deficiency from bleeding, folate deficiency, or anemia of chronic disease. Hemolysis may occur with hyperlipemic states. Thrombocytopenia may be a direct result of ethanol or secondary to hypersplenism. Similarly, leukopenia can result but is less likely to be a direct consequence of ethanol. In alcoholic hepatitis, the peripheral white blood cell count is increased to 12,000 to 14,000/mm^3 in 50% of patients. A leukemoid response can also be observed.

Hypoprothrombinemia, if present, is typically a result of severe alcoholic liver disease or of vitamin K deficiency. Aqueous vitamin K therapy can be administered.

Serum Tests: In the patient who lacks significant liver injury, liver tests may be normal. An elevation of serum aspartate aminotransferase (AST) typically two or more times higher than alanine aminotransferase (ALT) levels is common in patients with alcoholic liver disease. If the ratio reverses with abstinence, underlying fatty liver is more likely present. The reason why an elevation of AST over ALT develops is unclear. Although both are pyridoxine-dependent enzyme systems, ALT may be more dependent on pyridoxine. In addition, ALT is mainly a cytosolic enzyme, whereas AST is associated with intracellular organelles. Because organelle injury is more common than frank hepatocellular necrosis, the release of AST from organelles may cause higher serum levels of AST. When the AST/ALT ratio is less than 2, other etiologies of liver injury in the alcoholic should be suspected.

Hyperbilirubinemia is uncommon in fatty liver, except when microvesicular steatosis is severe. Alcoholic hepatitis is a cholestatic disease and elevation of total bilirubin to more than 85 μmol (5 mg/dL) is associated with increased mortality. A reduction of serum albumin and elevation of the prothrombin time can be indicative of advanced liver disease in either alcoholic hepatitis or alcoholic cirrhosis.

Hypergammaglobulinemia is common in end-stage alcoholic liver disease with elevations of both IgG and IgA. Nonorgan–specific autoantibodies (antinuclear, antismooth muscle antibodies) may be present at a low titer. Approximately 10% to 15% of patients with chronic alcoholic liver disease are anti–HCV positive.

The presence of a serum bilirubin higher than 85 μmol, an elevated prothrombin time, abnormal blood urea nitrogen, and a reduction of serum albumin have been associated with a poor prognosis for patients with alcoholic hepatitis.

RADIOLOGIC FINDINGS

If an abdominal x-ray is obtained, hepatomegaly, splenomegaly, and ascites may be observed. Intestinal loops will be central in a supine film, because the bowel floats in ascites.

The most useful radiologic test in the alcoholic is the abdominal ultrasound. Fatty infiltration of the liver, increased hepatic density due to advanced fibrosis, lobulation from cirrhosis, splenomegaly, and ascites can be assessed. Gallstones are increased in prevalence in end-stage liver disease, including alcoholic liver disease. The lack of dilated intra- or extrahepatic ducts plus the other findings of liver disease can help to exclude bile duct obstruction. Nonspecific thickening of the gallbladder wall can be seen with ascites. With Doppler ultrasound, the patency of the portal and hepatic veins and the direction of portal vein flow can be determined. The hepatic artery in the patient with alcoholic cirrhosis also tends to be larger than that of other forms of liver disease. Increased fibrosis and formation of regenerative nodules can reverse the flow of the portal vein. A mass may also be observed due to coexistent hepatocellular carcinoma.

Computed tomography (CT) will assist in the diagnosis of tumors, cirrhosis, ascites, and also pancreatic disease. Magnetic resonance imaging (MRI) is useful in patients with suspected hemochromatosis or secondary iron overload or liver tumors and in assessment of flow in hepatic vessels. With injection of contrast, there is a longer interval to peak enhancement than in those with normal livers.

Hepatic venography may be needed if coexistent Budd-Chiari syndrome is suspected and to determine wedged hepatic venous pressures to see if portal hypertension is present.

THERAPY AND PROGNOSIS

Cessation of the consumption of ethanol is the most important therapy for the patient with alcoholic liver disease, because long-term abstinence improves the survival of all alcoholic patients. Patients with alcoholic cirrhosis who lack clinical signs of portal hypertension may have a normal life expectancy with continued abstinence. It is also imperative to identify the potential of alcoholism as a cause for liver disease when any patient with abnormal liver tests is observed. Unfortunately, up to 25% of alcoholic patients will continue to drink regardless of previous intervention.

Uncomplicated fatty liver is a completely reversible lesion with ethanol abstinence. It may take up to 30 to 45 days to improve. Administration of anabolic steroids will hasten improvement in hepatic steatosis. Fatty liver can be a hallmark of a patient who is likely to progress to cirrhosis, thus *vigilance* in continued abstinence is necessary. Microvesicular steatosis can be associated with severe cholestasis and hepatic failure. Support and control of complications related to hepatic encephalopathy, administration of enteral supplementation, and correction of prothrombin time elevations with vitamin K administration are indicated.

The patient with alcoholic hepatitis often requires urgent care. In those with bilirubin levels greater than 85 μmol, prothrombin time elevation, and complications of portal hypertension such as ascites, the mortality may approach 50%. Coexistent azotemia of any cause is also associated with a high mortality. Many of these patients require hospitalization. Caloric supplementation with enteral or parenteral nutrition seems to improve survival. This should be started immediately upon admission or diagnosis. Both parenteral nutrition and enteral feeding seem equally effective. Correction of vitamin deficiencies should also be undertaken. Thiamine absorption will be abnormal for approximately 2 weeks after ethanol cessation, and parenteral supplementation should be given.

Coexistent HCV infection may prompt treatment with interferon-α. A reduced responsiveness has been observed in the alcoholic, and cessation of ethanol should be accomplished before interferon is administered.

The pharmacologic therapy of alcoholic hepatitis continues to be debated. Propylthiouracil (PTU), colchicine, S-adenosyl-L-methionine (SAMe), anabolic steroids, and corticosteroids have all been extensively evaluated. Infusion of insulin and glucagon has also been attempted to increase hepatocyte regeneration but with no success. Because the hypermetabolic state described in patients with alcoholic hepatitis is similar to that of hyperthyroidism, PTU has been evaluated. No significant effect on acute alcoholic hepatitis has been observed, although one long-term study has suggested that PTU will improve liver function in those outpatients who have advanced alcoholic liver disease and who continue to consume ethanol. Additional studies are needed before a recommendation of PTU can be made. Similarly, colchicine therapy has not been effective in acute alcoholic hepatitis, although a potential role in alcoholic cirrhosis (see later) has been suggested. SAMe may decrease lipid peroxidation, normalize methionine metabolism, and prevent depletion of hepatic glutathione to prevent progression of alcoholic liver injury. Preliminary results are encouraging. Oxandrolone, an anabolic steroid, will reduce steatosis and may have a beneficial role in the long-term outcome of very sick patients with acute alcoholic hepatitis based on one trial. Additional study seems warranted.

Corticosteroids may be the most promising therapy in acute alcoholic hepatitis. Numerous trials utilizing pred-nisone or prednisolone have been accomplished with varying results. However, at meta-analysis of the trials, there is a correlation with improved survival with use of corticosteroids, especially in those with coexistent spontaneous hepatic encephalopathy. In this group, short-term administration of prednisone at 40 mg/day seems warranted. Adequate nutrition must also be provided.

In patients with alcoholic cirrhosis, pharmacologic studies are more limited. Colchicine therapy has been advocated to reverse the fibrotic process. In one long-term trial over many years, improved survival of those with alcoholic cirrhosis has been observed. There seem to be few side effects, and the purported mechanism is colchicine's antifibrotic properties.

Liver transplantation for alcoholic liver disease has been debated for some time. Some argue that it is a self-inflicted disease and that the priority of the alcoholic patient should be downgraded over other patients on the transplant list. Others argue that medicine provides continuing care for patients who have developed other self-inflicted illnesses and that the alcoholic should fare no worse. Furthermore, the outcome and survival of the patient with alcoholic liver disease after liver transplantation is comparable to patients with other liver diseases. However, there is still reluctance to give a transplant to the patient with acute alcoholic hepatitis because of continued ethanol consumption up to admission and also because of poorer clinical results. For those with alcoholic cirrhosis, sustained abstinence (typically more than 6 months), a recognition by the patient of the cause of his or her liver disease, and good family support, often with active involvement in a treatment program, are prerequisites for consideration of liver transplantation. The patient with alcoholic cirrhosis will have similar long-term survival as others and may have less overall acute rejection. Recidivism does occur but is higher in those with shorter intervals of abstinence before transplantation (40% versus 6% to 11%) compared with those with abstinence for longer than 6 months. Because up to 30% of patients may resume ethanol consumption, all patients who undergo liver transplantation should be carefully followed; early intervention should be provided if the patient starts to drink again.

SUGGESTED READINGS

Beresford TP, Blow FC, Hill E, et al: Comparison of CAGE questionnaire and computer-assisted laboratory profiles in screening for cover alcoholism. Lancet 25:482–485, 1990.

Bosma A, Seifert G, Van Thiel-de Ruiter C, et al: Alcohol in combination with malnutrition causes increased liver fibrosis in rats. J Hepatol 21:394–402, 1994.

Casini A, Galli G, Salazano R, et al: Acetaldehyde induces c-fos and c-jun proto-oncogenes in fat-storing cell cultures through protein kinase C activation. Alcohol Alcohol 29:303–314, 1994.

Chedid A, Mendenhall CL, Garside P, et al: Prognostic factors in alcoholic liver disease. Am J Gastroenterol 82:210–216, 1991.

De la Hall P: Factors influencing individual susceptibility to alcoholic liver disease. In Alcoholic Liver Disease, Pathology and Pathogenesis, 2nd ed. London: Paston Press, 1995, pp 299–316.

De la Hall P: Pathological spectrum of alcoholic liver disease. In Alcoholic Liver Disease, Pathology and Pathogenesis, 2nd ed. London: Paston Press, 1995, pp 41–68.

Diehl AM: Alcoholic liver disease. Med Clin North Am 73:815–830, 1989.

Flier JS, Underhill LH: The cellular basis of hepatic fibrosis. N Engl J Med 328:1828–1835, 1993.

Flier JS, Underhill LH: Medical disorders of alcoholism. N Engl J Med 333:1058–1065, 1995.

Gassó M, Rubio M, Varela G, et al: Effects of S-adenosyl-methionine on lipid peroxidation and liver fibrogenesis in carbon tetrachloride-induced cirrhosis. J Hepatol 25:200–205, 1996.

Harris D, Brunt P: Prognosis of alcoholic liver disease. Alcohol Alcohol 30:591–600, 1995.

Ishak KG, Zimmerman H, Mukunda RB: Alcoholic liver disease: Pathologic, pathogenetic and clinical aspects. Alcohol Clin Exp Res 15:45–65, 1991.

Kearns PJ, Young H, Garcia G, et al: Accelerated improvement of alcoholic liver disease with parenteral nutrition. Gastroenterology 102:200–205, 1992.

Kershenobich D, Vargas F, Garcia-Tsao G, et al: Colchicine in the treatment of cirrhosis of the liver. N Engl J Med 318:1709–1713, 1988.

Leevy CM, Leevy CB: Liver disease in the alcoholic. Gastroenterology 105:294–296, 1993.

Lieber CS: Alcohol and the liver: 1994 update. Gastroenterology 106:1085–1105, 1994.

Liver Transplantation Consensus Conference. JAMA 25:351–355, 1983.

Mendenhall CL, Anderson S, Weesner RE, et al: Protein-calorie malnutrition associated with alcoholic hepatitis. Am J Med 76:211–222, 1984.

Okuda K, Ohnishi K: The role of viral infections in alcoholic liver disease. In Alcoholic Liver Disease, Pathology and Pathogenesis, 2nd ed. London: Paston Press, 1995, pp 147–159.

Olivera MA, Menéndez C, Kershenobich D: Tratamiento de la hepatitis alcoholica severa con S-adenosil-L-metionina (Abstract). Rev Gastroenterol Mex 59 (Suppl):69S, 1994.

Savolainen V, Perola M, Lalu K, et al: Early perivenular fibrogenesis: Pre-cirrhotic lesions among moderate alcohol consumers and chronic alcoholics. J Hepatol 23:524–531, 1995.

Schiff ER: Hepatic fibrosis—New therapeutic approaches. N Engl J Med 324:987–989, 1991.

Sherlock S: Alcoholic liver disease. Lancet 28:228–230, 1995.

Sorrell MF, Zetterman RK, Donovan J: Alcoholic hepatitis and liver transplantation: The controversy continues. Alcohol Clin Exp Res 18:222–223, 1994.

Thomson AD, Bird GL, Saunders JB: Alcoholic liver disease. Gut. Suppl:S97–S103, 1991.

Weiner FR, Esposti SD, Zern M: Ethanol and the liver. In The Liver and Pathobiology, 3rd ed. New York: Raven Press, 1994, pp 1383–1411.

Zetterman RK: Alcoholic liver disease. Curr Hepatol 13:159–177, 1993.

10

Fatty Liver, Nonalcoholic Steatohepatitis

Brent A. Neuschwander-Tetri

The accumulation of fat in hepatocytes, or hepatic steatosis, is a common histologic finding. As specific causes of liver disease have been identified and characterized, more attention has focused on the causes and consequences of hepatic steatosis, and especially nonalcoholic steatohepatitis (NASH), because these syndromes remain relatively enigmatic.

This chapter reviews the current knowledge about hepatic steatosis and its more worrisome variant, NASH. Because the inciting factor or factors that cause steatohepatitis and NASH are not presently known, the cumulative clinical knowledge is necessarily descriptive. As specific causes of these disorders are identified, we will most likely recognize steatosis and NASH as histologic manifestations of diverse metabolic defects, nutritional deficiencies, or even unrecognized infections.

EPIDEMIOLOGY

Benign Steatosis

Body habitus is the primary predictor of the presence of benign hepatic steatosis. Whereas hepatic steatosis is found in 21% of lean healthy males, almost all morbidly obese individuals will have hepatic steatosis. In the less obese, including those with body mass higher than 10% above lean body weight, about 75% have some degree of hepatic steatosis. How fat is distributed on the body predicts the presence of hepatic steatosis. In a curious analogy to coronary artery disease risk, body fat distributed about the hips is probably not a risk factor; however, a high ratio of abdominal fat to hip fat is a significant risk factor for hepatic steatosis. Youth is not protective; hepatic steatosis is found in obese children and just as frequently in adults.

Nonalcoholic Steatohepatitis

The risks factors for developing NASH are similar to the risks for benign steatosis. Because little is known of the underlying causes of NASH, efforts have been directed to characterize the recognizable risk factors for developing NASH. Although patients with NASH were once characterized as being obese, diabetic, female, and hyperlipidemic, not all patients fit this description. In fact, recent surveys have underscored the relatively high prevalence of NASH in patients without these "classic" risk factors (Table 10–1).

Obesity

Obesity is clearly the most significant risk factor for the development of NASH. The overall prevalence of NASH in obese patients has been estimated in both surgical series and autopsy studies. *Lobular hepatitis* (which in retrospect probably represents NASH) was found in 8.7% of patients in a large series of morbidly obese individuals about to undergo surgical small bowel bypass as a treatment for obesity; however, at autopsy, NASH was found in 18.5% of obese patients. Careful exclusion of coexisting risks (e.g., alcohol use, diabetes, protein malnutrition, and drug toxicity) has confirmed that obesity alone is a major risk for the development of this syndrome.

Diabetes

Diabetes mellitus is also frequently associated with hepatic steatosis. Steatosis is found in about one third of nonobese persons with type II diabetes at autopsy. As a group, patients found to have hepatic steatosis by sonography are more likely to have glucose intolerance and elevated baseline insulin levels than patients without ultrasonographic evidence

Table 10–1 Risk Factors for Hepatic Steatosis and Nonalcoholic Steatohepatitis

	Steatosis	NASH	Cirrhosis
Obesity (centripetal)	+++	++	++
Type II diabetes mellitus	++	+/−	+/−
Drugs	++	++	+/−
Female gender	+	−	−
Hypertriglyceridemia	+/−	+/−	−
Hypercholesterolemia	−	−	−

NASH, nonalcoholic steatohepatitis; +, minor risk factor; ++, moderate risk factor; +++, major risk factor; −, no risk.

Table 10–2 Causes of Macrovesicular Steatosis

Obesity (centripetal only)
Type II diabetes
Drugs
  Corticosteroids
  Estrogens
  Tamoxifen (weak estrogen agonist)
  Amiodarone
  Chloroquine
  Nifedipine and dilitiazem (case reports)
Metabolic
  Wilson's disease
Nutritional
  Starvation
  Protein deficit (kwashiorkor, eating disorders)
  Choline deficiency
  Excess carbohydrate
Infections
  Chronic hepatitis C
Miscellaneous
  Indian childhood cirrhosis
Jejunoileal bypass

of hepatic steatosis. Chronically elevated circulating insulin levels typically found in type II diabetic patients may be at least partly responsible for the accumulation of fat in the liver because of insulin's role in regulating intrahepatic fat synthesis and metabolism. In contrast, hepatic steatosis is relatively uncommon in type I diabetes, a condition characterized by episodes of hyperglycemia and low to normal insulin levels even with the best management. When steatosis is present in patients with type I diabetes, it seems to correlate with consistently poor glycemic control.

The role of diabetes as a cause of NASH, liver fibrosis, and ultimately cirrhosis in the absence of risk factors such as obesity continues to be debated. Arguments persist that diabetes alone is a risk factor for the development of cirrhosis, yet there is no strong evidence to implicate diabetes in the development of chronic liver disease in the absence of other risk factors. Many have concluded that coexistent obesity in patients with type II diabetes is the true risk factor for the development of liver disease.

Hyperlipidemia and Lipodystrophies

Hyperlipidemia, a condition that broadly includes elevations of serum cholesterol, serum triglycerides, or both, has been thought to be a risk factor or clinical marker for the development of hepatic steatosis and NASH. In reality, this association lacks solid epidemiologic evidence because establishing hypertriglyceridemia as a risk for the development of NASH has been confounded by the dominant effects of obesity and dietary habits. Nonetheless, genetic disorders of serum lipid metabolism are often characterized by hepatic steatosis. Additionally, the lipodystrophies are definitely associated with the development of NASH and the progression to end-stage liver disease. These rare diseases are characterized by abnormal mobilization of fat from peripheral stores, which greatly increases the flux of fatty acids through the liver. Whether the liver demonstrates abnormal fat metabolism in the lipodystrophies or is a passive target of the unusually high traffic of fatty acids is not known.

Gender

Of the risk factors for NASH identified in early surveys, female gender may have been overemphasized and remains unconfirmed. In fact, the prevalence of NASH is equal among men and women at autopsy and the prevalence of hepatic steatosis found by computed tomography (CT) im-

aging is equal among men and women. More recent surveys of patients with NASH have accordingly not shown an overwhelming predilection for the syndrome among women.

Drugs

Several drugs have been implicated in the development of benign steatosis and NASH (Table 10–2). The most common drugs involved corticosteroids and estrogens. Estrogens increase hepatic triglyceride synthesis, possibly outpacing the secretory capacity. Seemingly paradoxic is the association between the use of tamoxifen and the development of NASH. Well-characterized cases have been described women using it as an estrogen antagonist and as adjuvant therapy for breast cancer. In addition to its efficacy as an estrogen antagonist in the treatment of breast cancer, tamoxifen also exerts weak estrogenic activity depending on the target tissue. This activity may be responsible for its association with NASH.

PATHOPHYSIOLOGY

Hepatic steatosis is caused by an imbalance between the delivery or synthesis of fat in the liver and its subsequent secretion or metabolism. In other words, fat accumulates when the delivery of fatty acids to the liver, either from the circulation or by de novo synthesis within the liver, exceeds that capacity of the liver to metabolize the fat by β-oxidation or secrete it as very low density lipoprotein (VLDL). These are the two major mechanisms of fat delivery and two major mechanisms of fat disposal. Derangements in any of these pathways alone or in combination cause fat to accumulate in the liver and are discussed later in detail. Figure 10–1 shows how fat cycles between the liver and peripheral stores and the influence of major regulatory factors in governing the flux between the liver and the peripheral sites.

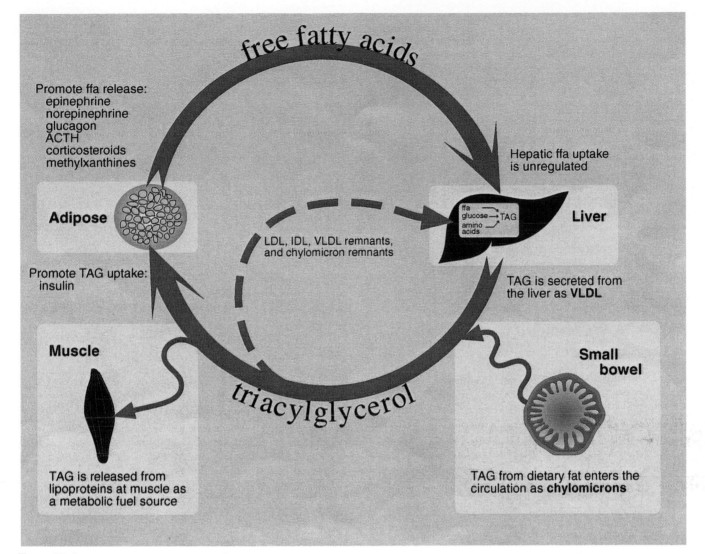

Figure 10–1
Fat cycles from peripheral stores to the liver as free fatty acids (ffa) bound to albumin and back to peripheral stores as triacylglycerol (TAG) bound to very low density lipoprotein (VLDL). TAG is also synthesized within the liver from excess glucose and amino acids. Dietary fat is converted to free fatty acids within the bowel lumen. Whereas short chain fatty acids (<11 carbon) can be delivered directly to the blood, longer chain fatty acids are re-esterified into TAG, incorporated into chylomicrons, and delivered to the circulation via the lymphatics. Fatty acids are removed from the TAG incorporated in circulating VLDL and chylomicrons by vascular lipoprotein lipases. In energy-requiring tissues such as muscle, the released fatty acids serve as a source of fuel whereas adipose tissue resynthesizes TAG for storage.

The flux through the cycle is highly dependent on the feeding state. During fasting, glucagon facilitates the release of TAG from peripheral fat stores. After a meal, insulin promotes the incorporation of fat into adipose tissue by locally upregulating vascular lipoprotein lipase activity. Insulin also promotes the formation of TAG from glucose within the liver and switches the trafficking of fatty acids from β-oxidation to TAG formation.

Delivery of Fatty Acids From Peripheral Stores to the Liver

Triglycerides, or triacylglycerol (TAG), are stored in adipose tissue and released as free fatty acids into the circulation through the actions of lipoprotein lipases. The hydrolysis of TAG in adipocytes is controlled by intracellular cyclic adenosine monophosphate (cAMP) levels. Therefore, hormonal and pharmacologic stimuli that increase adipocyte cAMP cause the release of free fatty acids from peripheral stores and increase the delivery of

fat to the liver. Epinephrine, norepinephrine, adrenocorticotropic hormone (ACTH), glucagon, corticosteroids, and methylxanthines (e.g., caffeine) are agents that stimulate adenyl cyclase and potently increase adipocyte lipolysis via a hormone-sensitive lipase. The increased lipolysis brought about by corticosteroids may reflect a protective response to prolonged starvation.

In the fed state, insulin exerts the opposite effect by increasing phosphodiesterase activity, thus depleting intracellular cAMP and preventing peripheral lipolysis. Insulin is also required for the reincorporation of fatty acids into triglyceride in both the liver and peripheral stores. Thus, after feeding, fat release from peripheral stores is inhibited and fat release from the liver is promoted.

Free fatty acids released from peripheral stores are hydrophobic and are strongly bound to circulating albumin. They are transported by albumin to tissues capable of taking up fatty acids and using them as metabolic substrates. The liver is the major site of fatty acid uptake, but the heart and skeletal muscle are also highly dependent on free fatty acids as a metabolic fuel and thus remove a fraction from the circulation.

Whereas the cAMP-mediated release of free fatty acids from the peripheral stores is highly regulated, the uptake of fatty acids by the liver is passive and unregulated. In the absence of feedback regulation, the liver cannot decrease fatty acid uptake even when the capacity to catabolize fatty acids or re-esterify them and secrete them back into the circulation as VLDL is overwhelmed. Derangements in peripheral lipolysis thus have a direct impact on the flux of fat through the liver.

Fatty Acid Synthesis Within the Liver

TAG is the most compact form of energy storage because of its inherent energy density. Conversion to fatty acids and then to TAG is thus the fate of most excess dietary carbohydrate and protein. Excess glucose is converted to fat by both the liver and adipocytes. In the liver, the backbone of most amino acids can be converted to pyruvate and then to acetyl-CoA, which feeds directly into cytosolic fatty acid synthesis.

Fate of Fatty Acids in the Liver

β-Oxidation

In the fasting state, adipocyte TAG is hydrolyzed to release free fatty acids, which are transported to the liver where they can serve as substrates for mitochondrial β-oxidation. β-Oxidation of fatty acids is a major source of energy needed to maintain liver viability during fasting. It is also the source of the ketone bodies, acetoacetate, acetone, and D-3-hydroxybutyrate. These are essential fuel sources for peripheral tissues, especially neurons, muscle, and brain when glucose is in short supply because of the inability of neural tissues to use free fatty acids as fuel. Defects in hepatic β-oxidation cause microvesicular steatosis of the liver, intolerance to fasting, and in some cases a myopathy because of the muscle's normal requirement for fatty acids as an energy source.

The first step in any pathway that metabolizes fatty acids is the formation of esters with coenzyme A, also called acyl coenzyme A (acyl-CoA). Because acyl-CoA cannot enter the mitochondria directly, the fat moiety is transferred to carnitine and the acyl conjugates with carnitine are selectively transported into the mitochondria. This carnitine shuttle requires three enzymes: (1) carnitine palmitoyl transferase I (CPTI), which forms the acyl carnitines; (2) a translocase, and (3) CPTII, which reverses the first step to form acyl-CoA from acylcarnitine within the mitochondria.

Once inside the mitochondria, acyl-CoA undergoes progressive shortening two carbons at a time to generate nicotinamide adenine dinucleotide in reduced form (NADH) and acetyl-CoA. This is the process of β-oxidation. The electrons carried by the NADH drive the production of adenosine triphosphate (ATP) and the acetyl-CoA produced is further catabolized by the Krebs cycle to form more ATP and other key metabolic intermediates, such as the ketone bodies. The enzymes required for the chain shortening have relative preferences for the newly delivered long chain fatty acids, the partly processed medium chain fatty acids, and the almost completely processed short chain fatty acids.

Defects in the function of the enzymes responsible for β-oxidation are increasingly recognized and associated with liver disorders that commonly present with some degree of microvesicular steatosis. Severe defects, such as CPTI deficiency, typically present during early childhood with fatty liver and intolerance to fasting. A defect in medium chain acyl-CoA dehydrogenase (MCHAD) has been found in some infants with sudden infant death. Other defects may manifest themselves during adulthood. One example is the association between acute fatty liver of pregnancy and a maternal partial defect in long chain hydroxyacyl-CoA dehydrogenase (LCHAD).

Certain drugs and toxins are known to impair mitochondrial β-oxidation and cause microvesicular steatosis. Valproic acid can undergo β-oxidation to intermediates that are toxic to mitochondria. Methylenecyclopropylalanine (hypoglycin) is a natural product found in unripe ackee fruit (*Blighia sapida*), which potently inhibits β-oxidation. Ackee is a popular fruit in Jamaica, and several deaths characterized by prodromal vomiting and hypoglycemia have been reported after the ingestion of unripe ackee.

The reason why impaired mitochondrial β-oxidation causes microvesicular steatosis has not been established. In general, the conditions under which β-oxidation is required (i.e., the nonfed state) are the same circumstances under which peripheral mobilization of fat is increased. Thus, there may be increased delivery of fatty acids to a liver, which is relatively energy deprived with respect to its ability to generate ATP. Potentially, the impaired mitochondrial function per se with the attendant ATP deficiency and other resulting metabolic abnormalities may impair the complex process of packaging and secreting TAG as VLDL.

An oxidation pathway of secondary importance in the flux of fatty acids through the liver is the peroxisomal pathway. Peroxisomes oxidize very long chain fatty acids (>22 carbon) and dicarboxylic acids to shorter chain lengths, which can then be managed by mitochondrial β-oxidation.

Formation and Secretion of VLDL

In the fed state, β-oxidation of fatty acids is not required as an energy source, and fatty acids delivered to the liver are mainly converted to TAG. Insulin regulates the metabolic path that fatty acids take in the liver. Without insulin, CPTI commits fatty acids to mitochondrial β-oxidation; when insulin levels are high, glycerol-3-phosphate acyltransferase commits fatty acids to the formation of TAG.

In the fed state, the liver also efficiently converts excess glucose and the backbone of many amino acids to TAG. Energy storage as TAG is probably preferred because of its compactness; TAG energy density is 9 kcal/g and can be stored as a relatively dehydrated mass. Carbohydrates and

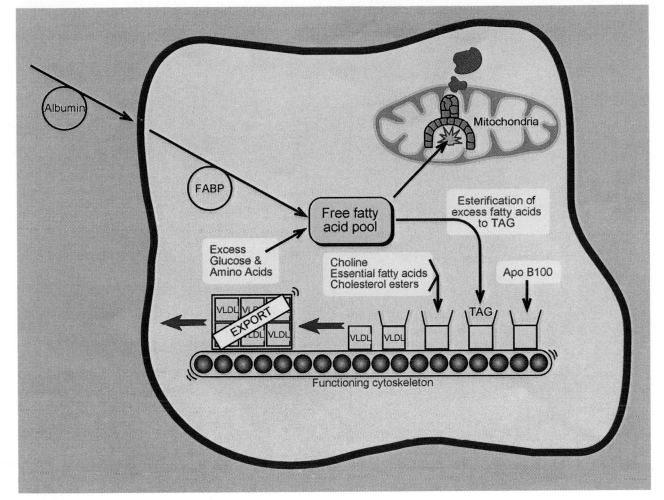

Figure 10–2
In hepatocytes, free fatty acids are either delivered from peripheral stores bound to albumin or synthesized from excess carbohydrate or amino acids. Fatty acids within hepatocytes are bound to a carrier protein fatty acid–binding protein (FABP). They are either shuttled to the mitochondria to generate energy (adenosine triphosphate [ATP]) and ketone bodies or esterified into TAG and packaged in VLDL for export. The packaging of TAG and the export of VLDL are complicated by numerous required components. An adequate supply of precursor amino acids and unimpaired protein synthesis are needed to make apolipoprotein B-100 (apoB-100); choline, essential fatty acids, and cholesterol esters are required to assemble VLDL. Finally, a functioning cytoskeletal network is then needed to export vesicles containing the VLDL particles from the hepatocyte. Defects or deficiencies in any one of these components will impair VLDL secretion and lead to fat accumulation within the cell.

amino acids are inherently less energy dense (3 and 4 kcal/g dry weight, respectively) and require solvation with a substantial amount of water, which only further reduces the energy density on a per weight basis.

Although delivery of fatty acids to the liver and fatty acid synthesis in the liver are the major contributors to liver TAG, not all liver TAG is derived from fatty acids. A fraction of liver TAG is taken up directly by endocytosis of lipoproteins and lipoprotein remnants such as low-density lipoprotein (LDL), intermediate-density lipoprotein (IDL), VLDL remnants, and chylomicron remnants. After binding to the LDL receptor and endocytosis, the TAG contained within these particles is released in a lysosomal compartment and mixed with newly synthesized TAG.

The secretion of TAG into the circulation in the form of VLDL is the only mechanism of disposing TAG from the hepatocyte. Because of its complexity, the synthesis and se-

cretion of VLDL from the liver is the rate-limiting step in the cycling of fat between the liver and peripheral stores. Through a process of combining TAG with apolipoprotein B-100, phosphatidyl choline, cholesterol, and cholesterol esters, functional VLDL is formed and secreted by exocytosis (Fig. 10–2). Much can go awry in the complex process of VLDL secretion. The result is TAG accumulation and its common clinical correlate, hepatic steatosis (Table 10–3). This simple fact explains why the many seemingly unrelated causes of steatosis have but this one clinical manifestation.

Although VLDL may acquire minor amounts of other lipoproteins once it enters the circulation, when it is secreted from the liver apolipoprotein B-100 (apoB-100) is the only protein component. ApoB-100 is coded by a single gene on chromosome 2, and the gene structure is defined by 29 exons (expressed sequences) and 28 introns (intervening se-

Table 10–3 Defects in VLDL Synthesis

Defect	Comments
ApoB gene defect	Homozygous abetalipoproteinemia is a severe disease of infancy; heterozygous hypobetalipoproteinemia varies in its phenotypic expression
Dietary protein deficiency	VLDL synthesis is especially sensitive to threonine deficiency
Choline deficiency	Required to form phosphatidylcholine, an essential component of VLDL
	Methionine may be able to replace choline as a methyl donor
	Major cause of TPN-induced steatosis
Essential fatty acid deficiency	Essential fatty acids are required for phosphatidylcholine synthesis
Cholesterol esterification defect	Cholesterol esters are required for VLDL assembly
Altered cytoskeleton	Impairs exocytosis

ApoB, apolipoprotein B; TPN, total parenteral nutrition; VLDL, very low density lipoprotein.

quences). The product mRNA translation is a 4536 amino acid protein with a molecular weight of 512 kD and an amino terminus LDL receptor–binding domain. Posttranslational processing includes *N*-glycosylation, acylation, and phosphorylation to achieve the functional protein. The synthesis of apoB-100 is rapid; protein synthesis requires less than 15 minutes and incorporation into VLDL followed by secretion requires another 30 minutes. Much newly synthesized apoB-100 never reaches the circulation and is instead subject to intracellular degradation. This excess synthesis may occur when the supply of TAG is inadequate to form VLDL. Conversely, the rate of apoB-100 synthesis can be overcome by excessive free fatty acid delivery to the liver.

Defects in apoB-100 synthesis and function cause TAG to accumulate in the liver. A simple deficiency of amino acids can prevent adequate apoB-100 synthesis, which may explain the steatosis commonly found in protein malnutrition (kwashiorkor). ApoB-100 is rich in threonine, and its synthesis is thus particularly sensitive to a deficiency of this amino acid. Certain apoB-100 gene mutations result in partial or complete loss of functional protein synthesis. Complete absence of functional protein (abetalipoproteinemia) presents in infancy with severe fat malabsorption and can lead to cirrhosis. The fat malabsorption associated with abetalipoproteinemia is probably due to the concomitant deficiency of apoB-48, the intestinal lipoprotein analogue of apoB-100 that is required for chylomicron assembly. ApoB-48 is required for intestinal fat absorption and is coded by the same gene as apoB-100 (see later). Partial loss of functional apoB-100, or hypobetalipoproteinemia, has a more diverse phenotypic expression depending on the degree of protein absence, but deficiencies have been identified in adults with NASH.

Sources of Plasma Triacylglycerol

In the fasted state, most plasma triglyceride is found within hepatically secreted VLDL, whereas the small remaining fraction is distributed among various VLDL degradation products (see later). In contrast, in the fed state, the majority of triglyceride is found within chylomicrons. There are two reasons for the dominance of chylomicron TAG over VLDL TAG in the fed state. Most obvious is that dietary fat absorbed from the small intestine is wholly incorporated into chylomicrons. In addition to the resultant increase in circulating chylomicrons, there is a decrease in hepatic VLDL secretion in the fed state because of the inhibitory effects of insulin on VLDL synthesis and secretion.

Chylomicron synthesis in the small bowel epithelial cells is analogous to hepatic VLDL synthesis and secretion in most respects. However, in humans, the predominant lipoprotein incorporated into nascent chylomicrons is apoB-48, whereas the liver incorporates apoB-100 into VLDL. Interestingly, apoB-48 is a protein with 2152 amino acids with a final molecular weight of 248 kD coded by the amino terminus of the apoB-100 gene; the 2153rd codon of the apoB-48 gene is a stop codon that leads to the smaller protein product. During the final assembly of chylomicrons, smaller amounts of the A lipoproteins are also incorporated, and the final product is secreted into the lymphatics. Short chain fatty acids less than 10 carbons can bypass this route of absorption and pass directly into the circulation.

Fate of Plasma Triacylglycerol

Lipoprotein Modification

Circulating lipoprotein complexes undergo several modifications before they release TAG at peripheral sites. Both VLDL and chylomicrons acquire C lipoproteins and apoE from circulating high-density lipoprotein (HDL). Neither VLDL nor chylomicrons lose apoB-100 or apoB-48 respectively to other lipoproteins, presumably because of the extensive hydrophobic interactions between these two lipoproteins and the lipid cores of the entire particles.

Release of Fatty Acids

Very little of the TAG in the circulation is absorbed by the liver. Depending on the levels of circulating insulin, circulating TAG is consumed either by adipose tissue or by energy-requiring tissues such as muscle. In the fed state, high insulin levels favor uptake by adipose tissue. In the fasted state, lower insulin levels favor utilization by muscle and other tissues able to release fatty acids from lipoprotein-bound TAG. The lack of direct uptake of TAG or fatty acids from VLDL or chylomicrons may explain the paradoxic lack of a strong correlation between hyperlipidemic states and hepatic steatosis.

The uptake of fat from lipoproteins requires release of free fatty acids from TAG by lipoprotein lipase (LPL) at the vascular endothelium. LPL is an enzyme that belongs to a multigene family, which includes pancreatic lipase. Although it is synthesized by many tissues, LPL is found predominantly in muscle and adipose tissue, which correlates with the major sites of TAG consumption. The enzyme attaches to vascular endothelial cells by its interaction with the glycoprotein heparan sulfate. The enzyme is not produced by vascular endothelial cells but instead is synthesized by adipocytes and myocytes. Because of their disparate roles in fat metabolism, fat and muscle express LPL under different conditions. LPL expression by the adipocyte is increased in the fed state by insulin, whereas expression in muscle is constitutively high and increases modestly with fasting.

Through the action of LPL, TAG is removed from VLDL and chylomicrons. Removal of TAG from VLDL sequentially generates VLDL remnants, IDL, and finally LDL in increasing order of density. The increasing density reflects the progressively decreasing TAG content. The removal of TAG from VLDL is relatively rapid; after 15 to 60 minutes, most TAG is removed from circulating VLDL. About half of VLDL is processed to LDL, whereas the other half is less fully defatted and generates VLDL remnants and IDL. Chylomicrons are depleted of their TAG even more rapidly, with a substantial fraction removed within 5 to 10 minutes after entering the circulation. The result is chylomicron remnants that contain 10% to 20% of their original TAG and all of the dietary cholesterol, which was originally carried by this gut-derived lipoprotein.

The end products after TAG is removed from VLDL and chylomicrons (namely VLDL remnants, IDL, LDL, and chylomicron remnants) are taken up by the liver. How much this uptake of relatively dense lipoproteins along with their residual TAG contributes to the fat pool in the liver is unknown but is probably minor compared with the intrahepatic synthesis of fatty acids and the delivery of fatty acids to the liver from peripheral stores. Uptake of lipoproteins is facilitated by the hepatic LDL receptor. The receptor interacts with apoE contained in VLDL remnants but in the more TAG-depleted and apoE–depleted LDL, the interaction is with apolipoprotein B-100. The LDL receptor has a relatively low affinity for LDL, and this weak interaction is probably one reason why LDL has a long circulating half-life of 3 days compared with the parent VLDL. The role of defects in LDL clearance as a cause of vascular disease remains controversial. ApoB-100 and apoE mutations have been identified; these decrease binding of LDL to the hepatic receptor and thus decrease the clearance of LDL. Although these mutations are associated with hypercholesterolemia and vascular disease, the relative importance of defects in each of the lipoproteins has not been resolved, and their role in contributing to hepatic steatosis is uncertain.

Other Forms of Hepatic Steatosis

Microvesicular Steatosis

Microvesicular steatosis is distinguished from macrovesicular steatosis on well-defined morphologic grounds and also by pathophysiologic mechanisms. Whereas macrovesicular steatosis is caused by an imbalance in the hepatic synthesis and export of TAG, all causes of microvesicular steatosis are related to defects in mitochondrial function (Table 10–4). The reason why the accumulated TAG of microvesicular steatosis is retained in smaller vesicles distributed pancellularly rather than coalescing into large droplets characteristic of macrovesicular steatosis is unknown.

Alcoholic Steatosis

The pathogenesis of alcoholic liver disease is reviewed in Chapter 9. The accumulation of TAG in the liver caused by alcohol, even in normal individuals with modest alcohol consumption, has not been fully explained. Hepatic TAG synthesis is increased after the consumption of alcohol. Fat may accumulate simply as a result of excessive TAG synthesis, or there may be a concomitant defect in the secretion of VLDL that contributes synergistically to the accumulation of fat in the liver. Alcohol is also a major mitochondrial toxin, which explains features seen in severe alcoholic hepatitis such as megamitochondria and microvesicular fat. Hepatic lipid peroxidation occurs during alcohol metabolism by the liver, and studies in many different organ systems have tied oxidant stress to the development of an inflammatory response.

Phospholipidoses

Phospholipid accumulation in the liver causes steatohepatitis and can cause a histologic picture similar to the steatosis caused by TAG accumulation. The phospholipidosis syndromes are caused by the accumulation of phospholipids in lysosomes. The expansion of membranes by excess phospholipids results in the development of enlarged lysosomes with a redundant membrane that is folded over repeatedly to form "lamellar bodies." These laminar bodies can be identified using electron microscopy because of their characteristic membranous whirl appearance.

The phospholipidoses are caused by impaired breakdown of phospholipids within lysosomes, leading to the accumulation of these amphipathic lipids in the lysosomal membranes. Genetic deficiencies of enzymes that metabolize phospholipids can cause a lethal accumulation of phospholipids within lysosomes. Wolman's disease occurs in childhood and is caused by the absence of lysosomal acid lipase. Cholesterol ester storage disease is caused by defective expression of the same enzyme, yet small residual activity can allow survival past childhood. Lysosomal sphingomyelinase is deficient in patients with Niemann-Pick disease.

Drugs that impair the lysosomal enzymes that metabolize phospholipids or diminish the lateral mobility of phospholipids within membranes are the major causes of the phospholipidoses (Table 10–5). Generally, drugs that cause phospholipidosis are polycationic (meaning that they have more than one positive charge) and amphipathic (meaning that in addition to the polar charged region of the molecule, much of the drug is nonpolar or hydrophobic). These properties allow such drugs to bind phospholipids within membranes and prevent their normal mobility and enzymatic degradation. The lysosomes are probably a target for such amphipathic drug accumulation because of their lower intraorganelle pH, which favors compartmental accumulation. The same mechanism is also responsible for mitochondrial accumulation of such drugs where they can be concentrated and impair mitochondrial function.

Because of the slow accumulation rate in the lysosomal membrane compartment, drugs that cause clinically apparent phospholipidosis are typically administered for prolonged periods before an a significant amount of phospholipid accumulates. Thus, antibiotics such as gentamicin, ketoconazole, and azithromycin, which cause phospholipi-

Table 10–4 Causes of Microvesicular Steatosis

Cause	Mechanism
Drugs	
Valproic acid	Depletion of mitochondrial CoA; β-oxidation and blockade of β-oxidation enzymes by P-450 drug metabolites
Tetracycline (high dose)	Inhibited β-oxidation; impaired hepatic triglyceride secretion
Aspirin	Uncoupling oxidative phosphorylation; depletion of extramitochondrial acetyl-CoA, which prevents transport of fatty acids into the mitochondria
2-Arylpropionate NSAIDS (pirprofen, naproxen, ibuprofen, ketoprofen)	Inhibit β-oxidation of medium and short chain fatty acids
Amineptine	Inhibit β-oxidation of medium and short chain fatty acids
Nucleoside analogues (zidovudine, didanosine, zalcitabine, fialuridine)	Inhibition of mitochondrial DNA replication
Toxins	
Ethanol	Diminished mitochondrial NAD^+ impairs β-oxidation; mitochondrial oxidant stress damages mtDNA
Hypoglycin (unripe ackee)	Impaired β-oxidation
Bacillus cereus emetoxin	Impaired β-oxidation
Toxic shock syndrome	Unknown bacterial toxins
Genetic Defects	
Acute fatty liver of pregnancy	Defects in the β-oxidation; LCHAD defect in a subset of patients
β-Oxidation defects:	
CPT I	Inadequate substrate for β-oxidation
CPT II	Inadequate substrate for β-oxidation
Others	Inadequate substrate for β-oxidation
Ornithine transcarbamylase deficiency	Inhibition of long and medium chain fatty acid β-oxidation by ammonium
Alper's disease	Unknown mitochondrial defect
Other	
Reye's syndrome	Combined acquired and genetic defects in β-oxidation or ureagenesis
Cholestasis (foamy degeneration)	Impaired mitochondrial function by bile acids

CoA, coenzyme A; CPT, carnitine palmitoyl transferase; NSAIDs, nonsteroidal anti-inflammatory drugs; LCHAD, long-chain hydroxyacyl-CoA dehydrogenase.

Table 10–5 Hepatic Phospholipidoses

Metabolic diseases
  Niemann-Pick disease
  Wolman's disease
  Cholesterol ester storage disease
Drugs
  Amantadine
  Amiodarone
  Amitriptyline
  Chloroquine
  Chlorphenteramine
  Chlorpromazine
  Dilitiazem
  Fenfluramine
  Imipramine
  Nifedipine
  Oral contraceptives
  Propranolol
  Thioridazine
  Gentamicin

dosis experimentally, are not major causes of clinically evident phospholipidosis, because of their typically short treatment regimens. By contrast, the now abandoned antianginal drug perhexiline maleate and the antiarrhythmic drug amiodarone cause clinically relevant phospholipidosis because of their need for prolonged use.

The relationship between phospholipidosis and injury to the liver is unclear. Although there are reports of idiosyncratic-type reactions to amiodarone with clinically evident liver injury, this occurs only in a few cases compared with the frequent development of phospholipidosis. Steatohepatitis, as distinguished from phospholipidosis, can be found concomitantly with amiodarone treatment but does not appear to be a direct consequence of phospholipidosis.

Steatosis and Inflammation

The inflammatory response characteristic of NASH appears to develop only in the setting of pre-existing steatosis. The converse—the development of the characteristic mixed cellular infiltrate throughout the acinus without steatosis—is not a known histopathologic condition. One hypothesis is that the fat within the steatotic liver serves as a readily available target for lipid peroxidation. Lipid peroxidation produces highly toxic intermediates that promote inflammation and directly compromise cellular integrity.

CLINICAL FEATURES

Symptoms

Hepatic steatosis is usually asymptomatic. The most common complaint in patients with benign steatosis or NASH, particularly in the obese, is dull right upper quadrant pain, which may be caused by a distended liver capsule. A variety of less common nonspecific constitutional symptoms such as weakness, fatigue, and malaise are offered by patients with NASH. The prevalence and severity of these same constitutional symptoms is much greater in patients with alcoholic hepatitis, despite the similarity of biopsy findings and aminotransferase elevations.

Physical Examination

Palpable hepatomegaly can signify a liver enlarged by benign steatosis or NASH. However, hepatomegaly can be difficult to detect by palpation in many patients because of the coexistent obesity. There are no other specific physical findings that would suggest hepatic steatosis. Findings such as jaundice, spider angiomata, muscle wasting, ascites, and palmar erythema point to the development of cirrhosis.

Laboratory Evaluation

Most patients who come to medical attention for the evaluation of subclinical liver disease do so because of incidental laboratory abnormalities. This fact biases all clinical surveys that attempt to establish the sensitivity of laboratory testing for identifying patients with NASH. Progression of NASH can occur with normal laboratory testing; this has been shown in reports of the preoperative evaluation of patients undergoing surgical treatment for obesity. Among the laboratory tests available, the aminotransferases provide the most useful information. Other biochemical abnormalities that are common in alcoholic hepatitis (e.g., hypoalbuminemia, hyperbilirubinemia, and prothrombin time elevations) are not observed in NASH unless the disease has progressed to cirrhosis.

Aminotransferases

Patients with NASH typically have serum aminotransferases that range from normal to a maximum of four times the upper limit of normal (Table 10–6). The prevalence of elevated aminotransferases in patients with NASH is unknown. This is mainly because the presence of liver disease is not routinely pursued in patients with normal aminotransferases, even when imaging studies suggest hepatic steatosis. The presence of elevated aminotransferases cannot be used to distinguish benign steatosis from NASH.

One way in which aminotransferase elevations can be useful in identifying patients with NASH is the ratio of alanine aminotransferase (ALT) to aspartate aminotransferase (AST) activities. Whereas patients with alcoholic hepatitis typically have serum AST levels that exceed the ALT, patients with NASH often have an ALT that is greater than the AST level in the absence of cirrhosis. Identification of the intracellular origin of serum aminotransferases has not proved helpful in distinguishing NASH from alcoholic hepatitis. In both diseases, the ratio of mitochondrial AST to total AST is elevated, possibly reflecting a shared pathogenetic mechanism of mitochondrial injury.

Other Biochemical Markers

γ-Glutamyltranspeptidase (GGT) elevations correlate with increases in hepatic fat content, yet elevations of this enzyme are rarely isolated when substantial and are rarely worth pursuing further when trivial. Serum triglyceride elevations are found in only a few adults with NASH but are common in children.

Imaging

The major abdominal imaging modalities—sonography, CT, magnetic resonance imaging (MRI), and radionuclide techniques—can each contribute to the identification of focal or diffusely distributed hepatic steatosis (Table 10–7). Each has the ability to indicate the presence of hepatic steatosis, yet none of these techniques has the ability to distinguish benign hepatic steatosis from NASH. Generally, NASH is nonfocal, and thus areas of focal fat or focal sparing primarily create problems when distinguishing these lesions from a malignancy. An exception to the rule that NASH is not fo-

Table 10–6 Laboratory Findings of Steatosis and NASH

Aminotransferases (ALT and AST)	Normal values do not exclude steatosis or NASH Typically one to four times the upper limit of normal ALT is greater than AST in most patients (helpful in distinguishing from alcoholic steatosis/steatohepatitis)
Alkaline phosphatase	Typically normal but can be up to two times the upper limit of normal
γ-Glutamyl-transpeptidase (GGT)	Can be elevated; the degree of elevation correlates with the extent of the steatosis
Triglycerides	Frequently elevated in children with steatosis and NASH but not consistently elevated in adults
Cholesterol	No correlation; abnormally low cholesterol may indicate hypobetalipoproteinemia as a cause of steatosis/NASH
Total bilirubin	Normal in the absence of cirrhosis
Prothrombin time, albumin	Normal in the absence of cirrhosis

ALT, alanine aminotransferase; AST, aspartate transaminase; NASH, nonalcoholic steatohepatitis.

Table 10–7 Imaging Findings of Steatosis and NASH

	Ultrasonography	Computed Tomography
Diffuse steatosis and NASH	Echogenic liver parenchyma Loss of contrast between the bile duct wall and liver parenchyma Hemangiomas may appear hypoechoic compared with the surrounding liver parenchyma	Low-density liver parenchyma compared with the spleen
Focal steatosis	Often a geometrically shaped echogenic area No mass effect Can be transient, absent on follow-up studies	Single or multiple low-density areas (often with the appearance of metastatic disease)
Focal sparing	Area of decreased echogenicity Often in caudate lobe or adjacent to the gallbladder	Regions of normal density in an otherwise low-density liver

NASH, nonalcoholic steatohepatitis.

cal may be found in diabetic patients. Diabetic patients receiving insulin in their peritoneal dialysis fluid can develop subcapsular steatosis, which can progress to NASH that is confined to the periphery of the liver. Such observations may provide important insights into the role of insulin in the accumulation of hepatic fat and the importance of fat as a precursor lesion to NASH.

Ultrasonography

Compared with the normal liver, the fatty liver is diffusely echogenic or "bright" (Fig. 10–3). Ultrasonography of the liver is a reliable technique for the detection of hepatic steatosis only when the degree of steatosis is substantial. Thus, when biopsy results are compared with ultrasonographic findings, a significant amount of fat must be present for the liver to appear sonographically dense. The finding of a diffusely echogenic liver is not entirely specific for steatosis, because cirrhosis can cause a similar appearance but with a subjectively coarser texture.

Computed Tomography

CT scanning of the fatty liver typically reveals an abnormally low-density liver parenchyma compared with the spleen (Fig. 10–4). A low-density liver is a relatively common finding, occurring in up to 10% of all abdominal CT scans. Most commonly, the low attenuation is diffuse. However, in up to one third of the patients, the involvement is focal and appears as one or more low-density lesions in an otherwise normal liver. Focal fat can be found anywhere in the parenchyma or can be localized only to the periportal region. Focal sparing in an otherwise fatty liver can also be seen, and it has the appearance of a high-density lesion that can be confused with a malignancy. A comparison of the density of the focal area of sparing with its surrounding liver and with the spleen is helpful to identify its nature.

Magnetic Resonance Imaging

MRI can detect diffuse hepatic steatosis with a similar sensitivity to CT. MRI may not be particularly useful for further evaluating focal lesions suspected to be fat by CT, although phase shifting can be used to identify focal fat by its loss of intensity on T_1-weighted images.

Radionuclide Imaging

Radionuclide imaging using ^{99m}Tc sulfur colloid identifies focal areas of fat within the liver as focal defects, a finding that contributes nothing to making the distinction between benign and malignant etiologies. On the other hand, areas of focal sparing in the otherwise diffusely fatty liver will absorb tracer, and this can be helpful when evaluating such lesions. One radionuclide technique that has not been used often is the measurement of hepatic ^{133}Xe retention. Although this test offers the most sensitive measure of hepatic steatosis, its clinical usefulness has not been extensively evaluated.

Imaging Problems

Focal Fat

The incidental discovery of lesions in the liver caused by focal fat or focal sparing can be challenging. Even after using more than one imaging modality, focal areas of fat in the liver can be difficult to distinguish from primary or metastatic malignancies. The resultant uncertainty can lead the clinician down a path of escalating diagnostic invasiveness in children and adults alike. A few clues can point to focal fat, such as the typically aspherical or geometric appearance of focal fat without exerting a mass effect on adjacent structures. However, this is not always the case, and fine-needle aspiration biopsy of problematic lesions may be required to definitively exclude malignancy, especially in patients with a history of prior malignancy. If the level of concern is lower, especially in children, then repeated sonographic imaging within 3 to 6 months is a reasonable and more conservative approach.

Focal Sparing

Focal sparing, representing focal areas of normal liver, can be seen occasionally in an otherwise fatty liver. Focal sparing appears as a relatively hyperdense region by CT with

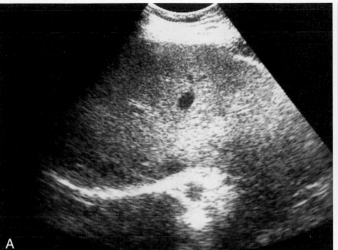

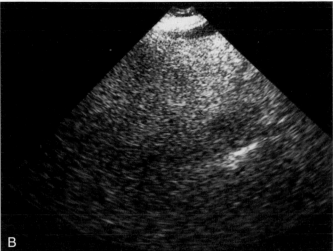

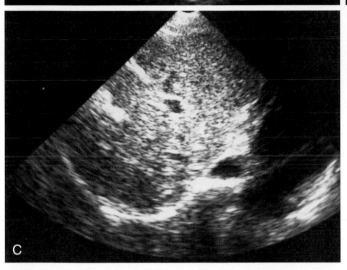

Figure 10–3
Sonographic images of the liver from patients with a biopsy-proven normal liver (*A*), severe steatosis (*B*), and cirrhosis caused by primary sclerosing cholangitis (*C*). Increased echogenicity is evident in both the steatotic and cirrhotic liver images compared with the normal liver.

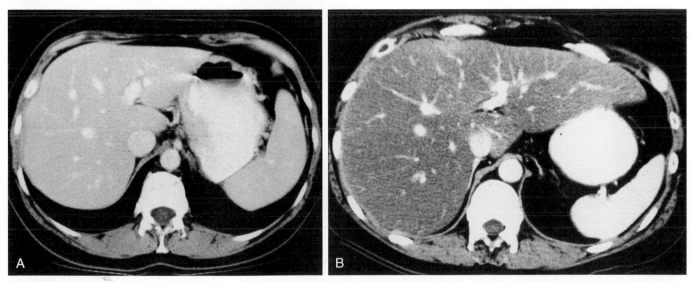

Figure 10–4
The abdominal computed tomography (CT) images demonstrate the appearance of a normal liver (*A*) and steatotic liver (*B*) after the administration of intravenous contrast solution. The normal liver density is comparable to the density of the spleen. The steatotic liver has a much lower radiographic density compared with the spleen, and the contrast-filled hepatic vasculature is accentuated by the surrounding low-density liver parenchyma. The image of the steatotic liver was obtained from a nondrinking woman who had received tamoxifen therapy for 3 years after the resection of a breast cancer. She complained of dull pain in the right upper quadrant of the abdomen. A liver biopsy showed severe steatosis, Mallory's hyaline, and the presence of inflammation characteristic of nonalcoholic steatohepatitis (NASH).

corresponding hypodense areas identified by sonography. These areas, such as the commonly spared caudate lobe, tend to receive aberrant portal venous drainage with isolation of the spared segments of the liver from intestinal venous blood. The location and geometric shape of focal sparing generally distinguishes focal sparing from malignancy in a fatty liver, but a fine-needle biopsy for histologic confirmation may be necessary in unusual circumstances.

Identification of Other Lesions in a Fatty Liver

Fat within the liver also creates problems in properly identifying other pathology, especially by ultrasonography. Hemangiomas are typically echodense, yet these benign lesions may appear as relatively hypodense lesions when surrounded by the much more echodense fatty parenchyma. Dynamic CT scanning and tagged red blood cell radionuclide imaging are the best tests for establishing the identity of such lesions when there is significant doubt. Detection of dilated intrahepatic bile ducts in the fatty liver can also present problems, because the usual contrast between the normal liver and the echodense bile duct wall is lost.

DIAGNOSIS

Liver Biopsy

The diagnosis of NASH can be established only by liver biopsy. The clinical setting, the risk factors, the laboratory data, and the imaging studies can only be suggestive. In fact, all of these together remain insensitive and nonspecific for the diagnosis. Moreover, none of these can distinguish benign steatosis from NASH.

Indications

Because biochemical abnormalities and imaging findings have poor sensitivity in signaling the presence of NASH, the threshold for obtaining a liver biopsy to evaluate patients suspected of having NASH should be low. Early recognition of NASH by biopsy can provide the necessary incentive to achieve sustained weight loss, which results in improved histology and prevention of progressive liver disease in selected patients.

Biopsy Findings

The histologic findings in NASH are substantially similar to those typically found in alcoholic hepatitis and are reviewed in detail in Chapter 5. Characteristic lesions in both conditions are hepatocellular steatosis and lobular inflammation; sometimes Mallory bodies and fibrosis are also found. The steatosis found in NASH is predominantly macrovesicular (>2 μm), with fat globules that laterally displace hepatocyte nuclei. By contrast, microvesicular fat is characterized by less than 1-μm globules that do not displace the nucleus peripherally. The lobular distribution of fat can vary in NASH, with panlobular and perivenular localization being the most common patterns. In situations where identification of fat is essential to convincingly identify microvesicular steatosis, a frozen section of the biopsy must be stained

with a fat-specific stain such as Oil red O. Oil red O specifically highlights fat as dark red globules on a pale background.

Inflammation is an essential component in NASH. The absence of the characteristic inflammation in a fatty liver is the hallmark of benign steatosis. The inflammatory cells of NASH are a mixture of neutrophils and mononuclear cells and are found throughout the lobule. Although the presence of neutrophils is a characteristic finding, neutrophils are not usually the predominant inflammatory cell type. Nonetheless, focal neutrophilic infiltrates can be found in areas of focal necrosis.

The presence of Mallory bodies and glycogen nuclei are variable findings in NASH biopsies. Mallory bodies are aggregates of cytoskeletal proteins and can be found in some NASH biopsies. Mallory bodies appear as eosinophilic, stranded structures in the hepatocyte cytoplasm and are identified most easily in ballooned hepatocytes. The presence of Mallory bodies is not a required histologic feature of NASH, and they are often small compared with the Mallory bodies found in alcoholic hepatitis. The presence of large or antler-shaped Mallory bodies should raise the suspicion of surreptitious alcohol abuse, because these more obvious accretions are typical of alcoholic liver disease. In contrast, glycogen nuclei are usually seen more frequently in NASH than in alcoholic liver disease. The central accumulation of glycogen in hepatocyte nuclei makes the nuclei appear ring-like around a clear central region. The cause of glycogen nuclei is uncertain, but the identity of the nuclear abnormality has been confirmed by electron microscopy. It is a nonspecific finding common in diabetes, Wilson's disease, and other disorders.

The identification of fibrosis in NASH is undoubtedly the most worrisome finding, because it predicts the potential for progression to cirrhosis in a given patient. The pattern of early fibrosis in NASH is similar to that seen in alcoholic liver disease, with collagen around the central vein and in the zone 3 perisinusoidal spaces producing a chicken-wire appearance. The overall prevalence of fibrosis in patients with NASH is uncertain; most earlier surveys were conducted before hepatitis C could be excluded serologically as a contributing factor; however, recent studies indicate that fibrosis is found in approximately 15% to 30% of patients.

TREATMENT AND PROGNOSIS

Weight Reduction

Weight loss can effectively normalize aminotransferases and reduce sonographically detectable liver fat in obese adults and children who present with elevated aminotransferases and hepatic steatosis. The benefit of reducing or eliminating hepatic steatosis is two-fold. If symptoms such as right upper quadrant abdominal pain are present, these can be improved or eliminated. More significantly in terms of overall prognosis is the potential to eliminate the risk of NASH and progressive liver disease.

The degree of weight loss needed to achieve normalization of serum aminotransferases and improvement in sonographically detectable hepatic steatosis has not been rigorously established. Several studies have shown that only modest weight reduction is needed, but exact numbers are hard to come by.

The means by which weight is lost is also very important. Gradual weight reduction achieved while providing adequate nutrients such as essential amino acids in the form of complete protein, essential fatty acids, and vitamins is crucial. Substantial caloric deficit can yield short-term weight loss, but the flux of fat from peripheral stores to the liver in the setting of inadequate essential amino acids and other key nutrients cause the delivery of fat to the liver to exceed its capacity to synthesize and secrete VLDL. The net result is worsening of the hepatic fat accumulation.

Management of Diabetes

Prevention of frequent hyperglycemic episodes is effective in reducing hepatic steatosis in patients with type I diabetes. However, NASH is not a significant problem for these patients, and thus the need for better glycemic control with respect to liver disease is to reduce symptomatic hepatomegaly caused by the benign accumulation of hepatic triglycerides. The role of improved glycemic control to prevent NASH and progressive liver disease in patients with type II diabetes has probably been overstated in the past. Weight reduction is much more important, and in the absence of significant weight reduction, type II diabetic patients typically fail to have improved liver enzymes despite treatment with insulin to achieve better control of blood glucose.

Liver Transplantation

Liver transplantation is an option for selected patients who progress to decompensated cirrhosis. One percent of transplants may be for patients with progressive liver disease caused by NASH. Even this figure may underestimate the true prevalence of end-stage liver disease caused by NASH, because the characteristic findings of NASH can resolve after the development of cirrhosis and patients may present with bland cryptogenic cirrhosis. Additional evidence linking abnormalities of hepatic fat metabolism and the development of cirrhosis is provided by studies showing a disproportionately high prevalence of mutations in the apoB-100 lipoprotein gene in patients with cryptogenic cirrhosis. Moreover, there are now case reports of NASH developing as a recurrent disease following liver transplantation, suggesting that peripheral metabolic abnormalities or infectious causes may contribute to NASH.

Unproved Treatment Strategies

The increasingly frequent identification of patients who are lean and do not have identifiable and correctable risk factors for NASH has led to the search for alternative treatment strategies with the aim of preventing progressive liver disease. There are reports that ursodiol may be beneficial, but these have not been corroborated by larger clinical trials or explained by the known pathophysiology of steatosis and NASH. Because of the complexity of fat secretion from the liver, there are likely to be many different causes of steatosis (and by inference NASH) that will each require its own specific treatment. For example, choline is required for the synthesis of lecithin, a phospholipid necessary for VLDL formation and triglyceride secretion. Choline deficiency was a major cause of hepatic steatosis during prolonged administration of parenteral nutrition before the solutions were routinely supplemented with additional choline. Pantothenic acid deficiency has also been proposed as a cause of hepatic steatosis. Pantothenic acid is a necessary nutritional precursor for the synthesis of coenzyme A, and coenzyme A is essential for hepatic fat metabolism. In one unblinded study, pantothenic acid supplementation was thought to cause histologic improvement in hepatic steatosis. Well-designed clinical studies are needed to define the people who might benefit from such therapeutic interventions.

SUGGESTED READINGS

Bacon BR, Farahvash MJ, Janney CG, Neuschwander-Tetri BA: Nonalcoholic steatohepatitis: An expanded clinical entity. Gastroenterology 107:1103–1109, 1994.

Baldridge AD, Perez-Atayde AR, Graeme-Cook F, et al: Idiopathic steatohepatitis in childhood: A multicenter retrospective study. J Pediatr 127:700–704, 1995.

Batman PA, Scheuer PJ: Diabetic hepatitis preceding the onset of glucose intolerance. Histopathology 9:237–243, 1985.

Carson K, Washington MK, Treem WR, et al: Recurrence of nonalcoholic steatohepatitis in a liver transplant recipient. Liver Transplant Surg 3:174–176, 1997.

Diehl AM, Goodman Z, Ishak KG: Alcohollike liver disease in nonalcoholics: A clinical and histologic comparison with alcohol-induced liver injury. Gastroenterology 95:1056–1062, 1988.

Fromenty B, Berson A, Pessayre D: Microvesicular steatosis and steatohepatitis: Role of mitochondrial dysfunction and lipid peroxidation. J Hepatol 26 (Suppl 1):13–22, 1997.

Galambos JT, Wills CE: Relationship between 505 paired liver tests and biopsies in 242 obese patients. Gastroenterology 74:1191–1195, 1978.

Gruffat D, Durand D, Graulet B, Bauchart D: Regulation of VLDL synthesis and secretion in the liver. Reprod Nutr Dev 36:375–389, 1996.

Itoh S, Yougel T, Kawagoe K: Comparison between nonalcoholic steatohepatitis and alcoholic hepatitis. Am J Gastroenterol 82:650–654, 1987.

Lee RG: Nonalcoholic steatohepatitis: A study of 49 patients. Hum Pathol 20:594–598, 1989.

Ludwig J, Viggiano TR, McGill DB, Ott BJ: Nonalcoholic steatohepatitis. Mayo Clin Proc 55:434–438, 1980.

Pinto HC, Baptista A, Camilo ME, et al: Nonalcoholic steatohepatitis: Clinicopathological comparison with alcoholic hepatitis in ambulatory and hospitalized patients. Dig Dis Sci 41:172–179, 1996.

Powell EE, Cooksley WG, Hanson R, et al: The natural history of nonalcoholic steatohepatitis: A follow-up study of forty-two patients for up to 21 years. Hepatology 11:74–80, 1990.

Van Ness MM, Diehl AM: Is liver biopsy useful in the evaluation of patients with chronically elevated liver enzymes? Ann Intern Med 111:473–478, 1989.

Wanless IR, Lentz JS: Fatty liver hepatitis (steatohepatitis) and obesity: An autopsy study with analysis of risk factors. Hepatology 12:1106–1110, 1990.

Zammit VA: Role of insulin in hepatic fatty acid partitioning: Emerging concepts. Biochem J 314:1–14, 1996.

Chapter

11

Hereditary Hemochromatosis

Bruce R. Bacon

Our understanding of several aspects of hereditary hemochromatosis (HH) has greatly expanded over the last few years with the identification and cloning of the hemochromatosis gene *(HFE)*, the introduction of a commercially available genetic test, and a new understanding of the normal physiology and pathophysiology of the hemochromatosis gene product. Additionally, it has become increasingly apparent that iron plays an important role in various liver diseases other than hemochromatosis. For example, it is well established that in about 40% to 50% of patients with alcoholic liver disease, chronic hepatitis C, and nonalcoholic steatohepatitis, there are abnormalities in various serum markers of iron metabolism. Furthermore, a high prevalence of heterozygosity for the hemochromatosis gene has been identified in patients with porphyria cutanea tarda and nonalcoholic steatohepatitis. This chapter focuses on new developments in the understanding and diagnosis of HH, the pathophysiologic mechanisms that have been elucidated by the newly identified gene, and the role of mild secondary iron overload in several additional liver diseases.

IRON OVERLOAD SYNDROMES (Table 11–1)

The term *hemochromatosis* should be reserved for the *HFE*-linked inherited disease that is determined by the inappropriately high absorption of iron by the gastrointestinal mucosa, which leads to the pathologic deposition of excessive iron in the parenchymal cells of the liver, heart, pancreas, and other organs. Eventually, the result is cell and tissue damage, fibrosis, and functional insufficiency. There are several other clinically distinct syndromes of iron overload that should be distinguished from *HFE*-linked hemochro-

matosis. These include *secondary iron overload* where there is an increase in absorption of intestinal iron that is promoted by an underlying condition other than HH. Examples of such underlying conditions are anemia from ineffective erythropoiesis such as in thalassemia, aplastic anemia, sideroblastic anemia, various liver diseases, excessive ingestion of medicinal iron, and congenital atransferrinemia. *Parenteral iron overload* is always iatrogenic and is caused by red blood cell transfusions or iron dextran injections. Some patients who have ineffective erythropoiesis and thus secondary iron overload on that basis can also have complications by having parenteral iron overload when they require blood transfusions. *Neonatal iron overload* is a rare disorder that has been recognized during the last 15 to 20 years. It is thought by some to be caused by an intrauterine hepatic viral infection that results in an excessive uptake of iron into the fetal liver, which in the absence of mature cytoprotective mechanisms can result in liver failure, and is often fatal without liver transplantation. *African iron overload* is presumed to be caused by an additional genetic factor that is not human leukocyte antigen (HLA)-linked in addition to the well-known dietary factor related to ingestion of iron-enriched home-brewed beer.

A brief review of certain aspects of the diagnosis and management of patients with HH, as well as the role of iron in other liver diseases, is timely given the recent discovery of the gene *(HFE)* for HH. The significance of this discovery relates to several major areas: (1) it has already led to improved accuracy in diagnosis; (2) it raises the possibility of a major public health effort in population screening for HH; and (3) it is beginning to result in an improved understanding of the pathophysiology of abnormal iron metabolism seen in HH as well as contributing to the understanding of normal iron absorption and metabolism.

Table 11–1 Classification of Iron Overload Syndromes

Hereditary Hemochromatosis

HFE-linked
    C282Y/C282Y
    C282Y/H63D
Non–*HFE*-linked, familial
African iron overload, inherited, non–*HFE*-linked

Secondary Iron Overload

Anemia caused by ineffective erythyropoiesis
    β-Thalassemia
    Sideroblastic anemia
    Aplastic anemia
    Pyruvate kinase deficiency
    Pyridoxine-responsive anemia
Liver disease
    Alcoholic liver disease
    Chronic viral hepatitis B and C
    After portocaval shunt
    Porphyria cutanea tarda
Miscellaneous
    Excessive iron ingestion
    Congenital atransferrinemia (rare)

Parenteral Iron Overload

Red blood cell transfusions
Iron dextran injections
Associated with long-term hemodialysis

Neonatal Iron Overload

HEREDITARY HEMOCHROMATOSIS

HH is a common disorder of iron metabolism that affects approximately 1 in 250 to 300 individuals of northern European descent. Methods are now available to allow for the detection of HH in asymptomatic probands and in presymptomatic relatives of patients with the disease; therefore, a diagnosis can be legitimately applied to individuals who have not yet developed any of the toxic consequences of iron overload in tissues. Thus, it is no longer justified to confine the diagnosis only to those individuals who are either symptomatic or who manifest organ damage such as cirrhosis, diabetes, heart failure, arthritis, or skin pigmentation. Rather, all individuals who have inherited both alleles of the mutant hemochromatosis gene and who have direct or indirect markers of iron overload should be regarded as homozygous for HH. Over the past several years, this concept has increased awareness of the disease, leading to early diagnosis and treatment, and undoubtedly has already led to reduced morbidity and increased survival.

Genetics

HFE encodes for a major histocompatibility complex (MHC) class I–like molecule that requires interaction with β₂-microglobulin (β₂M) for normal presentation on the surface of cells. The protein has a peptide-binding domain, an immunoglobulin-like domain, a single transmembrane region, and a short cytoplasmic tail (Fig. 11–1). Two missense mutations have been identified in *HFE*. One results in a change of cysteine to tyrosine at position 282 (C282Y); the second results in a change in histidine to aspartate at amino acid position 63 (H63D). In the original study by Feder and associates, 83% of typical phenotypic patients (148 of 178) with HH were homozygous for the C282Y mutation. There were an additional eight patients (4%) who are compound heterozygotes in whom one allele contained the C282Y mutation and the other allele contained the H63D mutation (Table 11–2). Numerous additional studies have now confirmed the original observations of Feder and associates showing homozygosity for the C282Y mutation in 64% to 100% of patients with typical phenotypic HH from the United States, France, Australia, Italy, Canada, Austria, and other parts of the world. In the series from Australia, 100% of patients with HH who had a family history of iron overload were homozygous for the C282Y mutation. Conversely, in the study from Italy, only 64% of patients were homozygous for C282Y; however, the patient population evaluated in this study included patients with thalassemia and with chronic liver disease due to hepatitis C and alcoholism, suggesting that perhaps some of these patients had secondary iron overload. Alternatively, the frequency of

Figure 11–1
Model of the HFE-protein based on its homology with major histocompatibility complex (MHC) class 1 molecules. The HFE protein is a single polypeptide with three extracellular domains that would be analogous to the α₁, α₂, and α₃ domains of the other MHC class-1 proteins. β₂-Microglobulin is a separate protein and would interact with the HFE gene product in a noncovalent manner in the α₃-homologous region. The approximate locations of the C282Y (Cys282Tyr) and H63D (His63Asp) mutations are shown (From Feder JN, Gnirke A, Thomas W, et al: A novel MHC class 1-like gene is mutated in patients with hereditary haemochromatosis. Nat Genet 13:399–409, 1996.)

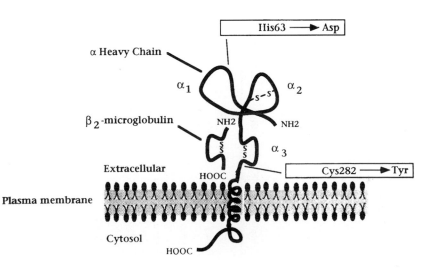

Table 11–2 *HFE* in Hereditary Hemochromatosis*

Study	Feder, et al	Beutler, et al	Jazwinska, et al	Jouanolle, et al	Carella, et al	Adams and Chakrabarti	UK Haem. Consort	Borot, et al	Bacon, et al	Total
Country	USA	USA	Australia	France	Italy	Canada	United Kingdom	France	USA	
No. of patients	178	147	112†	65	75	128	115	94	66	980
Genotype n (%)										
C282Y / C282Y	148 (83)	121 (82)	112 (100)	59 (91)	48 (64)	122 (95)	105 (91)	68 (72)	60 (91)	843 (86)
C282Y‡ / H63D	8 (4)	8 (5)	0	3 (5)	5 (7)	0	3 (2.6)	4 (4.2)	2 (3)	33 (3.3)
C282Y / Wild type	1 (0.5)	2 (1)	0	0	2 (2.7)	2 (1.6)	1 (0.9)	4 (4.2)	1 (1.5)	13 (1.3)
H63D / H63D	1 (0.5)	2 (1)	0	1 (1.5)	1 (1.3)	0	1 (0.9)	2 (2.1)	0	8 (0.8)
H63D / Wild type	7 (4)	4 (3)	0	2 (3)	3 (4)	0	0	8 (8.5)	2 (1.5)	26 (2.6)
Wild type / Wild type	13 (7)	10 (7)	0	0	16 (21)	4 (3.1)	5 (4.3)	8 (8.5)	1 (1.5)	57 (5.8)

*For these nine studies, hemochromatosis was diagnosed clinically, usually with a liver biopsy demonstrating increased hepatic iron concentration and an elevated hepatic iron index, with exclusion of patients with various causes of secondary iron overload.
†All patients had a positive family history of iron overload.
‡Compound heterozygote.

C282Y may not be as high in southern Italian populations. Compound heterozygotes comprise approximately 3% to 5% of patients in most studies suggesting that the H63D mutation has some importance in the development of clinically significant iron overload, at least when found in conjunction with the C282Y mutation. Further studies are necessary to determine the significance of the compound heterozygous condition. In these studies from around the world, there are still approximately 10% to 15% of patients who have a clinical syndrome that is phenotypically similar to HH but who do not have the C282Y mutation. Possible explanations for these patients are that some were misdiagnosed and actually had one of the various causes of secondary iron overload or that they have another syndrome of iron overload that is indistinguishable phenotypically from what is typically called HH.

Pathophysiologic Mechanisms

When the *HFE* gene was first described in 1996, some investigators questioned how an MHC class I-like molecule could be involved in iron absorption and metabolism. They raised the possibility that the actual hemochromatosis gene was just closely linked to the "candidate" gene but that *HFE* was not really the gene responsible for hemochromatosis. The recent demonstration of a *HFE* knockout mouse that exhibits a phenotype identical to patients with hemochromatosis (elevated transferrin saturation, increased parenchymal hepatic iron loading) provides irrefutable evidence for *HFE* being the hemochromatosis gene. Nonetheless, the mechanisms by which the HFE protein regulates iron absorption and the way in which the abnormal protein resulting from the C282Y mutation results in a failure of regulation of iron absorption are still unknown. However, the requirement for intact β_2M for normal iron uptake and cellular distribution has been demonstrated. It has been shown that β_2M-deficient mice become iron loaded with elevated plasma iron levels, transferrin saturation, and hepatic iron concentration. Furthermore, as has been shown in humans with HH, there is an increase in mucosal transfer of iron from the gastrointestinal tract with preferential hepatocellular (rather than the Kupffer cell) deposition of hepatic iron.

Immunohistochemical staining has shown that the HFE protein has a unique cellular distribution in the normal human gastrointestinal tract. Studies have shown that staining for the HFE protein was seen in some epithelial cells in every segment of the alimentary tract; however, cellular and subcellular expression in the small intestine was distinctly different from that seen in other segments. In the stomach and colon, staining was polarized and restricted to the basolateral cell surface, whereas in the epithelial cells of the esophagus and submucosal leukocytes, nonpolarized staining of the plasma membrane was evident. In contrast, the staining in the small intestine was mainly intracellular and perinuclear and limited to cells in deep crypts. Because iron absorption occurs primarily in the villi of the small intestine, the localization of the HFE protein in crypt cells suggest that it may be involved in predetermining the iron-absorptive capacity of intestinal cells before they migrate up the villi.

Recent studies have shown that HFE appears to have some type of physical association with transferrin receptor (TfR). Because the C282Y mutant HFE is not expressed at the cell surface, it has been speculated that it could not bind with TfR and, thus, had no effect on the affinity of TfR for transferrin. The binding site of HFE to TfR has not yet been identified, and the stoichiometry of the HFE-TfR-transferrin complex remains to be determined. Finally, it appears that the C282Y mutation may decrease the rate of TfR-dependent iron accumulation by decreasing the rate of recycling of endocytosed TfR. This could well result in cells in the deep crypts sensing to be iron deficient with the resultant upregulation of the recently identified divalent metal transporter-1 (DMT-1), which transports iron at the villus tip. It is anticipated that additional studies will be completed over the next several years and that these pathways will be clearly delineated.

Clinical Features

HH is still unrecognized and underdiagnosed mainly because physicians often feel that it is a rare disorder manifested by the classical triad of clinical findings consisting of increased skin pigmentation, diabetes, and cirrhosis. In fact, numerous studies have shown that HH is found in about 1 in 250 individuals of northern European descent and the heterozygote frequency occurs approximately 1 in 10 individuals. Thus, hemochromatosis is the most common inherited abnormality in white populations. In the early 1990s, HH was increasingly identified by evaluating patients who have abnormal iron studies on routine serum chemistry panels or by performing iron studies in a patient who has a family history of HH. When patients are identified in this way, the majority of them (approximately 75%) are asymptomatic and do not exhibit any of the end-stage manifestations of hemochromatosis. For the most part, they do not have diabetes, cirrhosis, skin pigmentation, or arthropathy. About 25% of them will have increased fatigue, which improves with treatment. Thus, it is important for clinicians to realize that because HH is so common that any patient with an elevated transferrin saturation or an elevated ferritin level should be considered to possibly have HH. When patients do present with symptoms, consideration of hemochromatosis should be given for symptoms of fatigue, right upper quadrant abdominal pain, arthralgias, impotence, decreased libido, symptoms of heart failure, or diabetes (Table 11–3). Similarly, findings of hepatomegaly, cirrhosis, extrahepatic manifestations of chronic liver disease, testicular atrophy, signs of congestive heart failure, skin pigmentation, and arthritis should raise the suspicion of HH (Table 11–4). Needless to say, many of the aforementioned symptoms and signs are indicative of disease processes other than HH, but when systematic studies of arthritis clinics or diabetes clinics have looked specifically for HH, previously undiagnosed cases have been identified, often to the surprise of the physician taking care of those patients. These studies illustrate the need to consider HH in patients who present with the symptoms and signs known to occur in established HH.

In older series of patients with HH, when patients were identified by symptoms or findings of the disease, women typically presented about 10 years later than men, presumably because of a "protective effect" of menstrual blood loss and iron loss during pregnancy. More recently, when greater proportions of patients were identified by screening blood

Table 11–3 Symptoms in Patients with Hereditary Hemochromatosis

Asymptomatic

Abnormal serum iron studies on routine screening chemistry panel
Evaluation of abnormal liver tests
Identified by family screening
Identified by population screening

Nonspecific, Systemic Symptoms

Weakness
Fatigue
Lethargy
Apathy
Weight loss

Specific, Organ-Related Symptoms

Abdominal pain (hepatomegaly)
Arthralgias (arthritis)
Diabetes (pancreas)
Amenorrhea (cirrhosis)
Loss of libido, impotence (pituitary, cirrhosis)
Congestive heart failure (heart)
Arrhythmias (heart)

samples or were discovered by family screening studies, the age of diagnosis for women is approximately equivalent to that for men. Additionally, young (younger than 30 years of age) multiparous women can definitely be iron loaded and should not be excluded from further work-up. Thus, in the face of abnormal iron studies, clinicians should not wait for

Table 11–4 Physical Findings in Patients with Hereditary Hemochromatosis

Asymptomatic

No physical findings
Hepatomegaly

Symptomatic

Liver
  Hepatomegaly
  Cutaneous stigmata of chronic liver disease
  Splenomegaly
  Liver failure (e.g., ascites, encephalopathy)
Joints
  Arthritis
  Joint swelling
Heart
  Dilated cardiomyopathy
  Congestive heart failure
Skin
  Increased pigmentation
Endocrine
  Testicular atrophy
  Hypogonadism
  Hypothyroidism

typical symptoms or findings of HH before considering the diagnosis of HH.

Diagnosis

Once the diagnosis of HH is considered, either by an evaluation of abnormal screening iron studies, in the context of family studies, in a patient with an abnormal genetic test, or in the evaluation of a patient with any of the aforementioned symptoms or clinical findings, definitive diagnosis is relatively straightforward. Delayed diagnosis most often comes as a result of a physician not considering HH as a possibility, thinking that it is rare disorder. Once considered, fasting transferrin saturation (TS) (serum iron divided by total iron-binding capacity [TIBC] or transferrin x 100%) and ferritin levels should be obtained; both of these will be elevated in a symptomatic patient (Table 11–5). Transferrin saturation should be obtained in the fasting state, because serum iron levels have a diurnal variation and can be increased after a meal. Unfortunately, the sensitivity and specificity of the TS and ferritin levels become problematic when young individuals are being evaluated or when patients have abnormal iron studies in the context of other diseases. Thus, as many as 30% of women with HH younger than 30 years of age may have a normal TS. Alternatively, in the absence of HH, serum iron studies (predominantly ferritin) can be abnormal in about 40% to 50% of patients with chronic viral hepatitis, nonalcoholic steatohepatitis, and alcoholic liver disease. Additionally, because ferritin is an acute phase reactant, other inflammatory disorders (e.g., rheumatoid arthritis) and various neoplastic diseases (e.g., lymphoma, other cancers) can cause elevated serum ferritin levels in the absence of iron overload. Thus, serum iron studies alone have many false-positive and false-negative results in predicting iron stores and reliance on these studies by themselves for diagnosis of HH can result in errors of diagnosis. The development of a widely available genetic test has already contributed to better characterization of those patients with underlying liver disease and abnormal serum iron studies. Nonetheless, in the absence of any other medical illness, the combination of an elevated transferrin saturation and an elevated ferritin level is approximately 90% sensitive and specific for the diagnosis of HH. However, it must be remembered that all that may be required is a TS higher than 55% and a ferritin of more than 300 ng/mL in a young woman. It is not necessary to have a TS of 90% to 100% or a ferritin level higher than 1000 ng/mL.

Currently, if either a fasting TS or ferritin level is elevated, regardless of what has led to it being obtained, a liver biopsy should be performed to establish a diagnosis by using histochemical iron stains (Perls' Prussian blue stain) and biochemical determination of HIC with calculation of the hepatic iron index (HII). Additionally, liver biopsy can provide an assessment of the degree of fibrosis and whether or not cirrhosis is present and of other histologic abnormalities such as steatosis. From a prognostic standpoint, the presence of fibrosis or cirrhosis is important to establish, and the risk of hepatocellular cancer is significantly increased in those who have established cirrhosis. Histologically, iron deposition is found in higher levels in periportal (zone 1) hepatocytes with a periportal to pericentral gradient (Fig. 11–2). On higher power iron is seen predomi-

Table 11–5   Laboratory Findings in Patients with Hereditary Hemochromatosis

Measurements	Normal Subjects	Patients with Hereditary Hemochromatosis	
		Asymptomatic	*Symptomatic*
Blood (fasting)			
Serum iron level (μg/dL)	60–180	150–280	180–300
Serum transferrin level (mg/dL)	220–410	200–280	200–300
Transferrin saturation (%)	20–50	45–100	80–100
Serum ferritin level (ng/mL)			
Men	20–200	150–1000	500–6000
Women	15–150	120–1000	500–6000
Genetic (*HFE* mutation analysis)			
C282Y/C282Y	Wt/wt	C282Y/C282Y	C282Y/C282Y
C282Y/H63D*	Wt/wt	C282Y/H63D	C282Y/H63D
Liver			
Hepatic iron concentration			
μg/g, dry weight	300–1500	2000–10,000	8000–30,000
μmole/g, dry weight	5–27	36–179	140–550
Hepatic iron index†	<1	1 to >1.9	>1.9
Liver histology			
Perls' Prussian blue stain	0–1+	2+ to 4+	3+, 4+

*Compound heterozygote
†Hepatic iron index (HII) is calculated by dividing the hepatic iron concentration (in μmole/g, dry weight) by the age of the patient (in years). With increased knowledge of genetic testing results in patients with iron overload, the specificity of HII has diminished.

nantly in parenchymal cells, with sparing of Kupffer cells (Fig. 11–3). When early diagnosis and treatment are not done, then patients can progress to micronodular cirrhosis and liver failure (Fig. 11–4). In symptomatic patients, the hepatic iron concentration will typically be above 10,000 μg/g dry weight (normal <1500 μg/g dry weight) and values as high as 40,000 μg/g can be seen. In patients with alcoholic siderosis or with secondary iron overload related to chronic viral hepatitis or NASH, the HIC is usually not higher than 10,000 μg/g. With the diagnosis of younger patients with earlier HH because of family studies or use of genetic screening tests, HIC levels at the time of diagnosis can be as low as 3000 μg/g.

The hepatic iron index (HII) has been a helpful method of establishing a diagnosis of HH and of distinguishing heterozygotes and patients with alcoholic liver disease with secondary iron overload from homozygotes. The HII is based on a concept that patients with HH have a progressive increase in HIC with age, whereas heterozygotes for HH or patients with various forms of secondary iron overload do not have a progressive increase with age; however, recent studies have challenged the concept that HIC increases with age. Nonetheless, the HII is calculated by taking the HIC (converted to micromoles per gram dry weight) and dividing by the patient's age (in years). Numerous studies from around the world have shown that a HII higher than 1.9 is

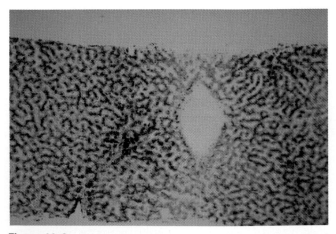

Figure 11–2
Liver histology in hereditary hemochromatosis. At low power, increased iron deposition can be seen in a periportal distribution (Perls' Prussian blue stain, original magnification ×40).

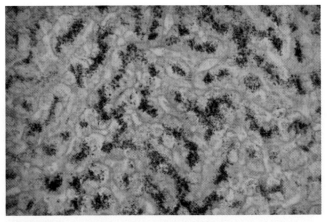

Figure 11–3
Liver histology in hereditary hemochromatosis. At higher power, the iron deposits can be seen predominately in hepatocytes in a pericanalicular distribution (Perls' Prussian blue stain, original magnification ×200).

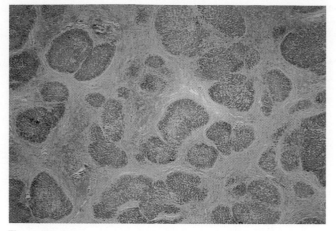

Figure 11–4
Liver histology in hereditary hemochromatosis. At low power, micronodular cirrhosis is seen in this sample from an explant liver from a patient who received an orthotopic liver transplant for complications of endstage liver disease due to hemochromatosis (Masson trichrome stain, original magnification ×10).

consistent with a diagnosis of homozygous HH. The HII is not meant to be used in patients with parenteral (or transfusional) iron overload. Recent studies have shown that as many as 15% of patients with HH (identified by genetic testing) will have a HII of less than 1.9. As additional experience with genotyping is obtained, it is anticipated that there will be many patients with a HII of less than 1.9 who are homozygous for the genetic defect.

Whether a liver biopsy needs to be performed in all patients to establish a diagnosis is controversial. Most hepatologists consider liver biopsy in this setting to be a relatively minor and safe outpatient procedure that gives definitive information about a diagnosis that has lifetime significance and important implications for family members. Alternatively, some physicians have suggested that an elevated TS or ferritin level provides sufficient information for diagnosis of iron overload and that therapeutic phlebotomy can be initiated on this basis alone. The rationale here is that phlebotomy is relatively harmless and if the patient does not have iron overload or HH, then he or she will become anemic after 4 to 6 units of blood (1 to 1.5 g of iron) have been removed; however, the amount of blood that needs to be removed to be certain of a diagnosis of HH when using this technique has not been definitively defined. Certainly, more than 20 units of blood (5 g of iron) would satisfy most physicians that the patient was significantly iron loaded; however, in a recent series of 40 patients with HH, as few as 8 to 11 units (2 to 2.75 g of iron) were required to deplete excess iron stores in four patients (all women, three of whom were younger than 30 years of age) with clearly defined HH who were homozygous for the C282Y mutation. How would these patients be characterized without an initial diagnostic liver biopsy? There is substantial concern that without a definitive liver biopsy, many patients would not be accurately diagnosed, and appropriate follow-up or family screening would not be initiated. HH is a diagnosis for a lifetime with important family implica-

tions, and the diagnosis should be accurate. Currently, liver biopsy should be an important component of making a definitive diagnosis of HH.

An exception to this approach may come when young individuals are identified, either as a result of family studies or by screening with a genetic test. For example, if a young (<40 years) individual is identified by genetic testing (C282Y homozygote) as part of a screening survey or as a relative of a well-defined proband and has an elevated TS or ferritin level and no clinical evidence of liver disease, it might be appropriate to proceed with therapeutic phlebotomy in the absence of a liver biopsy. In this setting, it is unlikely that the patient will have cirrhosis or a significant increase in hepatic fibrosis, and with a positive genetic test or an appropriate family history, the accuracy of the diagnosis would be very high. It is hoped that prospective studies evaluating all of the parameters used for diagnosis (i.e., TS, ferritin, genetic test, HIC, HII, liver biopsy findings) will be performed over the next several years to clearly delineate the relative predictive power of each parameter. We have developed an algorithm for when to use liver biopsy in the diagnosis of HH (Fig. 11–5).

Treatment

Once the diagnosis of HH is established, physicians must turn their responsibility to ensuring that patients are adequately treated and that family screening is performed. Treatment is simple, inexpensive, and safe. Patients should be encouraged to have weekly therapeutic phlebotomy of 500 mL of whole blood. This is equivalent to approximately 200 to 250 mg of iron, depending on the hemoglobin concentration of the blood removed. Some patients can tolerate twice weekly phlebotomy, and reports from older literature describe patients who tolerated phlebotomy three times per week; however, this is tedious and often inconvenient. Monthly phlebotomy should not be recommended unless patients cannot tolerate phlebotomy more frequently. Therapeutic phlebotomy should be performed until patients develop iron-limited erythropoiesis, which is identified by the failure of the hemoglobin or hematocrit to recover before the next phlebotomy. It is reasonable to monitor TS and ferritin levels periodically to predict the return to normal iron stores and to provide a method of encouragement to patients who are undergoing phlebotomy. However, some physicians treat patients until they are anemic and then reorder iron studies. I prefer to continue therapeutic phlebotomy until the TS is less than 50% and serum ferritin levels are less than 50 ng/mL. Some clinicians favor bringing the ferritin level down to 20 ng/mL. I think that it is not necessary for patients to become anemic (hematocrit <30% to 33%); rather, the desired endpoint is for them to be depleted of their excess iron stores. Most patients tolerate therapeutic phlebotomy quite well and actually have a sense of improved well-being after the initial phlebotomies have been completed. If liver enzymes have been abnormal, they will characteristically return to normal once iron stores have been depleted; however, established cirrhosis will not reverse. There are some reports of portal fibrosis improving with phlebotomy therapy. Other benefits of therapeutic phlebotomy include reduction of skin pigmentation, improvement in cardiac function, reduction in insulin requirements

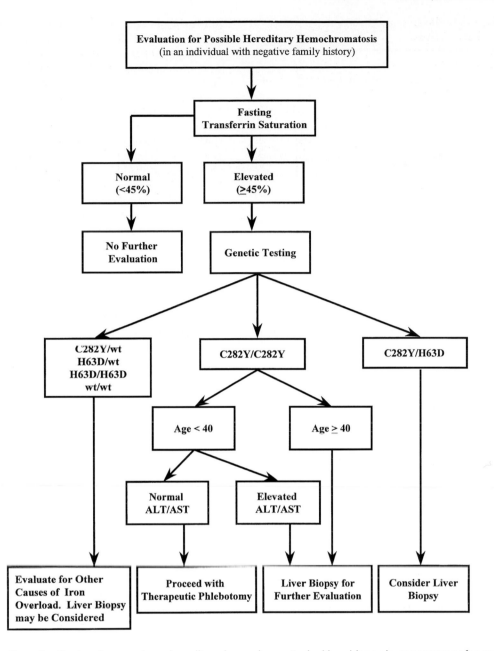

Figure 11–5

Algorithm for evaluation of patients who may have hereditary hemochromatosis. Liver biopsy is unnecessary for young subjects (<40 years old) with normal liver enzymes, who are C282Y homozygotes with indirect evidence of increased iron stores (i.e., elevated transferrin saturation or ferritin). Treatment with therapeutic phlebotomy should be initiated.

in those patients who are diabetic, reduction in abdominal pain, and an improved energy level and sense of well-being (Table 11–6). Conditions that characteristically do not reverse with phlebotomy include testicular atrophy, established cirrhosis, and arthropathy.

Once the initial therapeutic phlebotomy has been completed and patients have been successfully depleted of their excess iron stores, then most patients will require maintenance phlebotomy of 1 unit of blood to be removed every 2 to 3 months. Because most patients with HH absorb approximately 3 mg/day of iron in excess of their daily requirements, they will accumulate an excess of approximately 270 mg of iron over a 3-month period. This is bal-

anced by the 250 mg of iron that is taken with a phlebotomy; thus, maintenance phlebotomy every 3 months is usually adequate. Some patients absorb more than the 3 mg/day of iron and thus require maintenance phlebotomy more often. It is unusual for patients to require maintenance phlebotomy more often than every 2 months. Occasionally, a few patients who have been accurately diagnosed (HII >1.9, homozygosity for the C282Y mutation) do not reaccumulate iron for reasons that are unclear. These patients have usually been older, and the presumption is that their efficiency of iron absorption has been diminished with age. When this situation occurs, patients should be evaluated for occult blood loss from the gastrointestinal tract.

Table 11–6 Response to Phlebotomy Therapy in Hereditary Hemochromatosis

Reduction to normal of tissue iron stores
Improved survival if diagnosis and treatment before the development of cirrhosis and diabetes
Improved sense of well-being and energy level
Improved cardiac function
Improved control of diabetes
Reduction in abdominal pain
Reversal of hepatic fibrosis (~30% of cases)
Reduction in skin pigmentation
Normalization of elevated liver enzymes
No reversal of established cirrhosis
No (or only minimal) improvement in arthropathy
No reversal of testicular atrophy

Screening

It is recommended that all first-degree relatives of an identified proband be screened for hemochromatosis, including siblings, parents, and children. Certainly, this recommendation could be extended to include aunts, uncles, and cousins as well. Currently, the minimum for screening would be fasting TS. For individuals who are older than 35 years of age, phenotypic expression should be present in all homozygous individuals, although the accuracy of TS has not yet been tested against the genetic test as a "gold standard." In the past, within a sibship, HLA studies could be used as a surrogate genetic test and individuals who shared an identical HLA-haplotype at the A and B loci with the proband were believed to be homozygous for the disease. This was probably accurate in most cases, but it will be of interest to see how these studies hold up now that a more specific genetic test is available. With the availability of a genetic test, the use of HLA typing has diminished and genetic testing has replaced HLA typing. Whether genetic testing should be used as a general population screening technique is under debate. Issues relate to the cost efficiency of such a program and problems with denial of medical insurance for patients with a diagnosis of a genetic disorder. Furthermore, it is still not clear how many C282Y homozygous patients will go on to develop iron overload; for example, there have been a few examples of C282Y homozygotes who are "nonexpressing homozygotes," who even in their 70s and 80s have not developed increased iron stores. Further studies will define the role of the genetic test in population screening. One study has predicted that general population screening using a genetic test would be cost effective if the cost of the genetic test was less than $20. Currently, C282Y and H63D DNA analysis by PCR is commercially available by one of the large reference laboratories, costing approximately $175, and by numerous DNA diagnostic laboratories in academic pathology departments.

In the context of family screening, an elevated TS or an elevated ferritin level in a family member warrants further evaluation by means of either a genetic test or probably a liver biopsy for histochemical and biochemical determination of hepatic iron stores. At the present time, the standard of care would be to perform a liver biopsy in a family member with an elevated TS or an elevated ferritin level to confirm or disprove a diagnosis of HH. This may change as more experience is gained with use of the genetic test. Thus, for siblings of a proband, who are C282Y homozygotes, who have an elevated TS, and who are young (younger than 40 years of age), a liver biopsy may not be necessary and proceeding to therapeutic phlebotomy would be reasonable. Clinical studies should be done to confirm that this is an appropriate and reasonable approach before it becomes widespread clinical practice. When patients are identified by the genetic test in population screening outside of the context of a family history and who do have an elevated TS or ferritin, liver biopsy should probably be performed to establish or disprove a diagnosis. Again, as experience with the genetic test is gained, treatment decisions on the basis of the genetic test and blood studies alone, without the need for liver biopsy, may be made.

IRON AND OTHER LIVER DISEASES

As mentioned previously, abnormal serum iron studies have been described in about 40% to 50% of patients with alcoholic liver disease, chronic viral hepatitis, and nonalcoholic steatohepatitis. Additionally, it has been known for years that iron plays a role in porphyria cutanea tarda. Only a few of these patients will have a mild increase in hepatic iron concentration, and this is usually not to the degree of iron loading seen in typical HH. Serum and hepatic iron studies are generally normal in patients with cholestatic liver diseases. The fact that serum ferritin levels are elevated in many patients with alcoholic liver disease in the absence of HH has been recognized for years. Liver biopsy with measurement of HIC and calculation of HII has been necessary in the past to distinguish HH from alcoholic siderosis. Now, with the advent of genetic testing, it will be of increasing interest to see if any of these alcoholic siderotic patients are heterozygous for the C282Y mutation. To date, there has been no known benefit from phlebotomy therapy to deplete iron stores in alcoholic siderotic patients.

It has been reported that 40% to 50% of patients with porphyria cutanea tarda have at least one allele with the C282Y mutation and that many patients are in fact C282Y homozygotes. Furthermore, in nonalcoholic steatohepatitis (NASH) about 40% of patients have at least one allele with the C282Y mutation, again, indicating the importance of genetic testing in this disorder. Of greatest importance in the NASH series is that those patients who are C282Y positive had a high frequency of fibrosis, indicating a possible synergistic effect between tissue iron stores and the development of fibrotic liver disease in patients with NASH. Similarly, a recent study in patients with chronic hepatitis C has shown that patients who were C282Y heterozygotes were found to have an increased incidence of fibrosis. These findings would raise the question of whether or not therapeutic phlebotomy would be beneficial for treatment of patients with nonalcoholic steatohepatitis and for patients with chronic hepatitis C. Phlebotomy therapy has been used as an adjunctive treatment in chronic hepatitis C in the past, and it has repeatedly shown to result in reduction in ALT levels, although this treatment does not have an antiviral effect. Whether phlebotomy has a beneficial effect on liver histology in chronic hepatitis C is unknown.

SUMMARY

In summary, the findings from the recent discovery of HFE have led to an enhanced ability for clinicians to accurately diagnose patients with hereditary hemochromatosis. It has resulted in the discovery that many patients who are C282Y homozygotes actually have hepatic iron indexes that are less than the typical cut-off of 1.9. Furthermore, a synergistic role of hepatic iron in C282Y heterozygotes has been found in patients with porphyria cutanea tarda, chronic hepatitis C, and NASH. A rational role for phlebotomy therapy in these diseases may become apparent with time. We are continuing to learn about the pathophysiologic mechanisms that occur in HH, and we will be able to apply this information to numerous other liver diseases.

SUGGESTED READINGS

Adams PC, Deugnier Y, Moirand R, Brissot P: The relationship between iron overload, clinical symptoms, and age in 410 patients with genetic hemochromatosis. Hepatology 25:162–166, 1997.

Adams PC, Gregor JC, Kertesz AE, Valberg LS: Screening blood donors for hereditary hemochromatosis: Decision analysis model based on a 30-year database. Gastroenterology 109:177–188, 1995.

Adams PC, Kertesz AE, Valberg LS: Clinical presentation of hemochromatosis: A changing scene. Am J Med 90:445–449, 1991.

Bacon BR: Diagnosis and management of hemochromatosis. Gastroenterology 113:995–999, 1997.

Bacon BR, Powell LW, Adams PC, et al. Molecular medicine and hemochromatosis: at the crossroads. Gastroenterology 116:193–207, 1999.

Bacon BR, Sadiq S: Hereditary hemochromatosis: Diagnosis in the 1990's. Am J Gastroenterol 92:784–789, 1997.

Bacon BR, Tavill AS: Hemochromatosis and the iron overload syndromes. In Zakim D, Boyer TD (eds): Hepatology: A Textbook of Liver Disease. Philadelphia: WB Saunders, 1996, pp 1439–1472.

Bassett ML, Halliday JW, Powell LW: Value of hepatic iron measurements in early hemochromatosis and determination of the critical iron level associated with fibrosis. Hepatology 6:24–29, 1986.

Bonkovsky HL, Poh-Fitzpatrick M, Pimstone N, et al: Porphyria cutanea tarda, hepatitis C, and HFE gene mutations in North America. Hepatology 27:1661–1669, 1998.

Bonkovsky HL, Slaker DP, Bills EB, Wolf DC: Usefulness and limitations of laboratory and hepatic imaging studies in iron-storage disease. Gastroenterology 99:1079–1091, 1990.

Burke W, Thomson E, Khoury MJ, et al: Hereditary hemochromatosis: Gene discovery and its implications for population-based screening. JAMA 280:172–178, 1998.

Chapman RW, Morgan MY, Laulicht M, et al: Hepatic iron stores and markers of iron overload in alcoholics and patients with idopathic hemochromatosis. Dig Dis Sci 27:909–916, 1982.

Di Bisceglie AM, Axiotis CA, Hoofnagle JH, Bacon BR: Measurement of iron status in patients with chronic hepatitis. Gastroenterology 102:2108–2113, 1992.

Edwards CQ, Griffen LM, Goldgar D, et al: Prevalence of hemochromatosis among 11,065 presumably healthy blood donors. N Engl J Med 318:1355–1362, 1988.

Feder JN, Gnirke A, Thomas W, et al: A novel MHC class 1-like gene is mutated in patients with hereditary haemochromatosis. Nat Genet 13:399–409, 1996.

Feder JN, Tsuchihashi Z, Irrinki A, et al: The hemochromatosis founder mutation in HLA-H disrupts beta(2)-microglobulin interaction and cell surface expression. J Biol Chem 272:14025–14028, 1997.

Jazwinska EC, Cullen LM, Busfield F, et al: Haemochromatosis and HLA-H. Nat Genet 14:249–251, 1996.

Jouanolle Am, Gandon G, Jezequel P, et al: Haemochromatosis and HLA-H. Nat Genet 14:251–252, 1996.

Olynyk JK, O'Neill R, Britton RS, Bacon BR: Determination of hepatic iron concentration in fresh and paraffin-embedded tissue: Diagnostic implications. Gastroenterology 106:674–677, 1994.

Parkkila S, Waheed A, Britton RS, et al: Association of the transferrin receptor in human placenta with HFE, the protein defective in hereditary hemochromatosis. Proc Natl Acad Sci U S A 94:13198–13202, 1997.

Parkkila S, Waheed A, Britton RS, et al: Immunohistochemistry of HLA-H, the protein defective in patients with hereditary hemochromatosis, reveals a unique pattern of expression in gastrointestinal tract. Proc Natl Acad Sci U S A 94:2534–2539, 1997.

Phatek PD, Guzman G, Woll JE, et al: Cost-effectiveness of screening for hereditary hemochromatosis. Arch Intern Med 154:769–776, 1994.

Santos M, Schilham MW, Rademahers LHPM, et al: Defective iron homeostatis in β_2-microglobulin knockout mice recapitulates hereditary hemochromatosis in man. J Exp Med 184:1975–1985, 1996.

Smith BC, Grove J, Guzail MA, et al: Heterozygosity for hereditary hemochromatosis is associated with more fibrosis in chronic hepatitis C. Hepatology 27:1695–1699, 1998.

Waheed A, Parkkila S, Zhou XY, et al: Hereditary hemochromatosis: Effects of C282Y and H63D mutations on association with β_2-microglobulin, intracellullar processing, and cell surface expression of the HFE protein in COS-7 cells. Proc Natl Acad Sci USA 94:12384–12389, 1997.

Zhou XY, Tomatsu S, Fleming RE, et al: HFE gene knockout produces a mouse model of hereditary hemochromatosis. Proc Natl Acad Sci U S A 95:2492–2497, 1998.

Chapter

12

Wilson's Disease

Peter Ferenci

Wilson's disease is an autosomal recessive inherited disorder of copper metabolism resulting in pathologic accumulation of copper in many organs and tissues. The hallmarks of the disease are the presence of liver disease, neurologic symptoms, and Kayser-Fleischer corneal rings. The familial nature of Wilson's disease was recognized in the original description of this disease by Samuel Alexander Kinnier Wilson.

EPIDEMIOLOGY

Until very recently, Wilson's disease was believed to be rare. By a population-based approach, the incidence of Wilson's disease was estimated to be at least 1:30,000 to 50,000 (Ireland: 17/100,000 live births; former East Germany: 29/100,000) with a gene frequency of 1:90 to 1:150. However, these estimates were based mainly on adolescents or adults presenting with neurologic symptoms. More recent data indicate that neurologic symptoms occur only in about half of the patients with Wilson's disease. Thus, the incidence of Wilson's disease was underestimated by these studies. Furthermore, in selected populations (e.g., Jews from Uzbekistan), Wilson's disease seems to be even more common. Among selected groups of patients, Wilson's disease is certainly more frequent. About 3% to 6% of patients transplanted for fulminant hepatic failure have fulminant Wilson's disease. Wilson's disease accounts for 16% of young adults with chronic active hepatitis of unknown origin.

PATHOGENESIS

The basic defect in Wilson's disease is the impaired biliary excretion of copper, resulting in the accumulation of copper in various organs including the liver, the cornea, and the brain. The consequence of copper accumulation is the development of severe hepatic and neurologic disease. Excess copper in tissues leads to the production of free radicals and to DNA cleavage. Probably the greatest source of damage is through the production of free radicals. Copper overload particularly affects mitochondrial respiration and causes a decrease in cytochrome C activity. Damage to mitochondria is an early pathologic effect in the liver. Damage to the liver has been shown to result in increased lipid peroxidation and abnormal mitochondrial respiration, both in copper-loaded dogs and in patients with Wilson's disease. The mechanisms triggering copper-induced lipid peroxidation are unknown. However, it is conceivable, that due to hepatic copper accumulation, patients with Wilson's disease are particularly sensitive to any oxidative stress.

The pathogenesis of neurologic disease is less clear. Neuronal damage is mediated by copper deposition in the brain. Copper may be directly toxic to neurons or may exert its effects by selective inhibition of brain monoamine oxidase A (MAO_A). Copper accumulation in the brain may be secondary to liver damage, but this hypothesis is inconsistent with the clinical observation that many patients with neurologic disease have only mild liver disease and that conversely patients with advanced liver failure have no neurologic symptoms. Furthermore, the preferential affection of basal ganglia cannot be explained. The discovery of Wilson's disease gene may help us to better understand the pathophysiology of copper metabolism. ATP7B is also expressed in the brain, but its function is unknown. It is conceivable that increased copper uptake into the brain is a direct result of a certain mutation, resulting in specific functional alterations of cerebral ATP7B.

Wilson's Disease Gene

Wilson's disease gene was localized to human chromosome 13 by cosegregation of the disease with the red cell enzyme marker, esterase D, in several large Middle Eastern kindreds. Further linkage analysis of additional families, using more polymorphic DNA markers, defined a region close to the retinoblastoma locus as the candidate region for Wilson's disease gene. By positional cloning strategies, Wilson's disease gene was identified by three independent groups in 1993. Final identification was established with the use of conserved regions of the previously discovered Menkes' disease (another disease with impaired copper metabolism) gene. Wilson's disease gene codes for a copper transporting P-type adenosine triphosphatase (ATPase), - ATP7B.

The functionally important regions of Wilson's disease gene are six copper-binding domains, a transduction domain (amino acid residues 837 to 864; containing a Thr-Gly-Glu motif) involved in the transduction of the energy of adenosine triphosphate (ATP) hydrolysis to cation transport, a cation channel and phosphorylation domain (amino acid residues 971 to 1035; containing the highly conserved Asp-Lys-Thr-Gly-Thr motif), an ATP-binding domain (amino acid residues 1240 to 1291), and eight hydrophobic regions predicted to span the cell membrane.

More than 60 mutations occurring throughout the whole gene have been documented to date. Mutations include missense and nonsense mutations, deletions, and insertions. Some mutations are associated with a severe impairment of copper transport, resulting in severe liver disease very early in life; other mutations appear to be less severe with disease appearance in midadulthood. Although most reported mutations occur in single families, a few are more common. The His1069Gln missense mutation occurs in 30% to 95% of patients of Eastern, Northern, and Central European origin. It is less frequent in patients of Mediterranean descent and is seen only rarely in patients of non-European origin. Approximately 10% of patients of French or British extraction have a Gly1266Lys mutation in the ATP hinge domain. The 2299insC mutation can be detected in some patients of European and Japanese descent. The Arg778Leu mutation is present in 27% of Taiwanese patients but is not found in non-Asian patients. In Sardinia, two frameshift mutations (1515insT and 2464delC) are found in approximately 20% of patients. These mutations were not found in other populations.

The study of genotype-phenotype correlation is hindered by the lack of clinical data, the rarity of some mutations, and the high frequency of the presence of two different mutations of Wilson's disease gene in individual patients (compound heterozygotes). Sufficient information is available only for the His1069Gln mutation. This mutation is associated with late-onset (Fig. 12–1) neurologic disease with a female preponderance (female-to-male ratio of 3:1).

Hepatic Copper Metabolism and the Role of ATP7B

A scheme of hepatic copper metabolism is shown in Figure 12–2. Copper is an essential component of important enzymes such as lysyl oxidase, superoxide dismutase, cytochrome C, tyrosinase, and DOPA-ß-monooxygenase (in-

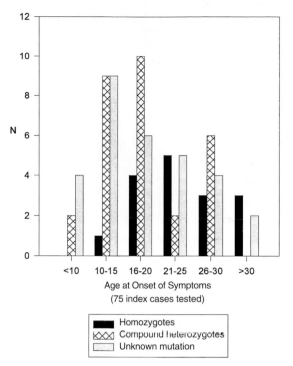

Figure 12–1
The His1069Gln mutation in Central European patients with Wilson's disease. The age of onset is defined by the time of the occurrence of the first symptoms. Sixty-four patients were Austrians. In the remaining patients, the countries of origin were: Croatia (three patients); Hungary (two patients); Germany, Czechoslovakia, Russia, Serbia, and Bosnia (each with one patient).

volved in catecholamine synthesis). Dietary copper intake (about 1 to 4 mg/day) far exceeds the trace amounts required. Dietary copper is absorbed in the upper intestine and binds loosely to albumin, certain amino acids (histidine, cystein, threonine), and peptides. Most of the ingested copper is taken up by the liver. The hepatic uptake of diet-derived copper appears to be an unsaturable, carrier-mediated, energy-independent mechanism. Another source of hepatic copper is derived from (desialyated) ceruloplasmin (AsCPN), the major copper transporting protein in plasma by a receptor-mediated process. Ceruloplasmin is produced in the liver. Copper is incorporated into apoceruloplasmin, possibly at the level of the Golgi compartment. Ceruloplasmin contains six tightly bound copper atoms. Its main function is to carry copper to various tissues. Another important physiologic role of ceruloplasmin is to act as a ferroxidase, converting Fe^{2+} to Fe^{3+}.

In the hepatocyte, glutathione (GSH) has an affinity for Cu^+ and stable Cu^+-GSH complexes are formed. Cu^+-GSH functions in intracellular copper transport and is an effective copper donor to metallothionein (MT) and superoxide dismutase. Metallothionein is a cytosolic, low molecular weight, cysteine-rich, metal-binding protein. The copper stored in metallothionein can be donated to other proteins, either after degradation in lysosomes or by exchange via GSH complexation.

Because hepatic uptake of dietary copper in not saturable, hepatic copper accumulation can easily be induced.

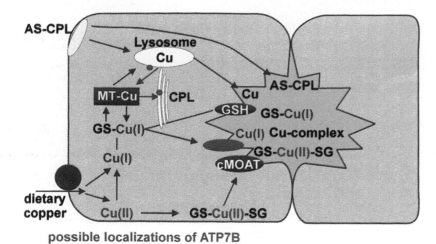

possible localizations of ATP7B

Figure 12–2
Model of hepatobiliary copper transport. (GSH, glutathione, MT, metallothioneine; CPL, ceruloplasmin; AS-CPL, asialoceruloplasmin; cMOAT, canalicular mixed organic anion transporter.) (Modified from Dijkstra M, Vonk RJ, Kuipers F: How does copper get into bile? New insights into the mechanism[s] of hepatobiliary copper transport. J Hepatol 24 [Suppl 1]:109–120, 1996. © 1996 EASL, the European Association for the Study of the Liver.)

Toxicity of copper, however, depends on its molecular association and subcellular localization rather than on its concentration in the liver. Metallothionein-bound copper is nontoxic. Several metals, including zinc, can induce metallothionein synthesis.

Excess copper is secreted into the bile. There are at least three pathways for hepatobiliary excretion of copper: (1) lysosomal exocytosis, (2) a GSH-dependent route at the canalicular membrane (probably by the mixed organic acid transporter c-MOAT), and (3) secretion by ATP7B. The localization of ATP7B within the hepatocyte and its precise role in hepatic copper transport is unknown at present. Biochemically, an ATP-dependent copper carrier was identified at the canalicular membrane (canalicular copper transporter [c-COP]). Wilson's disease protein is present in cells in two forms, the 160-kDa and the 140-kDa products. The 160-kDa product is located in the trans-Golgi network, the 140-kDa product is in mitochondria. Wilson's disease protein may function in copper transport combined with the synthesis of ceruloplasmin, and the Golgi apparatus is the likely site for the Wilson's disease protein to manifest its function.

CLINICAL PRESENTATIONS

Wilson's disease may present with various clinical conditions, the most common ones being liver disease and neuropsychiatric disturbances. None of the clinical signs is typical or diagnostic. One of the most characteristic features of Wilson's disease is that no two patients, even within a family, are ever quite alike. With increased awareness of Wilson's disease, patients are generally diagnosed earlier, thus "late" consequences of the disease like Kayser-Fleischer rings or severe neurologic symptoms are less frequently seen. Early symptoms, if present at all, may be uncharacteristic and nonspecific. Patients presenting with acute or chronic hepatic Wilson's disease are indistinguishable from patients with liver diseases of other etiology. Early neurologic symptoms are also quite untypical and may progress slowly over many years before a diagnosis is made based on "typical signs." About half of the patients are referred for psychological testing because of poor performance in school or behavioral problems. Year-long psychotherapy is

not uncommon in such patients before the diagnosis is finally made.

Kayser-Fleischer Rings

Characteristically, the ring starts as a small crescent of golden brown granular pigment seen at the top of the limbus. This is followed by the appearance of a lower crescent, and these two crescents gradually broaden, meet laterally, and form complete rings (Fig. 12–3). The finding of a complete ring, therefore, suggests long-standing disease and is a useful indicator of severe copper overload. The ring is not always detected by clinical inspection. If doubt exists, the cornea should be examined under a slit lamp by an experienced ophthalmologist. Kayser-Fleischer rings are present in 95% of patients with neurologic symptoms, in 50% to 60% of patients without neurologic symptoms, and only in 10% of asymptomatic siblings.

Liver Disease

Most patients with Wilson's disease, whatever their clinical presentation or presymptomatic status, have some degree of

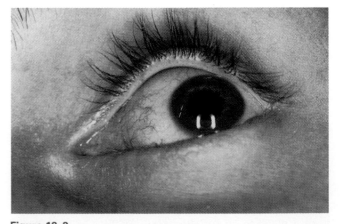

Figure 12–3
Kayser-Fleischer ring in a 15-year-old patient with neurologic Wilson's disease.

Table 12–1 Liver Biopsy Findings in 64 Patients with Wilson's Disease

Liver Histology	Hepatic Presentation	Neurologic Presentation	Siblings	Total
Cirrhosis	19	7	1	27
Fibrosis	3	3	2	8
Chronic hepatitis, active	6	3	2	11
Chronic hepatitis, mild	1	6	3	10
Steatosis	–	2	1	3
Minimal changes	1	3	1	5
Total	30	24	10	64

All biopsies were obtained before the initiation of therapy.

liver disease (Table 12–1). Chronic liver disease (if undiagnosed and untreated) may precede manifestation of neurologic symptoms for more than 10 years. Patients can present with liver disease at any age. The most common age of hepatic manifestation is between 8 and 18 years, but cirrhosis may already be present in children younger than 5 years of age. On the other hand, Wilson's disease is also diagnosed in patients presenting with advanced chronic liver disease in their 50s or 60s without neurologic symptoms and without Kayser-Fleischer rings.

Depending on referral patterns, the proportion of patients presenting with liver disease alone varies from 20% to 46%. Liver disease may mimic various forms of common liver conditions, ranging from asymptomatic elevated aminotransferase to acute hepatitis, fulminant hepatic failure (about one of six patients with hepatic presentation), chronic hepatitis, and cirrhosis (about one of three patients) with all of its complications (Table 12–2).

Acute Wilsonian Hepatitis and Fulminant Wilson's Disease

Acute wilsonian hepatitis is indistinguishable from other forms of acute (viral or toxic) liver diseases. It should be suspected in young patients with acute non-A–E hepatitis. Liver histology often reveals the presence of cirrhosis. This initial episode of liver damage may be self-limiting and may resolve without treatment, and diagnosis is often made retrospectively, when neurologic symptoms occur years later.

On the other hand, the disease may rapidly deteriorate and resemble fulminant hepatic failure with profound jaundice, hypoalbuminemia, ascites, severe coagulation defects, hyperammonemia, and hepatic encephalopathy. Hepatocellular necrosis results in the release of large amounts of stored copper. Hypercupriemia results in hemolysis, and severe hemolytic anemia complicates acute liver disease. Although Wilson's disease is rare, it is not uncommon in patients presenting with fulminant hepatic failure and accounts for 6% to 12% of patients with fulminant hepatic failure referred for emergency liver transplantation.

Although fulminant and subfulminant liver failure due to Wilson's disease has several distinctive features, rapid diagnosis may be very difficult. Serum aminotransferase activity is usually not increased above 10 times normal, and thus alanine aminotransaminase (ALT) and serum aspartate aminotransferase (AST) levels are much lower than the values commonly recorded in fulminant hepatitis. The combination of anemia, marked jaundice, and relatively low aminotransferase activities in young patients should always raise the suspicion of acute Wilson's disease. The conventionally used parameters of copper metabolism are of little use. Kayser-Fleischer corneal rings and neurologic abnormalities are absent in most patients presenting with acute liver disease. An alkaline phosphatase-total bilirubin ratio below

Table 12–2 Clinical Symptoms in Patients with Wilson's Disease who Present with Liver Disease

Author (Country)	Walshe (UK)	Stremmel (Ger)	Schilsky (USA)	Scott (UK)	Ferenci (Austria)
No. with liver disease (out of)	87 (>250)	? (51)	20* (320)	17* (45)	30 (64)
Presenting symptom					
Jaundice, anorexia, vomiting (%)	44	14	15	41	37
Ascites/edema (%)	26	14	50	24	23
Variceal hemorrhage (%)	6		10	6	3
Hemorrhagic diathesis (%)	8				3
Hemolysis (%)	20	10	5		10
Hepatomegaly/splenomegaly (%)	16	49	15	29	17
Fulminant hepatic failure (%)	NA	NA	NA	NA	17
Asymptomatic† (%)		18	5		23

*Only cases with chronic hepatitis.
†Elevated alanine aminotransferase at routine testing, or the incidental finding of cirrhosis or of Kayser-Fleischer rings.
NA, not available.

2.0 has been claimed to provide 100% sensitivity and specificity to diagnose wilsonian fulminant liver failure, but the usefulness of this test has not been confirmed in larger series. The best diagnostic test is the quantification of copper in biopsy material or in the explanted liver. One puzzling feature of fulminant Wilson's disease is the preponderance of female sex (female-to-male ratio of 5:1).

Chronic Hepatitis due to Wilson's Disease

Wilson's disease may present, particularly in young patients, with a clinical syndrome indistinguishable from chronic hepatitis of other etiology. Symptoms include malaise, fatigue, anorexia, and vague abdominal complaints. Arthralgias, amenorrhea, delayed puberty, and low-grade jaundice may be present. Frequently, Kayser-Fleischer rings are absent, and plasma ceruloplasmin is in the normal range. Liver biopsy shows severe chronic hepatitis; however, the diagnosis can be missed if hepatic copper content is not measured. Suspicion for Wilson's disease should be high in young persons with chronic hepatitis of unclear etiology. In this group, Wilson's disease is a common diagnosis. Without treatment, patients progressively deteriorate with ascites, edema, and occasionally jaundice within a few months and eventually die of liver failure.

Patients presenting with neurologic symptoms may also have significant liver disease. In a substantial proportion of patients, symptomatic liver disease predates the occurrence of neurologic signs. Previously, it was believed that "cirrhosis is present in all patients with neurologic disturbances." In most patients, cirrhosis was clinically asymptomatic and was only diagnosed by liver biopsy. However, if a liver biopsy is performed in all patients presenting with neurologic symptoms at diagnosis, the proportion of patients with cirrhosis is only about 25%, and about half of the patients have only minimal liver disease (see Table 12–1).

Neurologic Presentation

Neurologic symptoms usually develop in adolescence or in the twenties. However, there are well-documented cases in whom neurologic symptoms developed much later (45 to 55 years). The initial symptoms may be very subtle abnormalities, such as mild tremor, speech, and writing problems and are frequently misdiagnosed as behavioral problems associated with puberty. The symptoms may remain constant or progress steadily. The hallmark of neurologic Wilson's disease is a progressive movement disorder. The most common symptoms are dysarthria, dysphagia, apraxia, and a tremor-rigidity syndrome (so-called "juvenile parkinsonism"). Because of increasing difficulty in controlling movement, patients become bedridden and unable to care for themselves. Ultimately, the patient becomes helpless—usually alert but unable to talk. In patients presenting with advanced liver disease, neurologic symptoms are mistaken as signs of hepatic encephalopathy.

Psychiatric Presentation

About one third of patients present initially with psychiatric abnormalities. Symptoms can include reduced performance in school or at work, depression, very labile mood, sexual exhibitionism, and frank psychosis. Frequently, adolescents with problems in school or work are referred for psychological counseling and psychotherapy. Among our patients, two were hospitalized in psychiatric institutions for psychosis, one committed several suicide attempts, and two had severe alcohol abuse, before the diagnosis of Wilson's disease was made. The delay in diagnosis in one case was 12 years.

Other Clinical Manifestations

Hypercalciuria and *nephrocalcinosis* are not uncommon in patients with Wilson's disease and may be the presenting signs. Hypercalciuria is possibly the consequence of a tubular defect in calcium reabsorption. Penicillamine therapy was accompanied by a decrease in urinary calcium excretion to normal values in half of the patients studied. Wiebers and associates observed renal stones in 7 of 54 patients with Wilson's disease.

Cardiac manifestations in Wilson's disease include arrhythmias, cardiomyopathy, cardiac death, and autonomic dysfunction. Of patients with Wilson's disease, 34% have electrocardiographic abnormalities. Two cases of cardiac death were reported (one died of repeated ventricular fibrillation; the other died of dilated cardiomyopathy). In one of them, copper content in the myocardium was measured and found to be very high.

The occurrence of *chondrocalcinosis and osteoarthritis* in Wilson's disease may be due to copper accumulation, similar to the arthropathy of hemochromatosis

DIAGNOSIS

The diagnosis of Wilson's disease is usually made on the basis of clinical findings and laboratory abnormalities (Table 12–3). According to Sternlieb, a diagnosis of Wilson's disease can be made if two of the following symptoms are present: Kayser-Fleischer rings, typical neurologic symptoms, and low serum ceruloplasmin levels.

Patients with Neurologic Disease

In a patient presenting with typical neurologic symptoms and Kayser-Fleischer rings, the diagnosis is straightforward. No additional tests are required, and routine laboratory parameters just confirm the diagnosis. Kayser-Fleischer rings are rarely absent in neurologically symptomatic patients. However, there are a few well-documented cases of neurologic Wilson's disease without demonstrable Kayser-Fleischer rings. In such patients, the diagnosis is usually made by a low serum ceruloplasmin level.

Clinical neurologic examination is more sensitive than any other method to detect neurologic abnormalities. No further diagnostic procedures are necessary to establish the diagnosis.

Brain magnetic resonance imaging (MRI) is useful to document the extent of changes in the central nervous system. The most common abnormalities are changes in signal intensity of gray and white matter (Fig. 12–4), and atrophy of the caudate nucleus, brain stem, cerebral, and cerebellar hemispheres. A characteristic finding in Wilson's disease is the "face of the giant panda" sign, but this is found only in a few patients. In Wilson's disease, an abnormal pontocer-

Table 12–3 Routine Tests for Diagnosis of Wilson's Disease

Test	Typical Finding	False-Negative Result	False-Positive Result
Serum ceruloplasmin	Decreased	Normal levels in patients with marked hepatic inflammation; overestimation by immunologic assay	Low levels in: Malabsorption Aceruloplasminemia Liver insufficiency Heterozygotes
24-hr urinary copper	>100 μg/24 hr	Normal: Incorrect collection Children without liver disease	Increased: Hepatocellular necrosis Contamination
Serum "free" copper	>10 μg/dL	Normal if ceruloplasmin overestimated by immunologic assay	
Hepatic copper	>250 μg/g dry weight	Due to regional variation In patients with active liver disease In patients with regenerative nodules	Cholestatic syndromes
Kayser-Fleischer rings by slit lamp	Present	In up to 40% of patients with hepatic Wilson's disease In most asymptomatic siblings	Primary biliary cirrhosis

ebellar tract correlates with pseudoparkinsonian, and an abnormal dentatothalamic tract with cerebellar signs. The presence of portosystemic shunt is strongly associated with abnormality of the globus pallidus. On treatment, some of the MRI abnormalities are fully reversible. Auditory evoked brain stem potentials are helpful to document the degree of

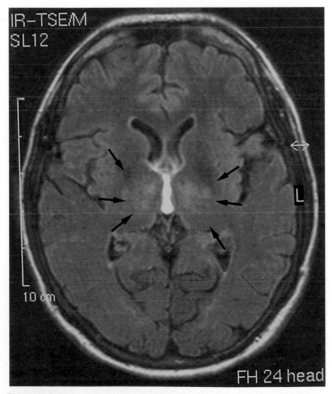

Figure 12–4
Cranial MRI (T2-weighted image, fluid attenuation inversion recovery [FLAIR], by courtesy of D. Prayer, MD) of a patient with Wilson's disease and neurologic symptoms. Signal hyperintensity in the thalamus (arrows) is shown.

functional impairment and the improvement by decoppering treatment.

Patients with Liver Disease and Hemolytic Anemia

Diagnosis is much more complex in patients presenting with liver disease. None of the commonly used parameters alone allows a certain diagnosis of Wilson's disease. Usually a combination of various laboratory parameters is necessary to firmly establish the diagnosis.

Kayser-Fleischer rings may be absent in up to 50% of patients with wilsonian liver disease and even in a higher proportion in fulminant Wilson's disease. On the other hand, patients with primary biliary cirrhosis may occasionally have Kayser-Fleischer rings.

Laboratory Parameters

Routine Laboratory Parameters of Liver Disease

In general, aminotransferases are only mildly increased, and deep jaundice combined with mild elevation of liver enzymes in nonsurgical patients should raise the suspicion for fulminant Wilson's disease. However, increases of aminotransferases may be indistinguishable from findings seen in acute hepatitis. Sometimes alkaline phosphatase activities are relatively low in patients with Wilson's disease. A ratio of total serum bilirubin concentration and alkaline phosphatase activity (>2) may differentiate fulminant Wilson's disease from other forms of fulminant hepatic failure. However, the usefulness of this test has not been confirmed in larger series.

Serum Ceruloplasmin

Serum ceruloplasmin can be measured by an immunologic assay or by the oxidase method. Because the immunologic ceruloplasmin assay can be automated by nephelometric methods, it is widely used in clinical laboratories. The oxi-

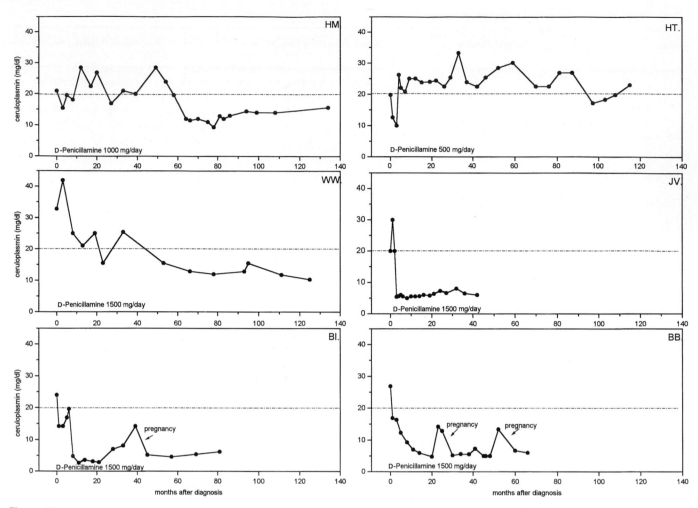

Figure 12–5
Effect of decoppering therapy on serum ceruloplasmin levels in patients with Wilson's disease with normal or borderline ceruloplasmin levels at diagnosis. On treatment, ceruloplasmin decreased in most patients to low levels, but in some (HT), it remained in the low-normal range. Note the effect of pregnancy on serum ceruloplasmin levels (BI and BB).

dase method is only performed in specialized centers. Whereas serum ceruloplasmin is decreased in most patients with neurologic Wilson's disease, it may be in the low normal range in up to 45% of patients with hepatic disease. On the other hand, even a low ceruloplasmin level is not diagnostic for Wilson's disease in the absence of Kayser-Fleischer rings. It may be low in subjects with familial hypoceruloplasminemia, in severely malnourished subjects, and in heterozygous carriers of the Wilson disease gene. Very low levels were found in a patient with autoimmune hepatitis, which increased after treatment with steroids. Thus, in patients with liver disease, a normal ceruloplasmin level cannot exclude, nor is a low level sufficient to make, the diagnosis of Wilson's disease.

There are several possible explanations for the high proportion of patients with hepatic Wilson's disease with ceruloplasmin levels in the normal range. In view of the multiple mutations of Wilson's disease gene, differences in the functional impairment of the gene product, a Cu-ATPase, may be associated with variations in clinical and laboratory findings. Second, apoceruloplasmin may interfere with the immunologic assay for ceruloplasmin. Its contribution to the results obtained in patients with low ceruloplasmin values is

negligible, but in those closer to the borderline, the additional apoceruloplasmin may push them into the normal range. An overestimation of serum ceruloplasmin can be suspected if the serum copper concentration is lower than expected by the measured ceruloplasmin (which contains 0.3% of copper) level (see later). Finally, ceruloplasmin is an acute phase reactant and its serum concentration increases as a consequence of inflammation. Most patients with normal ceruloplasmin levels had marked liver disease. The decrease of ceruloplasmin after initiation of decoppering treatment (Fig. 12–5) in parallel with the improvement of liver disease supports this concept. Similarly, serum ceruloplasmin may increase in pregnancy to high normal values.

Serum Copper

In general, serum copper values parallel those of ceruloplasmin. Therefore, serum copper is frequently low in patients with Wilson's disease. However, about half of patients have serum copper levels in the normal range. Patients with fulminant Wilson's disease or hemolytic anemia may even have greatly increased levels. Most of the copper in serum is bound to ceruloplasmin and under normal conditions less than 5% circulates as "free copper." In normal subjects, it does not exceed 10 μg/dL. The "free" copper concentration can be calculated by subtracting the ceruloplasmin-bound copper (ceruloplasmin times 3.3) from the total copper concentration. An increased free copper level (>10 μg/dL) is considered as a useful diagnostic test for Wilson's disease (providing the measured ceruloplasmin level is correct, see earlier).

Urinary Copper Excretion

Urine copper excretion is markedly increased in patients with Wilson's disease (88% in one study); however, its usefulness in clinical practice is limited. The estimation of urinary copper excretion may be misleading due to incorrect collection of 24-hour urine volume or to copper contamination. In presymptomatic patients, urinary copper excretion may be normal but may increase after D-penicillamine challenge. On the other hand, urinary copper excretion is also increased in any disease with extensive hepatocellular necrosis.

Hepatic Copper Content

Hepatic copper content is increased in most patients with Wilson's disease and usually exceeds 250 μg/g dry weight (normal: up to 50 μg/g). In the absence of other tests suggestive for abnormal copper metabolism, a diagnosis of Wilson's disease cannot be made based on an increased hepatic copper content alone. Patients with chronic cholestatic diseases, neonates, and young children and possibly also subjects with exogenous copper overload have increased hepatic copper concentration higher than 250 μg/g. On the other hand, hepatic copper content may be normal or borderline in about 10% of patients with unquestionable Wilson's disease due to sampling, given the great regional differences in hepatic copper distribution, especially in the cirrhotic liver. In one study, multiple biopsies taken from the explanted livers of two patients with fulminant hepatic failure revealed an up to 500-fold variation in copper content. Only 2 of 14 and 3 of 16 specimens, respectively, were within the diagnostic range for Wilson's disease, but in a cirrhotic liver all the specimens tested yielded diagnostic results. Thus, estimates from a single biopsy specimen may be misleading.

Liver Biopsy

Light Microscopy

Liver biopsy findings are generally nonspecific and not directly helpful to make the diagnosis of Wilson's disease. Liver pathology (Fig. 12–6) includes early changes like fatty intracellular accumulations, which often proceed to marked steatosis. At later stages, hepatic inflammation with portal and periportal lymphocytic infiltrates, the presence of necrosis and fibrosis may be indistinguishable from other forms of hepatitis. Some patients have cirrhosis without any inflammation. The detection of focal copper stores by the Rhodanin stain is a pathognomonic feature of Wilson's disease but is only present in a few patients (approximately 10%).

Electron Microscopy

Ultrastructural abnormalities in Wilson's disease include pathologic changes of mitochondria and peroxisomes. Hepatocellular mitochondria are pleomorphic, with varying combinations of abnormalities including enlargement, bizarre shapes, increased matrix density, separation of the normally apposed inner and outer membranes, widened intercristal spaces, enlarged granules, and crystalline, vacuolated, or dense inclusions. Sometimes peroxisomes are abnormally enlarged, rounded, or misshapen and contain a granular or flocculent matrix of varying electron density.

Magnetic Resonance Imaging of the Liver

Hepatic T_2-weighted MRI changes include multiple tiny low-intensity nodules surrounded by high-intensity septa in about 60% of patients. Some patients also have low-intensity nodules in T_1-weighted images. Patients with abnormal MRI findings have liver cirrhosis or fibrosis. In contrast, patients without pathologic MRI findings on liver morphology had only slight histopathologic changes in the parenchyma and normal laboratory data. In patients with low-intensity nodules of the liver by MRI and unknown causes of liver cirrhosis, laboratory data and histopathology should be checked when searching for disorders of copper metabolism.

Radiocopper Test

The basis of this test is the biphasic plasma kinetics of copper. An oral dose of ^{64}Cu is given, and the blood radioactivity at 1, 2, 24, and 48 hours is determined. Initially, labeled copper is taken up by the liver and is completely removed from the serum. Later, the label reappears bound to ceruloplasmin. This second peak is absent in patients with Wilson's disease. Usually, the ratio of the 24- or 48-hour peak to the early (2 hours) peak is calculated. The test is only useful in patients and siblings with ceruloplasmin levels in or close to the normal range. The usefulness of this test is further limited by the considerable overlap between affected patients and heterozygotes. Several modifications of the radiocopper test (intravenous instead of oral administration, measurement of radiocopper incorporation into ceruloplasmin) did not improve the sensitivity of the radiocopper test. Today, the radiocopper test is replaced by molecular genetic testing. In unclear atypical cases, the presence of an abnormal test may support the diagnosis of Wilson's disease.

Mutation Analysis

Direct Mutation Analysis

Direct molecular genetic diagnosis is difficult because of the occurrence of many mutations, each of which is rare. Furthermore, most patients are compound heterozygotes (i.e., carry two different mutations). Screening for mutations is typically done by single-strand conformation polymorphism analysis. Those samples showing a shift of one or both bands can then be sequenced to identify the exact mutation. This approach is quite useful as a research tool but is impractical for clinical diagnosis. In contrast, using allele-specific probes, direct mutation diagnosis is rapid and clini-

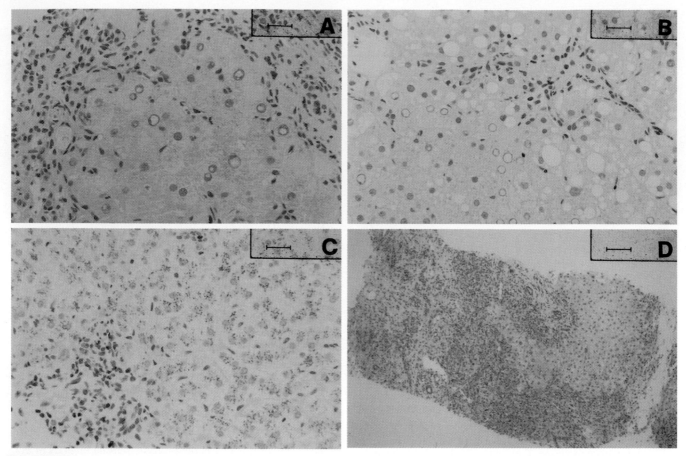

Figure 12–6
Liver histology in Wilson's disease. *A,* Vacuolated nuclei (H & E, ×400), and portal infiltration (grade 2) extending into the lobules in a 32-year-old asymptomatic sibling. *B,* Marked steatosis, vacuolated nuclei (H & E, ×400), and mild lobular infiltration (grade 1) in the 18-year-old asymptomatic sibling (His1069Gln homozygote). *C,* Copper granules in hepatocytes (Rhodanine, ×200), mild portal infiltration (grade 1), and fibrosis (stage 2) in a 15-year-old girl (compound heterozygote for His1069Gln) with neurologic Wilson's disease. No biochemical evidence of liver disease is present. *D,* Severe chronic active hepatitis (grade 4) with bridging necrosis and fibrosis stage 4 in a 24-year-old man (unknown mutation) presenting as severe acute hepatitis (H & E, ×100). (All photographies courtesy of K. Kaserer, MD.)

cally very helpful, if a mutation occurs with a reasonable frequency in the population. In Austria, the His1069Gln mutation is present in 61% of patients with Wilson's disease, and a two-step PCR based test for this mutation has become very useful. For example, the large family of an index patient homozygous for this mutation with more than 40 members was examined within 2 days. An asymptomatic affected sibling and several heterozygotes were detected, even if first degree relatives were not available for testing (Fig. 12–7). Eventually, a multiplex PCR for the most frequent mutations in Wilson's disease should make direct mutation analysis for diagnosis feasible.

Haplotype Analysis

Because of the complexity in identifying the numerous mutations in Wilson's disease, haplotypes can be used to screen for mutations and to examine asymptomatic siblings of index patients. Several highly polymorphic microsatellite markers have been described that closely flank the gene and are highly variable: D13S316, D13S314, D13S301, and D13S133. Where the markers are different at each locus in a patient, testing of at least one parent or child of the patient is necessary to obtain the haplotype. The identification of unusual haplotypes can lend support but is not sufficient to confirm the diagnosis of Wilson's disease.

Microsatellite markers are also useful to study the segregation of the Wilson disease gene in most families. By this approach, diagnostic dilemmas in differentiating heterozygote gene carriers and affected asymptomatic siblings can be solved. For such analysis, at least one first-degree relative and the index patient is required. Haplotype analysis and restriction fragment length polymorphism of flanking genes (before the discovery of the Wilson disease gene) proved to be extremely useful for prenatal testing and for providing a firm diagnosis of affected siblings in families with Wilson's disease (Fig. 12–8).

Family Screening

Once a diagnosis of Wilson's disease has been made in an index patient, an evaluation of his or her family is manda-

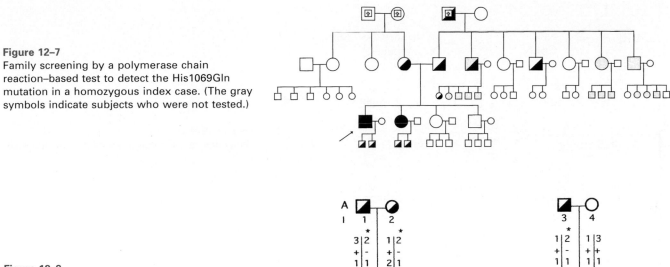

Figure 12-7
Family screening by a polymerase chain reaction–based test to detect the His1069Gln mutation in a homozygous index case. (The gray symbols indicate subjects who were not tested.)

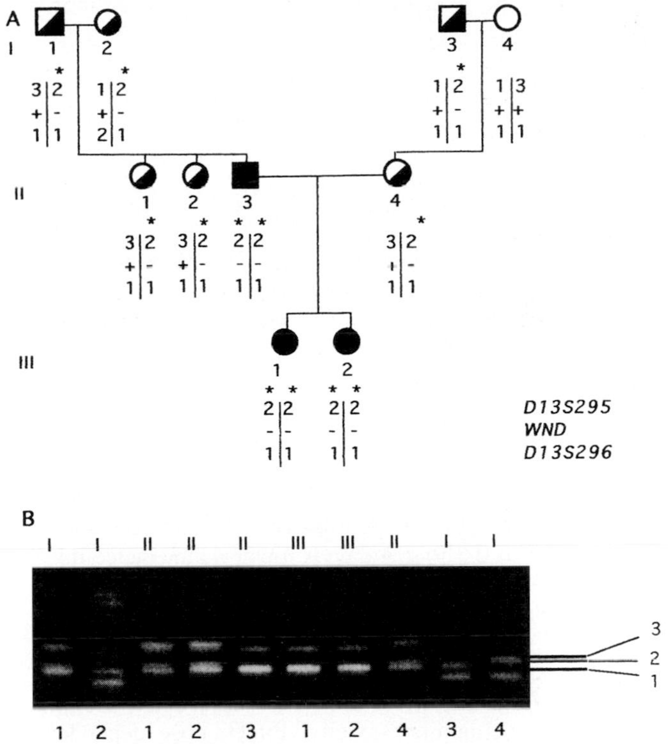

Figure 12-8
Application of haplotype analysis in family screening. *A*, Pedigree with DNA haplotypes of microsatellite marker analysis. The numbers indicate allelic designations at microsatellite marker loci. (*, mutant alleles.) *B*, Separation of the polymorphic dinucleotide microsatellites on a polyacrylamide gel. The index case (II/3) was a 39-year-old man presenting with cirrhosis, Kayser-Fleischer rings, and neurologic symptoms. His elder daughter (III/1, 10 years) had elevated alanine aminotransferase (ALT) and a liver biopsy diagnostic for Wilson's disease (WND). Her 4-year-old sister (III/2) was healthy and had normal ALT, normal ceruloplasmin, and normal urinary copper excretion. By haplotype analysis, she was identified as homozygous carrier of the Wilson disease gene. The diagnosis was confirmed by liver biopsy. (From Maier-Dobersberger TH, Rack S, Granditsch G, et al: Diagnosis of Wilson's disease in an asymptomatic sibling by DNA linkage analysis. Gastroenterology 109:2015–2018, 1995.)

tory. The likelihood to find a homozygote among siblings is 25%, among children 0.5%. Testing of second-degree relatives is only useful if the gene was found in one of the immediate members of his or her family. No single test is able to identify affected siblings or heterozygote carriers of the Wilson disease gene with sufficient certainty. Today, mutation analysis is the only reliable tool for family screening.

Algorithm for Diagnosis of Wilson's Disease

A diagnostic algorithm is suggested in Figure 12–9. In the absence of typical clinical findings, measurement of hepatic copper content is mandatory in every patient with unexplained elevations of liver enzymes and some abnormal parameters of copper metabolism. In patients without any signs of altered copper metabolism, it should also be measured, if the level of suspicion is high. Furthermore, patients with ceruloplasmin levels in the normal range should be referred for a radiocopper test or PCR-based mutation analy-

sis. In selected patients with still unclear findings or in whom a liver biopsy cannot be performed because of impaired coagulation, a "test" treatment with decoppering agents can be initiated for 6 to 12 months.

TREATMENT

Penicillamine

Penicillamine was first reported to be effective in treating Wilson's disease by Walshe in 1956 and has since been the "gold standard" for therapy. Penicillamine acts by reductive chelation: It reduces copper bound to protein and thus decreases the affinity of the protein for copper. Reduction of copper thus facilitates the binding of copper to the drug. The copper mobilized by penicillamine is then excreted in the urine. Within a few weeks to months, penicillamine brings the level of copper to a subtoxic threshold and allows tissue repair to begin. Most symptomatic patients, whether he-

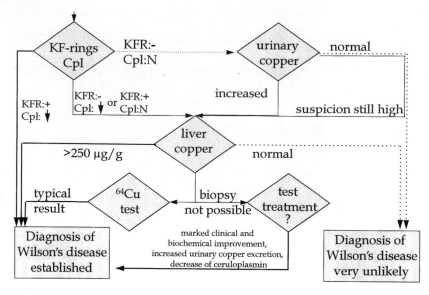

Figure 12–9
Flow diagram for diagnosis of Wilson's disease.

patic, neurologic, or psychiatric, respond within months of starting treatment. Among neurologic patients, a significant number may experience an initial worsening of symptoms before they get better.

The usual dose of penicillamine is 1 to 1.5 g/day. Initially, this dose will cause a large cupriuresis, but copper excretion later decreases to 0.5 mg/day. To prevent deficiency induced by penicillamine, pyridoxine (vitamin B_6) should be supplemented (50 mg/week). Once the clinical benefit has been established, it is possible to reduce the dosage of penicillamine to 0.5 to 1 g/day. A lower maintenance dose will decrease the likelihood of late side effects of the drug.

A major problem of penicillamine is its high level of toxicity. In our series, 20% of patients had major side effects and were switched to other treatments. Other series report even higher frequencies of side effects. There are two broad classes of penicillamine toxicity: direct, dose dependent side effects and immunologically induced lesions. Direct side effects are pyridoxine deficiency and interference with collagen and elastin formation. The latter results in skin lesions like cutis laxa and elastosis perforans serpingiosa. By routine skin biopsies 1 year after the initiation of treatment, we found signs of elastic and collagen fiber abnormalities in every patient; however, none developed symptomatic skin disease to date. These side effects can be prevented or mitigated by decreasing the dosage of penicillamine. More recently, it was suggested that that total absence of holoceruloplasmin as a result of intensive decoppering is associated with impaired iron mobilization from the liver. Hepatic iron concentrations in the range seen for patients with hemochromatosis were found in a few patients with Wilson's disease after year-long high-dose penicillamine treatment. Immunologic-mediated side effects include leukopenia and thrombocytopenia, systemic lupus erythematosus, immune complex nephritis, pemphigus, buccal ulcerations, myasthenia gravis, optic neuritis, and Goodpasture's syndrome. Immunologic-mediated side effects occur within the first 3 months of treatment and require immediate cessation of penicillamine. To diagnose these side effects as soon as possible, patients should be monitored during the first 6 weeks

of therapy. If the drug is well tolerated, control intervals can be gradually prolonged.

Trientine

Trientine is a copper chelator that acts primarily by enhancing urinary copper excretion. Trientine is licensed for treatment of Wilson's disease and is now generally available. Experience with trientine is not as extensive as with penicillamine. It seems to be as effective as penicillamine with much fewer side effects. Its efficacy was evaluated in patients with intolerance to penicillamine. Discontinuation of penicillamine resulted in death from hepatic decompensation or fulminant hepatitis in 8 of 11 patients who stopped their own treatment after an average survival of only 2.6 years. In contrast, 12 of 13 patients with intolerance to penicillamine switched to trientine (1 to 1.5 g/day) were alive at 2 to 15 years later. The remaining patient died from an accidental cause. However, the efficacy of trientine was not compared with penicillamine as the initial treatment of Wilson's disease. Uncontrolled anecdotal reports and our own experience, indicate that trientine is a satisfactory first-line treatment for Wilson's disease. In the early phase of treatment, trientine appears to be more potent in mobilizing copper than penicillamine, but cupriuresis diminishes more rapidly than with penicillamine. The cupriuretic power of trientine may be disappointing, but it is sufficient to keep the patient clinically well.

Ammonium Tetrathiomolybdate

This drug has two mechanisms of action. First, it complexes with copper in the intestinal tract and thus prevents absorption of copper. Second, the absorbed drug forms a complex with copper and albumin in the blood and renders the copper unavailable for cellular uptake. There is very limited experience with this drug. Tetrathiomolybdate appears to be a useful form of initial treatment in patients presenting with neurologic symptoms. In contrast to penicillamine therapy, treatment with tetrathiomolybdate does not result in initial neurologic deterioration. This agent is particularly effective at removing copper from the liver. Because of its effectiveness, continuous use can cause copper deficiency. Bone marrow depression has been described in a few patients treated with this drug.

Zinc

Zinc interferes with the intestinal absorption of copper by two mechanisms. Both metals share the same carrier in enterocytes and pretreatment with zinc blocks this carrier for copper transport. This effect of zinc has a half-life of about 11 days. Second, zinc induces metellothionein in enterocytes, which acts as an intracellular ligand binding zinc, copper, and other metals thus rendering them unavailable for systemic absorption. Instead, these metals are excreted in the feces with desquamated epithelial cells. Increased fecal excretion of copper has been demonstrated in patients with Wilson's disease on treatment with zinc. Furthermore, zinc also induces metallothionein formation in hepatocytes and binding of copper to metallothionein protects hepatocytes against copper toxicity.

Data on zinc in the treatment of Wilson's disease are derived mainly from uncontrolled studies using different zinc preparations (e.g., zinc sulfate, zinc acetate) at different doses (75 to 250 mg/day).

The efficacy of zinc was assessed by four different approaches. First, patients successfully decoppered by D-penicillamine were switched to zinc treatment and the maintenance of their asymptomatic condition was monitored. Most patients maintained a negative copper balance, and no symptomatic recurrences occurred. Hepatic copper levels remained unchanged over treatments periods of 12 to 20 months. In two patients, D-penicillamine was reinstituted because of progressive disease, both patients eventually died soon thereafter. Another patient died of liver failure. Stremmel observed the occurrence of severe neurologic symptoms in a 25-year-old asymptomatic sibling 4 months after switching from D-penicillamine to zinc. Hoogenrad reported three patients who died of liver failure after treatment was switched to zinc therapy.

A second group are symptomatic patients switched to zinc as alternate treatment due to intolerance to D-penicillamine. Sixteen case histories have been published to date. Liver function and neurologic symptoms improved in three and five patients, respectively. One patient further deteriorated neurologically and improved on retreatment with D-penicillamine. The remaining patients remained in stable condition.

In a third group, zinc was used as first-line therapy. About one third were asymptomatic siblings of patients with Wilson's disease; two thirds presented with neurologic or hepatic symptoms. Most patients remained free of symptoms or improved. In 15%, neurologic symptoms worsened and then improved on D-penicillamine. Three patients died of progressive liver disease.

Finally, in a prospective study, Czlonkowska compared the results of treatment with D-penicillamine or zinc sulfate in 67 newly diagnosed cases of Wilson's disease. This was not a randomized study, every other patient was treated with zinc. The effectiveness of long-term treatment with D-penicillamine and zinc was similar in those patients who were able to continue the initial therapy. Zinc was better tolerated than D-penicillamine. However, two patients who were treated with zinc therapy died of progressive liver disease.

It is unknown whether a combination of zinc with chelation therapy is useful or not. Theoretically, these drugs may have antagonistic effects. Interactions in the maintenance phase of zinc therapy with penicillamine and trientine were investigated by Cu balance studies and absorption of orally administered ^{64}Cu as endpoints. The result on Cu balance was about the same with zinc alone as it is with zinc plus one of the other agents. Thus, there appear to be no advantages to concomitant administration.

Antioxidants

As discussed earlier, the main mechanism of hepatocellular injury by excess copper is the formation of free radicals resulting in lipid peroxidation and impaired mitochondrial respiration. Thus, antioxidants, such as α-tocopherol, may be important adjuncts in the treatment of Wilson's disease. There are no large experiences with α-tocopherol. A few observations indicate that this therapeutic adjunct may be useful in the severe liver disease.

Liver Transplantation

Liver transplantation is the treatment of choice in patients with fulminant Wilson's disease and in patients with decompensated cirrhosis. The selection criteria for fulminant Wilson's disease and of decompensated wilsonian cirrhosis are similar to those for fulminant hepatic failure or decompensated cirrhosis of other etiology, respectively. Besides improving survival, liver transplantation also corrects the biochemical defect underlying Wilson's disease. However, the role of this procedure in the management of patients with neurologic Wilson's disease in the absence of hepatic insufficiency is still uncertain.

Schilsky retrospectively analyzed data obtained on 55 transplants performed in patients with Wilson's disease at centers in the United States and Europe. Indication for orthotopic liver transplantation included 33 patients with hepatic insufficiency and 21 with wilsonian fulminant hepatitis. One patient had intractable neurologic Wilson's disease. The mean and median survival after orthotopic liver transplantation were 2.7 and 2.5 years, respectively; the longest survival time after transplantation was 20 years. Survival at 1 year was 79%. Nonfatal complications occurred in five patients.

Fifty-one orthotopic liver transplants were performed on 39 patients (16 pediatric patients and 23 adults) with Wilson's disease at the University of Pittsburgh. Twenty-two patients had fulminant hepatic failure, and 17 had chronic advanced liver disease (nine with and eight without associated neurologic dysfunction). The rate of primary graft survival was 73%, and patient survival rate was 79.4%. Survival was better for those with a chronic advanced liver disease presentation (90%) than it was for those who presented with fulminant hepatic failure (73%).

The outcome of neurologic disease after liver transplantation is uncertain. In the retrospective survey, four of the seven patients with neurologic or psychiatric symptoms due

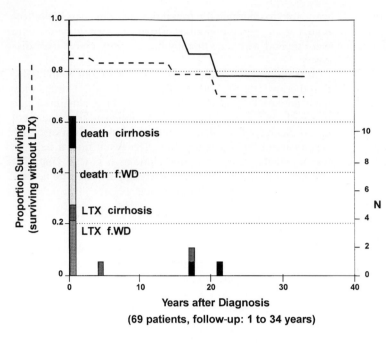

Figure 12–10
Cumulative survival in 69 Austrian patients with Wilson's disease. The *broken lines* indicate "survival rates," if death or liver transplantation are chosen as endpoints. The *bars* refer to the number of patients dying of or transplanted for fulminant Wilson's disease or decompensated cirrhosis.

to Wilson's disease improved afterwards. A few case reports either document dramatic improvement in neurologic function over a period of 3 or 4 months after orthotopic liver transplantation or the development of postoperative central pontine and extrapontine myelinolysis and new extrapyramidal symptoms 19 months after the liver transplant.

PROGNOSIS

If left untreated, symptomatic Wilson's disease progresses to death in all patients. Most patients will die of complications of advanced liver failure, some of progressive neurologic disease. The overall mortality from Wilson's disease treated medically (in most cases by D-penicillamine) has not been assessed prospectively. The mortality in 33 patients followed for 21 years by Scheinberg and Sternlieb was approximately 20%. This figure is close to the cumulative mortality in 69 Austrian patients (Fig. 12–10). In this group there was a substantial early mortality due to liver failure within the first 2 months after diagnosis. Only two patients died during the follow-up period; one of them developed liver failure after a 2-year period of noncompliance. About an equal number of patients with severe liver failure survived after orthotopic liver transplantation. In a German study, in 51 patients the cumulative survival was slightly reduced during the early period of follow-up but was not different from an age- and sex-matched control population after 15 years of observation (96%).

Liver Disease

In general, prognosis depends on the severity of liver disease at diagnosis. In patients without cirrhosis or with compensated cirrhosis, liver disease does not progress after the initiation of decoppering therapy. Liver function improves gradually (Fig. 12–11), and liver function parameters (serum albumin, prothrombin time) will become normal in

most patients within 1 to 2 years. In compliant patients treated with D-penicillamine or trientine, liver function remains stable and no progressive liver disease is observed.

Schilsky followed 20 patients with wilsonian chronic hepatitis. Treatment with D-penicillamine was promptly initiated in 19 patients. One patient refused treatment and died 4 months later. Treated patients received D-penicillamine or trientine for a total of 264 patient-years (median of 14 years). In 18 patients, there was symptomatic improvement and virtually normal levels of serum albumin, bilirubin, aspartate aminotransferase, and alanine aminotransferase fol-

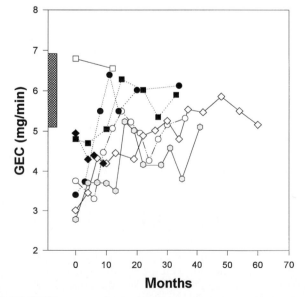

Figure 12–11
Serial determination of galactose elimination capacity (GEC) in seven patients with hepatic Wilson's disease.

Table 12–4 Prognostic Index in Wilson's Disease

	0*	1*	2*	3*	4*
Serum bilirubin (μmol/L)	<100	100–150	151–200	201–300	>301
AST (× ULN)	<2.5	2.5–3.5	3.6–5	5.1–7.5	>7.5
PT (sec over control)	<4	4–8	9–12	13–20	>21

Slightly modified according to Nazer H, Ede RJ, Mowat AP, et al: Wilson's disease: Clinical presentation and use of prognostic index. Gut 27:1377–1381, 1986. A score ≥7 is associated with high probability of death.
AST, aspartate aminotransferase; PT, prothrombin time; ULN, upper limit of normal; *, score points.

lowed within 1 year. One woman died after 9 months of treatment. Two patients, who became noncompliant after 9 and 17 years of successful pharmacologic treatment, required liver transplantation.

In patients presenting with fulminant Wilson's disease, medical treatment is rarely effective. Without emergency liver transplantation, mortality is very high. In a group of 34 patients, a prognostic index based on serum bilirubin levels, aspartate aminotransferase activity, and prothrombin time (Table 12–4) was developed. A score of more than 7 was always associated with death. However, this prognostic score has not been validated prospectively. Nevertheless, it is a useful guide to assess short-term mortality in the setting of liver transplantation.

Hemolytic Anemia

If diagnosed and treated early, hemolysis subsides within a few days after the initiation of D-penicillamine therapy. Spontaneous remissions may occur even without treatment, but relapse occurs usually within a few months. Hemolysis associated with active liver disease may progress rapidly to fulminant Wilson's disease.

Neurologic Disease

Patients presenting with neurologic symptoms have a better prognosis than do those presenting with liver disease. None of our patients died; two required liver transplantation. In Brewer's series, 2 of 54 patients died of complications attributed to their impaired neurologic function.

Neurologic symptoms are partly reversible. Improvement of neurologic symptoms occurs gradually over several months. Initially, neurologic symptoms may worsen, especially on treatment with D-penicillamine. In some patients, neurologic symptoms disappear completely, and abnormalities documented by evoked responses or MRI may completely resolve within 18 to 24 months.

Ten of our patients were followed for 5 years prospectively after diagnosis. Brain function was assessed by repeated recording of short latency sensory potentials, auditory brain stem potentials, and cognitive P300-evoked potentials. Electrophysiologic and clinical improvement was observed as early as 3 months after the initiation of chelation therapy and continued until final assessment after 5 years. Three patients became completely normal, but residual symptoms were detectable in seven patients. Such permanent deficits are unlikely to be improved by liver transplantation.

SUGGESTED READINGS

Overviews

Brewer GJ, Yuzbasiyan-Gurkan V: Wilson disease. Medicine 71:139–164, 1992.
Hoogenraad TU: Wilson's Disease. Philadelphia: WB Saunders, 1996.
Scheinberg IH, Sternlieb I: Wilson's Disease. Vol 23: Major Problems in Internal Medicine. Philadelphia: WB Saunders, 1984.

Hepatic Copper Transport

Dijkstra M, Vonk RJ, Kuipers F: How does copper get into bile? New insights into the mechanism(s) of hepatobiliary copper transport. J Hepatol 24 (Suppl 1):109–120, 1996.

Mutations of Wilson's Disease Gene

Cox DW: Molecular advances in Wilson disease. Prog Liver Dis 10:245–263, 1996.

Diagnosis

Figus A, Angius A, Loudianos O, et al: Molecular pathology and haplotype analysis of Wilson's disease in Mediterranean populations. Am J Hum Genet 57:1318–1324, 1995.
Grimm G, Madl CH, Katzenschlager R, et al: Detailed evaluation of brain dysfunction in patients with Wilson disease. Electroencephalogr Clin Neurophysiol 82:119–124, 1992.
Maier-Dobersberger TH, Ferenci P, Polli C, et al: The His1069Gln mutation in Wilson s disease: Detection by a rapid PCR-test, clinical course and liver biopsy findings. Ann Intern Med 127:21–26, 1997.
Maier-Dobersberger TH, Rack S, Granditsch G, et al: Diagnosis of Wilson's disease in an asymptomatic sibling by DNA linkage analysis. Gastroenterology 109:2015–2018, 1995.
Oder W, Grimm G, Kollegger H, et al: Neurological and neuropsychiatric spectrum of Wilson disease: A prospective study in 45 cases. J Neurol 238:281–287, 1991.
Petrukhin KE, Fischer SG, Pirastu M, et al: Mapping, cloning and genetic characterization of the region containing the Wilson disease gene. Nat Genet 5:338–343, 1993.
Petrukhin KE, Lutsenko S, Chernov I, et al: Characterization of the Wilson disease gene encoding a P-type copper transporting ATPase: Genomic organization, alternative splicing, and structure/function predictions. Hum Mol Genet 3:1647–1656, 1994.
Steindl P, Ferenci P, Dienes HP, et al: Wilson's disease in patients presenting with liver disease: A diagnostic challenge. Gastroenterology 113:212–218, 1997.
Sternlieb I, Scheinberg IH: The role of radiocopper in the diagnosis of Wilson s disease. Gastroenterology 77:138–1342, 1979.
Tanzi RE, Petrukhin K, Chernov I, et al: The Wilson disease gene is a copper transporting ATPase with homology to the Menkes' disease gene. Nat Genet 5:344–350, 1993.
Thomas GJ, Forbes JR, Roberts EA, et al: The Wilson disease gene: Spectrum of mutations and their consequences. Nat Genet 9:210–217, 1995.
van Wassenaer-van Hall HN, van den Heuvel AG, Algra A, et al: Wilson disease: Findings at MR imaging and CT of the brain with clinical correlation. Radiology 198:531–536, 1996.

Treatment

Brewer GJ, Dick RD, Johnson V, et al: Treatment of Wilson's disease with ammonium tetrathiomolybdate. I: Initial therapy in 17 neurologically affected patients. Arch Neurol 51:545–554, 1994.

Czlonkowska A, Gajda J, Rodo M: Effects of long-term treatment in Wilson's disease with D-penicillamine and zinc sulphate. J Neurol 243:269–273, 1996.

Prognosis

Scheinberg IH, Jaffe ME, Sternlieb I: The use of trientine in preventing the effects of interrupting penicillamine therapy in Wilson's disease. N Engl J Med 317:2009–2013, 1987.

Schilsky ML, Scheinberg IH, Sternlieb I: Liver transplantation for Wilson disease: Indications and outcome. Hepatology 19:583–587, 1994.

Schilsky ML, Scheinberg IH, Sternlieb I: Prognosis of wilsonian chronic active hepatitis. Gastroenterology 100:762–767, 1991.

Stremmel W, Meyerrose KW, Niederau C, et al: Wilson s disease: Clinical presentation, treatment, and survival. Ann Intern Med 115:720–726, 1991.

Walshe JM, Yealland M: Chelation treatment of neurological Wilson disease. Q J Med 86:197–204, 1993.

Chapter

13

The Porphyrias, α_1-Antitrypsin Deficiency, Cystic Fibrosis, and Other Metabolic Diseases of the Liver

James H. Reichheld
Herbert L. Bonkovsky

etabolic disease of the liver may be protean and may be profound. Historically, a poorly understood group of diseases because of their elusive molecular bases, metabolic diseases of the liver have been the subject of intense and fruitful study in recent years.

Advances in molecular medicine have provided perhaps the greatest potential for understanding the epidemiology and pathophysiology of these disorders and are leading to promising new diagnostic and therapeutic interventions. Organ (liver and bone marrow) transplantation has already found its way into the therapy of some of these disorders. Identification of single enzyme defects has allowed for replacement enzyme therapy in Gaucher's disease and for avoidance of enzyme substrates in hereditary fructose intolerance. Gene localization and cloning have allowed for appropriate genetic counseling, prenatal screening, and potential recombinant enzyme replacement therapy for several metabolic diseases of the liver. Capacity for curative treatment has been demonstrated in animal models of gene therapy, some of which are now leading to human trials.

In this chapter, we review the major disorders of hepatic metabolism that result in liver disease. Taken together, the diseases comprise a diverse group and involve virtually every organ system. These disorders have in common the ability to cause profound hepatic and systemic disease, and they now have the potential to be treated effectively and even cured as a result of recent advances in our understanding of their molecular subtleties.

THE PORPHYRIAS

The porphyrias are diseases caused by defects in heme synthesis. They have been implicated in the popularized "mad-

ness" of King George III, in Vincent van Gogh's bouts with psychiatric illness, and as a biologic basis for the legend of vampires. In all the porphyrias, specific enzyme defects in the biosynthetic pathway of heme result in the accumulation of toxic metabolites, manifested variably as disorders of the skin, nervous system, and liver, depending on the enzyme affected. Although hepatic effects may be minimal, systemic effects may be marked and varied. Indeed, the porphyrias may deceivingly mimic other clinical syndromes, and porphyria was considered to be "the little imitator" almost 70 years ago by Jan Waldenstrom, in deference to syphilis, known then as "the big imitator." Only those disorders with major hepatic manifestations are considered here.

The porphyrias are classified as *hepatic* or *erythropoietic* based on the organ in which the major overproduction of heme precursors occurs. The *acute hepatic porphyrias* may be associated with acute neurologic crises. Such crises can be exacerbated and even precipitated by an array of medications, such that many porphyric crises are unwittingly induced or essentially iatrogenic. Although generally rare, the porphyrias are more common in specific populations, and in certain areas they have been associated with an increased risk of hepatocellular carcinoma.

The diagnosis is based first on detection of porphyrin precursors in blood or urine, and further distinction is based on the examination of urine or stool for the accumulation of specific precursors. High concentrations of porphyrins within urine may impart a purple or red color, justifying the name "porphyria," from the Greek (porphyra) for "purple." Porphyric crises may be minimized by avoiding precipitants, and the symptoms of acute attacks can be managed by suppressing the synthesis of toxic compounds.

Epidemiology and Pathophysiology

Different porphyrias may predominate in specific geographic areas. For example, among the acute porphyrias, variegate porphyria is the most common type found in South Africa, whereas the acute intermittent type is the predominant acute porphyria in Europe and the United States. Some are autosomal dominant, whereas others are recessive; and, for protoporphyria, the pattern of inheritance is apparently variable. Symptomatic porphyria typically presents only after the onset of puberty and crises of acute porphyria affect women more frequently than men. Drugs are the most common precipitants of attacks in the acute hepatic porphyrias, inciting symptomatic disease in predisposed individuals. Although the list of potential offenders is extensive, common precipitants include barbiturates, hydantoins, sulfonamides, oral contraceptives, carbamazepine, and valproic acid. Ethanol may exacerbate the acute porphyrias and porphyria cutanea tarda (PCT) and protoporphyria as well.

An understanding of the pathophysiology of the porphyrias follows study of the biosynthetic pathway of heme (Fig. 13–1). Eight enzymatic steps are involved, and seven main defects are described. Deficiencies of enzymatic activities result in overproduction of toxic precursors by feedback derepression of δ-aminolevulinic acid (ALA) synthase, the first and rate-controlling enzyme of the pathway. ALA synthase condenses glycine and succinyl coenzyme A to form δ-aminolevulinic acid, a probable neurotoxin. Heme normally provides repression of this enzyme (Fig. 13–2A); a deficiency of intracellular heme in hepatocytes results in elevated ALA production (see Fig. 13–2B). Porphobilinogen, the metabolite following ALA, which is also produced in excess in several of the acute porphyrias (Table 13–1), may

similarly be neurotoxic, but there is less evidence for this than for ALA. Neurologic effects may be partly caused as well by heme deficiency in neuronal tissue. The cutaneous features of the porphyrias are secondary to photosensitization by porphyrins, although the specific cutaneous effects of excess protoporphyrin differ from those of the other porphyrins.

In the acute hepatic porphyrias, the chief site of porphyrin production is the liver. Other than the enzyme defect, however, there is little structural or functional liver pathology. Nonetheless, with progressive disease, porphyrins may be directly hepatotoxic. Alcohol can have a cooperative role in effecting liver disease. Iron overload associated with PCT may be responsible for hepatocellular damage, particularly in association with hepatitis C virus. An increased risk of the development of hepatocellular carcinoma has been associated with acute intermittent porphyria in Scandinavia and recently in France, but has not, to date, been noted in the United States. PCT is also associated with an increased risk of development of hepatocellular carcinoma, although it is not yet clear whether such risk can be attributed to the accumulation of hepatic uroporphyrin per se or to other causes of chronic hepatitis or cirrhosis associated with PCT (e.g., alcohol, iron overload, or chronic hepatitis C).

Clinical Features

Hepatic Porphyrias

There are five hepatic porphyrias, four associated with acute neurologic crises, called *acute hepatic porphyrias.* They include δ-*aminolevulinic acid dehydrase deficiency, acute in-*

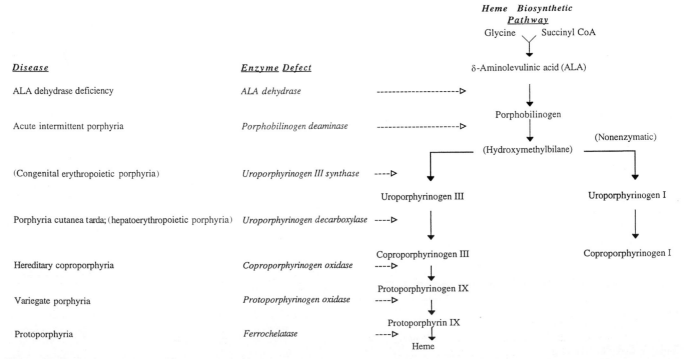

Figure 13–1
The porphyrias—heme biosynthesis and enzymatic defects. (ALA, δ-Aminolevulinic acid. *Open-headed [horizontal] arrows* indicate the site of enzymatic defect; *solid [vertical] arrows* represent the normal synthetic pathway. Diseases in parentheses are erythropoietic porphyrias and are not discussed in this chapter.)

A. _Normal Hepatic Heme Metabolism_

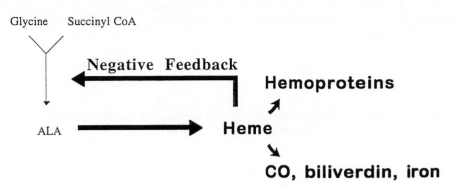

Figure 13–2
Regulation of hepatic heme metabolism and defects in manifest acute porphyria.

Normal heme biosynthesis results in feedback repression of ALA synthesis.

B. _Hepatic Heme Metabolism in Manifest Acute Porphyria_

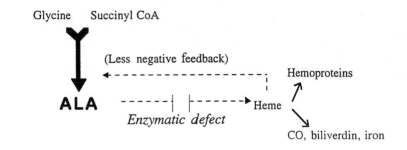

Enzymatic defect results in ↓ heme biosynthesis and, therefore, in derepression (induction) of ALA synthesis.

termittent porphyria, hereditary coproporphyria, and variegate porphyria (see Table 13–1 and Fig. 13–1). PCT involves hepatic accumulation of porphyrins and may be associated with liver disease, but it is not associated with acute crises. A syndrome resembling acute hepatic porphyria may be induced by lead toxicity. As discussed elsewhere in this chapter, hereditary tyrosinemia type 1, which is associated with overproduction of succinylacetone, a potent inhibitor of ALA dehydrase, may also be associated with porphyric crises. Acute attacks are generally more common in women, usually after the onset of puberty, and are associated with the luteal phase of menstruation, such that some women suffer attacks monthly.

Acute Hepatic Porphyrias

Severe Deficiency of ALA Dehydrase

Deficiency of ALA dehydrase results in decreased conversion of ALA to porphobilinogen and, therefore, in greatly increased ALA formation without increased porphobilinogen (PBG) formation. For unclear reasons, increased excretion of coproporphyrin may also occur. Recurrent, severe neurologic attacks may occur, marked by abdominal pain and even respiratory and bulbar paralysis. Some paresis may be permanent. In order for clinical manifestations to occur, a profound deficiency of ALA dehydrase must be present, because normally the activity of this enzyme in the liver is

present in great excess, compared with ALA synthase or PBG deaminase. Fortunately, profound deficiency of ALA dehydrase is rare. It may be hereditary (homozygous or compound heterozygous deficiency) or acquired (due to inhibitors such as succinylacetone or lead).

Acute Intermittent Porphyria

The most common form of acute porphyria in the United States, acute intermittent porphyria (AIP) is an autosomal dominant disorder of variable penetrance, which is characterized by a deficiency of PBG deaminase. The gene (located on chromosome 11q24.1-2) has been cloned and sequenced. Two closely similar forms of mRNA have been identified. The housekeeping form is larger than the erythroid form. The two forms differ in that exon 2 is skipped in the former, whereas exon 3 is skipped in the latter. The housekeeping form is slightly larger than the erythroid form. Numerous genetic defects, including point mutations, splice defects, and exon deletions have been identified, all of them leading to the AIP phenotype. To date, no clear phenotypic manifestations have been related to specific genotypic abnormalities.

The defective gene is carried by 5 to 10 per 100,000 individuals. Most commonly, women present in the third decade of life, men in the fourth, and attacks are precipitated by medications. ALA and PBG accumulate in association with colicky abdominal pain that may last days and is fre-

Table 13–1   The Porphyrias with Major Hepatic Manifestations—Classification and Features

Disease	Enzyme Defect	Autosomal Inheritance	Clinical Features	Metabolite Profile with Overt Disease		
				Urine	*Stool*	*Blood*
ACUTE HEPATIC PORPHYRIAS						
ALA dehydrase deficiency (severe)	ALA dehydrase	Recessive	Neurovisceral	**ALA** **PBG** (URO) **COPRO**	Normal	**PROTO**
Acute intermittent porphyria	Porphobilinogen deaminase	Dominant	Neurovisceral	**ALA** **PBG** (URO) (COPRO)	(URO) (COPRO) **PROTO**	(URO) (COPRO) (PROTO)
Hereditary coproporphyria	Coproporphyrino-gen oxidase	Dominant	Neurovisceral cutaneous	**ALA** **PBG** (URO) **COPRO**	(URO) **COPRO**	(COPRO)
Variegate porphyria	Protoporphyrino-gen oxidase	Dominant	Neurovisceral cutaneous	**ALA** **PBG** (URO) **COPRO**	(URO) **COPRO** **PROTO**	(PROTO)
OTHER HEPATIC PORPHYRIAS						
Porphyria cutanea tarda	Uroporphyrinogen decarboxylase	Dominant or sporadic	Cutaneous	(ALA) **URO** (COPRO)	**URO** **COPRO**	(URO)
Protoporphyria	Ferrochelatase	Dominant or recessive	Cutaneous	(URO) (COPRO)	(COPRO) **PROTO**	(COPRO) **PROTO**

ALA, δ-aminolevulinic acid; URO, uroporphyrin; COPRO, coproporphyrin; PROTO, protoporphyrin; PBG, porphobilinogen. Bold type indicates an elevated level; parentheses indicate that the level may be normal or slightly elevated. When a metabolite is not listed, its level is typically not elevated.

quently accompanied by constipation, nausea, and vomiting. Pain and paresthesias over the trunk and extremities are common symptoms. Despite these sensations, examination more typically reveals a motor neuropathy. An array of other neurologic abnormalities may be found on examination, including tachycardia and hypertension, bulbar findings, and areflexia. Psychological effects may be manifested subtly as depression or anxiety or may rage as frank psychosis and delirium. Hyponatremia may represent hypothalamic disease, which, along with the neurologic crisis, may result in seizures or coma. Death may follow infection associated with recurrent aspiration or pulmonary paralysis.

Hereditary Coproporphyria

Estimates of the incidence and prevalence of hereditary coproporphyria (HCP) are made difficult by its more benign course and less severe presentation than AIP. Deficiency of coproporphyrinogen oxidase results in elevated coproporphyrin III, excreted in stool and less so in urine. The gene for HCP has been cloned and sequenced, localized to chromosome 9, and numerous mutations have been described. Acute attacks, similar to those in AIP, may present as a vesiculobullous dermatitis covering the face, hands, or other exposed skin. Coproporphyrin III is excreted in bile, and any cholestatic process will increase blood levels and promote active disease.

Variegate Porphyria

Also called South African porphyria because of its high incidence there, variegate porphyria (VP) is caused by deficiency of protoporphyrinogen oxidase. The gene for protoporphyrinogen oxidase has been localized to chromosome 1q22. Approximately 3 in 1000 South Africans of Dutch ancestry are affected by a single point mutation traced to a common founder who emigrated from the Netherlands to Cape Town in 1688. VP is usually dominantly inherited. Symptoms and signs are variable, as its name suggests, and patients may suffer attacks similar to AIP, photosensitivity similar to HCP, or may be entirely asymptomatic. Liver tissue fluoresces under ultraviolet light but shows no other characteristic changes. Recent data from South Africa suggest an association between VP and hepatocellular carcinoma.

Chronic Hepatic Porphyrias

Porphyria Cutanea Tarda

Because its principal enzymatic defect is in the liver, PCT is classified as a hepatic porphyria but not an acute porphyria because it lacks acute neurologic attacks. The enzymatic deficiency is of uroporphyrinogen decarboxylase. Three types of PCT have been identified. Type I is the most common, comprising about 75% of cases. It is caused by an apparently acquired or sporadic and potentially reversible deficiency of hepatic uroporphyrinogen decarboxylase activity. The causes of the deficiency are often unclear and probably multifactorial. Recognized associations include heavy exposure to alcohol, halo-aromatic chemicals such as polychlorinated biphenyls or tetra-chloro dibenzo-p-dioxin, exposure to estrogens, iron overload, and chronic hepatitis C.

Type II PCT is a form in which activity of uroporphyrinogen decarboxylase is decreased 50% in all tissues, including the liver. The cause of this deficiency is a hereditary defect. However, this degree of decrease per se is not sufficient to cause clinical or biochemical features of active PCT. This is not surprising because hepatic activity of uroporphyrinogen decarboxylase is much higher than that of PBG deaminase or ALA synthase. Thus, even a 50% decrease in uroporphyrinogen decarboxylase would not generally be sufficient to limit the rate of heme biosynthesis. Other factors, including those already listed for type I, are also important in the pathogenesis of clinical illness in type II PCT.

Type III PCT is a rare form in which an apparently inherited defect in uroporphyrinogen decarboxylase occurs, but only in the liver. Subjects with type III PCT thus have positive family histories, normal erythrocyte uroporphyrinogen decarboxylase, and decreased hepatic uroporphyrinogen decarboxylase. Because there is apparently only one gene for uroporphyrinogen decarboxylase in all tissues, it is far from clear how or why type III PCT occurs. The gene for uroporphyrinogen decarboxylase has been cloned and sequenced, localized to the short arm (q) of chromosome 1, and numerous mutations have been identified, all of which may give rise to a PCT phenotype. No clear phenotypic-genotypic associations have emerged to date.

PCT is the most common hepatic porphyria and has classically been associated with the Bantus of South Africa who used to drink an iron-laden "Kaffir" beer that had been brewed in iron pots. Indeed, iron overload is both a common finding and an important exacerbant of hepatic pathology, and there is an association between sporadic PCT and heterozygous hemochromatosis. Clinical findings include photosensitivity (Fig. 13–3A) similar to that in HCP or VP, and

hepatic disease is consistently present, often in association with alcohol ingestion, iron overload, or exogenous estrogens. Deposition of uroporphyrin may itself be toxic. Moderate aminotransferase elevations are typical, whereas cholestatic indices are usually normal or mildly elevated. Glucose intolerance is common, although frank diabetes is unusual.

Liver biopsy demonstrates moderate siderosis and may show steatosis, fibrosis, and necrosis. The tissue fluoresces brightly under ultraviolet light (Fig. 13–4). An association has been elucidated between patients with sporadic (versus familial) PCT and hepatitis C virus (HCV) infection, such that 60% to 90% of PCT patients test positive for HCV antibody or RNA. There is an association between both persistent serum aminotransferase elevation and the severity of liver disease in PCT and the presence of HCV infection. It remains unclear whether HCV is a precipitant of PCT. Iron overload seems to potentiate liver disease in patients with either HCV or PCT, and hepatic iron overload in patients with PCT may predispose those with concurrent HCV infection to more severe hepatocellular disease. The main reason for increased hepatic iron in PCT is the C282Y mutation of the *HFE* gene (see Chapter 11). In some studies, the H63D mutation has also occurred with increased frequency in PCT patients compared with controls.

Erythropoietic Porphyrias

Our discussion is limited to protoporphyria; congenital erythropoietic porphyria, erythropoietic coproporphyria, and hepatoerythropoietic porphyria are quite rare.

Protoporphyria (Erythropoietic Protoporphyria)

Protoporphyria (PP) is caused by a hereditary deficiency in the activity of ferrochelatase (see Figs. 13–1 and 13–2 and Table 13–1). Although this deficiency is present in all tissues, the major overproduction of PP occurs chiefly within developing erythrocytes. The gene for ferrochelatase has

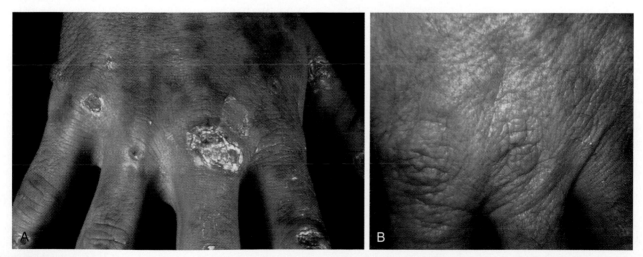

Figure 13–3
The porphyrias: cutaneous findings. *A,* Severe ulceration of the hands in a patient with porphyria cutanea tarda (PCT). The cutaneous changes of PCT are not typically at such an advanced stage. *B,* The hand of a patient with protoporphyria, showing subtle but characteristic thickening of the skin over the knuckles, so-called "peau d'orange" (orange skin–like change).

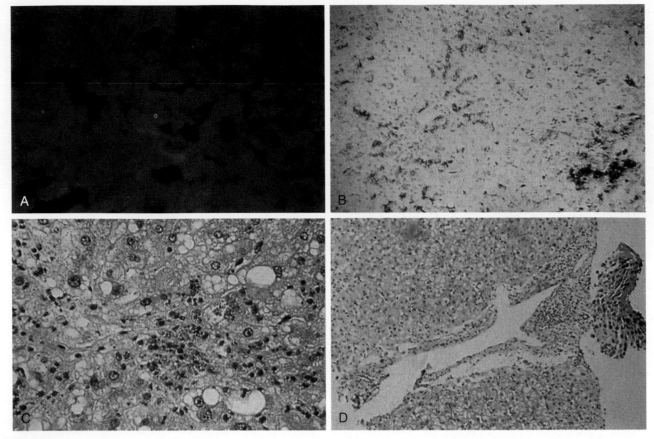

Figure 13–4
Porphyria cutanea tarda (PCT): liver histopathology. *A,* Unstained liver biopsy from a patient with PCT, viewed under fluorescence microscopy. *B,* Photomicrograph of a liver biopsy from a patient with PCT showing siderosis, an early finding (H & E, ×250). *C,* Photomicrograph of a liver biopsy from a patient with PCT showing fatty infiltration of the liver. *D,* Low-power photomicrograph showing fibrosis and the development of hepatoma in a liver biopsy from a patient with PCT (H & E, ×100; *A–D* provided courtesy of J Bloomer, MD).

been cloned and sequenced, localized to chromosome 18q22, and numerous mutations have been described, all of which give rise to a PP phenotype. Some of these appear to be more severe than others, with greater risks for development of liver damage, which is the most serious potential complication of the disease.

The inheritance of PP is complicated and variable among affected kindreds. It is autosomal dominant in some, autosomal recessive in others; and it has been attributed in some to a genetic defect in the ferrochelatase gene coupled to a second genetic defect at another locus. Even in those with apparently autosomal dominant inheritance, the activity of ferrochelatase, measured in liver, fibroblasts, or lymphocytes, is much less than the 50% of normal that would be predicted for a defect in one of two alleles. This suggests that the active enzyme is a dimer and that only dimers of two normal subunits retain activity. Evidence for this model has come from studies involving ultraviolet inactivation of ferrochelatase.

Within a single kindred, some members with reduced ferrochelatase activity have few clinical or biochemical manifestations, whereas others have marked manifestations, suggesting that factors other than reduced ferrochelatase activity are important in the pathogenesis of disease. Indeed,

this is a feature typical of all the common forms of porphyria.

PP was not clearly characterized until the 1960s despite its relative frequency. Although likely the second most common porphyria after PCT, PP may be missed because an excess of protoporphyrin, the biochemical hallmark, is detectable only in blood or stool, not urine. Therefore, testing, if limited to the urine, will miss the diagnosis.

Skin photosensitivity is acutely manifested by stinging, burning, or itching of exposed skin, followed within several hours by erythema, edema, and, chronically, by scarring hypertrophic changes (see Fig. 13–3B). The chronic changes in PP are usually less severe than in PCT, HCP, or VP. Marrow accumulation of protoporphyrin results in characteristic stem cell fluorescence. Marrow toxicity is commonly associated with mild anemia and rarely with frank hemolysis. Pigmented gallstones, laden with protoporphyrin, are frequently found even in young patients. Deposition of protoporphyrin crystals is found in hepatocytes and Kupffer cells, resulting in liver fluorescence and, under polarized light, in a characteristic birefringence (Fig. 13–5). Hepatic pigment deposition also causes the disease's most severe effects. Nonfatal hepatic fibrosis, cirrhosis, or unremitting cholestasis and liver failure are uncommon but severe sequelae.

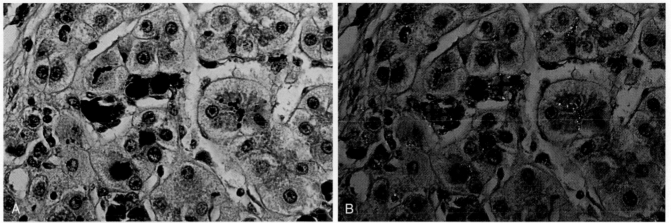

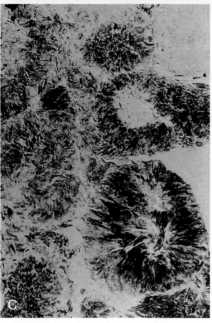

Figure 13–5
Protoporphyria: liver histopathology. *A,* Photomicrograph of a liver from a patient with protoporphyria, showing brown deposits of protoporphyrin IX within Kupffer cells, canaliculi, and hepatocytes (H & E, ×400, regular light). *B,* The same tissue as *A,* visualized under polarized light, showing characteristic birefringence of protoporphyrin IX (H & E, ×400, polarized light; *A* and *B* courtesy of G Klatskin, MD). *C,* Electron microscopy of protoporphyrin IX crystals within the liver of a patient with protoporphyria. (Courtesy of J Bloomer, MD.)

Diagnosis

The porphyrias are difficult, if not impossible, to diagnose on the basis of clinical findings alone because of their protean manifestations, as outlined earlier. Still, while porphyria is often diagnosed only after an extensive clinical evaluation, most patients referred to centers specializing in the evaluation and care of patients with porphyria do not have the disease. It is important to think of the diagnosis of porphyria in patients with consistent clinical features. However, it is especially important not to jump to an unwarranted diagnostic conclusion unless biochemical findings are fully supportive. In this regard, the most important confounding entities are the secondary porphyrinurias.

Screening tests for porphyria rely on rapid detection of excess PBG or porphyrins in urine, blood, or stool. The Hoesch and Watson-Schwartz tests detect urinary porphobilinogen, which reacts with Ehrlich's reagent to form a visible red pigment. The Hoesch test is easy to perform and interpret at the bedside. One or two drops of urine are added to 2 to 3 mL of Ehrlich's reagent (2 g p-dimethylaminobenzaldehyde [DMAB] in 100 mL 6M HCl). The immediate development of a cherry red color on top of the solution is a positive test. Both the Hoesch and Watson-Schwartz tests may be confounded by pH indicators that are red in acid, by indoles, and by methyldopa metabolites, each of which may lead to false-positive results. Then, too, conditions in which ALA dehydrase is greatly reduced will not produce an increase in urinary porphobilinogen. Quantitative measurements should, therefore, follow all positive qualitative test results.

The urine talc test and amyl alcohol test are qualitative tests for increased urinary porphyrins in which a Wood lamp is used to visualize a porphyrin-laden pink or red fluorescent phase. Quenchers of porphyrin fluorescence or dilute urine may cause a false-negative test result, and some nonporphyrin compounds may fluoresce. Positive test results are, therefore, confirmed by HPLC or similar quantification tests of uroporphyrins and coproporphyrins.

PP does not result in increased urine porphyrin excretion and, therefore, cannot be diagnosed by examination of the urine. Through an acid extraction technique, erythrocyte protoporphyrin can be identified under a Wood lamp. PP and the other erythropoietic porphyrias will test positive, as will conditions such as lead poisoning or iron deficiency, in which erythrocytic zinc protoporphyrin levels are increased. This is because acids remove zinc from the chelate, leaving free portoporphyrin. Direct fluorescence microscopy of erythrocytes can identify erythrocytes that contain increased porphyrin levels, though rapid fading, a problem particularly with protoporphyrin, may result in false-negative results. Stool porphyrins can be identified under a Wood lamp after extraction with amyl alcohol, glacial acetic acid, and ether. Bacterial heme metabolism may result in false-positive results as may gastrointestinal bleeding. All such positive screening test results for porphyrins should be confirmed by specific quantitative testing. Similarly, with patients in whom the index of suspicion is high, apparently negative screening tests should also be confirmed by such testing.

Treatment

Acute Porphyrias

The treatment of acute porphyria involves the careful avoidance of exogenous precipitants between attacks while giving supportive care and vigorously attempting to curb the production of heme precursors during acute crises. There are therapies beneficial to treatment of all the porphyrias, and others specific to a particular porphyria (Table 13–2).

Treatment of Acute Attacks

Initial management typically requires narcotic control of pain, which may be enhanced with the use of a phenothiazine, such as chlorpromazine. Tachycardia and hypertension may be controlled with β-blockade (propranolol), and the patient should be monitored carefully for possible progression of neuromuscular dysfunction, particularly the onset of respiratory paralysis.

By modifying enzyme activity, the production of heme precursors can be minimized. Through suppression of ALA synthase activity, administration of glucose intravenously may help to diminish symptoms. This "glucose effect" takes advantage of observations in rodents and humans that fast-ing increases ALA synthase activity and that, to the contrary, carbohydrate administration reduces activity. A goal of 300 g/day or more of glucose or carbohydrate therapy is recommended in the acutely ill patient. Because of nausea or vomiting, this may need to be given parenterally.

If, despite the aforementioned measures, the patient's status worsens, or if improvement does not ensue within the first 36 hours, heme infusion is indicated. Indeed, if promptly available, there is no reason not to give heme immediately to any patient with acute porphyria who is sufficiently ill to require hospital admission. Treatment of porphyria with exogenous heme infusion first began more than 25 years ago. By increasing the regulatory pool of heme and consequently promoting feedback repression of ALA synthase, administration of exogenous heme (as hematin) reduces ALA synthase activity. Whereas the biochemical effect on ALA and PBG synthesis suppression is fleeting, the clinical benefits are usually more lasting. The usual dose is 3 to 4 mg/kg/day for 3 to 5 days. Potential side effects include thrombophlebitis, coagulopathy, and reversible renal tubular damage. The presently available hematin preparations must be given within 1 hour to preclude degradation if prepared in sterile water, as the manufacturer suggests. However, when prepared as a 1:1 molar complex with human serum albumin, hematin is stable for at least 24 hours and has fewer side effects as well.

Women susceptible to luteal phase disease recurrence may benefit from a luteinizing hormone–releasing hormone (LHRH) analogue, which is typically continued for over a year. Side effects include an initial worsening of symptoms and osteopenia, for which the patient should prophylactically receive calcium supplements and, if warranted, bisphosphonates. Oral contraceptives have been used in place of LHRH analogues but have the potential disadvantage of promoting ALA synthase activity and consequently precipitating attacks.

Prevention of Attacks

Factors known to be capable of precipitating or exacerbating acute attacks of disease should be avoided. The most

Table 13–2 The Porphyrias: Therapy for Acute Attacks and Chronic Disease

Acute Attacks	• Control pain with narcotics as warranted; consider phenothiazine. • Control hypertension and tachycardia with β-blockade. • Monitor for neuromuscular/respiratory dysfunction. • Remove exacerbating drugs or chemicals. • Glucose/carbohydrate therapy, at least 300 g/day glucose. • Heme therapy as intravenous hematin, 3–4 mg/kg for 3–5 days. • LHRH analogue for women with luteal phase recurrence.		
Chronic or Recurrent Disease	**General Interventions** • Avoid alcohol, exacerbating drugs, or chemicals. • Wear sunscreen, opaque clothing. • Treat skin infection promptly.	**Porphyria Cutanea Tarda** • Diminish iron stores with phlebotomy. • Use chloroquine, hydroxychloroquine, or alkalization of urine to increase urinary porphyrin excretion. • Treat hepatitis C, if present.	**Protoporphyria** • Oral β-carotene • Erythrocyte transfusion, iron therapy • Cholestyramine, activated charcoal • Liver transplantation

LHRH, Leuteinizing hormone–releasing hormone.

important of these are alcohol (anything more than two drinks per day), other inducing drugs or chemicals (any agent capable of inducing hepatic cytochrome[s] P-450), intercurrent infections, starvation, severe dieting, or any dieting regimen that does not provide adequate daily intake of carbohydrate and protein.

All first-degree relatives of known patients should be evaluated carefully, with specific molecular testing (if the genomic abnormality has been identified in the index case of the family), with measurement of enzymatic activities in appropriate tissues (if such a defect has been characterized in the index case), or with quantitative measurement of urinary, fecal, and plasma porphyrins (and, for urine, of the porphyrin precursors ALA and PBG). Such evaluations are best performed in a specified center, because reliable assays and kindred analysis are not widely available. These studies are best done in prepubertal children, because acute attacks are rare before puberty, attesting to the role played by sex hormones in the pathogenesis of disease.

Reliable, validated assays of enzymatic activities deficient in the acute porphyrias are available only for ALA dehydrase and PBG deaminase, both of which are cytoplasmic and, therefore, present even in adult erythrocytes. In contrast, coproporphyrinogen and protoporphyrinogen oxidase are located in mitochondria and, therefore, are not present in mature erythrocytes. Reliable assays for the latter thus require the use of cells containing mitochondria (e.g., leukocytes or cultured skin fibroblasts).

All members of affected kindreds found to harbor the relevant enzymatic deficiency should be counselled to avoid the potential triggers of acute attacks (vide supra).

Porphyria Cutanea Tarda and Protoporphyria

Overt symptomatic PCT should be treated by removal of potential offending drugs and chemicals (e.g., estrogens, iron, alcohol). Although not clearly shown to exacerbate human PCT, P-450-inducing drugs such as barbiturates or hydantoins clearly exacerbate the uroporphyria that occurs in experimental models of PCT and are also best avoided.

The cornerstone of therapy of PCT continues to be the removal of iron from the liver, accomplished most rapidly and economically by therapeutic venesection, usually 1 unit of blood per week, continued until a mild degree of anemia and iron deficiency have been achieved. Typically, patients with PCT have a mild-to-moderate degree of iron overload; some are heterozygous for hereditary HLA-linked hemochromatosis; and a few are homozygous for this disease. Removal of 8 to 16 units of blood (2 to 4 g iron) are generally needed. However, iron depletion induces remission of PCT even when iron stores are normal. Patients with anemia and PCT can often be venesected if erythropoietin is given. This is particularly useful in the growing numbers of subjects with PCT complicating chronic renal failure and dialysis.

An antimalarial agent (chloroquine, hydroxyquine) may be added if the patient is severely affected. By forming water-soluble complexes with uroporphyrins, chloroquine and hydroxychloroquine increase urinary porphyrin excretion. Treatment with these agents should be instituted slowly (125 mg bid), and the patient should be monitored for retinopathy. Alkalization of the urine also promotes urinary excretion of porphyrins.

The association between HCV and PCT described earlier suggests potential new interventions, and resolution of PCT after antiviral therapy of chronic hepatitis C has been reported in a few subjects. Iron reduction for HCV-infected PCT patients with liver pathology may prove to be particularly important because iron reduction in hepatitis C patients without PCT has shown potential benefit in initial studies.

Active skin disease in PCT should be treated by avoidance of light exposure (opaque clothing and sunscreens) and trauma (because the skin is abnormally fragile). Typical sun-block products (e.g., PABA) are ineffective, because they do not block light of 400 to 415 nm, which is the type of light that excites cutaneous porphyrins and, with oxygen, gives rise to the cutaneous manifestations of all the cutaneous porphyrias.

The management of PP chiefly involves efforts to: (1) minimize PP overproduction, (2) ameliorate cutaneous symptoms and protect the skin from damage, (3) remove symptomatic PP-rich gallstones, and (4) avoid hepatic injury caused by excess accumulation of PP. Because iron deficiency exacerbates PP overproduction, it is important to be sure that such deficiency is not present. Most patients with PP are mildly anemic, due to the inborn error in heme synthesis. Thus, serum ferritin and transferrin saturation must be used to assess iron status. Hypertransfusion also reduces PP overproduction, but its use is limited to the minority of patients with PP with unusually severe disease.

Amelioration of the cutaneous manifestations involves the avoidance of sunlight, the use of wide-brimmed hats and clothing opaque to light, the use of opaque, barrier sunscreens, and administration of β-carotene. The latter must be used in large doses (120 to 180 mg/day), which impart a yellowish tinge to patients' complexions. Most patients feel that they do benefit from high doses of β-carotene; some take it only in the summer. Sunscreen products that use PABA as the active ingredient are ineffective in the porphyrias, because they do not block light of 400 to 415 nm. Secondary infection of skin should be treated promptly to avoid further complications.

Protoporphyrin-laden gallstones occur frequently in patients with PP, often at young ages. Stones causing symptoms should be removed by cholecystectomy.

The serious potential complication of PP is the development of pigmentary cirrhosis and liver failure. Anything that can cause or exacerbate cholestasis may potentiate and accelerate these processes. Therefore, all patients with PP who are not already immune should be vaccinated against hepatitis A and B, should be strongly counseled not to drink alcohol to excess (>2 drinks/day) and not to use drugs that have a high propensity to cause cholestasis (e.g., 17-alkylated androgens, phenothiazines). Although it was hoped that high doses of oral charcoal or cholestyramine would enhance fecal excretion of PP and reduce its enterohepatic circulation, there is scant evidence for the benefit of such therapy, and its chronic use is difficult for most patients. Similarly, administration of bile salts (cheno- or ursodeoxycholic acid) has not led to convincing evidence of increased fecal excretion of PP or clinical benefit.

Patients with PP and cirrhosis should be considered for liver transplantation. They may unpredictably develop rapidly accelerating cholestasis and liver failure. Intravenous infusions of heme have led to the stabilization of a few such patients. Any confounding causes of cholestasis should be corrected. Transplantation of such patients poses formidable challenges due to their severe light sensitivity: operating lights should have filters that screen out light of 380 to 420 nm; some patients have developed severe neuropathy in the postoperative period. Because transplantation does not correct the erythropoietic enzyme defect, these patients require continued surveillance for recurrent liver disease. In theory, bone marrow transplantation should be curative, but has only rarely been performed in PP.

Prevention of PCT and PP involves avoidance of potential triggering factors and careful evaluation of relatives of index cases. Subjects at risk for development of PCT may be detected by assay of erythrocytic Uro-D, although, as already described, only about 25% of patients have a familial form in which activity of this enzyme is reduced. All first-degree relatives should be screened with at least a random urine measurement of porphyria concentration.

Prevention of overt PP involves kindred evaluation with measurement of erythrocytic and fecal PP concentrations. If they are elevated, such subjects should be checked for iron deficiency (which is to be avoided), should be counseled to avoid exposure to hepatotoxins (e.g., alcohol), and should be vaccinated to prevent viral hepatitis (A&B). This is because any intercurrent cholestatic liver disease may precipitate severe hepatic decompensation due to toxic effects of retrained PP.

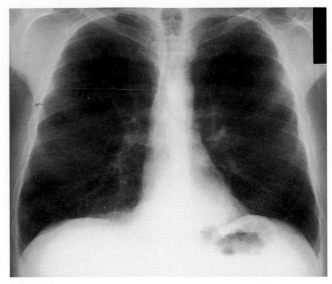

Figure 13–6
α_1-Antitrypsin deficiency: chest roentgenogram. Chest x-ray of a 39-year-old man with α_1-antitrypsin deficiency showing advanced chronic obstructive pulmonary disease, with hyperinflated lungs and flattened diaphragms. This 41-year-old man developed clinical emphysema and cirrhosis in his 30s.

α_1-ANTITRYPSIN DEFICIENCY

α_1-Antitrypsin (α_1-AT) deficiency is a relatively common autosomal disease of Caucasians that may cause pulmonary disease and less frequently, hepatic disease. By altering its tertiary structure, a single amino acid substitution causes disruption of normal cellular α_1-AT transport in hepatocytes, and the ensuing accumulation of the defective protein results in potentially severe liver disease and liver failure. The diagnosis is made by serum α_1-AT quantification, protease inhibitor typing, and histologic analysis. Orthotopic liver transplantation is the definitive therapy for progressive disease but fortunately is required for only a few affected patients. It is important to consider α_1-AT deficiency in the differential diagnosis of any patient with chronic hepatitis, cirrhosis, or hepatocellular carcinoma of unclear etiology.

Epidemiology and Pathophysiology

The deficiency of α_1-AT is most commonly associated with pulmonary disease but is also an important cause of hepatic disease, particularly in children and young adults. α_1-AT is a protease inhibitor that opposes the activity of trypsin and other proteases, most notably neutrophil elastase. α_1-AT is normally synthesized in the liver and its deficiency results in low serum levels. In the lung, low serum α_1-AT prevents the normal repression of tissue elastase, resulting in diminished elastic recoil and abnormally high lung compliance as elastase is destroyed. Ultimately, the patient suffers progressive obstructive pulmonary disease (emphysema) as the critical elastic component of lung recoil is diminished (Fig. 13–6). Whereas the likelihood of developing pulmonary disease is predictable from a patient's genotype, liver disease is less reliably predicted. Indeed, for unclear reasons, it is rare for

patients to have both pulmonary and hepatic manifestations of disease.

A better understanding of the epidemiology of α_1-AT deficiency can be gained by further examining the genetic basis for the disease. The α_1-AT gene is on chromosome 14 and may be represented by several different alleles. These alleles have been identified by studying electrophoretograms of serum α_1-AT, with comparison of relative rates of migration of the peptides. Each allele confers a different probability of developing clinical pulmonary or hepatic disease. Of more than 70 alleles, M (for "main") is the most common normal allele, and S and Z are the most common mutant alleles. Homozygosity for the S ("slow") allele (P_iSS [protease inhibitor SS]) results in approximately half the normal serum level of α_1-AT, with no associated disease. The most common Z ("slowest") mutant is caused by a point mutation resulting in a single base substitution (glutamine to lysine at amino acid 342), which produces profound deficiency of serum α_1-AT and pulmonary and hepatic disease in the homozygous patient, P_iZZ (protease inhibitor ZZ). The P_iSZ genotype carries little risk of clinical disease.

Approximately 1 in 40 adult Caucasians (of North American or Northern European origin) carry the Z allele for α_1-AT, such that approximately 1 in 1600 live white births are P_iZZ genotype. However, only 10% to 20% of patients homozygous for the Z allele will develop hepatic disease. This discrepancy may well be related to the underlying mechanism of disease. The serum deficiency of α_1-AT is likely not responsible for associated liver disease. Murine transgenic studies have shown that the *accumulation* of abnormal α_1-AT in hepatocytes, not the *absence* of protease repression, leads to hepatic disease. The mutant amino acid sequence results in abnormal protein folding and thus ad-

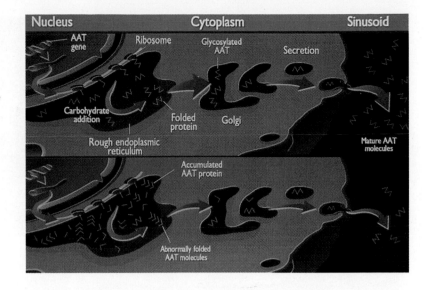

Figure 13–7
α_1-Antitrypsin deficiency: accumulation of defective protein. Schematic showing, *above,* normal α_1-antitrypsin gene and protein synthesis with prompt glycosylation and unhindered secretion of normal protein. *Below,* patient with P_iZZ genotype and synthesis of abnormal protein; transport from the rough endoplasmic reticulum is hindered, resulting in accumulation of the defective protein and hepatotoxicity.

versely affects post-translational processing of α_1-AT. The P_iZZ genotype appears to cause the reactive center of one α_1-AT molecule to bind the β-pleated sheet of another, resulting in polymerization of α_1-AT molecules. The transport of α_1-AT from its site of synthesis, the hepatocellular rough endoplasmic reticulum, through the Golgi apparatus and into the circulating blood is severely impaired (Fig. 13–7). Polymerized α_1-AT accumulates in the cells and mediates damage through as yet unclear means.

Studies of transduced human skin fibroblasts have demonstrated a marked delay in degradation of the abnormal protein in cells from P_iZZ patients with liver disease, compared with the protein from cells of patients without liver disease. This suggests that both a defect in export of abnormal protein and also a delay in its degradation are required for the development of hepatic disease. Similar transgenic studies may provide prognostic information for patients with P_iZZ genotype in the future.

Clinical Features

Hepatic disease occurs in 10% to 20% of individuals homozygous for the Z allele (P_iZZ) and is commonly first manifested in infancy. In the first few months of life, jaundice and hepatomegaly may accompany direct hyperbilirubinemia and mild serum aminotransferase elevations. More rarely, splenomegaly and ascites are present and synthetic function may be impaired.

This cholestatic picture is typically not fatal and may mark the individual's only liver disease until early adulthood. Indeed, a decade after initial presentation, a deficient individual may show no signs of clinical or biochemical disease. However, a subpopulation of individuals with clinical disease in infancy will present in late childhood or early adulthood with ascites, hepatosplenomegaly, variceal hemorrhage, or other signs of portal hypertension. Risk factors for progression to cirrhosis have not been clearly defined.

Upon inquiry, patients presenting with hepatic disease as children or young adults frequently report a history of neonatal jaundice. Adult patients, in particular, may present with chronic hepatitis or with signs of portal hypertension.

Whereas a quarter of cirrhotic individuals die during childhood, the decline of hepatic function is more typically slow, such that cirrhotic children or adults may survive many years before significant hepatic failure ensues.

There is a strong correlation between liver disease associated with α_1-AT deficiency and primary hepatocellular carcinoma, and α_1-AT deficiency should be considered as a possible predisposing factor for any patient with hepatocellular carcinoma.

Diagnosis

A serum quantitative α_1-AT level should be measured in jaundiced neonates or in any patient with chronic hepatitis, cirrhosis, or other liver disease of unclear etiology. Because it is an acute phase reactant, falsely high ("normal") α_1-AT levels may accompany inflammatory states. After the first few months of life, deficient individuals will have liver histology marked by periportal hepatocytes with diastase-resistant, PAS-positive intracellular globules (Fig. 13–8). These globules are not specific to α_1-AT deficiency, but in this disease they represent an intracellular accumulation of α_1-AT, as evidenced by specific immunoperoxidase staining. They may also be found in Kupffer cells. Inflammation, periportal fibrosis, or cirrhosis may be present. Accretion of α_1-AT within the rough endoplasmic reticulum is evident on electron microscopy. α_1-Antitrypsin deficiency and extrahepatic biliary atresia have similar clinical presentations in neonates, but liver biopsy in α_1-AT deficiency reveals a marked paucity of intrahepatic bile ducts.

Subjects with low serum α_1-AT levels should undergo phenotyping by isoelectric focusing or agarose gel electrophoresis. Although both P_iZZ and P_iSZ patients are predisposed to hepatic disease, specific genotyping may be important for genetic counseling. Quantitative serum α_1-AT may be helpful in determining heterozygosity in such patients, although parental phenotyping may be necessary. Prenatal diagnosis and phenotyping are possible by amniotic fluid analysis. In the future, diagnostic studies involving DNA will likely provide diagnostic and genotypic information.

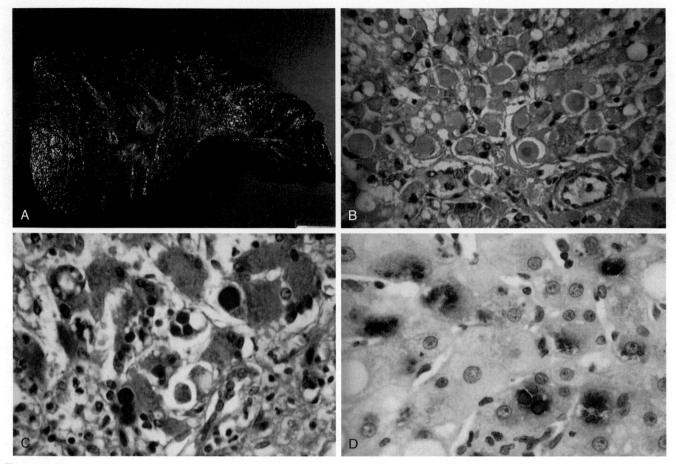

Figure 13–8

α_1-Antitrypsin deficiency: liver pathology. *A,* Cut surface of a liver from a patient who was transplanted for cirrhosis due to α_1-antitrypsin deficiency. The entire surface consists of relatively small, closely packed regenerative nodules encompassed by fibrous bands. This appearance is typical of cirrhosis and is nonspecific with regard to etiology. *B,* Photomicrograph of a liver biopsy showing prominent eosinophilic dense globules in the cytoplasm of many hepatocytes (H & E, ×250). *C,* Photomicrograph showing that the cytoplasmic globules are PAS-positive and diastase-resistant (PAS-diastase, ×250). *D,* Liver biopsy immunostained using α_1-antitrypsin as primary antibody. A positive reaction is indicated by the brown color (ABC immunostain technique ×400; courtesy of Barbara Banner, MD, University of Massachusetts Medical Center).

Treatment

Several established and experimental therapies exist for pulmonary disease, including cessation of tobacco use and avoidance of other potentially toxic inhalants, and infusion or inhalation of purified plasma α_1-AT. Surgical shunting has been used to maintain patients with moderate histologic liver disease complicated by severe portal hypertension. Orthotopic liver transplantation has remained the definitive intervention for patients with progressive liver failure and portal hypertension. Hepatic decline may proceed slowly, however, and patients may be maintained for years with conservative measures before surgical intervention is warranted. Survival of subjects with α_1-AT deficiency who have undergone orthotopic liver transplantation is similar to that of patients with other liver diseases, with 1- and 5-year survival rates of approximately 80% and 70%, respectively. The donor liver synthesizes normal protein and, therefore, the disease does not recur in the new liver, and serum levels of α_1-AT become normal.

Gene therapy does not at this time seem promising for the treatment of hepatic disease in α_1-AT deficiency. Such therapy aims for the re-expression of a normal α_1-AT protein but will not prevent the accumulation of mutant protein within hepatocytes. Moreover, expression of the normal gene may be associated with actual upregulation of the synthesis of mutant protein, possibly promoting and accelerating the development of liver disease. By stimulating expression of abnormal protein, gene therapy of *pulmonary* disease might also promote the development of hepatic disease, as may treatment of pulmonary disease with purified plasma α_1-AT. It appears that successful gene therapy of hepatic disease will mandate prevention of mutant protein expression while normal protein synthesis is vigorously promoted. Recent studies in a murine model of another metabolic liver disease, hereditary tyrosinemia type 1, have suggested a possible strategy for gene therapy providing adequate synthesis of normal protein and suppression of mutant protein. By conferring a genetic, selective advantage upon retrovirally corrected cells, in vivo propagation of corrected cells (producing normal protein) to the exclusion of

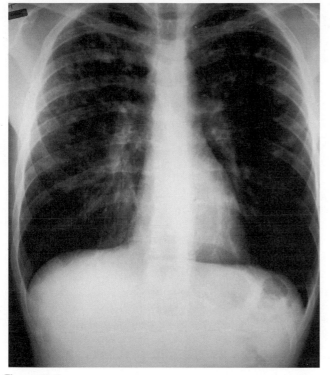

Figure 13–9
Cystic fibrosis: chest roentgenogram. Twenty-year-old man with cystic fibrosis showing early cystic changes as well as "train tracking," parallel lines representing thickened, dilated bronchi. Patchy densities are evident in the upper lung fields, consistent with bronchiectasis. (Courtesy of the Department of Radiology, University of Massachusetts Medical Center.)

mutant cells might be accomplished for α_1-AT deficiency. Such strategies are discussed further in this chapter in the section on hereditary tyrosinemia type 1.

CYSTIC FIBROSIS

Cystic fibrosis (CF) is a chronic disease of deficient chloride conductance manifested by tenacious, often obstructive epithelial secretions that result in clinical disease in several organ systems. Although pulmonary disease is frequently the most visible consequence of the disease (Fig. 13–9), CF is the most common cause of pancreatic insufficiency in young adults in the United States and is associated as well with hepatobiliary disease. As a result of improved management, more than half of patients with CF now live well into adulthood, and it is increasingly likely that the hepatic manifestations of this disease will be encountered.

Epidemiology and Pathophysiology

CF is inherited as an autosomal recessive trait, affecting more than 1 in 2000 white births, making it the most common autosomal recessive disease expressed clinically in white children. Much has been learned over the past decade about underlying defects in CF. The disease is associated with a defect of the CF transmembrane conductance regulator (CFTR), a cAMP-activated chloride channel that is predicted to be a protein of 1480 amino acids coded for by a gene located on chromosome 7q31. The CFTR has 12 membrane-spanning segments clustered into two regions, two nucleotide binding folds, and a regulatory region. Mutations causing clinical disease are chiefly found in the nucleotide binding folds, and more than 70% of North American and Northern European CFTR mutations involve a deletion of a single phenylalanine, at position 508 (ΔF508) of the first nucleotide binding fold (Fig. 13–10).

Within the liver, the CFTR is located along the apical membrane of biliary epithelial cells. Defective CFTR results in severely diminished chloride conductance, insufficient luminal fluid and, consequently, viscous, inspissated bile. Bile flow is reduced; secretion of protective mucin is decreased; and the concentrations of bile acids in bile are increased. Pancreatic insufficiency is associated with changes in bile acid absorption, and the intraluminal bile acid pool is shifted from hydrophilic, taurine-conjugated bile acids to hydrophobic, glycoconjugated bile acids, which are hepatotoxic. The result is ductal obstruction and oxidative ductal injury, leading to disease of the intra- and extrahepatic biliary system.

Clinical Features

Hepatobiliary complications of CF may present as disease of the liver, biliary tract, or gallbladder (Table 13–3).

Figure 13–10
Cystic fibrosis: the transmembrane conductance regulator (CFTR). Schematic showing *(left)* normal transmembrane transport of chloride, mediated by active transport, requiring binding of adenosine triphosphate (ATP) at the nucleotide binding region of the CFTR. Water molecules follow chloride conductance. Deletion *(right)* of a single phenylalanine at position 508 (ΔF508) of the nucleotide binding site of the CFTR results in inadequate ATP binding and diminished chloride conductance. As a result, little water follows and secretions are inspissated.

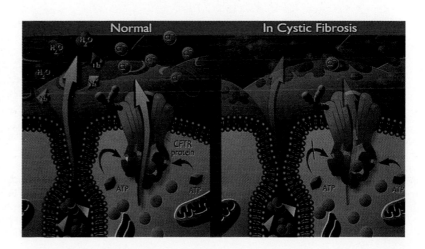

Table 13–3 Hepatobiliary Features of Cystic Fibrosis

Liver	Biliary Tract	Gallbladder
Only 10% symptomatic although > half affected	May present independently of hepatic disease	Most disease asymptomatic
Fatty Liver Common in infancy and adulthood, most common cause of hepatomegaly	*Common Duct Stricture* Caused by pancreatic fibrosis	*Microgallbladder* Gallbladder atrophied and collapsed
Biliary Fibrosis Hepatocytes spared; architecture preserved	*Choledocholithiasis*	*Cholecystic Dyskinesia* Gallbladder filled with thick bile
Multilobular Cirrhosis 2–5% of patients, may be accompanied by portal hypertension and splenomegaly	*Sclerosing Cholangitis* 1% of patients, ?chronic inflammation causative	*Cholelithiasis* 10–25% of patients, most asymptomatic, calcium bilirubinate
Neonatal Jaundice Not predictive of adult disease		
Comments: Liver chemistries neither sensitive nor specific Uneven distribution of disease → sampling error on liver biopsy	*Comments:* Alkaline phosphatase likely most sensitive test but must be fractionated; ultrasound may be helpful	*Comments:* Ultrasound helpful

Liver

More than half of patients with CF may have hepatic involvement, but only about 10% of patients with hepatic disease are symptomatic. Fatty liver is common, particularly in infancy. Chronic ductal obstruction is eventually accompanied by ductal proliferation, inflammatory infiltrate, and periportal fibrosis, known as biliary fibrosis (Fig. 13–11A). Hepatocytes are spared at this point, and the architecture of the liver is mostly preserved. Involved portal tracts may be unevenly distributed, such that liver biopsy is subject to

sampling error. With persistent insult, fibrosis progresses and multilobular biliary cirrhosis develops, initially leaving spared foci of structurally uninvolved hepatic tissue, but ultimately leading to a hard and nodular cirrhotic liver. Approximately 2% to 5% of patients, during their lifetimes, will develop cirrhosis as a complication of CF.

Although hepatic involvement in CF more typically presents in children with concurrent respiratory and pancreatic insufficiency, liver disease may be the first clinical feature, particularly in infants. More commonly, hepatomegaly is

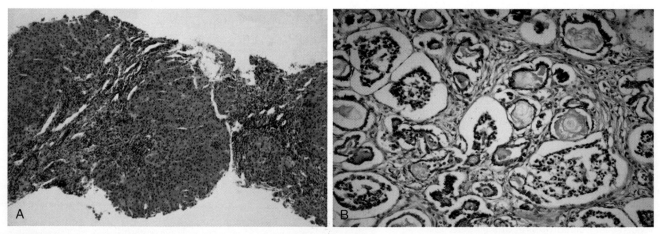

Figure 13–11
Cystic fibrosis: liver and pancreatic histopathology. *A,* Photomicrograph of a liver needle biopsy from a patient with cystic fibrosis showing portal triads greatly expanded as bands that extend across the biopsy and delineate nodules of residual parenchyma. These changes are typical of secondary biliary cirrhosis in cystic fibrosis (H & E, ×40). *B,* Photomicrograph of a pancreas from a child with cystic fibrosis. The pancreatic acini have been replaced by fibrosis. Dilated ducts are filled with inspissated eosinophilic secretions. The islets remain untouched but are closer together than normal because of the loss of parenchyma between them (H & E, ×100; courtesy Barbara Banner, MD, University of Massachusetts Medical Center).

noted in an otherwise asymptomatic adolescent or young adult. Fatty liver is the most common cause of hepatomegaly in CF, but hepatomegaly may also be falsely suggested if the liver is displaced inferiorly by pulmonary hyperinflation. Alternatively, hepatomegaly may be caused by passive congestion secondary to pulmonary hypertension in CF. A hard, nodular liver is suggestive of cirrhosis. Associated splenomegaly may be present and may cause left upper quadrant pain. Peripheral stigmata of portal hypertension are not frequently seen, and the first presenting sign of portal hypertension may be variceal hemorrhage. The risk of developing portal hypertension increases with age and, interestingly, shows familial clustering.

Biliary Tract and Gallbladder

Biliary tract involvement is common and may present independently of hepatic disease. In infants, CF may be manifested as jaundice as a result of obstructive liver disease, presenting similarly to biliary atresia. It is intriguing that neonatal jaundice does not seem to be predictive of future hepatic disease for patients with CF. As patients age, pancreatic fibrosis (see Fig. 13–11B) can result in common bile duct stricture. Approximately 10% to 25% of patients with CF have gallstones, most of which remain asymptomatic. Although they were thought in the past to be composed of cholesterol, the stones are believed now to consist chiefly of calcium bilirubinate. The gallbladder may be dyskinetic and filled with thick, mucoid bile or may be atrophied and collapsed, ("microgallbladder"). Almost a third of patients may have such a gallbladder. Finally, about 1% of patients with CF develop sclerosing cholangitis, possibly as a result of chronic inflammatory changes within the biliary system.

Diagnosis

The laboratory detection of early liver disease in CF may be difficult. More than 85% of patients with hepatomegaly will have abnormal liver chemistry test results, but the remainder may have entirely normal tests. Conversely, approximately 13% of patients with CF *without* histologic liver disease will have abnormal liver chemistries. Liver chemistry tests, therefore, are neither highly sensitive nor specific for underlying hepatic disease in CF. Alkaline phosphatase is probably the most sensitive chemistry for underlying cholestasis but must be fractionated because nonhepatic alkaline phosphatase may also be elevated in CF.

Underlying biliary disease may be revealed by diagnostic imaging. Ultrasound or oral cholecystography may demonstrate cholelithiasis, cholecystitis, or microgallbladder. ERCP can additionally reveal common duct stricture or sclerosing cholangitis. Hepatic scintigraphy may be helpful in detecting early liver involvement, even when ultrasound has been unrevealing. Liver biopsy serves as an important method for staging intrahepatic disease and for following progression, despite the recognized possibility of sampling error since intrahepatic disease is typically irregularly distributed, even when multilobular cirrhosis has developed. Sweat testing in the young adult or adolescent with unexplained cholestatic disease or portal hypertension may reveal CF and should always be performed in young patients with hepatobiliary disease of unclear origin.

Attempts to identify patients with CF at risk for developing liver disease have identified some predisposing factors. Foremost, hepatobiliary complications occur almost exclusively in patients with pancreatic insufficiency, although the degree of pancreatic insufficiency seems to have little significance. The prevalence of hepatobiliary disease is higher among males than females. Although a history of meconium ileus carries an increased risk, neonatal jaundice does not. Although some studies have suggested a possible association between hepatobiliary disease in CF and certain HLA types (e.g., DQ6), no characteristic genotype has been identified. Non-CF genes and exogenous factors may serve as important determinants in whether liver disease will develop and how severe it will be. The familial clustering of portal hypertension in CF-related liver disease suggests such factors may play a key role in its pathogenesis.

Treatment

Primary care is supportive. Avoidance and prompt, vigorous treatment of infection are continual challenges in patients with CF. Maintaining nutrition is of fundamental importance, with high-calorie, vitamin-enriched (particularly fat-soluble vitamins D, E, and K), elemental dietary supplementation as well as pancreatic enzyme administration. Vitamin A may be toxic to the liver in CF and should be supplemented with caution.

Ursodeoxycholic acid (UDCA) has emerged as an important therapy in patients with CF with hepatobiliary disease. UDCA is the major component of bear bile, found in much lower concentrations in human bile as a derivative of chenodeoxycholic acid. It is hydrophilic and may have a cytoprotective effect on biliary epithelium by displacing more toxic hydrophobic bile acids. In addition, micelles of UDCA are smaller and facilitate choleresis. Administration of UDCA in CF has been associated with improved liver chemistries, suggesting diminished cholestasis and reduced hepatotoxicity. Improvement in nutritional status is observed, perhaps by way of increasing fat absorption. UDCA has been associated with delayed progression of other cholestatic liver diseases such as primary biliary cirrhosis, and long-term prospective trials in patients with CF are underway. It is possible that, because of impaired bile acid absorption, higher doses of UDCA will be necessary to effect a clear change in the clinical course of CF-related liver disease. Patients receiving UDCA are given taurine supplementation, because therapy with UDCA exacerbates chronic CF-associated taurine deficiency. Taurine administration has also been associated with augmented fat absorption in patients with CF.

In patients who have developed advanced liver disease, management of portal hypertension becomes critical. Ultimately, orthotopic liver transplantation (OLT) may be considered. Liver transplantation in CF presents particular challenges because of the multiorgan, systemic nature of CF. In such patients, pulmonary disease and nutritional deficiency may affect outcome, and subsequent immunosuppressive therapy must be managed especially carefully so as to balance the risk of infection with that of graft rejection. One- and 5-year survival rates of patients with CF who have undergone OLT have been approximately 85% and 70%, respectively.

There are promising potential therapeutic advances under development. Because heterozygosity for defective CFTR function is not associated with clinical hepatobiliary disease, it has been postulated that fewer than half of functional CFTR receptors are needed for normal hepatobiliary phenotype and that homozygous disease might thus be amenable to gene therapy. Unlike gene therapy for other genetic diseases of the liver, gene therapy for CF must target not hepatocytes primarily, but the biliary epithelial cells, which divide infrequently. Recombinantly attenuated adenoviral vectors can infect nondividing cells and have been used successfully for gene transfer to biliary epithelial cells in animal models and are promising for future application in human CF therapy. Endoscopic retrograde biliary access might be used to distribute adenoviral or similar vectors of normal CFTR genes to biliary epithelial cells.

HEREDITARY TYROSINEMIA TYPE 1

The hereditary tyrosinemias represent a diverse group of clinical syndromes involving a spectrum of defects of tyrosine metabolism. Hereditary tyrosinemia type 1 is associated with severe liver disease. It is an autosomal recessive disorder of enzymatic deficiency resulting in hepatic and renal tubular toxicity and neurologic crises. There is a very high risk of developing hepatocellular carcinoma and, although the disease is rare worldwide, there are populations in which the gene is common and where complications of hereditary tyrosinemia account for almost one in three liver transplantations. Until recently, treatment has been limited to variably effective conservative measures such as dietary changes and liver transplantation. Now, directed enzyme repression may serve as an important modality of nonsurgical intervention and promising advances in gene therapy are being examined.

Epidemiology and Pathophysiology

Hereditary tyrosinemia type 1 presents early in life as either an acute disease of infants, which results in fatal liver failure within several months if left untreated, or as a chronic syndrome marked by progressive cirrhosis, renal tubular dysfunction, severe neurologic symptoms, and failure to thrive. The disease is geographically clustered and is notably prevalent in the Netherlands and French Canada. In one area of the province of Quebec more than 20% of individuals carry the defective gene.

This autosomal recessive mutation results in defective fumaryl acetoacetate hydrolase activity, promoting the accumulation of toxic metabolites in hepatocytes and renal tubular cells. The defective enzyme's substrate, fumarylacetoacetate, and the precursor maleylacetoacetate increase in plasma concentration as do tyrosine, methionine, and sometimes phenylalanine (Fig. 13–12). Succinylacetone (4,6-dioxoheptanoic acid) urinary concentrations are increased by the shunted metabolism of fumarylacetoacetate and maleylacetoacetate. Several different mutations of fumaryl acetoacetate hydrolase have been identified. Interestingly, members of the same family may have either the acute or chronic form, such that individuals with the same mutation may have different clinical disease. This variable phenotypic expression suggests that other factors—environmental influences or the influences of other genes—may affect the severity and course of the illness.

An accumulation of δ-aminolevulinic acid occurs as enzymatic shunting results in increased succinylacetone, which is a potent inhibitor of δ-aminolevulinic acid dehydrase. Increased δ-aminolevulinic acid is likely responsible for marked neuropathy resembling that seen with elevated δ-aminolevulinic acid in the hepatic porphyrias.

Clinical Features

Whereas the acute form of hereditary tyrosinemia type 1 results in hepatic failure over the first several months of life, the chronic form presents with more gradually progressive disease. Failure to thrive may be followed by more focal findings, such as hepatomegaly and, as cirrhosis develops, splenomegaly, ascites, jaundice, bruisability, and peripheral edema may ensue. Vitamin D-resistant, hypophosphatemic rickets may develop, and peripheral neuropathy may occur. The risk of hepatocellular carcinoma increases monthly such that, by 2 years of age, the risk of hepatocellular carcinoma is approximately 40%.

Diagnosis

Hereditary tyrosinemia may be anticipated from a family history or genetic screening, or the diagnosis may be made prenatally. Postgestationally, the diagnosis is typically made

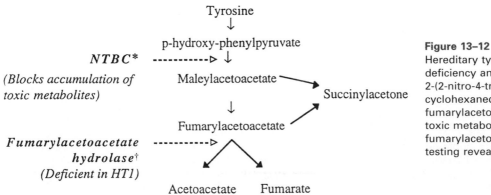

Figure 13–12
Hereditary tyrosinemia type 1—enzymatic deficiency and treatment with NTBC. (*NTBC = 2-(2-nitro-4-trifluoro-methylbenzoyl)-1,3-cyclohexanedione. †As a result of fumarylacetoacetate hydrolase deficiency, the toxic metabolites maleylacetoacetate and fumarylacetoacetate accumulate. Diagnostic testing reveals elevated succinylacetone.)

by the detection of biochemical abnormalities, including elevated urinary succinyl acetone and increased serum and urinary tyrosine, phenylalanine, and methionine. Decreased fumaryl acetoacetate hydrolase activity may also be detected in cultured skin fibroblasts. α-Fetoprotein elevation may reflect development of hepatocellular carcinoma, and more moderate elevations may also precede the development of neurological disease.

Treatment

Traditionally, hereditary tyrosinemia type 1 has been treated by eliminating dietary intake of tyrosine or related precursors so as to prevent the production of toxic metabolites. By this means, variable control of the disease is obtained, and some patients may not respond. Until recently, OLT has been the only means for more definitive treatment. Because of the progressive risk for hepatoma, transplantation in the first 2 years of life has been recommended to avoid progression to metastatic disease. The new liver has no defect in tyrosine metabolism, and hepatic manifestations thus do not recur. However, the renal defect in fumaryl acetoacetate hydrolase persists as does renal tubular dysfunction. Surprisingly, renal tubular defects persisting after hepatic transplantation do not appear to be clinically significant. Neurologic sequelae of hereditary tyrosinemia type 1 may resolve gradually but entirely after successful liver transplantation.

A novel and specific inhibitor of an early enzymatic step in tyrosine degradation has been used to decrease the rate and severity of liver damage. 2-(2-nitro-4-trifluoro-methylbenzoyl)-1,3-cyclohexanedione (NTBC) selectively inhibits 4-hydroxy-phenylpyruvate dioxygenase, preventing the development of toxic metabolites and reducing hepatotoxicity (see Fig. 13–12). It has improved and ultimately eliminated peripheral neuropathy, reduced the need for liver transplant, and may reduce significantly the risk of hepatocellular carcinoma.

Promising possibilities for new, effective modes of gene therapy are being investigated and may have important implications for the treatment of hereditary tyrosinemia and other diseases subject to hepatic gene therapy. It has been observed that the resected livers of patients with hereditary tyrosinemia type 1 are often a mosaic of cells, with cells expressing normal fumaryl acetoacetate hydrolase existing in regenerative nodules alongside mutant cells. It was postulated that this apparent spontaneous reversion to a normal allele might confer a selective advantage to these cells and promote their repopulation of the liver. The possibility of initiating and accelerating the repopulation of normal liver cells became a focus of attention.

In a study reported in 1996 that used a murine model of hereditary tyrosinemia type 1, transplantation of normal hepatocytes resulted in their seeding and repopulation of the liver, to the exclusion of mutant cells. Similarly, repeated portal vein infusion of retrovirus carrying the normal fumaryl acetoacetate hydrolase gene afforded complete repopulation of the liver with normally functioning, retrovirally transduced cells. In this model, it appears that normal differentiated hepatocytes preferentially multiply and replace cells carrying the mutant enzyme. By improving the efficiency of gene transfer, similar manipulations may be practical for repopulating mutant human liver with genotypically normal cells. By combining within the retroviral vector both the gene for transfer and also a second gene that affords a selective advantage for hepatocytes, it may eventually be feasible to both initiate and promote the repopulation of human liver with functional hepatocytes and overcome or eliminate the enzymatic defect without the need for OLT.

ACID LIPASE DEFICIENCY (WOLMAN'S DISEASE AND CHOLESTEROL ESTER STORAGE DISEASE)

Epidemiology and Pathophysiology

Deficiency of acid lipase results in two phenotypically distinct syndromes, Wolman's disease and cholesterol ester storage disease (CESD), each inherited as an autosomal recessive disorder. They are marked by diffuse deposition of cholesterol esters, resulting in hepatic and multiorgan disease. Wolman's disease presents with severe acute decline in early infancy, whereas CESD has a more benign course throughout adulthood (Table 13–4).

The gene coding for acid lipase has been localized to chromosome 10 and has recently been cloned. Acid lipase is a widely distributed lysosomal enzyme that normally hydrolyzes cholesterol esters of low-density lipoproteins (LDLs). While other lysosomal enzymes metabolize the protein component of LDLs to peptides and amino acids, acid lipase frees LDL cholesterol from esterification, making it available for cellular metabolism and for feedback repression of extrahepatic cholesterol synthesis. Therefore, deficiency of the enzyme results in an accumulation of cholesterol esters as well as increased cellular cholesterol synthesis. The liver, spleen, lymph nodes, and intestine are typically laden with cholesterol esters and triglycerides. In

Table 13–4   Acid Lipase Deficiency—Wolman's Disease and Cholesterol Ester Storage Disease

Enzyme Defect	Lysosomal acid lipase
Clinical Features	*Wolman's disease:* infant with abdominal pain and distention, vomiting, diarrhea, hepatosplenomegaly, mental retardation, adrenal calcification, and enlargement.
	CESD: may be asymptomatic; child/adult with hepatomegaly, cirrhosis, premature atherosclerosis, adrenal enlargement.
Diagnosis	Acid lipase deficiency in cultured leukocytes or skin fibroblasts. Liver biopsy with cholesterol ester–laden Kupffer cells, fibrosis, cirrhosis. Birefringent hepatocytes in CESD.
Treatment	*Wolman's disease:* supportive care, death by age one. Bone marrow transplant under investigation.
	CESD: 3-hydroxy-3-methylglutaryl-CoA (HMG-CoA) reductase inhibitors, supportive care of liver disease

CESD, cholesterol ester storage disease.

Wolman's disease, the adrenal glands are invariably affected as well.

Clinical Features

For unclear reasons, Wolman's disease and CESD have different clinical courses despite an apparently similar enzyme deficiency. Wolman's disease is characterized in early infancy by abdominal pain and distention, vomiting and diarrhea, and hepatosplenomegaly. Growth and neurologic development are retarded. Progressive hepatosplenomegaly and distention are accompanied by profound malabsorption, and death usually occurs within the first year of life. CESD has a more benign course and usually presents in childhood, although some patients present as young adults. The patient may be asymptomatic, but hepatomegaly is universal and typically progressive, with hepatic fibrosis leading ultimately to cirrhosis and complications of portal hypertension. Premature atherosclerosis accompanies hyperlipoproteinemia.

Liver chemistries (conjugated bilirubin and serum aminotransferases) are typically elevated in Wolman's disease but are usually normal in CESD. Plasma cholesterol and triglycerides are normal in Wolman's disease but usually elevated in CESD. Serum LDL may be elevated in CESD, whereas low hepatic synthesis in Wolman's disease likely accounts for low LDL levels. Without exception, patients with Wolman's disease have distinctive granular calcification diffusely involving enlarged adrenal glands, which is easily seen on an abdominal roentgenogram. The adrenal glands are enlarged but not calcified in CESD.

Liver biopsy demonstrates steatosis with cholesterol ester–laden Kupffer cells that are swollen and vacuolated. Fibrosis and, ultimately, cirrhosis may be evident. In CESD, hepatocytes show birefringent lipid globules. Kupffer cells do not show birefringence, probably owing to peroxidation of the Kupffer cell cholesterol esters.

Diagnosis and Treatment

A diagnosis is made from the characteristic clinical findings and from the demonstration of lysosomal acid lipase deficiency in cultured leukocytes or skin fibroblasts. Traditionally, intervention has been limited to supportive care. Inhibitors of 3-hydroxy-3-methylglutaryl-CoA reductase, such as lovastatin, may be used to diminish intracellular cholesterol synthesis. Recently, bone marrow transplantation has shown promise for patients with Wolman's disease, and cloning of the gene for acid lipase has engendered new potential for eventual recombinant enzyme replacement therapy and gene therapy.

HEREDITARY FRUCTOSE INTOLERANCE

Hereditary fructose intolerance (HFI) is an autosomal recessive defect of aldolase B, an isozyme of fructose biphosphate aldolase. The enzyme is found in liver, intestine, and kidney, where it normally cleaves fructose-1-phosphate into dihydroxyacetone phosphate and glyceraldehyde. Deficiency results in cytoplasmic accumulation of fructose-1-phosphate (Fig. 13–13).

The gene for aldolase B (ALDOB) is located on chromo-

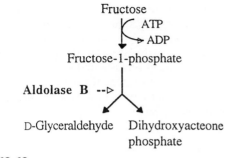

Figure 13–13
Hereditary fructose intolerance—enzymatic defect.

some 9q; more than 20 mutations have been described to date. More than half of North American and European allelic defects are accounted for by the A149P mutation. A strong founder effect is shown by linkage studies, suggesting that the distribution of the A149P mutation was likely by way of genetic drift, rather than by recurrent de novo mutation. HFI is most prevalent among northern Europeans.

Clinical findings include marked abdominal pain and vomiting after the ingestion of fructose, sucrose, or sorbitol (Table 13–5). Hypoglycemia may follow and can be fatal. Chronic effects include growth retardation, hepatomegaly, renal tubular damage, and hypophosphatemia. The diagnosis has traditionally been made by intravenous fructose challenge or by liver biopsy. However, as most enzymatic defects are coded for by just a few mutations, molecular diagnostic methods, such as analysis of DNA by RFLP and SSCP, are leading to less invasive diagnosis. Genetic screening of affected kindreds may be accomplished by similar means. Treatment involves the avoidance of fructose or sugars metabolized to fructose, and patients typically develop a strong distaste for sweet foods. Patients without chronic fructose exposure may anticipate a normal lifespan.

HEPATIC GLYCOGENOSES (GLYCOGEN STORAGE DISEASES)

Epidemiology and Pathophysiology

The glycogenoses, or glycogen storage diseases (GSDs), are caused by defects of glycogen metabolism, resulting in tis-

Table 13–5 Hereditary Fructose Intolerance

Enzyme Defect	Aldolase B (fructose-1-phosphate aldolase)
Inheritance	Autosomal recessive
Clinical Features	Hypoglycemia, abdominal pain, vomiting, hepatomegaly, renal tubular damage, hypophosphatemia, growth retardation
Diagnosis	Intravenous fructose challenge, liver biopsy, molecular diagnosis (DNA analysis)
Treatment	Avoidance of fructose-containing sugars; normal lifespan if treated

sue accumulation of normal or abnormal glycogen molecules and impaired conversion of glycogen stores to glucose. In most types, hypoglycemia ensues and may be severe or even fatal. Their inheritance is autosomal recessive, except for type VI, which is sex-linked. We limit our discussion to those affecting the liver (Table 13–6), which include all but type V, which affects muscle, and type VII, which affects erythrocytes.

Type I Glycogen Storage Disease

Type 1, or GSD 1 (Von Gierke's disease), affects the liver and kidney. There are three subtypes. Type 1a is caused by deficiency of hepatic microsomal glucose-6-phosphatase. The gene coding for glucose-6-phosphastase has been cloned and is located on chromosome 17. Type 1b is caused by a defective translocase required for glucose-6-phosphatase activity at the endoplasmic reticulum, and type 1c by defective microsomal phosphate/pyrophosphate translocase T-2 (Fig. 13–14).

Clinical Features

Clinical findings in infants include difficulty feeding and hypoglycemic seizures. Children have short stature and adiposity. Marked hepatomegaly is universal (Fig. 13–15A), but the absence of splenomegaly is a distinguishing feature from other storage diseases. Adults are short, often anemic, with proteinuria, microalbuminuria, renal calcifications, and chronic renal failure. Osteopenia and related fractures are not uncommon. Hyperlipidemia may be manifest as xanthomata, and hyperuricemia as gout. Adult liver findings commonly include adenomas (as many as 75% of patients), and there is an increased incidence of hepatocellular carcinoma. In contrast to hepatic adenomas in the general population, there is a strong male predominance in GSD 1. Notably, cirrhosis does not occur.

Type 1a (as well as types III, VI, and IX) is associated with polycystic ovarian disease, which is found in almost all female patients older than 5 years of age and is likely a consequence of hyperinsulinemia. Type 1b is associated with

defective neutrophil glucose-6-phosphatase transport and, as a result, bacterial infections and gingivitis are frequent problems. Platelet dysfunction can be seen in all subtypes. Hypoglycemia is evident on laboratory testing, as is metabolic acidosis. Aminotransferases are usually normal, but alkaline phosphatase and γ-glutamyl transferase may be elevated. Increased triglycerides, cholesterol, and uric acid levels are typical.

Diagnosis

Glucagon challenge and liver biopsy have traditionally been used to make the diagnosis. Intramuscular glucagon results in poor blood glucose response and elevated lactate levels. Liver biopsy shows hepatocytes filled with glycogen (see Fig. 13–15B), and special care must be taken to forward the sample to a diagnostic center for glycogen and specific enzyme quantification. Interestingly, Mallory bodies are found in adenomas of GSD 1 patients, in contrast with most other adenomas. Perhaps this suggests their potential for malignant degeneration, as Mallory bodies are often found in hepatocellular carcinomas.

The gene for glucose-6-phosphatase, the enzyme deficient in type 1a, has been cloned. Although many different mutations have been identified, they are clustered by ethnic background. Through DNA-based analysis, type 1a may be diagnosed noninvasively, and prenatal diagnosis is being developed as well. Similar noninvasive molecular diagnosis will likely follow for the other glycogenoses.

Treatment

Management focuses on maintaining adequate blood glucose levels (Table 13–7). Continuous nocturnal high-carbohydrate enteral feeding and frequent daytime feedings of a diet rich in carbohydrates are the mainstays of therapy. Raw cornstarch serves as a delayed-release source of glucose and may supplement feedings. Medical treatment is given as warranted for hyperlipidemia, gout, infections, and osteopenia. Granulocyte colony–stimulating factor has been used to boost neutrophil number and function in GSD 1b.

Table 13–6   The Hepatic Glycogen Storage Diseases—Enzyme Defects, Clinical Features

Glycogenosis	Enzyme Defect	Clinical Features
Type I (von Gierke's)		Hypoglycemia, acidosis, seizures, short stature, adiposity, hepatomegaly without cirrhosis and without splenomegaly. Adults with renal failure, anemia, osteopenia, hyperlipidemia, hepatic adenoma/adenocarcinoma, platelet dysfunction, gout, polycystic ovaries—type Ia, bacterial infection—type Ib
Type Ia	Glucose-6-phosphatase	
Type Ib	Translocase	
Type Ic	Phosphate/pyrophosphate translocase T-2	
Type II (Pompe's)	Lysosomal acid maltase	No hypoglycemia, macroglossia, cardiomegaly, hepatomegaly without cirrhosis and without splenomegaly
Type III (Cori's)	Amylo-1,6 glucosidase	Hypoglycemia, myopathy, cardiomyopathy, hepatomegaly without cirrhosis or splenomegaly, polycystic ovaries
Type IV (Andersen's)	Amylo-1,4→1,6 transglucosidase	Cirrhosis, death from liver failure
Type VI (Her's)	Hepatic phosphorylase	Polycystic ovaries
Type IX	Hepatic phosphorylase-b-kinase	Mild course, growth retardation, hepatomegaly, polycystic ovaries

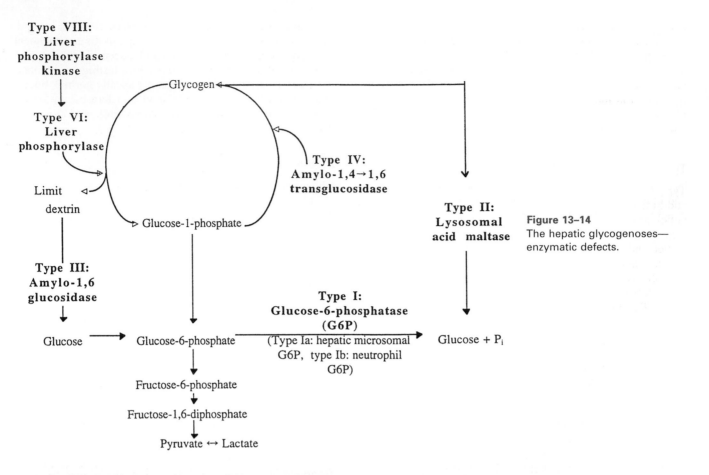

Figure 13–14
The hepatic glycogenoses—enzymatic defects.

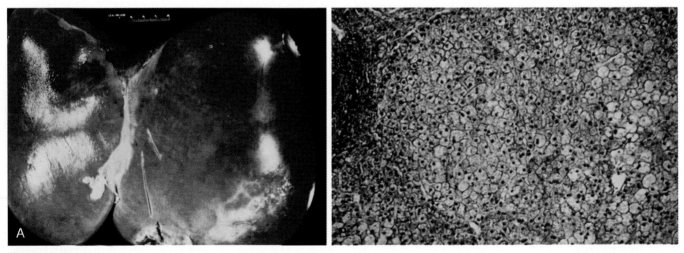

Figure 13–15
Glycogen storage disease Ia (von Gierke's disease): liver pathology. *A,* Capsular surface of a liver from a patient with glycogen storage disease Ia (von Gierke's disease). The liver is enlarged, and the capsule appears smooth and shiny, with the liver edges rounded rather than sharp. *B,* Photomicrograph of a liver from a patient with glycogen storage disease type Ia. All of the hepatocytes are expanded and pale due to glycogen-laden cytoplasm. Unlike fatty liver, in which the nucleus is pushed to the side by a single large cytoplasmic vacuole, glycogen storage is more diffuse within the cytoplasm and the nucleus remains in the center of the cell. The cells appear pale because much of the glycogen dissolves during processing (H & E, ×40; courtesy of Joseph Alroy, MD, Tufts University School of Veterinary Medicine, and Barbara Banner, MD, University of Massachusetts Medical Center).

Table 13–7   The Hepatic Glycogen Storage Diseases—Inheritance, Diagnosis, Treatment

Inheritance	Autosomal recessive, except type IV, which is sex-linked, and type IX, which has sex-linked forms
Diagnosis	Glucagon challenge → low blood glucose, high lactate
	Liver biopsy → glycogen-laden hepatocytes
	Molecular diagnosis becoming available
Treatment	Continuous nocturnal high-carbohydrate feeds, raw corn starch; supportive care of hyperlipidemia, gout, infection, osteopenia; potential gene therapy

Liver transplantation may be required for treatment of adenomas, although adenomas may regress upon commencement of enteral feedings. Whereas most patients survive to adulthood, many die as children. The cloning of the gene for glucose-6-phosphatase has paved the way for potential gene therapy of this condition.

Types II-IX GSD
(see Tables 13–6 and 13–7 and Fig. 13–14)

Type II GSD (Pompe's disease) results from deficiency of lysosomal acid maltase (α-1,4 glucosidase). Glycogen accumulates within lysosomes of all tissues in this generalized glycogenosis, but hypoglycemia does not occur. Onset may be in infancy or adulthood, the former typically more severe. Patients have hepatomegaly without splenomegaly, macroglossia, and cardiomegaly. Hyperlipidemia is evident and liver biopsy shows vacuolated lysosomes, packed with glycogen, as do all organs. The gene for lysosomal acid maltase has also been localized to chromosome 17, and gene therapy is being investigated as a therapeutic option.

Type III GSD (Cori's disease) involves a defect of amylo-1,6 glucosidase, a debranching enzyme, and is marked by myopathy, cardiomyopathy, hepatomegaly without splenomegaly, and pronounced hypoglycemia. Patients develop polycystic ovaries. Serum aminotransferases may be elevated, and creatinine kinase may be increased secondary to myopathy. Treatment may involve enteral glucose feedings but, because gluconeogenesis is enhanced, glucose levels may be maintained with high-protein supplementation as well. The course of the disease is less virulent than GSD I or II and patients usually live to adulthood.

Type IV GSD (Andersen's disease) is rare and differs from other GSDs in that cirrhosis is prevalent, and, consequently, splenomegaly is as well. Deficiency of amylo-1,4→1,6 transglucosidase results in structurally abnormal glycogen which affects all tissues and which is found in liver biopsies as PAS-positive intracellular aggregates. The course is usually one of progressive liver failure with death or transplantation usually by 5 years of age. Neuromuscular and cardiac disease may also predominate. For unclear reasons, liver disease does not progress in some patients. Curiously, liver transplant recipients may not suffer progression of the neuromuscular or cardiac effects of extrahepatic enzyme deficiency.

Type VI GSD (Her's disease) involves a sex-linked deficiency of phosphorylase and causes isolated hepatic disease marked by hepatomegaly without splenomegaly, hypoglycemia, and subsequent acidosis. Polycystic ovaries are commonly found. Type VIII is caused by deficient phosphorylase activation and presents similarly. Type IX involves deficiency of phosphorylase kinase as detected in erythrocytes. Its course is typically mild, with some growth retardation, hepatomegaly, and polycystic ovaries. Sex-linked forms exist.

GALACTOSEMIA

There are three key enzymes in the metabolism of galactose: galactokinase, galactose-1-phosphate uridyl transferase (GALT), and uridine diphospho-glucose 4-epimerase (Fig. 13–16). Classic galactosemia involves a hepatic and erythrocytic deficiency of GALT, inherited as an autosomal recessive trait. Galactose accumulation ensues and is toxic to tissues throughout the body, although the mechanism of toxicity remains unclear. The disease may be severe and result in childhood death or have a more moderate course, such that patients may survive through adulthood. This may depend on whether the enzyme deficiency is complete or partial (Table 13–8).

Accumulation of galactose is found within the fetus by 10 to 20 weeks' gestation, and toxic effects in utero are evidenced by early cataract development, low birth weight, and probable prenatal liver pathology. Newborns have difficulty feeding, with vomiting and diarrhea, malnutrition, and growth retardation. Hepatosplenomegaly is followed by development of macronodular cirrhosis, portal hypertension and ascites. Mental development is poor, with retardation and speech deficits. Ovarian failure is seen in most girls surviving to puberty. Patients with partial enzyme deficiency may survive well into adulthood, and the diagnosis should be considered in young cirrhotic patients as well as adult cirrhotic patients with other characteristic findings.

Screening tests will detect the presence of a glucose-oxidase negative urinary reducing agent; diagnosis is made definitively by measuring erythrocyte GALT levels. Prenatal diagnosis can be made by culturing cells from amniotic fluid and measuring enzyme levels. Liver biopsy reveals

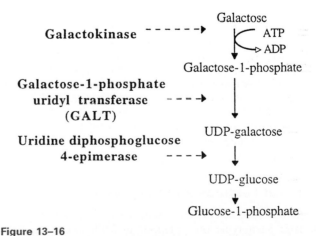

Figure 13–16
Galactosemia—enzymatic defects.

Table 13–8 Galactosemia

Enzyme Defect	Clinical Features	Diagnosis	Treatment
Galactose-1-phosphate uridyl transferase (GALT)	*Prenatal:* cataract-like corneal changes, liver disease *Newborns:* vomiting, malnutrition, hepatosplenomegaly, macronodular cirrhosis, portal hypertension, mental and growth retardation, death *Adults:* ovarian failure, cirrhosis	*Screening:* glucose-oxidase negative urinary reducing agent *Confirmation:* erythrocyte GALT deficiency *Prenatal:* GALT levels in cultured amniotic cells	Avoidance of galactose and lactose Estrogen replacement therapy for ovarian failure
Galactokinase	Cataracts, mild course	Erythrocyte enzyme deficiency	Avoidance of galactose/lactose
Uridine diphosphoglucose 4-epimerase	Clinical picture similar to GALT deficiency (above), severe course	Erythrocyte enzyme deficiency	Avoidance of galactose/lactose

fatty deposition in newborns and later shows regeneration, giant cells, and cirrhotic changes.

Dietary intervention is the mainstay of treatment. Avoidance of galactose or lactose products can result in significant improvement and even recovery. For unclear reasons, however, dietary-independent deficits may persist and progress. These can include mental deficits, speech pathology, and growth retardation. Ovarian failure almost invariably occurs in women and may be treated with exogenous estrogen and progesterone to promote the development of secondary sex characteristics and manage postmenopausal sequelae.

Deficiencies of the other key enzymes of galactose metabolism are rare. Galactokinase deficiency is mild and results in cataract formation; uridine diphosphoglucose 4-epimerase deficiency is severe and presents like classic galactosemia. Dietary intervention is the pillar of treatment.

THE MUCOPOLYSACCHARIDOSES

Epidemiology and Pathophysiology

The mucopolysaccharidoses (MPSs) are a group of lysosomal storage disorders leading to the lysosomal accumulation of mucopolysaccharides (glycosaminoglycans), resulting in a variety of mental and physical abnormalities. With one exception, their inheritance is autosomal recessive (type II is sex-linked recessive). Ten known enzymatic deficiencies account for six distinct syndromes that are classified by clinical features, urinary mucopolysaccharide analysis, and are identified by historical eponyms. Each enzyme deficiency results in defective metabolism of heparan sulfate, dermatan sulfate, chondroitin sulfate, or keratan sulfate (Table 13–9).

Clinical Features and Diagnosis

Although specific enzyme deficiencies may produce characteristic phenotypic presentations in MPS, there are many similarities among the several forms of MPS. Hepatosplenomegaly is a prominent feature, as are coarse facial features, skeletal defects, mental retardation, corneal clouding, joint stiffness, and cardiac disease.

Type IH (Hurler syndrome) is most frequently encountered and involves a deficiency of L-iduronidase, with an accumulation of dermatan sulfate and heparan sulfate. Its inheritance is autosomal recessive, and it is marked by dwarfism as well as the findings described earlier. Skeletal disease includes lumbar gibbus (hunchback) and clawhand. The adult Scheie variant, type IS, presents without mental retardation.

Type II, Hunter syndrome, involves deficiency of iduronosulfate sulfatase with an accumulation of dermatan sulfate and heparan sulfate. It is sex-linked recessive and seen only in males. Less severe than type I, patients typically survive well into adulthood. The remaining MPSs have autosomal recessive inheritance, including type III (Sanfilippo syndrome). There are four enzymatic deficiencies classified as Sanfilippo variants, each resulting in accumulation of heparan sulfate. They all cause severe mental retardation and moderate skeletal deformity. Skeletal abnormalities (Fig. 13–17) are most severe in type IV, Morquio syndrome, in which keratan sulfate aggregates are found as a result of N-acetylgalactosamine-6-sulfate sulfatase deficiency. Corneal clouding is typical. In both types III and IV, there is less liver or spleen enlargement than types I and II. In the Maroteaux-Lamy variant, type VI, N-acetylhexosamine-4-sulfate sulfatase causes an accumulation of dermatan and presents with the characteristic MPS findings already described.

Hepatosplenomegaly is a characteristic finding on examination in all types, and liver biopsy may demonstrate fibrosis and, ultimately, cirrhosis. Vacuolation of hepatocytes and Kupffer cells is produced by glycosaminoglycan-laden lysosomes, most evident on colloidal iron staining. Electron microscopy shows membrane-bound inclusions within hepatocytes, Kupffer cells, and hepatic stellate (Ito) cells.

Treatment

Until recently, treatment has been supportive. However, animal models of enzyme replacement therapy seem promis-

Table 13–9   The Mucopolysaccharidoses

Type of MPS	Enzyme Defect → Stored MPS	Inheritance	Clinical Features
Type IH (Hurler's)	α-L-Iduronidase → dermatan sulfate	Autosomal recessive	Hepatosplenomegaly, coarse facial features, skeletal defects (gibbus, clawhand), mental retardation, cardiac disease, corneal disease
Type IS (Scheie's)	α-L-Iduronidase → heparan sulfate	Autosomal recessive	Same as type 1H, but no mental retardation
Type II (Hunter's)	Iduronosulfate sulfatase → dermatan and heparan sulfate	Sex-linked recessive	Similar to type 1, but mental retardation less severe, retinal degeneration, no corneal disease
Type III (Sanfilippo's)	(4 Subtypes) → heparan sulfate	Autosomal recessive	Severe mental retardation, coarse facial features, little hepatosplenomegaly, moderate skeletal disease, eyes uninvolved
Type IV (Morquio's)	N-acetylgalactosamine-6-sulfate sulfatase → keratan sulfate	Autosomal recessive	Severe skeletal deformity, corneal disease, cardiac disease, little hepatosplenomegaly, mental status unaffected
Type VI (Maroteaux-Lamy)	N-acetylhexosamine-4-sulfate sulfatase → dermatan sulfate	Autosomal recessive	Corneal disease, cardiac disease, coarse facial features, mental status unaffected

MPS, mucopolysaccharidoses.

ing, and bone marrow transplantation has been successfully carried out with halting of disease progression and improvement in skin, joint, heart, and liver manifestations. Models for gene therapy are now being explored. Presently, life expectancy for type IH is less than 10 years, normal for type IS, and nearly normal for types II and IV. Patients with type III disease live into the second or third decade. For reasons as yet unclear, there is a great variation in the penetrance of each MPS and, therefore, in life expectancies.

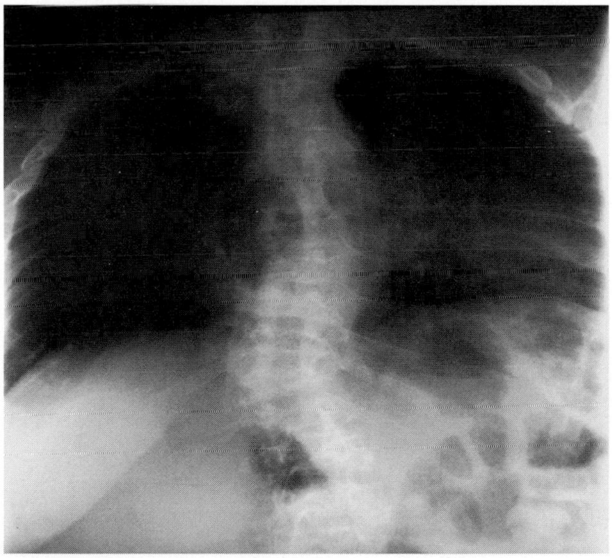

GAUCHER'S DISEASE

Epidemiology and Pathophysiology

The most common lysosomal storage disease and most frequent inborn error of lipid metabolism, Gaucher's disease is a paramount example of the profound implications of genetic mutation and the tangible benefits of advances in molecular medicine. The disease is caused by a defect in β-glucocerebrosidase (glucosylceramidase), which catalyzes the cleavage of glucocerebroside (glucosylceramide) to glucose and ceramide (Fig. 13–18). The gene of this enzyme has been cloned and localized to chromosome 1q21. Deficiency results in the accumulation of glucocerebroside in tissue macrophages, known as Gaucher cells (Fig. 13–19B), with subsequent toxicity to these tissues. Affected macrophages are present in the liver as Kupffer cells, in bone as osteoclasts, and are present in the spleen and lung as well.

Clinical Features

The clinical syndrome was first described by Charles Earnest Gaucher in 1882, although he erroneously believed an unidentified malignancy caused this multiorgan disease. As

Figure 13–17
Mucopolysaccharidosis (MPS) type IV (Morquio's syndrome): chest roentgenogram. This 59-year-old woman has several findings typical of MPS IV, including spinal shortening, marked kyphoscoliosis (together contributing to dwarfism), and widening of the ribs anteriorly but narrowing posteriorly. (Courtesy of the Department of Radiology, University of Massachusetts Medical Center.)

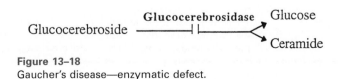

Figure 13–18
Gaucher's disease—enzymatic defect.

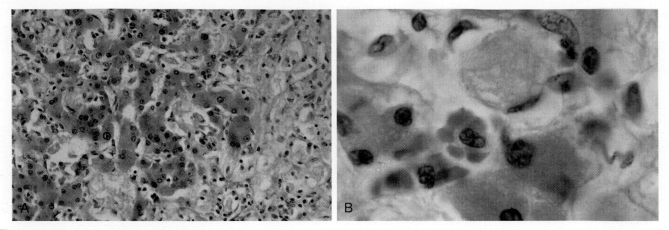

Figure 13–19

Gaucher's disease: liver histopathology. *A,* Photomicrograph of a liver biopsy from a patient with Gaucher's disease showing infiltration of the sinusoids and compression of the hepatic cords by glucocerebroside-laden Kupffer cells, known as Gaucher cells (H & E, ×200). *B,* High-power photomicrograph of a liver biopsy from a patient with Gaucher's disease. A Gaucher cell with the characteristic "wrinkled tissue paper" cytoplasmic appearance is seen in a sinusoid, adjacent to hepatocytes (H & E, ×1000; courtesy of Barbara Banner, MD, University of Massachusetts Medical Center).

would be predicted from the distribution of tissue macrophages, the primary syndrome is of hepatosplenomegaly, bone pain and fractures, hematopoietic disease, and pulmonary compromise. Three clinical syndromes are described (Table 13–10), classified by whether the nervous system is affected and by the age and rate of the onset of nervous system disease. Type I (non-neuronopathic) is without central nervous system (CNS) involvement. Type II is marked by early and rapid CNS affliction (acute neuronopathic), and type III (subacute neuronopathic) by CNS involvement that is delayed and more slowly progressive.

Type I is the most common. Its inheritance is autosomal recessive, with a particularly high prevalence (1 in 500 to 1 in 1000) among the Ashkenazi Jewish population. The incidence among all Jews is about 1 in 60,000 and is 1 in 100,000 among the general population of the United States.

Onset is in childhood or adulthood, and disease severity is variable. In children, growth retardation may be subtle or severe. In advanced disease, hepatomegaly may be massive, with the sinusoidal sequestration of glucocerebroside-laden Kupffer cells (see Fig. 13–19). Fibrosis is not unusual, but hepatocytes are not involved. Similarly, marked splenomegaly may develop, with Gaucher cell aggregation and fibrosis. Although spleen enlargement is usually asymptomatic, infarction may cause pain. Pulmonary disease is rare and suggests poor prognosis. The degree of bone involvement may vary widely; osteoporosis, cortical rarefaction, erosions and even avascular necrosis and collapse are all possible. Painful infarcts, known as pseudo-osteomyelitis or "bone crises" are common. The head and shaft of the femur are commonly affected with characteristic "Erlenmeyer flask" deformity, and the humerus, vertebrae, and pelvis may be

Table 13–10 Gaucher's Disease—Inheritance, Incidence, Clinical Features, and Treatment

Disease Type	Inheritance and Incidence	Clinical Features	Treatment
Type I	• Autosomal recessive • 1/500–1/1000 Ashkenazi Jewish • 1/60,000 general Jewish • 1/100,000 general United States	• Onset as a child or an adult • Hepatosplenomegaly • No neurologic disease • Growth retardation • Bone involvement • Pulmonary disease (poor prognosis)	• Hydration, analgesia • Enzyme replacement therapy • Calcium, vitamin D, bisphosphonates, orthopedic repair • Splenectomy if symptomatic • Bone marrow transplantation
Type II	• Autosomal dominant • Less than 1/100,000 • No ethnic predisposition	• Onset in infancy • Rapidly progressive neurologic decline • Hepatosplenomegaly • Growth retardation • Pulmonary involvement	• As for type I disease
Type III	• Autosomal dominant • Incidence unclear, ? 1/50,000 • No ethnic predisposition	• Onset in childhood • Slowly progressive neurologic disease	• As for type I disease

involved (Fig. 13–20). Thrombocytopenia and anemia secondary to splenic sequestration are common, and patients may have a history of easy bruising or bleeding. By definition, type I disease spares the CNS.

Type II is much less prevalent, likely less than 1 in 100,000. The incidence of type III may be as high as 1 in 50,000 live births, but no clear estimates are available. The inheritance of both types II and III is autosomal dominant, and there is no ethnic predilection. Rapidly progressive CNS disease in infancy is the hallmark of type II, which is also associated with poor growth, hepatosplenomegaly, and pulmonary disease. Death may occur early, with an average lifespan of just 2 years. In type III disease, neurologic disease progresses slowly; hepatosplenomegaly is prominent. Onset is in childhood, with the expected lifespan varying from infancy to adulthood.

Diagnosis

Diagnosis should be suspected in anyone with the features just described. A careful family history may further suggest the diagnosis. Marrow, liver, spleen, or lung may demonstrate glucocerebroside-packed Gaucher macrophages. These are seen in other diseases, however, such as hematopoietic malignancies, and definitive diagnosis is made by demonstration of deficient β-glucocerebrosidase activity in leukocytes. Increased glucocerebroside levels are found but are not specific. Prenatal testing in gestations at risk can be carried out via amniocentesis or chorionic villus sampling.

With the localization and cloning of the gene for Gaucher disease, mutations have been identified which may be prognostic of the type and severity of disease. Although more than 50 mutations have been characterized, a small number constitute the majority, and a few presently have specific prognostic value. Hence, more than 95% of Ashkenazi heterozygotes can be identified by screening for just five mutations. Indeed, a single alanine to guanine point mutation at nucleotide 1226, which codes for an asparagine to serine substitution at amino acid 370, is responsible for almost ¾ of affected Ashkenazis. Homozygosity predicts moderate type I disease, but compound heterozygosity with another Gaucher allele causes type I disease with more severe enzymatic deficiency and a more severe course.

Treatment

Traditional conservative therapy for symptomatic disease involves hydration, analgesia, and surgery as warranted for bone disease. Calcium, vitamin D, and bisphosphonates are helpful in delaying bone afflictions. Splenectomy is sometimes carried out but is of little benefit for the asymptomatic patient. Bone marrow transplantation has been successful but carries significant risk.

Recent advances in the therapy of Gaucher's disease have, at once, begotten hope and controversy. Enzyme replacement therapy, first proposed decades ago, has become a reality in recent years and provided remarkable benefit. By targeting a mannose receptor on the plasma membrane surface of macrophages, exogenous β-glucocerebrosidase, which has been modified to expose mannose residues, is directed selectively to macrophages. In type I disease, this therapy has been shown to halt the progression of and actu-

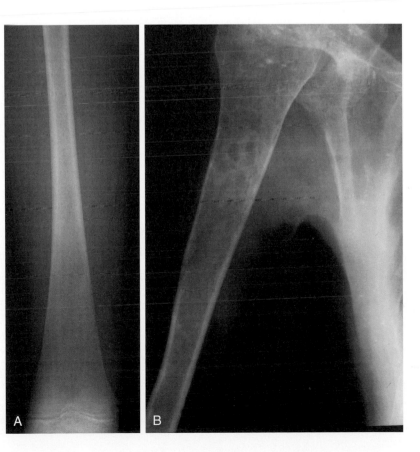

Figure 13–20
Gaucher's disease: extremity roentgenograms. *A,* Femur of a 12-year-old male who presented with dull bone pain and splenomegaly and was found to have Gaucher's disease, type I. The distal end of the femur has lost its normal concavity, resulting in the characteristic "Erlenmeyer flask" deformity. *B,* Humerus of a 26-year-old woman with Gaucher's disease, type I. There is marked osteopenia with cortical rarefaction and erosions. Painful infarcts, known as pseudo-osteomyelitis, may accompany advanced disease. (Courtesy of the Department of Radiology, University of Massachusetts Medical Center.)

ally reverse hepatosplenomegaly, hypersplenism, and pulmonary disease. Marrow composition, osteoporosis, and other bone lesions may improve. The therapy has not been shown effective for neurologic involvement in types II and III disease.

By targeting macrophages, replacement therapy has been made more efficient but is still very expensive. One year of therapy can cost more than $200,000. Controversy has therefore arisen over the dose and duration of therapy necessary to evoke and maintain an adequate response, and dose-response clinical trials continue. Development of methods for mass production of the enzyme by cells containing its cDNA, to replace placenta-derived enzyme, is not expected to dramatically decrease cost. Of note, animal models of gene therapy have been promising in vivo as have been in vitro studies with human cells, and human trials of gene therapy for Gaucher's disease are now underway.

SUGGESTED READINGS

General

Ghishan FK, Greene HL: Inborn errors of metabolism that lead to permanent liver injury. In Scriver C et al (eds): The Metabolic and Molecular Bases of Inherited Disease. New York: McGraw Hill, 1995, pp 1084–1137.

The Porphyrias

Bonkovsky HL: Porphyrin and heme metabolism and the porphyrias. In Zakim D, Boyer TD (eds): Hepatology, 2nd ed. Philadelphia: WB Saunders, 1990, pp 378–424.

Bonkovsky HL: Porphyria cutanea tarda and hepatitis C. Viral Hepatitis Reviews 4:75–95, 1998.

Bonkovsky HL, Banner BF, Lambrecht RW, Rubin RB: Iron in liver diseases other than hemochromatosis. Semin Liver Dis 16:65–82, 1996.

Bonkovsky HL, Healey JF, Lourie AN, Gerron GG: Intravenous heme-albumin in acute intermittent porphyria: Evidence for repletion of hepatic hemoproteins and regulatory heme pools. Am J Gastroenterol 86:1050–1056, 1991.

Hahn M, Bonkovsky HL: Disorders of porphyrin metabolism. In Wu G, Israel J (eds): Diseases of the Liver and Bile Ducts: A practical guide to Diagnosis and Treatment. Totowa, NJ: Humana Press, 1998, pp 249–272.

α_1-Antitrypsin Deficiency

Askari FK: Molecular mechanism of hepatocellular injury in alpha 1 antitrypsin deficiency. Hepatology 21:1745–1747, 1995.

Carrell RW, Whisstock J, Lomas DA: Conformational changes in serpins and the mechanism of alpha 1-antitrypsin deficiency Am J Respir Crit Care Med 150:S171–175, 1994. (Published erratum appears in Am J Respir Crit Care Med 151:926, 1995.)

Perlmutter DH: Clinical manifestations of alpha 1-antitrypsin deficiency. Gastroenterol Clin North Am 24:27–43, 1995.

Cystic Fibrosis

Colombo C, Crosignani A, Assaisso M, et al: Ursodeoxycholic acid therapy in cystic fibrosis-associated liver disease: A dose-response study. Hepatology 16:924–930, 1992.

Tanner MS, Taylor CJ: Liver disease in cystic fibrosis. Arch Dis Child 72:281–284, 1995.

Yang Y, Raper SE, Cohn JA, et al: An approach for treating the hepatobiliary disease of cystic fibrosis by somatic gene transfer. Proc Natl Acad Sci U S A 90:4601–4605, 1993.

Hereditary Tyrosinemia Type 1

Gibbs TC, Payan J, Brett EM, et al: Peripheral neuropathy as the presenting feature of tyrosinaemia type I and effectively treated with an inhibitor of 4-hydroxyphenylpyruvate dioxygenase. J Neurol Neurosurg Psychiatry 56:1129–1132, 1993.

Kvittingen EA, Rootwelt H, Berger R, Brandtzaeg P: Self-induced correction of the genetic defect in tyrosinemia type I. J Clin Invest 94:1657–1661, 1994.

Laine J, Salo MK, Krogerus L, Karkkainen J, et al: The nephropathy of type I tyrosinemia after liver transplantation. Pediatr Res 37:640–645, 1995.

Overturf K, Al-Dhalimy M, Tanguay R, et al: Hepatocytes corrected by gene therapy are selected in vivo in a murine model of hereditary tyrosinaemia type I. Nat Genet 12:266–273, 1996.

Acid Lipase Deficiency (Wolman's Disease and Cholesterol Ester Storage Disease)

Krivit W, Freese D, Chan KW, Kulkarni R: Wolman's disease: A review of treatment with bone marrow transplantation and considerations for the future. Bone Marrow Transplant 10(Suppl 1):97–101, 1992.

Leone L, Ippoliti PF, Antonicelli R: Use of simvistatin plus cholestyramine in the treatment of lysosomal acid lipase deficiency. J Pediatr 119:1008–1009, 1991.

Wolman M: Wolman disease and its treatment. Clin Pediatr 34:207–212, 1995.

Hereditary Fructose Intolerance

Cox TM: Aldolase B and fructose intolerance. FASEB J 8:62–71, 1994.

Tolan DR: Molecular basis of hereditary fructose intolerance: Mutations and polymorphisms in the human aldolase B gene. Hum Mutat 6:210–218, 1995.

Hepatic Glycogen Storage Diseases

Bianchi L: Glycogen storage disease I and hepatocellular tumours. Eur J Pediatr 152(Suppl 1):S63–S70, 1993.

Lei KJ, Chen YT, Chen H, et al: Genetic basis of glycogen storage disease type 1a: Prevalent mutations at the glucose-6-phosphatase locus. Am J Hum Genet 57:766–771, 1995.

Talente GM, Coleman RA, Alter C, et al: Glycogen storage disease in adults. Ann Intern Med 120:218–226, 1994.

Galactosemia

Beutler E: Galactosemia: Screening and diagnosis. Clin Biochem 24:293–300, 1991.

Holton JB: Effects of galactosemia in utero. Eur J Pediatr 154:S77–S81, 1995.

Sardharwalla IB, Wraith JE: Galactosaemia. Nutr Health 5:175–188, 1987.

Mucopolysaccharidoses

Resnick JM, Whitley CB, Leonard AS, et al: Light and electron microscopic features of the liver in mucopolysaccharidosis. Hum Pathol 25:276–286, 1994.

Wraith JE: The mucopolysaccharidoses: A clinical review and guide to management. Arch Dis Child 72:263–267, 1995.

Gaucher's Disease

Balicki D, Beutler E: Gaucher disease. Medicine 74:305–323, 1995.

Brady RO, Murray GJ, Barton NW: Modifying exogenous glucocerebrosidase for effective replacement therapy in Gaucher disease. J Inherit Metab Dis 17:510–519, 1994.

Gaucher disease: Current issues in diagnosis and treatment. NIH Technology Assessment Panel on Gaucher Disease. JAMA 275:548–553, 1996.

Rosenthal DI, Doppelt SH, Mankin HJ, et al: Enzyme replacement therapy for Gaucher disease: Skeletal responses to macrophage-targeted glucocerebrosidase. Pediatrics 96:629–637, 1995.

14

Primary Biliary Cirrhosis

Raoul Poupon
Renée Eugénie Poupon

Primary biliary cirrhosis is a chronic cholestatic disease of unknown cause, most often diagnosed in middle-aged women. Morphologically, primary biliary cirrhosis is characterized by portal inflammation and necrosis of cholangiocytes in the small- and medium-sized bile ducts. The disease is characterized biochemically by a cholestatic pattern and immunologically by the almost constant presence of mitochondrial antibodies and less often by that of nuclear antibodies. Although primary biliary cirrhosis is a progressive disease, the rate of progression varies greatly from one patient to another. The terminal phase is characterized by hyperbilirubinemia and morphologically by cirrhosis.

EPIDEMIOLOGY

According to epidemiologic studies, estimates of the prevalence range from 100 to 200 per million, with a strong female predominance (10:1) and a median age at diagnosis between 50 and 55 years. The disease, to our knowledge, has never been described during childhood or adolescence.

Prevalence of primary biliary cirrhosis in families with one affected member is about 4% (which is much higher than in the general population). Similarly, the occurrence of other immune-related disorders is common in first-degree relatives of patients with primary biliary cirrhosis. There is a weak association between the disease and the HLA DR8 antigen. An excess frequency of haplotype C4AQ0 has also been reported.

PATHOGENESIS AND IMMUNOLOGIC ABNORMALITIES (Fig. 14–1)

The initial lesion is a focal and segmental destruction of interlobular bile ducts. This results in chronic cholestasis, which progresses toward "biliary" cirrhosis. Numerous immunologic abnormalities are found in primary biliary cirrhosis. The most characteristic are an increase in serum IgM levels, the presence of circulating autoantibodies (in particular antimitochondrial and antinuclear antibodies), a defective suppressor T cell activity, and abnormalities of macrophage function.

Antimitochondrial Antibodies and Other Antibodies (Fig. 14–2)

Antimitochondrial antibodies (AMAs) are present in approximately 90% of patients with primary biliary cirrhosis. They are nonorgan and nonspecies–specific antibodies. The AMAs in primary biliary cirrhosis were shown initially to react with a trypsin-sensitive antigen (M2) of the internal mitochondrial membrane. Using Western immunoblotting, it was then shown that M2 contains several antigenic determinants with molecular masses of about 75 to 70, 56 to 50, 48 to 43, and 36 kD. The identity of this nonorgan and nonspecies–specific autoantigen was unknown until 1988, when two groups independently found that the M2 antigen of 70 to 75 kD (which was cloned by Gershwin and coworkers in 1987) was the E2 component of the pyruvate dehydrogenase complex. It later became clear that the antigenic determinants of M2 identified by Western blotting were all components of pyruvate dehydrogenase or the 2-oxoacid dehydrogenase complex located on the mammalian inner mitochondrial membrane. The enzyme subunits of the complexes of

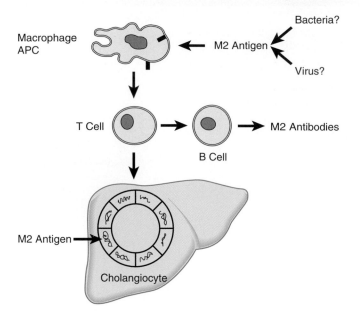

Figure 14–1
Pathogenesis. Macrophages present the M2 antigen or the cross-reactive peptide to CD4 lymphocytes by means of a class II antigen. CD4 T cells help CD8 T cells to become cytotoxic effector cells for cholangiocytes expressing the M2 antigen. CD4 cells also activate B cells to produce M2 antibodies.

the two oxoacid dehydrogenases and mitochondrial M2 antigens, together with the prevalence of the antibodies in primary biliary cirrhosis, are indicated in Table 14–1. Anti-M2 mainly reacts with the 74-kD antigen of pyruvate dehydrogenase, because approximately 95% of sera are positive by immunoblotting.

Other nonorgan and nonspecies specific antibodies are frequently detected in AMA-positive and AMA-negative patients with primary biliary cirrhosis. These include antinuclear, antismooth muscle, rheumatoid factor, and antithyroid antibodies.

Antinuclear antibodies are observed in up to 70% of patients with primary biliary cirrhosis (Table 14–2). In 10% to 15% of cases, they are anticentromere antibodies and are generally associated with the CREST (calcinosis cutis, Raynaud's phenomenon, esophageal dysfunction, sclerodactyly, telangiectasia) syndrome. In certain cases, anticentromere antibodies are found despite the absence of clinical signs of scleroderma.

Anti–M2

- Are present in 90% of patients with primary biliary cirrhosis

- Titer does not correlate with disease severity

- Are found in about 10% of healthy relatives of patients with primary biliary cirrhosis

- Are constantly present after liver transplantation

Figure 14–2
Link between anti-M2 antigens and pathogenesis.

Table 14–1   Enzyme Subunits of the 2-Oxoacid Dehydrogenase Complexes and M2 Mitochondrial Autoantigens

	MW (kD)	Prevalence of Antibody in PBC
Pyruvate Dehydrogenase		
PDC-E1a pyruvate decarboxylase	41	41–66%
PDC-E1b pyruvate decarboxylase	36	2–7%
PDC-E2 acetyltransferase	74	95%
E3 lipoamide dehydrogenase	55	38%
Protein X	52	95%
2-Oxoglutarate Dehydrogenase		
OGDC-E1 2-oxoglutarate decarboxylase	110	Low
OGDC-E2 succinyl transferase	48	39–88%
Branched-Chain 2-Oxoacid Dehydrogenase		
BCOADC-E1a acyl decarboxylase	46	
BCOADC-E1B acyl decarboxylase	38	
BCOADC-E2 acyl transferase	50	53–55%

From Gershwin ME, Rowley M, Davis PA, et al: Molecular biology of the 2-oxo-acid dehydrogenase complexes and anti-mitochondrial antibodies. In Boyer JL, Ockner RK (eds): Progress in Liver Diseases. Philadelphia: WB Saunders, 1992, pp 47–61.
BCOAD, branched-chain 2-oxoacid dehydrogenase; PBC, primary biliary cirrhosis; PDC, pyruvate dehydrogenase complex.

Approximately 30% of patients with primary biliary cirrhosis have autoantobodies, which give a nuclear rim pattern in immunofluorescence studies. In a few patients with primary biliary cirrhosis, these antibodies are directed against the receptor for lamin B, a constitutive protein of the inner nuclear membrane. These antibodies are more frequent in autoimmune hepatitis and systemic lupus erythematosus. In a larger number of patients with primary biliary cirrhosis (20% to 30%), these autoantibodies are directed against a nuclear pore protein of 210 kD. Clinical disease expression in such patients does not differ from that in patients without this antibody.

Table 14–2   Antinuclear Antibodies and the Diseases in Which They Are Found

Antibody Specificity	Disease (%, Prevalence)
Anticentromere	Scleroderma, CREST, primary biliary cirrhosis (10%)
Antilamins	SLE, scleroderma, autoimmune hepatitis, occasionally primary biliary cirrhosis (<5%)
Anti-Gp210	Primary biliary cirrhosis (20–30%)
Anti-Sp100	Primary biliary cirrhosis (20–30%)

CREST, calcinosis cutis, Raynaud's phenomenon, esophageal dysfunction, sclerodactyly, telangiectasia; SLE, systemic lupus erythematosus.

A third type of antinuclear antibody observed in primary biliary cirrhosis gives a speckled aspect by immunofluorescence, but nucleoli and condensed chromosomes are not stained. These autoantibodies react with a nuclear protein of 100 kD, which is known as Sp 100. These antibodies are present in approximately 20% to 30% of patients with primary biliary cirrhosis, regardless of whether they also have AMA.

Immune Effectors Involved in Cholangiocyte Necrosis

The main targets of the immune reaction are cholangiocytes. Several arguments suggest that mitochondrial antibodies are not cytotoxic and are not responsible for this phenomenon. In effect, they are not always present in primary biliary cirrhosis. The severity of the disease is unrelated to the antibody titer. After liver transplantation, the antibodies persist in the absence of evidence of disease recurrence. The mitochondrial antibodies may be present in the absence of any lesion suggestive of biliary necrosis. Bile duct destruction is linked directly to the cytotoxicity of T lymphocytes or to cytokines produced by CD4 and CD8 cells in contact with biliary lesions. Data on cytokines network are poorly documented, and available results are controversial.

Epitopes Involved in the Immune Reaction Leading to Cholangiocyte Necrosis

Several lines of evidence suggest that the antigens recognized by the AMAs could be the target for T lymphocytes on cholangiocytes. In effect, the pyruvate dehydrogenase complex E2, or a cross-reactive molecule, is overexpressed on cholangiocytes, predominantly at the luminal domain, independent of the presence or not of circulating AMAs. The T lymphocytes of patients with primary biliary cirrhosis have cytotoxicity activity against autologous cholangiocytes. CD4 T cells, specific for pyruvate dehydrogenase, are present in the portal inflammatory infiltrate. The mechanisms leading to the hyperexpression of the M2 epitope at the luminal domain of epithelial cells are unknown.

Hypotheses Explaining the Immune Response

As in other autoimmune diseases, environmental factors have been incriminated in the genetically susceptible hosts. One such factor is bacterial infection, the main argument being cross-reactivity between AMAs and antigens of *Escherichia coli* or other mycobacteria *(Mycobacterium gordonii)*. The data indicate that these bacteria express an epitope in common with pyruvate dehydrogenase. In rabbits, injection of a lysate of *Salmonella minnesota* R-mutants elicits antibodies against mitochondrial antigens of 50 to 70 kD. As in primary biliary cirrhosis, these antibodies recognize the lipoyl domain of the E2 component of pyruvate dehydrogenase. In patients with primary biliary cirrhosis, mutants of *E. coli* represent a large proportion of bacteria found in the urine and the intestine. One characteristic of these mutants is a liposaccharide defect of the bacteria membrane, leading to an increased immunogenicity. Some experimental data suggest that the liposaccharide of the R-mutant forms, and

lipid A associated with it, might escape the reticuloendothelial system and be excreted in bile in patients with primary biliary cirrhosis. In other words, these compounds could be the target of the immune reaction and explain the production of AMAs through molecular mimicry, by a mechanism somewhat similar to that observed in HLA B27–positive ankylosing spondylarthritis.

Mycobacteria have been implicated in the pathogenesis of other granulomatous diseases. In one study, the presence of antibodies to *M. gordonii* was found in patients with primary biliary cirrhosis, but not in controls or in patients with other chronic liver diseases. These antibodies cross-react with the M2 autoantigens. The same authors subsequently reported the presence of mycobacterial DNA in the liver of patients with primary biliary cirrhosis. However, these findings have not been confirmed by other groups.

More than 80% of patients with primary biliary cirrhosis show abnormal sulfoxidation, compared with only 20% to 25% of healthy controls. Sulfoxidation is one step in the metabolization of certain drugs, especially chlorpromazine. Patients who develop cholestatic hepatitis on chlorpromazine have defective sulfoxidation. It is also one of the metabolic pathways leading to the production of endogenous sulfate. It has been postulated that this deficit could make patients with primary biliary cirrhosis more susceptible to the toxicity of certain endogenous compounds or some drugs.

Mechanisms of Progression of the Disease
(Fig. 14–3)

Disease progression is characterized by periportal lesions, ductular proliferation, fibrous and necroinflammatory septa, which progress between portal triads leading gradually to nodule formation, then to cirrhosis. The severity of bile duct inflammatory lesions and of ductopenia and the degree of severity of periportal lesions are highly related to the degree of fibrosis. By contrast, the degree of severity of biliary le-

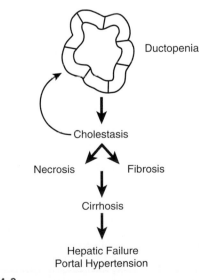

Figure 14–3
Progression of liver injury.

sions and the degree of periportal or lobular lesions are poorly correlated. Periportal lesions could be the consequence of immune aggression or the consequence of the cholestasis resulting from bile duct destruction.

DIAGNOSIS AND CLINICAL COURSE

Symptoms and Physical Examination

Before 1970, the diagnosis of primary biliary cirrhosis was often made relatively late. Patients presented in the terminal phase with cholestasis, signs of portal hypertension, and hepatocellular insufficiency. Now, most patients are diagnosed before the terminal phase; many are asymptomatic, whereas others have symptoms such as pruritus (Table 14–3).

Pruritus is seen in approximately 50% of patients at the time of diagnosis. It is generally intermittent, occurring mainly in the evening and at night. In 5% to 10% of patients, pruritus starts during the last 3 months of pregnancy, and this can lead to the diagnosis of cholestasis of pregnancy. The arguments against this diagnosis are the persistence of pruritus and laboratory test abnormalities after delivery, features that are never observed in cholestasis of pregnancy. Jaundice rarely precedes pruritus. A precise cause for the rise in serum bilirubin level should be identified in such a setting (e.g., drug-induced hepatitis, hyperthyroidism, migration of gallstones, and intercurrent diseases). The jaundice of primary biliary cirrhosis is usually a sign of poor prognosis, because it reflects the severity of the disease.

Currently, in about one half of cases, primary biliary cirrhosis is diagnosed in the absence of symptoms, but in the presence of abnormal liver test results, in particular increased serum activity of aminotransferases, γ-glutamyltranspeptidase (GGT) or alkaline phosphatase. In some patients, the diagnosis of primary biliary cirrhosis is made during the work-up for an associated autoimmune disease such as Sicca syndrome, Raynaud's phenomenon, or thyroid disease. In fewer than 10% of cases, primary biliary cirrhosis is now diagnosed in the terminal phase.

The physical examination is very important in primary biliary cirrhosis, because certain signs have prognostic

value and thus reflect the severity of the disease. Jaundice, hepatomegaly, splenomegaly, ascites, and edema point to advanced or progressive disease. Hyperpigmentation, cutaneous exfoliation, lichenification, xanthelasmata, and xanthomata have little or no prognostic value. Hyperpigmentation is most evident on the trunk, arms, and areas of exfoliation and lichenification related to pruritus. Xanthelasmata are frequent in female patients with marked hypercholesterolemia. Xanthomata are generally observed in patients with persistent hyperbilirubinemia. Bone pain resulting from osteopenia is now rarely observed at the time of diagnosis. Signs of peripheral neuropathy are frequent but must be carefully sought; they are most common in patients with Sjögren's syndrome.

Laboratory Tests

Most patients with primary biliary cirrhosis have abnormal liver tests characterized by mild elevation of aminotransferases (alanine aminotransferase [ALT] or aspartate aminotransferase [AST]) activity, frank elevation of GGT and alkaline phosphatase activities, and increased levels of immunoglobulins (mainly IgM). The increased erythrocyte sedimentation rate is constant. The changes in biochemical tests are strongly related to the stage of the disease and to histologic lesions. In our experience, the degree of elevation in alkaline phosphatase and in GGT is strongly related to the severity of ductopenia. The increase in aminotransferase activity and IgG levels reflects the degree of periportal and lobular necrosis and inflammation. Hyperbilirubinemia reflects the existence of cirrhosis. Thrombocytopenia is usually indicative of portal hypertension.

As in other cholestatic diseases, serum cholesterol levels—with a frank increase in high-density lipoprotein (HDL) cholesterol—are often elevated. In patients with severe disease, an increase in low-density lipoprotein (LDL) cholesterol, associated with the presence of lipoprotein X, is usually found.

Measurement of serum markers of fibrosis may be helpful. Hyaluronic acid level has been shown to be a marker of extensive fibrosis. Serum bile acid levels are not routinely determined. Serum bile acid levels are correlated with the degree of severity of histologic lesions, in particular with the degree of ductopenia and fibrosis. The main interest of repeated measurements of serum bile acids is the evaluation of the compliance to ursodeoxycholic acid (UDCA) treatment, and thus its efficacy.

Histopathology

Primary biliary cirrhosis is characterized by chronic, nonsuppurative cholangitis that mainly affects interlobular and septal bile ducts. The inflammatory infiltrate consists essentially of lymphocytes and mononuclear cells in close contact with the basal membrane of cholangiocytes undergoing necrosis. In some cases, the infiltrate consists of plasma cells, macrophages, and polymorphonuclear cells (especially eosinophils). The inflammation can take the form of epithelioid granulomas. They are present more often in the early stage of disease. There are few (if any) arterial lesions. In contrast, portal venules are often compressed and occluded by the inflammatory reaction. Bile duct destruction and pau-

Table 14–3   Clinical Features of 100 Consecutive Patients with Primary Biliary Cirrhosis at the Time of Presentation

Sign or Symptom	% Affected
Insidious onset of pruritus	57
Simultaneous onset of pruritus and jaundice	20
Postpartum persistence of pruritus of pregnancy	5
Jaundice preceding pruritus	2
Jaundice without pruritus	6
Portal venous hypertension	4
Hepatosplenomegaly	3
Discovery during an evaluation of another condition	4

Data from Sherlock S, Scheuer PJ: The presentation and diagnosis of 100 patients with primary biliary cirrhosis. N Engl J Med 289:674, 1973.

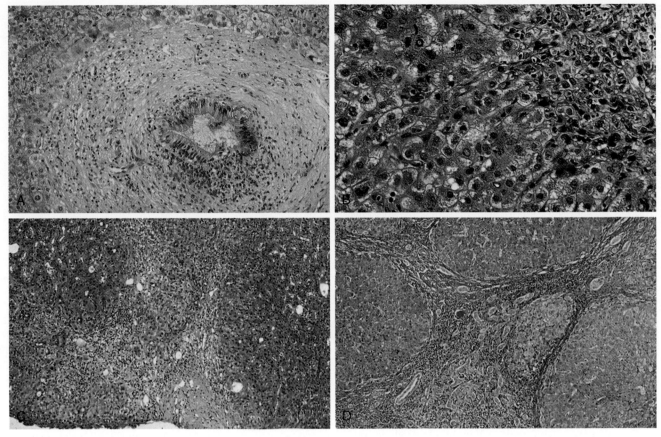

Figure 14–4
Histologic staging. *A, Stage I.* Nonsuppurative destructive cholangitis affecting a medium-sized interlobular bile duct. Biliary epithelium is partially destroyed. (Original magnification ×50.) *B, Stage II.* Proliferating ductules with rupture of the limiting plate. (Original magnification ×100.) *C, Stage III.* Inflammatory fibrous septa with aggregates of lymphoid cells. (Original magnification ×25.) *D, Stage IV.* Cirrhosis. Several regenerative nodules are seen. (Original magnification ×25.)

city are best assessed by determining the presence (or absence) of a bile duct relative to the presence of a branch of the hepatic artery. In normal liver, 70% to 80% of the portal arteries are accompanied by bile ducts. Bile duct paucity is usually defined by a percentage less than 50%.

Histologic lesions are classically divided into four stages (Fig. 14–4A–D). Stage I is characterized by portal inflammation and florid bile duct lesions. In this stage, inflammation remains confined to the portal triads. Disease progression is characterized by the gradual increase of periportal lesions, ductular proliferation, and periportal hepatitis (stage II). Periportal regions become focally irregular, and the lesion is characterized by cellular necrosis, separation of hepatocytes by inflammatory cells, and macrophages. Piecemeal necrosis is usually moderate, but, in some cases, it may be as severe as that observed in autoimmune hepatitis. Ductular proliferation is characteristic of stage II disease. It seems to be caused by metaplasia of periportal hepatocytes and their gradual acquisition of phenotypic characteristics of cholangiocytes. Stage III is characterized by a distortion of the hepatic architecture with numerous fibrous septa and periportal cholestasis. Cirrhosis (i.e., the existence of regenerative nodules) defines stage IV in the three classifications established by Scheuer, Popper, and Schaffner and by Ludwig and coworkers.

It is often difficult to distinguish these stages from each other. In fact, the lesions develop progressively at different rates in the different parts of the liver, such that an overlap between stages is usual.

Diagnosis (Fig. 14–5)

Diagnosis of primary biliary cirrhosis is usually very easy to make. To establish the diagnosis of primary biliary cirrhosis, the following criteria are mandatory: (1) biochemical evidence of cholestasis based usually on the elevation of both alkaline phosphatase and GGT activities; (2) presence of

Criteria Mandatory for Diagnosis

- Cholestasis

- M2 antibodies
  and/or
  Anti Sp100–Gp210

- Destructive cholangitis

Figure 14–5
Diagnosis of primary biliary cirrhosis.

M2 antibodies at a titer of 1/100 or higher when using immunofluorescence techniques; (3) histopathologic evidence of nonsuppurative cholangitis and destruction of small- or medium-sized bile ducts. The size of the liver biopsy specimen is critical. The probability of observing cholangitis and bile duct destruction increases with the number of portal tracts because of the patchy distribution of the lesions. At least 15 portal tracts should be present, and multiple sections should be reviewed to adequately appreciate or rule out cholangitis and ductopenia.

In approximately 5% to 10% of the patients, M2 antibodies are absent or present at a low titer ($\geq$1/100), when immunofluorescent techniques are used. In most, but not all, of the patients, antinuclear antibodies, anti-GP210, or anti-SP100 are present; in some of the AMA negative patients antibodies against the major M2 components (PDC E2, OGDC E2) are present using enzyme-linked immunosorbent assay (ELISA) or Western blotting techniques and finally elevated IgM levels are usually observed. In other words, in the absence of M2 antibodies, the diagnosis of primary biliary cirrhosis can still be made if GP210 or SP100 antibodies or frank elevation of IgM coexists with biochemical cholestasis and histopathologic evidence of bile duct lesions.

Differential Diagnosis

Some patients have characteristics of both *primary biliary cirrhosis* and *autoimmune hepatitis*. In those patients, the following features are found: strikingly elevated aminotransferase activity, moderate to severe piecemeal necrosis lesions, marked increase in IgG levels and sometimes anti-actin or antinuclear antibodies with homogeneous pattern by immunofluorescence. Patients who present with the characteristics of both diseases have been called "overlap syndrome" or "autoimmune cholangiopathy." In some patients, autoimmune hepatitis features occur in patients who initially have typical primary biliary cirrhosis. This mixed form must be identified, because in addition to UDCA treatment, they have to be treated with corticosteroids or even with cyclosporine.

Several drugs have been reported to induce cholestasis, cholangitis, and ductopenia. The most frequently incriminated drugs are phenothiazines, haloperidol, imipramine, amoxicillin, and clavulanic acid. Acute onset of cholestasis (sometimes associated with pruritus) is usually observed and resolves completely after several weeks or months after the medication is discontinued. AMAs are absent. Ductopenia, fibrosis, or even cirrhosis may occur.

Primary sclerosing cholangitis is characterized by chronic inflammation and fibrosis of intra- or extrabiliary ducts. In this setting, AMAs are absent. Cholangiography shows the classic stricturing and beading of the extra- and intrahepatic bile ducts. Liver biopsy shows the concentric periductular fibrosis that leads to progressive atrophy or even to the disappearance of bile ducts.

Sarcoidosis can cause real diagnostic difficulty. Characteristics of these two diseases are compared in Table 14–4. Sarcoidosis and primary biliary cirrhosis usually have distinct characteristics that allow clear distinction between the entities. However, sarcoidosis may be complicated by severe chronic cholestatis and portal hypertension, a clinical form that can mimic primary biliary cirrhosis. Finally, sarcoidosis and primary biliary cirrhosis may coexist in a single patient.

Idiopathic adulthood ductopenia is a term proposed by Ludwig and coworkers to describe a form of chronic cholestatis of unknown origin with clinical onset in adulthood, and associated with loss of intrahepatic bile ducts. In these patients, antimitochondrial antibodies are absent; there is no drug history; and cholangiographic findings show a normal biliary tree.

Associated Disorders

Associated disorders and their frequencies are given in Table 14–5. Scleroderma, especially minor forms, may be observed in approximately 10% of patients (sclerodactyly or CREST syndrome). Systemic forms are often limited to a

Table 14–4 Cholestatic Sarcoidosis Compared with Primary Biliary Cirrhosis

	Sarcoidosis	Primary Biliary Cirrhosis
Sex	Equal	80% Female
Age of onset	Young	Middle age
Pruritus	Yes (rare)	Yes (frequent)
Erythema nodosum	Yes	No
Respiratory symptoms	Yes (frequent)	Yes (rare)
Hepatosplenomegaly	Yes	Yes
Hilar adenopathy	Usual	Rare
Pulmonary infiltrate	Yes	Rare
Positive mitochondrial antibody	No	90%
Elevation of angiotensin converting enzyme	50%	10%
Positive Kveim-Siltzbach test	70%	No

Table 14–5 Prevalence of Associated Manifestations of Primary Biliary Cirrhosis

Disease	Prevalence (%)
Scleroderma	6.5
Sjögren's syndrome	42
Raynaud's phenomenon	21.7
Skin lesions	7.8
Hyperpigmentation	26
Xanthomas	13
Arthropathies	36
Pulmonary disease	6
Osteopenia	8.3
Renal dysfunction	3.2
Urinary tract infections	2.3
Thyroiditis	7.4
Diabetes	6
Gallstones	7.8
Cancer (extrahepatic)	5

From a cohort of 217 patients with primary biliary cirrhosis followed from 2 to 6 years.

minor esophageal motor disorder or to a reduction in carbon dioxide diffusion capacity. Raynaud's phenomenon is usually observed in 10% to 20% of patients. Anticentromere antibodies, characteristic of CREST syndrome, are found in 10% to 20% of patients. Sjögren's syndrome, most often in its minor form, is frequent in primary biliary cirrhosis. Arthropathies and arthralgias are noted in 5% to 50% of patients with primary biliary cirrhosis. The clinical significance varies greatly. Thyroid abnormalities and antithyroid antibodies are observed in approximately 15% of patients with primary biliary cirrhosis. The most frequent forms are hyperthyroidism and Hashimoto's disease. Hyperthyroidism may be associated with a rise in serum bilirubin and aggravation of cholestasis.

Several cases of villous atrophy due to gluten intolerance have been reported in patients with primary biliary cirrhosis. The number of cases reported indicates more than a random association. Primary biliary cirrhosis should be suspected in a patient in whom celiac disease is discovered and liver test results are abnormal. A similar association has been reported in patients with sclerosing cholangitis. In this setting, contrary to primary biliary cirrhosis, a gluten-free diet led to an improvement in liver test results. Villous atrophy is sometimes asymptomatic.

The frequency of gallstones can reach 30% to 50% according to the duration and severity of the disease. It is higher in patients with cirrhosis. Migration of stones through the bile ducts can aggravate cholestasis. Treatment of hypercholesterolemia with clofibrate can lead to the formation of gallstones, which disappear when the drug is withdrawn. Supersaturation of the bile by calcium has been reported during long-term treatment with cholestyramine.

Pancreatic abnormalities have been reported in primary biliary cirrhosis, with pancreatogram alterations, mainly at the tail. A marked functional abnormality is rare. It does not generally explain steatorrhea, when present. This is usually observed in patients with marked cholestasis.

Lung involvement is frequent in primary biliary cirrhosis but is generally subclinical. Pulmonary fibrosis occurs most frequently in patients with CREST syndrome or Sjögren's syndrome. The hepatopulmonary syndrome, characterized by hypoxemia, and intrapulmonary vascular dilatation can also be observed in patients with advanced primary biliary cirrhosis. Pulmonary hypertension can occur in primary biliary cirrhosis, as in other forms of cirrhosis. The distinction between sarcoidosis and primary biliary cirrhosis is usually easy to make (see Differential Diagnosis).

Renal tubular acidosis, due to abnormal renal tubule function, is frequent but usually subclinical. An increased susceptibility to urinary tract infections has been reported but has not been confirmed in other studies. It has been suggested that neuropathies of both the peripheral and autonomic nervous systems are frequent in primary biliary cirrhosis and could be secondary to liver damage. Neuropsychiatric problems (e.g., anxiety, fatigue, depression) are frequent in women with primary biliary cirrhosis, especially those with Sjögren's syndrome.

The incidence of breast cancer would be higher in women with primary biliary cirrhosis. In contrast, the incidence of other cancers does not differ from expected rates.

The onset of pregnancy in patients with primary biliary cirrhosis has rarely been reported, because the disease usually occurs after menopause or causes amenorrhea. Pregnancy, especially in the last few weeks, induces cholestasis. Some cases of pregnancy have been reported in patients with primary biliary cirrhosis. It generally leads to an aggravation in cholestasis.

Complications of Primary Biliary Cirrhosis

Pruritus is present in approximately 70% to 80% of patients with primary biliary cirrhosis. It is usually moderate but can be severe in approximately 8% of cases. Pruritus is correlated with the degree of elevation of serum bile acid concentrations and the degree of severity of ductopenia. The pathogenesis of pruritus is unknown. Opiate antagonists (naloxone and namelfen) modulated the perception of pruritus and induced a withdrawal opiate syndrome, suggesting a possible role of endorphins.

In primary biliary cirrhosis, osteopenia is mainly caused by osteoporosis, whereas osteomalacia is rare. Osteopenia is present in 10% to 35% of the patients at the time of diagnosis. This frequency does not differ from that observed in other chronic liver diseases, such as sclerosing cholangitis, hemochromatosis, or chronic hepatitis.

Vitamin A, D, E, and K deficiencies can occur in primary biliary cirrhosis, especially in advanced or severe forms. This deficiency is mainly caused by malabsorption. The clinical manifestations of this deficiency are rare. Vitamin A deficiency must be corrected with care, because overdosage can lead to liver damage, particularly fibrosis. Vitamin D deficiency should be corrected, given the risk of osteopenia.

Portal hypertension is frequent in the course of primary biliary cirrhosis and develops generally after the onset of cirrhosis. In fewer than 5% of cases, portal hypertension or gastrointestinal bleeding may reveal the disease. Portal hypertension can occur in the absence of cirrhosis and may be caused by portal inflammation, compression of small portal venules, and regenerative nodular hyperplasia. Patients with primary biliary cirrhosis and portal hypertension complicated by gastrointestinal bleeding should first be treated with β-blockers and, in case of failure, with sclerosis or ligation of varices. If these treatments fail, liver transplantation should be preferred to a portacaval shunt.

Hepatocellular carcinoma appears to be a rare complication of primary biliary cirrhosis. When hepatocellular carcinoma occurs, the liver is cirrhotic. The low incidence of hepatocellular carcinoma is usually explained by the relatively late formation of regenerative nodules in the course of the disease.

PROGNOSIS AND TREATMENT

Most patients in whom primary biliary cirrhosis was diagnosed when asymptomatic will develop symptoms in the following years (Fig. 14–6). In a 40-month period, 10% to 30% of asymptomatic patients become symptomatic. The mean duration of the asymptomatic phase is extremely variable but is on the order of 6 years. The 5-year survival rate of asymptomatic patients is approximately 90%. After 5 years of progression, the proportion of survivors is significantly lower than in a paired control population. The duration of the symptomatic phase varies greatly but can last for

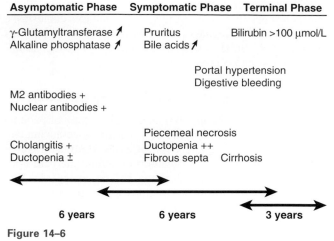

Asymptomatic Phase	Symptomatic Phase	Terminal Phase
γ-Glutamyltransferase ↗	Pruritus	Bilirubin >100 μmol/L
Alkaline phosphatase ↗	Bile acids ↗	
		Portal hypertension
		Digestive bleeding
M2 antibodies +		
Nuclear antibodies +		
	Piecemeal necrosis	
Cholangitis +	Ductopenia ++	
Ductopenia ±	Fibrous septa	Cirrhosis

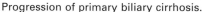

6 years   **6 years**   **3 years**

Figure 14–6
Progression of primary biliary cirrhosis.

10 years. The mean 5-year survival rate among symptomatic patients is 50%, with a range of 30% to 70%.

The terminal phase of the disease is defined when serum bilirubin level is higher than 100 μmol/L (6 mg/dL), with or without signs of portal hypertension (gastrointestinal bleeding, ascites, or encephalopathy). The disease progression is summarized in Table 14–6.

In 1979, Shapiro and coworkers showed the importance of serum bilirubin as a prognostic factor for survival in primary biliary cirrhosis. They noted that, after a relatively stable phase, serum bilirubin increased sharply in the months preceding death. In patients with serum bilirubin levels above 34 μmol/L (2 mg/dL), the mean survival was 4 years; in those with values above 102 μmol/L (6 mg/dL) 2 years, and in those with values above 170 μmol/L (10 mg/dL) 1.4 years. The extraordinary importance of bilirubin for short-term and long-term survival was confirmed in all later studies. Several prognostic models have been proposed to improve the prognostic value of serum bilirubin. These models are complex or are not highly superior to serum bilirubin alone. The Mayo Risk Score has been used as a prognostic index in patients with primary biliary cirrhosis (Table 14–7).

It is important to emphasize that the prognostic value of serum bilirubin level for survival free of liver transplantation is similar in UDCA-treated patients as in nontreated patients.

Medical Treatments

As primary biliary cirrhosis is known to be an autoimmune disease, most drugs used for its treatment have been selected on the basis of their immunosuppressive or anti-inflammatory properties. Figure 14–7 lists the main drugs and their therapeutic targets.

As with all chronic diseases, the most difficult choice for assessing efficacy is the endpoints. Survival is clearly a valid criterion of efficacy but creates a number of problems; for example: (1) the need for long-term follow-up of a large number of patients; and (2) ethical considerations if the treatment is ineffective or carries a high risk of side effects. One way of shortening the study period is to use surrogate markers. Given the lack of validated surrogate markers in primary biliary cirrhosis, survival free of liver transplantation appears to be one of the best endpoints. Finally, with a long-term treatment, the balance between benefit and adverse effects is of crucial importance.

Azathioprine, an immunosuppressive drug that is frequently used to prevent allograft rejection, was evaluated in two trials. Azathioprine had little clinical value and a slight benefit in terms of survival. Azathioprine is no longer used in the treatment of primary biliary cirrhosis.

D-Penicillamine was selected for its anticupr, eretic properties because copper accumulates in the liver of patients with primary biliary cirrhosis as much as in those with Wilson's disease, and it has immunosuppressive and antifibrotic properties. D-Penicillamine (tested in a total of 748 patients) had no therapeutic benefit on primary biliary cirrhosis but was associated with a high incidence of serious side effects (up to 30%). It has now been abandoned for the treatment of primary biliary cirrhosis.

In a 1-year trial, 36 symptomatic patients, who had no complications of cirrhosis were randomized to receive either prednisolone (30 mg/day, progressively reduced over 8 weeks to 10 mg/day maintenance dose) or a placebo. Pred-

Table 14–6 Progression of Primary Biliary Cirrhosis with Time (Cumulative Percentage of Patients with the Sign After 4 Years of Follow-up)

0 → 4 Years	%
Hepatomegaly	+30
Splenomegaly	+28
Ascites	+25
Gastrointestinal bleeding	+22
Cirrhosis	+50
Bilirubin >105 μmol/L (>6.2 mg/dL)	+25
Albumin <29 g/L	+35

From Christensen E, Crowe JP, Doniach D, et al: Clinical pattern and course of disease in primary biliary cirrhosis based on an analysis of 236 patients. Gastroenterology 78:236–246, 1980.

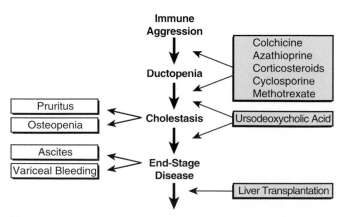

Figure 14–7
Main drugs for the treatment of primary biliary cirrhosis and their therapeutic targets.

Table 14–7   Calculation and Interpretation of the Mayo Risk Score for Primary Biliary Cirrhosis

Step 1: Calculate R
R = 0.871 × $\log_e$ (bilirubin in mg/dL) + (−2.53 $\log_e$ [albumin in g/dL]) + 0.039 age in years + 2.38 $\log_c$ prothrombin time in sec) = 0.859 (if edema is present).

Step 2: To obtain the probability of survival for at least t more years, one reads ($S_0(t)$ from the table below and computes $S(t) = [S_0(t)]^{\exp(R-0.57)}$

t(years)	1	2	3	4	5	6	7
$S_0(t)$	0.970	0.941	0.883	0.833	0.774	0.721	0.651

nisolone treatment improved aminotransferase and alkaline phosphatase activities, procollagen III peptide, and IgG but not serum bilirubin, pruritus, and fatigue in the first weeks; there was a trend to an improvement in liver histology. These beneficial effects were offset (in addition to the usual adverse effects of corticosteroids) by increased bone loss.

In a randomized clinical trial, 19 precirrhotic patients received cyclosporine (4 mg/kg/day) and 10 patients received a placebo. After 1 year, cyclosporine therapy improved pruritus, bilirubin levels, ALT and alkaline phosphatase activities, γ-globulin, and AMA titer. In a subgroup of 20 patients who have completed the 2-year study period, cyclosporine therapy apparently had a beneficial effect on liver histology; however, changes in liver morphology in such a small group of patients should be interpreted cautiously. Most patients had renal toxic effects and hypertension. In a large European trial (346 patients with a median follow-up of 2.5 years), cyclosporine therapy had similar effects on laboratory parameters but had no significant effect on histologic progression. The survival rate improved in the cyclosporine group by a multivariate analysis but not in a univariate analysis. This discrepancy could be explained by an imbalance between the groups at the time of randomization. Cyclosporine therapy has a very modest therapeutic effect and causes severe adverse effects.

Colchicine has been used for its antifibrotic and antiinflammatory properties. In a trial by Kaplan and coworkers, colchicine (0.6 mg twice daily) improved serum levels of bilirubin, albumin, alkaline phosphatase, cholesterol, and aminotransferase but not the severity of symptoms or histologic features at 2 years. At 4 years, there was a trend toward a decrease in mortality from liver disease but not from all causes. Similar results in terms of biochemical liver tests were reported in two other trials.

Although colchicine treatment was associated with an improvement in a number of liver tests, a beneficial long-term effect on disease progression remains to be established. Drug toxicity was minimal in all three studies.

The efficacy of colchicine combined with UDCA versus UDCA alone was evaluated in the treatment of patients with nonadvanced primary biliary cirrhosis in a 2-year controlled study. This study suggests that colchicine appears to provide a slight benefit relative to UDCA alone in these patients.

In 1988, Kaplan and coworkers first reported an improvement in symptoms and liver tests in two primary biliary cirrhosis patients treated with low-dose oral pulse methotrexate (15 mg/wk). In an open pilot study, these results were extended to nine women with symptomatic precir-

rhotic primary biliary cirrhosis who were treated for an average of 17 months. Liver histology improved in five patients and was stable in the remaining four patients. The improvement in histology was caused primarily by decreased portal inflammation and bile duct injury.

The combination of UDCA and methotrexate has been reported to improve alkaline phosphatase activity better than UDCA alone, but these results have not been confirmed. In one pilot study comprising 32 patients treated for 2 years, the UDCA-methotrexate combination was associated with substantial toxicity but had no additional benefit over UDCA alone.

The mechanism of action of methotrexate in primary biliary cirrhosis is unclear. At first, the choice of methotrexate seemed paradoxical, because long-term methotrexate therapy has been reported to be associated with liver toxicity. Kaplan and coworkers observed no hepatotoxicity of methotrexate, but the number of patients was small and the duration of treatment short. The potential hepatotoxicity of long-term, low-dose methotrexate administration is in fact controversial. Interstitial pneumonitis is an infrequent complication of low-dose methotrexate therapy in patients with psoriasis, but occurs in 3% to 5% of patients with rheumatoid arthritis. A higher incidence (14%) has been reported in patients with primary biliary cirrhosis. The use of methotrexate must be restricted to clinical trials until its safety and efficacy have been demonstrated.

In 1987, we postulated that long-term treatment with UDCA might displace endogenous bile acids from the enterohepatic circulation and thus reverse their suspected cytotoxicity. Several lines of evidence suggest that UDCA protects the liver by increasing the intrinsic ability to secrete bile acids and other organic anions into bile. Other possible mechanisms involve immune modulation—UDCA reduces both cholestasis and abnormal expression of HLA class I molecules on hepatocytes, and also possibly on biliary cells—and stabilization of hepatocellular membranes.

In a pilot study of patients with primary biliary cirrhosis, UDCA led to major sustained improvements in liver function tests. To determine whether UDCA would slow the progression of primary biliary cirrhosis toward the terminal phase, 73 patients with primary biliary cirrhosis were randomized to receive UDCA (13 to 15 mg/kg/day) and 73 the placebo for 2 years. After 2 years of treatment with UDCA, the proportion of patients with clinically overt disease had fallen significantly; in particular, there was a clear improvement in the severity of pruritus. Patients receiving UDCA showed significant improvements in serum bilirubin levels, alkaline phosphatase, aminotransferase and GGT activities, cholesterol and IgM levels, the AMA titer, and the Mayo risk score. There was a significant improvement in the mean histologic score and in all histologic features except fibrosis in the treated group.

Because of the patient selection criteria and the short duration of follow-up, there were few liver transplantations, thus preventing any comparison between the two groups on this criteria. Given the benefit of UDCA, all patients completing the study received UDCA in open label fashion and were monitored for a further 2-year period. The incidence of liver transplantation or liver transplantation/death was significantly lower in the patients who received UDCA for 4 years than in those initially receiving the placebo (Fig. 14–8).

By contrast, in two other large trials UDCA delayed the progression of the disease but did not reduce the need for liver transplantation. We therefore analyzed the combined

data of these three trials (548 patients) to determine the effect of UDCA on survival free of transplantation after 4 years of treatment in patients with primary biliary cirrhosis, no matter what the severity of the disease. We showed that long-term UDCA therapy improves survival free of transplantation.

Two important questions about UDCA therapy of primary biliary cirrhosis remain unanswered: (1) which patients are most likely to benefit from UDCA treatment? and (2) at which stage should UDCA be introduced? In our combined study, subgroup analysis showed that UDCA survival free of transplantation was improved in patients with moderate or severe disease. In patients with mild disease (serum bilirubin level <20 μmol/L, 1.2 mg/dL) an effect was not shown. However, these patients do not have time to progress to end-stage disease in 4 years; thus, longer follow-up studies will be needed.

Liver Transplantation

Orthotopic liver transplantation is the only therapeutic option for end-stage primary biliary cirrhosis. Most centers consider patients with primary biliary cirrhosis to be excellent candidates for liver transplantation, because they are usually young to middle-aged women without other major organ disease.

One-year survival following liver transplantation for primary biliary cirrhosis now exceeds 75% in most centers. An excellent 5-year survival rate of 71% was reported in the largest series (194 patients). Most deaths occur in the first 3 months and are caused by primary nonfunction, rejection, or infection.

Rehabilitation is usually excellent and as many as 94% of survivors return to work (at least part time). After liver transplantation, patients with primary biliary cirrhosis may expect prompt resolution of the symptoms and complications related to liver disease. Osteodystrophy tends to worsen in the first 3 to 4 months after transplantation, and then bone loss stops and bone mass is restored almost to normal within 2 to 3 years.

The effect of liver transplantation on extrahepatic manifestations of the autoimmune phenomena is more controversial. After liver transplantation, 90% of patients show some improvement in keratoconjunctivitis sicca, and approximately 50% show complete remission of these symptoms. Eighty percent to 90% experience an improvement in arthropathy and Raynaud's phenomenon. These effects may be caused by immunosuppression rather than by liver grafting itself.

There is significant controversy as to whether primary biliary cirrhosis recurs after transplantation. Serologic abnormalities in the form of raised IgM levels and AMA persist in most patients receiving transplant for primary biliary cirrhosis, but levels tend to decrease. Liver test abnormalities after transplant are nonspecific and cannot reliably differentiate the numerous causes of cholestasis in the liver allograft. Thus, considerable emphasis has been placed on histologic findings. However, even with biopsy, the risk of recurrence of primary biliary cirrhosis following transplant remains unclear. On the basis of histologic features "compatible with primary biliary cirrhosis," the rate of recurrence varies from 0% to 90%. The reasons for these varying re-

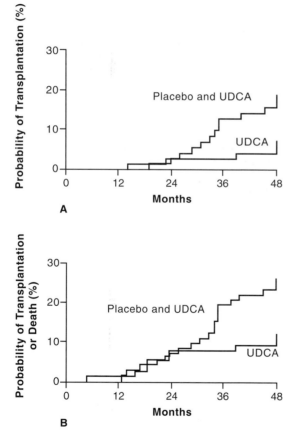

Figure 14–8

Probabilities of liver transplantation *(upper panel)* and liver transplantation or death *(lower panel)* in patients treated with ursodeoxycholic acid (UDCA).

During the first 24 months, patients were randomly assigned to receive UDCA or placebo; thereafter, all patients were treated with UDCA. The probabilities of liver transplantation, or transplantation, or death were significantly lower in patients treated 4 years with UDCA than in those who first received placebo (P = .003, RR 0.21, 95% CI 0.07–0.66; P = .005, RR 0.32, 95% CI 0.0.14–0.74, respectively). (From Poupon RE, Poupon R, Balkau B, the UDCA-PBC Study Group: Ursodiol for the long-term treatment of primary biliary cirrhosis. N Engl J Med 330:1342–1347, 1994. Copyright © 1994 Massachusetts Medical Society. All rights reserved.)

sults are probably related to the criteria used for diagnosis. The Mayo Clinic group has concluded that recurrent primary biliary cirrhosis can be diagnosed unequivocally only if the hallmark of the condition (i.e., granulomatous bile duct destruction) is found. Using this strict morphologic criterion, recurrence rates range from 0% to 8%. Recurrent primary biliary cirrhosis seems to have a good prognosis.

The efficacy of liver transplantation in patients with primary biliary cirrhosis was demonstrated definitively in 1989. The observed survival of 161 primary biliary cirrhosis patients who had undergone liver transplantation was compared with the predicted survival (Mayo model) of these same patients if they had been treated conservatively. Six months after liver transplantation, the survival probabilities in the liver transplant recipients were significantly higher than the Mayo predictions. These findings have been confirmed in additional studies.

The most difficult question to answer is not which treatment to choose but when to transplant. Liver transplantation should be performed while the patient is well enough to tolerate the operation, yet sufficiently late in the course of the disease to make it cost effective. The two current criteria for liver transplantation in primary biliary cirrhosis are progressive hyperbilirubinemia (above 100 to 150 μmol/L, 5.9 to 8.8 mg/dL) and/or ascites. A less common criterion is uncontrolled recurrent gastrointestinal bleeding. Intolerable pruritus or intractable fatigue is a highly subjective criterion and must remain an exceptional indication for liver transplantation.

Our approach to treatment is as follows: (1) to recommend UDCA for patients at an early stage of the disease, or (2) to refer patients in the terminal phase for transplantation. The stage at which UDCA becomes ineffective remains to be determined (onset of cirrhosis, extreme bile duct paucity?). Further studies are needed to define the patients who are most likely to respond to UDCA therapy and to assess the benefit of combined medical treatments.

SUGGESTED READINGS

Berg PA, Doniach D, Roitt IM: Mitochondrial antibodies in primary biliary cirrhosis: Localisation of the antigen to mitochondrial membranes. J Exp Med 126:277–290, 1967.

Christensen E, Crowe JP, Doniach D, et al: Clinical pattern and course of disease in primary biliary cirrhosis based on an analysis of 236 patients. Gastroenterology 78:236–246, 1980.

Flannery GR, Burroughs AK, Butler P, et al: Antimitochondrial antibodies in primary biliary cirrhosis recognize both specific peptides and shared epitopes of the M2 family of antigens. Hepatology 10:370–374, 1989.

Gershwin ME, Mackay IR, Sturgess A, Coppel RL: Identification and specificity of a cDNA encoding the 70-kD mitochondrial antigen recognized in primary biliary cirrhosis. J Immunol 138:3525–3531, 1987.

Hopf U, Stemerowicz R, Rodloff A, et al: Relation between *Escherichia coli* R (rough)-forms in gut, lipid A in liver, and primary biliary cirrhosis. Lancet 2:1419–1421, 1989.

Kaplan MM: Primary biliary cirrhosis. N Engl J Med 316:521–528, 1987.

Kaplan MM, Alling DW, Zimmerman HJ, et al: A prospective trial of colchicine for primary biliary cirrhosis. N Engl J Med 315:1448–1454, 1986.

Kaplan MM, Knox TA, Arora S: Primary biliary cirrhosis treated with low-dose oral pulse methotrexate. Ann Intern Med 109:429–431, 1988.

Lombard M, Portmann B, Neuberger J, et al: Cyclosporin A treatment in primary biliary cirrhosis: Results of a long-term placebo controlled trial. Gastroenterology 104:519–526, 1993.

Markus BH, Dickson ER, Grambsch PM, et al: Efficacy of liver transplantation in patients with primary biliary cirrhosis. N Engl J Med 320:1709–1713, 1989.

Mitchison HC, Palmer JM, Bassendine MF, et al: A controlled trial of prednisolone treatment in primary biliary cirrhosis: Three-year results. J Hepatol 15:336–344, 1992.

Popper H: The problem of histologic evaluation of primary biliary cirrhosis. Virchows Arch [Pathol Anat] 379:99–102, 1978.

Portmann BC, MacSween RNM: Diseases of the intrahepatic bile ducts. In MacSween RNM, Anthony PP, Scheuer PJ (eds): Pathology of the Liver. Edinburgh: Churchill Livingstone, 1987, pp 424–453.

Poupon R, Chrétien Y, Poupon RE, et al: Is ursodeoxycholic acid an effective treatment for primary biliary cirrhosis? Lancet 1:834–836, 1987.

Poupon RE, Balkau B, Eschwège E, Poupon R, the UDCA-PBC Study Group: A multicenter, controlled trial of ursodiol for the treatment of primary biliary cirrhosis. N Engl J Med 324:1548–1554, 1991.

Poupon R, Huet P-M, Poupon R, et al: A randomized trial comparing colchicine and ursodeoxycholic acid combination to ursodeoxycholic acid in primary biliary cirrhosis. Hepatology 24:1098–1103, 1996.

Poupon R, Poupon RE: Primary biliary cirrhosis. In Zakim D, Boyer TD (eds): Hepatology: A Textbook of Liver Disease, 3rd ed. Philadelphia: WB Saunders, 1996, pp 1329–1365.

Poupon RE, Poupon RE, Balkau B, the UDCA-PBC Study Group: Ursodiol for the long-term treatment of primary biliary cirrhosis. N Engl J Med 330:1342–1347, 1994.

Shapiro JM, Smith H, Schaffner F: Serum bilirubin: A prognostic factor in primary biliary cirrhosis. Gut 20:137–140, 1979.

Szostecki C, Will H, Netter HJ, Guldner HH: Autoantibodies to the nuclear Sp100 protein in primary biliary cirrhosis and associated diseases: Epitope specificity and immunoglobulin class distribution. Scand J Immunol 36:555–564, 1992.

Van de Water J, Turchany J, Leung PSC, et al: Molecular mimicry in primary biliary cirrhosis: Evidence for biliary epithelial expression of a molecule cross-reactive with pyruvate dehydrogenase complex-E2. J Clin Invest 91:2653–2664, 1993.

Vierling JM: Primary biliary cirrhosis. In Zakim D, Boyer TD (eds): Hepatology: A Textbook of Liver Disease, 3rd ed. Philadelphia: WB Saunders, 1990, pp 1158–1205.

Walker JG, Doniach D, Roitt IM, Sherlock S: Serological tests in diagnosis of primary biliary cirrhosis. Lancet 1:827–831, 1965.

Worman HJ, Courvalin JC: Autoantibodies against nuclear envelope proteins in liver disease. Hepatology 14:1269–1279, 1991.

Yeaman SJ, Fussey SPM, Danner DJ, et al: Primary biliary cirrhosis: Identification of two major M2 mitochondrial autoantigens. Lancet 1:1067–1070, 1988.

15

Primary Sclerosing Cholangitis

Denise M. Harnois
Russell H. Wiesner
Nicholas F. LaRusso

Primary sclerosing cholangitis (PSC) is a chronic cholestatic liver disease of unknown etiology characterized by fibrosing inflammation and destruction of the extrahepatic or intrahepatic bile ducts. PSC is a progressive disease, and over time the bile ducts become narrowed and obliterated. Patients are often asymptomatic at diagnosis, but in most, the disease progresses slowly over a 10- to 15-year period, leading to fibrosis and biliary cirrhosis, portal hypertension, and liver failure. Before 1980, no more than 100 cases of PSC had been reported. In contrast, PSC is currently one of the most common adult cholestatic liver diseases and is the fourth leading indication for liver transplantation in adults in the United States.

Seventy-five percent of patients with PSC are male, and the average age at diagnosis is 40 years. The disease is typically associated with inflammatory bowel disease (IBD) (at least 70%). The majority have ulcerative colitis (90%), and a smaller percentage have Crohn's colitis (~10%).

There is no effective treatment for PSC at this time, although several drugs have been evaluated in both controlled and uncontrolled trials. Preliminary data on ursodeoxycholic acid (UDCA), tacrolimus, and methotrexate show improvement in liver biochemistries with little benefit in histology, survival, or time to transplantation. Liver transplantation is the treatment of choice in patients with end-stage liver disease related to PSC. This chapter will review the epidemiology, pathogenesis, clinical presentation, and treatment modalities available in PSC.

EPIDEMIOLOGY

The prevalence of PSC in the United States is unknown; however, estimates can be made based on the close associa-tion of PSC and ulcerative colitis. Studies have shown a 2.4% to 7.5% prevalence of PSC in patients with chronic ulcerative colitis. Therefore, because there are 40 to 225 cases of ulcerative colitis per 100,000 population, it is estimated that the prevalence of PSC is two to seven cases per 100,000 population. An epidemiologic study from Sweden in 1991 supported this estimate and noted a prevalence of ulcerative colitis and PSC per 100,000 population of 171 and 6.3 cases, respectively. These estimates probably understate the actual prevalence because 20% to 30% of patients with PSC do not have coexistent ulcerative colitis, and patients with PSC may go undiagnosed since many are asymptomatic.

DISEASE ASSOCIATIONS

IBD occurs in 50% to 75% of patients with PSC, the majority of whom have ulcerative colitis. In addition, PSC is associated with an increased prevalence of autoimmune disorders and with a variety of other conditions (Table 15–1).

Table 15–1 Associated Diseases in Primary Sclerosing Cholangitis

Riedel's thyroiditis	Celiac disease
Retroperitoneal fibrosis	Chronic pancreatitis
Vasculitis	Sjögren's syndrome
Porphyria cutanea tarda	Immune thrombocytopenia purpura
Pyoderma gangrenosum	Lupus anticoagulant
Bronchiectasis	Systemic sclerosis

PATHOGENESIS

The cause of PSC is unknown; however, a number of possible mechanisms have been proposed including chronic portal bacteremia, toxic bile acid metabolites, chronic viral infections, and ischemic vascular damage. Genetic predisposition and immunologic abnormalities have been postulated to contribute to the pathogenesis and progression of PSC and are generally accepted as the most important etiologic factors.

Nonimmune Factors

Bacteria, Cytokines, and Toxins

Approximately 70% of patients with PSC also have IBD, more commonly ulcerative colitis than Crohn's disease. This close relationship led to speculation that portal bacteremia or absorption of toxins from an inflamed colon may have a major role in the pathogenesis of PSC. Early investigators described portal bacteremia in patients with ulcerative colitis who came to surgery and proposed that the primary event in PSC was chronic low-grade portal vein bacteremia that caused chronic biliary tract inflammation and fibrosis. Other investigators, however, were unable to demonstrate portal vein bacteremia in patients undergoing surgery for ulcerative colitis. Additionally, experimental portal bacteremia did not result in development of classic PSC. Support for this theory was also weakened by the fact that sclerosing cholangitis can develop before the diagnosis of colitis is made and the natural history of PSC is unaffected by colectomy. Furthermore, PSC is diagnosed in a substantial number of patients who have no histologic evidence of ulcerative colitis. All of this evidence suggests that portal bacteremia is not a major factor in the pathogenesis of PSC.

There is evidence to support the theory that a proinflammatory bacterial peptide may cause sclerosing cholangitis. In an experimental animal model, the toxic bacterial peptide product (N-formyl L-methionine-L-leucine 125-L-tyrosine, fMLT) was introduced into the colon of healthy rats and rats with experimental colitis, and an enterohepatic circulation of fMLT was demonstrated. Experimental colitis was associated with an 8-fold increase in biliary excretion of this proinflammatory peptide. A second study by Yamada and associates demonstrated that transrectal administration of fMLT in rats induced a marked inflammation in the portal triad and mild hepatocyte necrosis, which appeared to be more prevalent in the epithelial cells in the smaller bile ducts. Lichtman and associates showed that intestinal bacterial overgrowth in rats was associated with hepatic inflammation similar to that seen in PSC. However, the relevance of these findings to the pathogenesis of PSC in humans is unclear.

Cytokines mediate inflammatory reactions and have been proposed to be involved in the pathogenesis of liver diseases that are characterized by inflammation and fibrosis. Tumor necrosis factor (TNF), which was administered intravenously to rats, resulted in bile duct proliferation and portal tract inflammation, supporting the theory that TNF is involved in hepatobiliary injury. In a second study, pentoxifylline suppressed TNF release by Kupffer cells, reduced plasma TNF levels in rats with bacterial overgrowth, and prevented liver injury. However, studies have been unable to demonstrate a difference in TNF production in patients with PSC. Because the TNF locus is located within the major histocompatibility complex (MHC), genetic differences in or near the TNF locus could theoretically account for the known HLA associations in PSC. Other investigators have postulated that potentially toxic bile acids, such as lithocholic acid, arising as a result of increased bacterial activity in the colon are responsible for the development of PSC. This hypothesis has been refuted by studies that have been unable to demonstrate abnormalities in bile metabolism in patients with PSC.

Clinical evidence suggests that absorption of toxins through an inflamed colon may not play a major role in the pathogenesis of PSC, because many patients with PSC have mild or quiescent IBD. PSC has been documented to occur years before the onset of symptoms of ulcerative colitis, and in many cases there is never any clinical or histologic evidence of IBD. These findings suggest that portal bacteremia, absorption of bacterial products, and toxic bile acid metabolites related to the presence of colonic disease may not contribute in a substantial way to the pathogenesis of PSC.

Vascular Ischemia

The bile ducts are richly supplied by the hepatic vasculature, and obstruction of this arterial supply leads to ischemic necrosis and ultimately to the disappearance of the bile ducts and fibrosis. Hepatic artery infusion of 5-fluorodeoxyuridine (5-FUDR) as a treatment of liver metastasis from colorectal adenocarcinoma may induce occlusion of small hepatic arteries, resulting in sclerosing cholangitis, which is similar to PSC both histologically and cholangiographically. Bile duct disappearance is also a feature of chronic rejection following liver transplantation. Although this may partially be of immunologic origin, vascular ischemia may also be involved, because intimal thickening of hepatic arterioles can be seen. However, careful histologic analysis of the recipient bile ducts, peribiliary arterioles, and arteries in patients with PSC undergoing liver transplantation has failed to reveal evidence of vascular injury.

Viral Infections

Viral agents have been postulated to be involved in the pathogenesis of PSC. Cytomegalovirus infection (CMV) has been implicated, because this agent can cause interlobular duct damage and a decreased number of interlobular bile ducts. However, fibrosis and obliterative cholangitis, which are characteristic of PSC, have never been shown to be associated with CMV. Additionally, inclusion bodies that are characteristic of CMV have never been demonstrated histologically in the bile duct cells of patients with PSC. A study evaluating the liver tissue of patients with PSC by a polymerase chain reaction–based assay detected human CMV DNA in only 1 of 37 patients, suggesting that CMV replication and reactivation are not responsible for PSC.

Early reports also suggested the possibility that reovirus type 3 may have a role in the pathogenesis of PSC. Two studies showed that the reovirus type 3 induced cholangitis and biliary atresia in weanling mice and primates. However, more recent information has shown that titers of antibodies to this virus do not differ between normal adult control patients and those with PSC. Thus, there is no definitive evidence to support the theory that viral agents have a major ongoing role in the pathogenesis of PSC.

Immune Factors

Genetic Factors

Genetic factors have been postulated to play a role in disease susceptibility. In a study of 25 patients with PSC, HLA-B8 was present in 60% of patients with PSC, compared with only 25% of control subjects. An independent study confirmed HLA-B8 to be present in 80% of patients with ulcerative colitis and liver disease; additionally, HLA-DR3 was found in 70% of these patients. Therefore, a patient with ulcerative colitis who possesses the HLA-B8,DR3 haplotype has a 10-fold increased risk of developing PSC. HLA-B8 and DR3 are associated with a number of other autoimmune diseases; therefore, their increased prevalence is strongly suggestive that there are immunologic factors involved in the pathogenesis of PSC. In patients who do not possess this haplotype, HLA-DR2 was discovered in 69% of those with PSC compared with 34% of control subjects. HLA-DR52 has also been shown to be present in 70% of patients with PSC compared with 30% of controls. Another independent study did not confirm this finding. HLA status may affect the natural history of the disease, because the presence of HLA-DR4 may be associated with a more rapid disease progression.

Humoral and Cellular Immune Factors

Several features of PSC suggest that humoral immune factors have a role in its pathogenesis. PSC is characterized by lymphocytic infiltration and bile duct destruction, hypergammaglobulinemia, and increased serum IgM levels, all suggestive of an immune mechanism. PSC is associated with classic antibodies such as antimitochondrial and antismooth muscle antibodies, although more commonly seen in primary biliary cirrhosis (PBC) than in PSC. Antineutrophil nuclear antibodies and antineutrophil cytoplasmic antibodies (ANCAs) have also been found in high titers in patients with PSC. These antibodies have also been identified in patients with IBD, supporting the theory of a common immunopathologic mechanism in patients with ulcerative colitis and PSC. Several apparently unique antibodies have recently been identified in patients with PSC. Das and colleagues have identified an unusual epitope (or epitopes) on biliary epithelial cells that cross-reacts with a 40-kD colonic epithelial protein isolated from the mucosa of patients with ulcerative colitis. Circulating IgG antibodies directed against this 40-kD peptide were detected in two thirds of patients with PSC. The clinical implication of this epitope remains unclear.

Plasma complement fragments C3 and C4d have been shown to be significantly elevated in patients with PSC compared with patients with extrahepatic obstructive cholestasis and with normal control subjects. These findings support the hypothesis that circulating immune complexes

are involved in the pathogenesis of PSC; however, whether these are primary or secondary events related to the liver disease is unknown.

Biliary epithelial cells aberrantly express class II HLA and ICAM-1 molecules in PSC. The significance of aberrant MHC class II expression is unclear but suggests that biliary epithelial cells may present autoantigens to CD4 T cells or be more readily recognized as targets by cytotoxic CD8 T cells. Autoreactivity of T lymphocytes in patients with PSC has been demonstrated. Quantitative abnormalities of T lymphocyte subsets have also been identified. However, CD8 T cells are infrequently found in a peribiliary distribution in precirrhotic disease. indicating that they are unlikely to be primary effector cells in disease pathogenesis. The proportion of CD4 T cells in inflamed portal tracts is also decreased in PSC compared with other cholangiopathies. These findings suggest that biliary epithelial cells are targets of an immune reaction in PSC. The factors that induce and regulate this MHC class II expression are unknown.

CLINICAL FEATURES AND DIAGNOSIS

Signs and Symptoms

PSC has a male predominance of $2:1$, with an average age of onset at 40 years but a wide age distribution of 1 to 90 years. Patients may be asymptomatic at the time of presentation; however, most have cholestatic biochemical profiles. Seventy-five percent of patients will present with progressive fatigue, pruritus, or jaundice. Ascending cholangitis secondary to bacterial infection of the biliary tree, characterized by pain, fever, and jaundice, is unusual unless the biliary tree has been previously violated by a stricturoplasty or choledochoenterostomy. Other symptoms are those associated with chronic liver disease, such as weight loss, ascites, variceal bleeding from an esophageal or stomal source, and hepatic encephalopathy (Table 15–2). On physical examination, one half of patients will have hepatomegaly or jaundice. Splenomegaly, hyperpigmentation, and xanthomas occur less often than in patients with PBC. The initial physical examination may be normal in up to 50% of patients.

Biochemical Abnormalities

Abnormalities in serum alkaline phosphatase levels occur in virtually all patients with PSC. Serum levels of aspartate aminotransferase (AST) are increased in 90% of patients,

Table 15–2 Clinical Symptoms and Physical Examination Findings Associated with Primary Sclerosing Cholangitis

Symptoms and Physical Findings	Frequency (%)
Fatigue	75
Pruritus	70
Weight loss	40
Fever	30
Hepatomegaly	55
Jaundice	50

and the mean increase is approximately three times the upper limits of normal. At the time of diagnosis, one half to two thirds of patients with PSC will have an increase in their total serum bilirubin. Bilirubin levels fluctuate considerably, and a sudden elevation may suggest disease progression but more likely represents the development of complications such as a dominant stricture, common duct stone, or cholangiocarcinoma. Serum albumin levels and prothrombin time are commonly normal at the time of diagnosis but will become abnormal as liver failure develops. Tests related to copper metabolism, including serum copper and ceruloplasmin levels, are commonly increased in patients with PSC. Hepatic tissue copper levels are also increased in most patients reflecting the cholestatic nature of the disease.

Cholangiography

Current criteria used to diagnose PSC are based on the characteristic intrahepatic and extrahepatic changes seen on cholangiography of the biliary tree. Visualization of the biliary tree with endoscopic retrograde cholangiopancreatography or transhepatic cholangiography is therefore necessary to confirm the diagnosis of classic PSC. Typical cholangiographic features include multifocal stricturing and irregularity involving either or both the intrahepatic and extrahepatic bile ducts (Fig. 15–1). The strictures are generally diffusely distributed; they are short and annular, with inter-

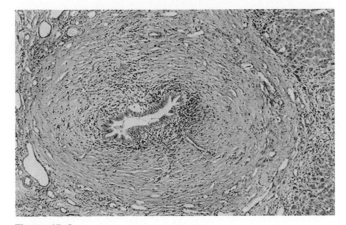

Figure 15–2
A liver biopsy specimen showing an intrahepatic bile duct with abnormal epithelium and concentric periductal fibrosis (H & E).

vening segments of normal or dilated bile ducts producing the classic "beaded" appearance. Diverticular outpouching occurs in 25% of patients with PSC. Pancreatic duct abnormalities are found in up to 15% of patients and resemble changes typically seen in chronic pancreatitis. However, PSC is rarely associated with clinical pancreatic insufficiency.

Histologic Appearance

The main features on liver biopsy specimens include periductal fibrosis and inflammation, bile ductular proliferation and biliary ductopenia. Fibrous obliterative cholangitis forming a classic "onion-skin" appearance is nearly diagnostic for PSC but is rarely present in biopsy specimens (Figs. 15–2 and 15–3). In patients with PSC, a liver biopsy is most helpful in disease staging, which in turn helps to determine the prognosis (Table 15–3).

There is a subset of patients who exhibit the biopsy and biochemical changes of PSC but do not have the classic

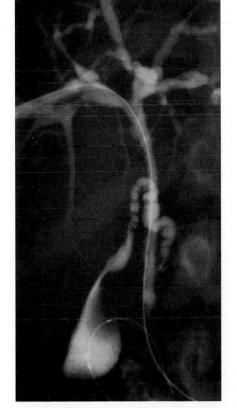

Figure 15–1
Typical cholangiographic features of primary sclerosing cholangitis include multifocal stricturing and irregularity involving both the intrahepatic or extrahepatic bile ducts.

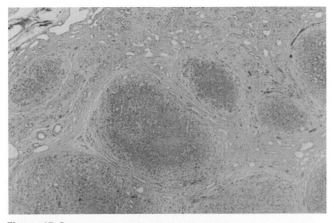

Figure 15–3
Liver biopsy specimen showing advanced fibrous obliterative cholangitis and cirrhosis in primary sclerosing cholangitis (H & E).

Table 15–3 Histologic Staging Criteria for Primary Sclerosing Cholangitis

Stage	Criteria
Stage 1 (portal stage)	Portal hepatitis or bile duct abnormalities, with little or no periportal inflammation and fibrosis
Stage 2 (periportal stage)	Periportal fibrosis with or without periportal hepatitis, or prominent enlargement of portal tracts with intact limiting plates
Stage 3 (septal disease)	Septal fibrosis or bridging necrosis, or both. Bile ducts are often absent or damaged. In the parenchyma, there is biliary and fibrosing piecemeal necrosis with associated copper deposition.
Stage 4 (cirrhotic stage)	Biliary cirrhosis. Bile ducts have often disappeared.

cholangiographic features. These patients are said to have "small duct PSC." Small duct PSC may occur alone or in combination with large duct PSC. The key lesion in the histopathology of small duct PSC is pleomorphic and fibrous obliterative cholangitis. The incidence, natural history, and pathogenesis of this variant remain unknown.

Differential Diagnosis

In the presence of IBD, PSC should be considered the probable diagnosis in a young to middle-aged patient who is found to have an elevated alkaline phosphatase. However, the differential diagnosis of liver disorders that can present with cholestasis include PBC, alcoholic hepatitis, drug-induced hepatitis, viral hepatitis, and autoimmune hepatitis. These disorders can generally be differentiated on the basis of clinical history, liver biochemistries, viral serologies, histology, and cholangiography.

Chronic cholestasis and bile duct paucity in adults, seen in PBC and PSC, are also associated with sarcoidosis, chronic graft-versus-host disease, and liver allograft rejection. The most useful test in distinguishing PBC from PSC is a cholangiogram. The extrahepatic ducts are not involved in PBC, and radiographic abnormalities present in the intrahepatic bile ducts in patients with PBC are usually easily distinguished from those in PSC. Other causes of chronic cholestasis include liver involvement in histiocytosis X and drug injury as described with phenothiazines and imipramine. Ductopenia in adults is labeled idiopathic when serum is negative for antimitochondrial antibody, the cholangiogram is normal, IBD is absent, and drug and viral injury can be eliminated. Investigation of human immunodeficiency virus (HIV)-infected patients has led to the recognition of a condition called acquired immunodeficiency syndrome (AIDS)–related sclerosing cholangitis. Typically, patients have pain in the right upper quadrant and an obstructive liver biochemistry profile. Ultrasound examination may show thickened bile ducts and less often bile duct stricturing or dilatation. The features on cholangiography are indistinguishable from those of PSC. In one study examining the natural history of AIDS-related sclerosing cholangitis, the median CD4 lymphocyte count was 240 (normal >500) with a range of 5 to 341. A potential infective cause has been identified in up to 75% of cases. Cryptosporidiosis has been most strongly linked to this disease entity and, to a lesser extent, cytomegalovirus.

TREATMENT

No specific therapy, except for orthotopic liver transplantation, has proved effective for PSC. Medical treatment strategies aimed at halting the progression of the disease have had disappointing results (Table 15–4).

D-Penicillamine

The finding of increased hepatic copper levels in patients with PSC provided the rationale for investigating the use of D-penicillamine therapy. A randomized placebo-controlled trial conducted at the Mayo Clinic and reported in 1988 showed no beneficial results on disease progression as measured by clinical, biochemical, histologic, radiographic, or survival parameters. In addition, 21% of patients receiving D-penicillamine reported side effects.

Methotrexate

Methotrexate was evaluated in a prospective placebo-controlled double-blind trial and reduced serum alkaline phosphatase levels but had no effect histologically on serial liver biopsies nor did it have an effect radiographically on endoscopic retrograde cholangiography (ERCP). There was also no appreciable effect on other biochemical parameters, such as bilirubin, aminotransferases, or albumin. There are currently no data to support the empirical use of methotrexate in treating PSC.

Corticosteroids

Trials utilizing corticosteroids have involved both topical application in the biliary tree and systemic administration. Most studies have been unable to demonstrate a long-term benefit from corticosteroid therapy. A prospective study of prednisone used in conjunction with colchicine demonstrated a temporary decrease in the serum levels of bilirubin and alkaline phosphatase at 6 and 12 months; however, these favorable effects had disappeared by 24 months. Additionally, use of corticosteroids for the treatment of PSC has been associated with enhanced loss of trabecular bone.

Table 15–4 Medical Therapy for Primary Sclerosing Cholangitis

D-Penicillamine
Methotrexate
Ursodeoxycholic acid
Corticosteroids
Azathioprine
Cyclosporine
Tacrolimus (FK-506)

This loss leads to an increased risk of developing osteoporosis and compression fractures.

Ursodeoxycholic Acid

The rationale for investigating the use of UDCA in the treatment of PSC includes evidence that it plays an immune modifying role by decreasing the expression of HLA antigens and inhibiting cytokine production. A second reason for using UDCA is based on the hypothesis that replacing the bile acid pool with a less toxic bile acid such as UDCA may decrease liver injury. Several small controlled trials have shown biochemical improvement in patients receiving UDCA. Recently, the results of a randomized, placebo-controlled trial of UDCA in the treatment of PSC were reported. In total, 105 patients with well-documented PSC were randomized to receive either UDCA (13 to 15 mg/kg/day) or placebo. The mean follow-up was 2.9 years. UDCA did not affect time until treatment failure defined by the endpoints of death, liver transplantation, or the development of cirrhosis. UDCA was associated with an improvement in liver biochemistries but not histology. UDCA is, therefore, not considered an effective therapy for patients with PSC when used as the sole treatment.

Other Immunosuppressive Agents

There are no controlled trials published using azathioprine or 6-mercaptopurine (6-MP) in the treatment of PSC. Azathioprine has been used sporadically, and anecdotal reports have been published showing both improvement and rapid deterioration in patients treated for PSC. Perhaps the most compelling data to support the contention that azathioprine and 6-MP are ineffective in the treatment of PSC is the fact that many centers have used these agents to treat IBD successfully but have noticed no improvement in associated PSC.

Cyclosporine therapy was also evaluated in a few patients in a controlled clinical trial. There was a significant decrease in serum alkaline phosphatase levels, but there was no effect on cholestatic symptoms, histologic progression, or progression to complications from end-stage liver disease.

Recently, the use of tacrolimus (FK-506) was reported in an open-label trial for the treatment of PSC. The study had a total of 10 patients, all of whom had a confirmed diagnosis of PSC and underwent pre-therapy evaluations, which consisted of serum liver biochemistries, percutaneous liver biopsy, and ERCP or percutaneous transhepatic cholangiography. After a 1-year follow-up, the alkaline phosphatase levels declined by more than 50%; the serum bilirubin levels returned to normal; and the AST and ALT levels both decreased. However, there were no observed changes in the cholangiographic findings, and there was little or no statistical difference between the pre and post therapy biopsies.

MANAGEMENT OF CHOLESTASIS AND ITS COMPLICATIONS

The complications that are commonly associated with a chronic cholestatic liver disease such as PSC include fatigue, pruritus, steatorrhea, fat-soluble vitamin deficiencies (vitamins A, D, and E), and metabolic bone disease. Fatigue, a common complaint of patients with PSC, may occur early in the disease and become more severe as the disease progresses. Little is known about the cause of fatigue, and short of liver transplantation, little can be done to relieve this symptom.

One of the most debilitating symptoms that occurs in PSC is the presence of pruritus. Despite the fact that pruritus is not clearly related to the accumulation of bile acid or its sequestration in the skin, most patients' symptoms can be effectively treated with bile acid-binding resins (e.g., cholestyramine). Other therapies that have been clinically effective in treating patients with pruritus include activated charcoal, methyltestosterone, ondansetron, UDCA, ultraviolet phototherapy, S-adenosylmethionine, phenobarbital, rifampin, plasmapheresis, and opiate antagonists such as naloxone hydrochloride and nalmefene.

Steatorrhea and malabsorption of fat-soluble vitamins are complications that occur in late PSC. Fat malabsorption in patients with cholestatic liver disease is generally related to a decreased secretion of conjugated bile acids into the small intestine. However, if steatorrhea develops in the absence of jaundice, then the presence of chronic pancreatitis or celiac disease should be considered. Asymptomatic vitamin A deficiency has been reported in 40% to 82% of patients with PSC; symptomatic vitamin A deficiency as manifested by night blindness has also been reported. Vitamin D and E deficiencies were only found in a few patients with early stage PSC. However, vitamin D deficiency was reported in 57% and vitamin E deficiency in 43% of patients with end-stage PSC undergoing evaluation for liver transplantation. This information suggests that these vitamin deficiencies may be more common than had been previously suspected. Additionally, elevated total serum cholesterol levels were reported in 41% of these patients. The clinical significance of this hypercholesterolemia and its impact on patient survival or the development of coronary artery disease is unknown.

Metabolic bone disease, and in particular osteoporosis, has been shown to be a frequent complication of patients undergoing evaluation for liver transplantation for PSC. Bone mineral density levels below the fracture threshold have been reported in 50% of patients with advanced PSC. Bone mineral densities did not correlate with serum levels of bilirubin, 25-hydroxyvitamin D, fecal fat excretion, or the presence or absence of chronic ulcerative colitis. Histomorphometric examination of bone from these patients showed increased bone reabsorption, reduced bone formation, and moderate to severe osteopenia with no evidence of osteomalacia. The pathogenesis and etiology of this osteopenia remains unknown, and there is currently no effective therapy to manage or prevent osteopenia associated with chronic cholestatic liver disease.

MANAGEMENT OF THE COMPLICATIONS OF PSC

Bacterial Cholangitis

Bacterial cholangitis generally occurs in patients who have had previous biliary surgical manipulation or in whom obstructing strictures of the large ducts have developed. The results of several open trials suggest that mechanical drainage techniques to relieve obstruction can improve symptoms. Many of these situations can be treated by endoscopic decompression, eliminating the need for surgery. Cholelithiasis and choledocholithiasis occur in up to 30% of patients with PSC. Transhepatic or endoscopic stone extraction and sphincterotomy or surgical intervention may be necessary to prevent the occurrence of bacterial cholangitis. The use of long-term prophylactic broad-spectrum antibiotics is controversial. Patients with a compromised biliary system (e.g., endoprosthesis in situ or hepaticojejunostomy) who are prone to develop recurrent cholangitis may benefit from antibiotic maintenance therapy given daily in lower than therapeutic doses. In these circumstances, use of ciprofloxacin and trimethoprim-sulfamethoxazole may reduce the risk of recurrent cholangitis.

Dominant Stricture

In approximately 20% of patients with PSC, a dominant stricture will develop. These strictures can occur at the hilum or anywhere along the common bile duct or common hepatic duct. Clinically, patients frequently present with fever, pruritus, and jaundice. If a dominant stricture is found on cholangiogram, a thorough investigation should be performed to rule out cholangiocarcinoma. If it is determined to be a benign stricture, then a balloon dilatation should be performed either endoscopically or transhepatically. It has been reported that 50% of patients with PSC who receive balloon dilatation of a dominant stricture will have improvement for up to 2 years. Dominant strictures may also be managed by surgical dilatation or choledochojejunostomy. One concern with biliary reconstructive surgery is that it may have an adverse impact on a patient's candidacy for orthotopic liver transplantation in the future. In a combined series from the University of Pittsburgh and the Mayo Clinic, prior biliary surgery was not found to adversely affect outcome. However, a study from France has shown that prior abdominal surgery increased transfusion requirements and hospital mortality at the time of transplantation. At UCSF and Johns Hopkins, prior biliary surgery increased operative time but had no impact on blood loss or mortality.

The difficulty in evaluating a dominant stricture is ruling out the possibility of cholangiocarcinoma. The incidence of cholangiocarcinoma in patients with PSC is between 10% and 30%. Patients with long-standing ulcerative colitis and cirrhosis on liver biopsy are at greatest risk. In patients with PSC, the diagnosis of cholangiocarcinoma is extremely difficult to confirm. This difficulty arises because biliary cytology and histologic analyses establish the diagnosis in only 50% of cases. Early reports suggested that serum concentrations of CA 19-9, a tumor-associated antigen, may be of value in detecting cholangiocarcinoma in patients with PSC. The sensitivity and specificity of a CA 19-9 value greater than 100 U/mL for cholangiocarcinoma in PSC were 89% and 86%, respectively. However, a subsequent paper reported that an elevated serum CA 19-9 level in a patient with stage IV PSC did not reliably predict coexisting cholangiocarcinoma. An index of two serum markers generated using the formula CA 19-9 + (CEA × 40) gave an accuracy of 86% in diagnosis of cholangiocarcinoma.

The prognosis of patients with cholangiocarcinomas is dismal. In the absence of treatment, life expectancy is less than 4 months. These tumors are insensitive to chemotherapy and radiation, and thus resection provides the greatest possibility for long-term survival. Even with resection, however, the prognosis is grim. In 1990, a collective series of 499 patients were reported to have a mean survival of 21 months following surgical resection. However, in a more recent study, Nagorney and associates reported a 5-year survival of 44% in a series of 49 patients without PSC undergoing a curative resection for cholangiocarcinoma.

Liver transplantation has been attempted for unresectable cholangiocarcinomas. Pichlmayr and associates reported the outcome of 50 patients with intrahepatic cholangiocarcinoma who underwent liver resection or liver transplantation. The median survival rates were 12.8 months in the group of patients after liver resection and 5 months after liver transplantation. The longest survival after transplantation was 25 months. Goldstein and associates reported a 1-year survival of only 53% and a disease-free survival rate of 40% in patients transplanted for cholangiocarcinoma. At this time, transplantation is reserved for a highly selected group of patients who have cholangiocarcinoma and should be done only in the context of experimental protocols.

Portal Hypertension

End-stage PSC is frequently complicated by portal hypertension. As with other causes of liver disease, esophageal variceal bleeding is best managed with banding or sclerotherapy. In patients in whom traditional endoscopic therapy fails to prevent bleeding, a transjugular intrahepatic portosystemic shunt (TIPS) should be considered. A TIPS procedure may also be helpful in managing patients with peristomal varices who have undergone a proctocolectomy for underlying IBD and who have an ileal stoma. Local measures such as ileostomy revision, venous ligation, and injection of sclerosants are generally unsuccessful. This complication may potentially be avoided by performing an ileoanal anastomosis procedure for patients with PSC who require a proctocolectomy for chronic ulcerative colitis.

Liver Transplantation

Liver transplantation is now considered the treatment of choice for patients with end-stage liver disease secondary to PSC. Indications for liver transplantation include intractable ascites, recurrent bacterial cholangitis, hepatic encephalopathy, failure to thrive, and complications of portal hypertension including hemorrhage due to esophageal or stomal varices. Results show that patients undergoing liver transplantation for PSC have a 1-year survival of 96.9% and a 5-year survival of 87.9%.

There is, however, an increased incidence of chronic ductopenic rejection, which results in graft loss, and an increased incidence of biliary strictures in patients posttransplantation for PSC. The Mayo Clinic has found evidence suggestive of recurrent PSC in 5 of 60 patients transplanted for PSC. The University of Pittsburgh reviewed the cholangiograms of 32 patients transplanted for PSC with biliary strictures and 32 non-PSC grafts with strictures. Both groups were matched for the type of biliary anastomosis (choledochojejunostomy) and for the time interval between transplantation and stricture diagnosis. The study revealed that mural irregularity and diverticulum-like outpouchings (findings that are suggestive of PSC) occurred more frequently in patients transplanted for PSC. In another study, liver allograft biopsies were examined from 22 patients transplanted for PSC, 185 patients transplanted without PSC, and 22 patients in whom a Roux loop was constructed for reasons other than PSC at the time of transplantation. Of the patients receiving transplants for PSC, 27% had biopsy specimens that showed fibrous cholangitis, and 14% showed classic fibro-obliterative lesions, compared with 5% and 0% in the Roux control group and 2% and 0% in the controls without PSC. However, the natural history of PSC following liver transplantation and the prevalence of recurrence is still uncertain.

A number of studies have confirmed that patients with PSC and ulcerative colitis have a significantly increased risk of developing colorectal neoplasia compared with patients with ulcerative colitis alone. In one study, the relative risk of colorectal cancer was elevated 10-fold compared with the general population for exposure to both sclerosing cholangitis and colitis but not cholangitis alone. Patients with IBD and PSC who undergo liver transplantation remain at increased risk for developing colon cancer. Therefore, even after transplantation, monitoring for colon cancer by annual screening colonoscopy and submission of biopsy specimens for evidence of dysplasia is recommended for patients who have had verified ulcerative colitis for 8 years or more.

PROGNOSIS

Natural History

Although many patients are asymptomatic at the time of diagnosis, prospective studies show that PSC is a progressive disease. The largest of these studies, from the Mayo Clinic, involved 174 patients with PSC with a mean follow-up of 6 years. The median survival from the time of diagnosis was 11.9 years, and both symptomatic and asymptomatic patients had a shorter life expectancy than did a US population matched for age, sex, and race. These results have also been confirmed at several other major centers with a median survival between 9 and 11 years. There is no relationship between the course of PSC and accompanying IBD.

Predicting patient survival on the basis of clinical, biochemical, and histologic features of PSC is important for determining the appropriate time for transplantation. The Cox multivariate regression analysis has facilitated the development of a prognostic model based on clinically useful variables. A survival score can be calculated and applied to individual patients. In a study of patients at five referral centers, age, serum bilirubin level, hepatic histologic stage, and the presence of splenomegaly were all variables that adversely affected survival (Table 15–5). In another model from King's College, patient age, serum alkaline phosphatase level, the presence of hepatomegaly or splenomegaly, and hepatic histologic stage were all independent prognostic variables. It is important, however, to remember that these models have not been evaluated prospectively, and additional studies are needed to test their application in the

Table 15–5   Prognostic Models for Primary Sclerosing Cholangitis

Multicenter group index = (0.535 × log e bilirubin mg/dL) + 0.486 × histologic stage + 0.041 × age (years) + 0.705 (if splenomegaly present)

King's College index = 1.81 (if hepatomegaly present) + 0.88 (if splenomegaly present) + 2.66 × log 10 (alkaline phosphatase IU/L) + 0.58 × histologic stage + 0.04 × age (years)

timing of liver transplantation and to refine their use in monitoring the effect of therapeutic intervention on disease progression.

SUGGESTED READINGS

Bergasa NV, Jones EA: The pruritus of cholestasis. Semin Liver Dis 13:319–327, 1993.

Beuers U, Spengler U, Kruis W, et al: Ursodeoxycholic acid for treatment of primary sclerosing cholangitis: A placebo controlled trial. Hepatology 16:707–714, 1992.

Brandt DJ, MacCarty RL, Charboneau JW, et al: Gallbladder disease in patients with primary sclerosing cholangitis. Am J Roentgenol 150:571–574, 1988.

Brentnall TA, Haggitt RC, Rabinovitch PS, et al: Risk and natural history of colonic neoplasia in patients with primary sclerosing cholangitis and ulcerative colitis. Gastroenterology 110:331–338, 1996.

Chapman RW, Varglese Z, Gaul R, et al: Association of primary sclerosing cholangitis with HLA-B8. Gut 24:38–41, 1983.

Das KM, Vecchi M, Sakamakis S: A shared and unique epitope(s) on human colon, skin, and biliary epithelium detected by monoclonal antibody. Gastroenterology 98:464–469, 1990.

Donaldson PT, Farrant JM, Wilkinson ML, et al: Dual association of HLA DR2 and DR3 with primary sclerosing cholangitis. Hepatology 13:129–133, 1991.

Duerr RH, Targan SR, Landers CJ, et al: Neurtrophil cytoplasmic antibodies a link between primary sclerosing cholangitis and ulcerative colitis. Gastroenterology 100:1385–1391, 1991.

Farges O, Malassagne B, Sebaugh M, Bismuth H: Primary sclerosing cholangitis: Liver transplantation or biliary surgery. Surgery 117:146–155, 1995.

Farrant JM, Hayllar KM, Wilkinson ML, et al: Natural history and prognostic variables in primary sclerosing cholangitis. Gastroenterology 100:1710–1717, 1991.

Forbes A, Blanshard C, Gazzard B: Natural history of AIDS related sclerosing cholangitis: A study of 20 cases. Gut 34:116–121, 1993.

Harrison RF, Davies MH, Neuberger JM, Hubscher SG: Fibrous and obliterative cholangitis in liver allografts: Evidence of recurrent primary sclerosing cholangitis? Hepatology 20:356–361, 1994.

Hay JE, Lindor KD, Wiesner RH, et al: The metabolic bone disease of primary sclerosing cholangitis. Hepatology 14:257–261, 1991.

Hay JE, Wiesner RH, Shorter RG, et al: Primary sclerosing cholangitis and celiac disease: A novel association. Ann Intern Med 109:713–717, 1988.

Heldwein W, Weinzier M, Pape GR, et al: Ursodeoxycholic acid for treatment of primary sclerosing cholangitis: A placebo controlled trial. Hepatology 16:707–714, 1992.

Jorgensen RA, Lindor KD, Sartin JS, et al: Serum lipid and fat soluble vitamin levels in primary sclerosing cholangitis. J Clin Gastroenterol 20:215–219, 1995.

Knox TA, Kaplan MM: A double blind controlled trial of oral-pulse methotrexate therapy in the treatment of primary sclerosing cholangitis. Gastroenterology 106:494–499, 1994.

Lichtman SN, Sartor RB, Kekee J, Schwab JH: Hepatic inflammation in rats with experimental small intestinal bacterial overgrowth. Gastroenterology 98:414–423, 1990.

Lindor KD, Wiesner RH, LaRusso NF, Hamburger HA: Enhanced autoreactivity of T-lymphocytes in primary sclerosing cholangitis. Hepatology 7:884–888, 1987.

Ludwig J: Small duct primary sclerosing cholangitis. Semin Liver Dis 11:11–1796, 1991.

Ludwig J, Kim CH, Wiesner RH, Krom RA: Floxuridine induced sclerosing cholangitis: An ischemic cholangiopathy. Hepatology 9:215–218, 1989.

Ludwig J, Wiesner RH, LaRusso NF: Idiopathic adulthood ductopenia: A cause of chronic liver disease and biliary cirrhosis. J Hepatol 7:193–199, 1988.

Mehal WZ, Hattersley AT, Chapman RW, Fleming KA: A survey of cytomegalovirus (CMV) DNA in primary sclerosing cholangitis (PSC) liver tissues using a sensitive polymerase chain reaction (PCR) based assay. J Hepatol 15:396–399, 1992.

Mehal WZ, Lo JM, Wordworth BP, et al: Hla DR4 is a marker for rapid disease progression in primary sclerosing cholangitis. Gastroenterology 106:160–167, 1994.

Minuk GV, Rascanin N, Paul RW, et al: Reovirus type 3 infection in patients with primary biliary cirrhosis and primary sclerosing cholangitis. J Hepatol 5:8–13, 1987.

Narumi S, Roberts JP, Emond JC, et al: Liver transplantation for sclerosing cholangitis. Hepatology 22:451–457, 1995.

Nichols JC, Gores GJ, LaRusso NF, et al: Diagnostic role of serum CA 19-9 for cholangiocarcinoma in patients with primary sclerosing cholangitis. Mayo Clin Proc 68:874–879, 1993.

Olsson R, Danielsson A, Jarnerot G, et al: Prevalence of primary sclerosing cholangitis in patients with ulcerative colitis. Gastroenterology 100:1319–1323, 1991.

Pichlmayr R, Lamesch P, Weimann A, et al: Surgical treatment of cholangiocellular carcinoma. World J Surg 19:83–88, 1995.

Porayko MK, Wiesner RH, Hay JE, et al: Bone disease in liver transplant recipients: incidence, timing, and risk factors. Transplant Proc 23:1462–1465, 1991.

Rosen CB, Nagorney DM, Wiesner RH, et al: Cholangiocarcinoma complicating primary sclerosing cholangitis. Ann Surg 213:21–25, 1991.

Sanaldi G, Donaldson PT, Magrin S, et al: Activation of the complement system in primary sclerosing cholangitis. Gastroenterology 97:1430–1434, 1989.

Sheng R, Campbell WL, Zajko AB, Baron RL: Cholangiographic features of biliary strictures after liver transplantation for primary sclerosing cholangitis: Evidence of recurrent disease. Am J Roentgenol 166:1109–1113, 1996.

Steckman M, Drossman DA, Lesesne HR: Hepatobiliary disease that precedes ulcerative colitis. J Clin Gastroenterol 6:425–428, 1984.

Van Thiel DH, Carroll P, Abu-Elmayd K, Rodriguez-Rilo H: Tacrolimus (FK506): A treatment for primary sclerosing cholangitis: Results of open label preliminary trial. Am J Gastroenterol 90:455–459, 1994.

van den Hazel SJ, Speelman P, Tytgat GN, et al: Role of antibiotics in the treatment and prevention of acute and recurrent cholangitis. Clin Infect Dis 19:279–286, 1994.

Vierling JM, Fennell RH Jr: Histopathology of early and late human hepatic allograft rejection: Evidence of progressive destruction of interlobular bile ducts. Hepatology 5:1076–1082, 1985.

White TT, Hart MJ: Primary sclerosing cholangitis. Am J Surg 153:439–443, 1987.

Wiesner RH, Grambsch PM, Dickson ER, et al: Natural history, prognostic factors and survival analysis. Hepatology 10:430–436, 1989.

Wiesner RH, LaRusso NF: Clinicopathologic features of the syndrome of primary sclerosing cholangitis. Gastroenterology 79:200–206, 1980.

Yamada S, Ishii M, Liang LS, et al: Small duct cholangitis induced by N-formyl L-methionine L-leucine L-tyrosine in rats. J Gastroeterol 29:631–636, 1994.

Chapter

16

Noncirrhotic Portal Hypertension

Kunio Okuda

Elevation of portal vein pressure (PVP) occurs in a number of disorders other than cirrhosis, and they are collectively called *noncirrhotic portal hypertension.* Although portal hypertension entails a serious sequela, such as variceal bleeding, mortality from variceal rupture is generally lower in noncirrhotic portal hypertension because of a better liver function compared with cirrhosis. The number of patients with an individual disease that causes noncirrhotic portal hypertension is relatively small, and our understanding of pathophysiology and epidemiology is limited at present.

Portal hypertension is generally defined as a PVP elevated above the upper normal limit of about 10 mm Hg. The mechanism of elevation of PVP and the pathologic changes causing portal hypertension vary with each disease. Portal hypertension is commonly classified according to the location of obstructive changes (i.e., prehepatic, intrahepatic, and posthepatic) along the vascular system, and intrahepatic portal hypertension is further subdivided into presinusoidal, sinusoidal, and postsinusoidal types. A typical example of prehepatic portal hypertension is extrahepatic portal vein thrombosis, and Budd-Chiari syndrome due to membranous obstruction of the inferior vena cava is a purely posthepatic portal hypertension. In this chapter, pathophysiology and clinical features related to noncirrhotic portal hypertension in individual disorders and management are discussed with less emphasis on the basic aspects of portal hypertension.

PATHOPHYSIOLOGY OF PORTAL HYPERTENSION

Changes in PVP is a function of the interplay between blood flow and vascular resistance. Resistance to the blood flow within a vessel is inversely proportional to the fourth power of the vessel radius, according to Poiseuille's law. Thus, theoretically, changes in the vessel diameter affect the PVP to a much greater extent than does the change in portal blood flow. The blood vessel systems that influence PVP encompass not only large portal vein branches but also the portal venules, sinusoids, hepatic venules, hepatic veins, and inferior vena cava. In clinical practice, wedged hepatic vein pressure (WHVP) and free hepatic vein pressure (FHVP) can be measured with relative ease by hepatic vein catheterization, but accurate determination of PVP is difficult because it requires an invasive technique such as portal vein catheterization. Measurement of splenic pulp pressure is less accurate, and it could cause intra-abdominal bleeding if the spleen is enlarged with increased PVP. It is generally assumed that in cirrhosis WHVP is close to PVP with a very small PVP-WHVP gradient, and the gradient between PVP or WHVP and FHVP is large. What WHVP represents, whether the sinusoidal pressure or the pressure in the portal inflow vessels, is still disputed. The wall of large vessels is an elastic structure that may undergo a hardening process, and the degree of loss of elasticity that also contributes to increased resistance is difficult to measure.

The reaction of the endothelium and intima of the portal vein wall to various chemical and mechanical stimuli and subsequent subendothelial changes are poorly understood. Injection of killed nonpathogenic colon bacilli into the portal vein in animals induces marked portal fibrosis without thrombotic changes and elevation of PVP within a short time. Although some investigators attempt to explain noncirrhotic portal hypertension by intrahepatic portal thrombosis, thrombosis is usually incited by endothelial damage and more likely by a secondary reaction to the primary change that occurs along the portal vein endothelium. There are many disorders with portal hypertension that are histologically characterized by portal fibrosis and sclerosis of the vein wall without evidence for thrombosis, such as schistosomiasis. Another difficulty that hinders full understanding of the pathophysiology of noncirrhotic portal hypertension is splenomegaly. Little is known about the function of the spleen and its influence on the portal hemodynamics. The size of the spleen is not correlated with PVP. Splenomegaly is milder in extrahepatic portal thrombosis compared with idiopathic portal hypertension (IPH), yet PVP is higher in the former. In a splenomegalic state, more lymphokines may be released from the spleen flowing into the portal vein system and affect the endothelium, but little information is currently available. Some patients with cirrhosis develop a huge splenomegaly, and others do not. Clearly, splenomegaly in cirrhosis is not a congestive spleen; some spleens weigh more than 1 kg in cirrhosis. Splenic blood flow is always increased in splenomegaly, and if it were caused by congestion, flow should be suppressed. In cirrhotic patients with splenomegaly, the difference between PVP and WHVP is much greater than that in patients without splenomegaly. Splenomegaly somehow increases intrahepatic presinusoidal resistance. In tropical splenomegaly syndrome, which is caused by chronic malaria, the hepatic vein pressure gradient is large, suggesting increased presinusoidal resistance.

It is now well established that in portal hypertension there is a hyperdynamic circulation within the splanchnic vascular bed. It is characterized by decreased arteriolar resistance that results in peripheral vasodilatation, and vasodilatation is accompanied by increased cardiac output. Such hyperdynamic flow is present not only in the splanchnic circulation but also in the systemic circulation. The mechanism for hyperdynamic circulation in portal hypertension is very complex and is not discussed in detail here. In the past, portal vein flow was thought to be reduced in liver cirrhosis, but we found by Doppler flowmetry that unless a hepatofugal flow occurs along the portal axis through a large collateral route, portal blood flow is not reduced. In fact, PVP somewhat decreases as portal systemic collaterals develop. In other words, portal blood flow and pressure are influenced by collateral circulation, which also contributes to the increased splanchnic blood flow. One of the questions is which contributes more to the development of portal hypertension—the increased portal resistance (backward theory) or increased blood flow (forward theory)? From the clinical point of view, the increased portal blood flow due to splenomegaly and reduced mesenteric vascular resistance seem to contribute to portal hypertension, just as much as does increased vascular resistance. Our national study in Japan found that splenectomy combined with devascularization reduced PVP from an average of 346 mm H_2O to 281 mm H_2O in patients (n = 321) with IPH. Without devascularization, the pressure drop would have been even greater.

The site of increased resistance influences portal hemodynamics to a varying extent. It is difficult to analyze the degree of contribution of sinusoidal changes to portal hypertension, because development of intrahepatic collateral circulation that originates in the lobule obscures the picture. Thus, the mechanism of intrahepatic portal hypertension is very complex, and there are very few purely presinusoidal or postsinusoidal morphologic changes. Even in IPH, which

is an example of presinusoidal portal hypertension, there are considerable sclerotic changes along the hepatic vein system, and WHVP is mildly to moderately elevated. The sinusoidal resistance within the hepatic lobule is perhaps subject to various humoral factors, structural changes along the sinusoid such as presinusoidal fibrosis and capillarization, and autonomic nervous control. Increased resistance in the hepatic vein system that includes the terminal hepatic venule also affects portal hemodynamics, elevating PVP and creating collateral circulation. In patients with veno-occlusive disease, WHVP is elevated considerably, but the pressure elevation is less remarkable as the site of resistance becomes more distal to the liver. Thus, splenomegaly is less pronounced in membranous obstruction of the inferior vena cava compared with IPH and noncirrhotic portal fibrosis. Encephalopathy, which is second to variceal bleeding as a major complication of portal hypertension, is rather uncommon in noncirrhotic portal hypertension, because the liver function is generally well preserved.

DIAGNOSIS OF PORTAL HYPERTENSION

A past history of gastrointestinal (variceal) bleeding and visible dilated abdominal veins, typically seen in Budd-Chiari syndrome, may be a hint for portal hypertension on physical examination. A more direct and practical diagnosis is provided by abdominal ultrasound. With ultrasound, the presence of ascites is recognized instantaneously, and splenomegaly is easily seen on the left lower intercostal scan (Fig. 16–1). The relative size of the spleen can also be measured. A dilated paraumbilical vein is easily recognized. Splenorenal shunts are identified as a multilocular structure near the splenic hilum, which on Doppler ultrasound is found to have a flow within it (Fig. 16–2). In the hands of an expert sonographer, an enlarged and winding left gastric vein supplying esophageal varices can be delineated (see Fig. 16–2). Portal vein thrombosis can be readily recognized and differentiated from an intraportal growth of tumor (mainly hepatocellular carcinomas [HCC]) by Doppler ultrasound. The blood flow is absent within a clot, or if present, it is hepatopetal (Fig. 16–3). In the case of HCC, flow in and around the thrombus is hepatofugal (Fig. 16–4).

Nonsurgical direct measurement of PVP is possible only by catheterization of the portal vein, which is achieved either via a percutaneous transhepatic route or by reopening the once occluded umbilical vein. Indirect measurement can be obtained by puncture of the spleen for splenic pulp pressure or of the liver parenchyma for hepatic pressure, which parallels PVP. Hepatic blood flow can be determined based on the Fick principle with a catheter in the hepatic vein using Bromsulphalein (BSP) or indocyanine green (ICG). Doppler flowmetry now permits measurement of portal blood flow volume, which is the product of the diameter of the portal vein and speed of flow, although the former is subject to considerable errors. The flow direction within the splenic vein can also be determined by Doppler ultrasound. It changes in the presence of a large splenogastrorenal shunt, which is frequently associated with hepatic encephalopathy, and Doppler can demonstrate it. A computed tomography (CT) scan is also useful, because it shows splenomegaly and large shunts, such as a dilated paraumbilical

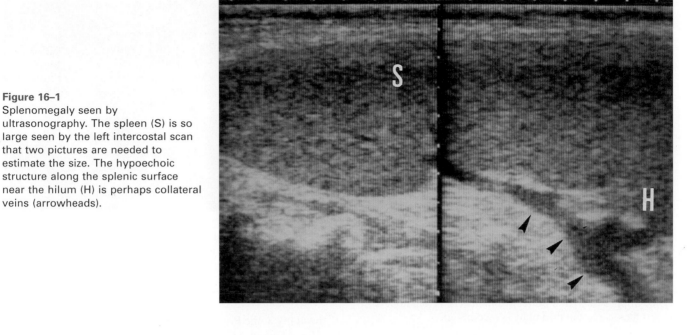

Figure 16–1
Splenomegaly seen by ultrasonography. The spleen (S) is so large seen by the left intercostal scan that two pictures are needed to estimate the size. The hypoechoic structure along the splenic surface near the hilum (H) is perhaps collateral veins (arrowheads).

vein (Fig. 16–5), paraesophageal varices (Fig. 16–6), and renal shunts. Magnetic resonance (MR) angiography is a new imaging modality that delineates collateral veins clearly without use of contrast medium (Fig. 16–7). Esophageal and gastric varices are seen indirectly by conventional barium swallow examination and more directly by endoscopy. Celiac arteriography delineates the portal axis (splenoportal) in its venous phase, and any hepatofugal collateral originating from the axis can be seen, such as left gastroesophageal varices. More direct and complete opacification of the portal vein system is possible by portal vein catheterization and contrast injection. It can be done after a pressure

measurement. If one can place one catheter in the hepatic vein and another in the portal vein, then Doppler measurement of portal flow speed and ultrasound measurement of the portal vein diameter permit calculation of portal venous resistance. The degree of intrahepatic and extrahepatic shunting can be measured by injecting two differently labeled radioactive particles at the splenic hilum and hepatic hilum within the portal vein and determining radioactivities retained by the liver and the lungs. The latter represents radioparticles that have bypassed the liver (extrahepatic shunts) and the intrahepatic collaterals. Several other methods can be used to estimate the degree of shunting.

Figure 16–2
Color Doppler ultrasonography for the diagnosis of portal hypertension.
A, markedly enlarged paraumbilical vein with flow within it. *B,* An enlarged left gastric vein flowing into the esophageal varices.
C, Splenorenal shunt at the splenic hilum. Doppler signal (colors) indicates winding blood channels.

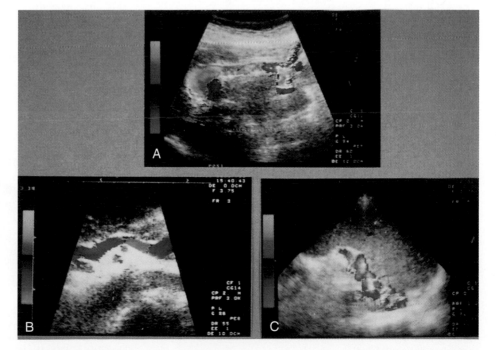

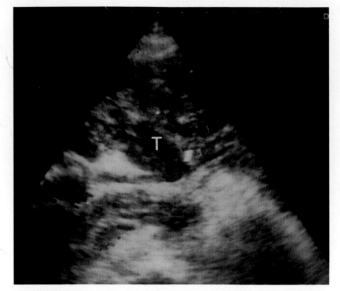

Figure 16–3
Color Doppler scan of a portal thrombus (T). A hepatopetal blood flow along the thrombus is recognized.

IDIOPATHIC PORTAL HYPERTENSION (HEPATOPORTAL SCLEROSIS, NONCIRRHOTIC PORTAL FIBROSIS)

This is an adult disease that corresponds to Banti's disease or syndrome, excluding known etiologies. The disease was first described toward the end of 19th century as a disorder characterized by splenomegaly and anemia with no hematologic or other causes. Subsequently, it was found that most such patients had a demonstrable etiology such as cirrhosis, schistosomiasis, and portal vein thrombosis. However, when Whipple analyzed 316 patients who underwent sple-

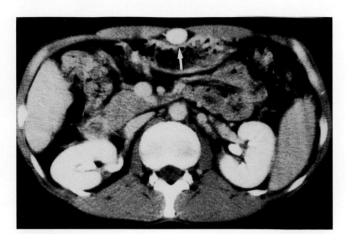

Figure 16–5
A large paraumbilical vein *(arrow)* in the midline of the abdomen is obvious in this contrast-enhanced computed tomography scan.

nectomy at the Presbyterian Hospital, New York, there were 26 patients in whom no obliterative factor was found along the portal vein system. In 1962 in Japan, Imanaga found that one third of his patients with portal hypertension were not cirrhotic at surgery and had intrahepatic presinusoidal obstruction. In the same year in India, Ramalingaswami noticed that a significant number of autopsy livers from patients with portal hypertension had no cirrhosis, but the portal tracts were very fibrosed. Indian investigators coined a term *noncirrhotic portal fibrosis* (NCPF) for this disease. Shortly thereafter in Los Angeles, Mikkelsen and his group, which included renowned pathologists Edmondson and Peters, described 36 patients with splenomegaly and noncirrhotic portal hypertension in whom marked phlebosclerosis was apparent in the intrahepatic and extrahepatic portal vein system. In more than one half of these patients, the portal vein was partially or completely occluded. They thought

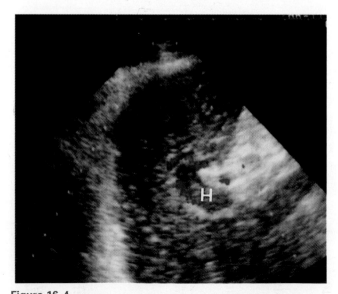

Figure 16–4
Color Doppler scan of a tumor thrombus (H, hepatocellular carcinoma) within the portal vein. Blood flow along the thrombus is hepatofugal.

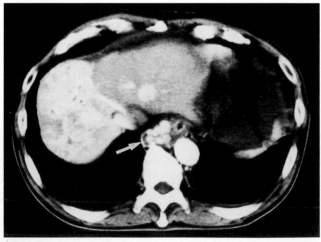
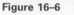

Figure 16–6
A widened paraesophageal structure was identified as paraesophageal varices (arrow) upon injection of contrast medium. The lobar attenuation difference is due to portal invasion of hepatocellular carcinoma.

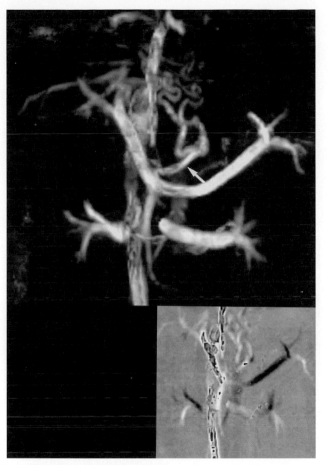

Figure 16–7
Magnetic resonance angiography by the phase-contrast technique (without contrast medium) clearly demonstrates the hepatofugal left gastric vein *(arrow)*. The black and white colors in the *inset* indicate the flow direction. The left gastric vein is flowing cephalad, away from the liver. (Courtesy of H. Abe, MD.)

that these cases shared the same unidentifiable etiology and that thrombosis was secondary to the sclerotic changes of the portal vein system, because portal thrombosis that frequently occurs in cirrhosis does not leave such severe phlebosclerosis. They called the disease *hepatoportal sclerosis*. It is not clear at the moment whether IPH of Japan, NCPF of India, and hepatoportal sclerosis of California represent the same disorder, but clinically they are very similar.

Diagnosis.   The definition adopted by the Japan IPH Study Committee (appointed by the Ministry of Health) has been a disorder characterized by splenomegaly, anemia, and portal hypertension without demonstrable diseases. The diagnostic criteria include: (1) splenomegaly, (2) normal to near-normal liver function tests, (3) demonstrable varices, (4) decrease of one or more of the formed elements of blood, (5) scintiscan not typical of cirrhosis and minimal bone marrow uptake of colloid, (6) patent portal and hepatic veins, (7) WHVP not as high as in cirrhosis, (8) grossly noncirrhotic, but frequently uneven liver surface, (9) marked portal fibrosis with no diffuse nodule formation, and (10) elevated PVP. Although not all of these criteria are necessary, portal hypertension must be unequivocal. In advanced cases, intrahepatic portal branches are frequently occluded in the periphery as seen by portography. However, in early cases, there is no evidence of portal thrombosis as shown in Figure 16–8.

Epidemiology.   It is generally believed that the so-called Banti disease was much more common in the past in Japan. When Banti first described the disease in northern Italy toward the end of last century, there must have been some cases corresponding to IPH, although his patients had various disorders. This disorder seems to have declined in incidence since then. There are no recent reports from north Italy. Of the 93 cases who were splenectomized by Whipple for Banti's syndrome cited earlier, 17 were caused by extrahepatic portal thrombosis and 50 by cirrhosis or schistosomiasis; 26 were idiopathic. At Los Angeles County Hospi-

Figure 16–8
An early case of idiopathic portal hypertension. Percutaneous transhepatic portogram shows a dilated splenic vein and portal trunk and unobturated portal vein branches. A large spleen is indirectly recognized from the size of the splenic vein in its hilum.

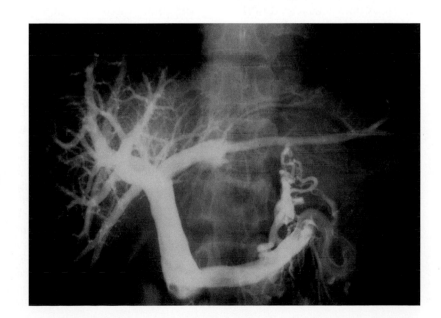

tal, a leading liver center in the world, there were 36 cases of hepatoportal sclerosis in 18 years (up to 1965). That means that it was very uncommon in California.

IPH has been designated in Japan as one of the intractable diseases, and the Japanese government pays the medical expenses for this disease if the patient is formally diagnosed as having IPH. Taking this unusual situation, an epidemiologic survey was carried out with the cooperation of major hospitals throughout Japan. It was estimated that there were 1376 patients with IPH in 1984 and that the incidence rate was $0.75/10^6$ population with an average morbidity of 12.5 years. In India, NCPF is more common in men with a reported male-to-female ratio of $2:1$ to $4:1$ and an average age of 30 to 35 years. In Japan, middle-aged women are more commonly affected and the female-to-male ratio is $3:1$ with an average age of 43 years (based on 624 cases). In the Mikkelsen series in the United States (US), 19 were women (48.7 years) and 17 were men (41.9 years). In a series in London in 1981, there were 16 women and 42 men with an average age of 46 and 36 years, respectively. These differences are perhaps due to the socioeconomic status of the population studied and to differences in diagnostic criteria, whether the material was autopsy or clinical, and how strictly portal vein thrombosis was excluded.

Pathophysiology. The liver is somewhat atrophic with shrunken areas and may have a wavy surface. The relative proportion of the left and right lobes may be grossly altered because of portal thrombosis and subsequent atrophy. At autopsy, large portal vein branches may have relatively fresh thrombi. Based on such findings, Wanless and Boyer suggest that intrahepatic portal thrombosis causes IPH. The IPH Study Group of Japan believes that thrombosis is secondary to sclerotic changes along the portal vein system, because early cases of IPH do not have portal thrombosis as studied by direct portography as shown in Figure 16–8. Some livers do not have demonstrable thrombosis at autopsy as in Figure 16–9. Splenomegaly is present from an early phase when there is no thrombosis, indicating that splenomegaly is not caused by congestion. It is well documented that portal venous flow is increased in IPH; it should be decreased in the presence of portal thrombosis. The onset is always insidious in IPH. If it is to be caused by large thrombosis, the onset is expected to be acute. There is no evidence of multiple thrombosis, which is common in patients with a hypercoagulable state.

The exact cause of IPH is still obscure, but the patients have a number of immunologic abnormalities. Autoantibodies are frequently demonstrable, and an ill-defined immunologic abnormality may underlie the disease. Experimentally, portal fibrosis mimicking IPH develops after intraportal injection of killed bacteria. Although suspected, there is no proof that repeated intra-abdominal infection causes IPH. Occasionally, patients with rheumatoid arthritis have splenomegaly and portal hypertension, but most patients with arthritis do not. It is a similar enigma. It is possible that some patients with IPH develop rheumatoid arthritis and are mistaken for having Felty syndrome, a subtype of rheumatoid arthritis. Histologically, there are no pathognomonic changes in the spleen, except for a marked hypertrophied red pulp. In the liver, the lobular architecture is maintained,

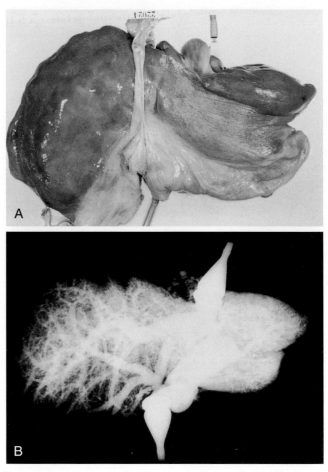

Figure 16–9

A, The liver in idiopathic portal hypertension. The surface is smoothly irregular but has no diffuse nodules. *B,* Postmortem portography and venography of a liver with idiopathic portal hypertension. The portal branches are seen all the way toward the periphery with no sign of thrombosis. (*A* and *B,* Courtesy of Prof. M. Okudaira.)

but the relationship between the portal and central areas is distorted in places. Collagen stain demonstrates irregularly distributed curly perisinusoidal fibers. The most marked changes involve sclerosis of the portal vein wall, which is thickened and sometimes hyalinized and is accompanied by perivascular fibrosis. The intrahepatic portal tracts are very fibrosed and expanded, and the small interlobular portal vein is so narrowed that its size may not be larger than that of the artery in the same portal tract (Fig. 16–10). Many aberrant vessels form around the portal tract. In peripheral portal vein branches, there may be obliterative changes caused by thrombosis, which Nayak and Ramalingaswami called *obliterative venopathy.* However, wedge biopsy from livers with IPH in Japan showed peripheral thrombosis in none of the 123 specimens studied by Kage and associates. Hemangiomatous changes in the Glisson capsule around large portal veins are secondary to thrombosis. The irregularly distributed parenchymal atrophy is clearly caused by reduced portal perfusion of the portal branch feeding that particular area; regenerative nodules of various sizes are commonly seen. If they are small, this may be an equivalent of nodular

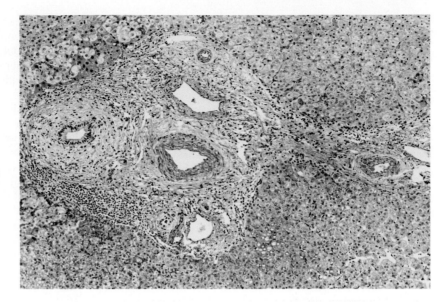

Figure 16–10
Portal fibrosis in idiopathic portal hypertension. The portal tract is markedly fibrosed with no evidence of cirrhosis. The size of the portal vein is about the same as an artery within the same portal area; normally, it should be five times the artery in diameter. The venous wall is also thickened.

regenerative hyperplasia, and a large regenerative nodule may form near the hepatic hilum, an equivalent of partial nodular transformation.

We studied the portal hemodynamics using the Doppler ultrasound and catheterization of the portal vein and the hepatic vein, and we measured various parameters in IPH in comparison with cirrhosis patients. The following were the results on average, IPH versus cirrhosis versus normal: liver volume (cm³), 912, 1102, 1328; portal flow (mL/min), 912, 660, 632; splenic volume (cm³), 688, 443, 143; splenic blood flow (mL/min), 407, 218, 120; PVP (mm Hg), 20.7, 22.3, 8.8; WHVP (mm Hg), 15.9, 23, 6.6; FHVP (mm Hg), 20.7, 22.3, 8.8; WHVP (mm Hg), 15.9, 23, 6.6; FHVP (mm Hg), 6.9, 7.1, 3.7; PVP-WHVP (mm Hg), no normal control, 6.3, 1.1; PVP-FHVP, 13.9, 17.3; PVP-FHVP, 9.1, 15.6; portal vascular resistance (mm Hg/mL/min/100 cm³ liver volume), 0.170, 0.320; presinusoidal resistance, 0.072, 0.021, postsinusoidal resistance 0.081 0.206, and intrahepatic shunt (%), 5.6 and 25.5. Thus, clearly hepatic blood flow is increased in IPH and so is splenic flood flow. The difference between WHVP and PVP is greater in IPH; the difference between WHVP and FHVP is greater in cirrhosis. Presinusoidal resistance is greater in IPH; postsinusoidal resistance is greater in cirrhosis; and cirrhosis has more intrahepatic shunt circulation. Thus, the site of portal resistance is mainly presinusoidal, but postsinusoidal resistance is just as much as presinusoidal in IPH, whereas in cirrhosis postsinusoidal resistance is 10 times the presinusoidal resistance.

Clinical Features. The most common clinical presentation is hematemesis, an incidentally found splenomegaly, anemia, and complaints associated with anemia. The physical examination demonstrates a large spleen and signs of anemia. Laboratory study shows pancytopenia compatible with hypersplenism. The weight of the spleen varies from 150 g to 2 kg with an average of 723 g in Japan. Colloid scintigraphy demonstrates a large spleen and a near-normal liver with no bone marrow uptake. Portography shows an enlarged portal vein axis with no thrombus and poor opacification of peripheral portal branches, suggesting narrowing

or occlusion. Venograms are unique in that the branches run smoothly with frequent vein-to-vein anastomoses. These venogram features are perhaps caused by parenchymal atrophy. The hepatic arteries are small, whereas the splenic artery is very enlarged and winding in its course, frequently forming an aneurysm at the splenic hilum.

Immunologic studies in IPH have shown that a significant number of patients are positive for various autoantibodies and less frequently have a coexistent autoimmune disease, such as thyroiditis, systemic lupus erythematosus, and Sjögren's syndrome; however, the test for lupus anticoagulant is negative. There is no evidence of coagulation factor deficiency or a hypercoagulable state. Hepatitis B and C are not associated etiologically

Treatment and Prognosis. The liver slowly undergoes atrophy, which is not necessarily progressive, and the liver's functional reserve is well maintained. The major cause of death is variceal bleeding. In rare cases, repeated uncontrollable bleeding may induce hepatic insufficiency. The survival curve for patients with IPH is somewhat between that for cirrhosis and for a healthy population of a comparable age. Management and prophylaxis of variceal bleeding are no different from those for cirrhotic patients. Because liver function is good, the risk of operative death is practically nonexistent, and some surgeons carry out a prophylactic operation for portal decompression or devascularization such as esophageal transection and Hassab operation. However, there has been no randomized prospective study on the efficacy of prophylactic surgery or sclerotherapy in IPH. Such studies are obviously needed; however, the difficulty is the small number of patients that each center encounters.

EXTRAHEPATIC PORTAL VEIN OBSTRUCTION

Definition, Epidemiology, and Pathophysiology. This disease is conventionally defined as obstruction in the prehepatic portion of the portal vein. The portal and splenic

Table 16–1 Past History in Extrahepatic Portal Obstruction

History	Age <20 yr (n = 93) %	Age ≧20 yr (n = 91) %
Hematemesis	24.7	36.3
Operation (not for portal hypertension)	8.6	34.1
Jaundice	5.4	14.3
Infectious disease	9.4	6.6
Disease of pancreas/biliary tract	1.1	14.3
Hepatitis	0	9.9
Alimentary tract disease	0	8.8
Trauma	2.2	2.2
Collagen disease	0	3.3
Blood disease	0	1.1
Parasitic disease	1.1	0
Neoplasm	0	1.1
Others	16.1	26.4
None	46.2	14.3

veins are continuous, but thrombosis within the splenic vein, not occluding the portal trunk, is not included in this disease. Splenic vein thrombosis is caused by a pancreatic disease or is associated with abdominal surgery, such as splenectomy and other abnormalities within the abdomen. The thrombus in the splenic vein or superior mesenteric vein may extend into the portal vein. Portal vein thrombosis is a common complication of liver cirrhosis, but it usually lacks a distinct clinical sign and is not included in extrahepatic portal vein obstruction (EHO). Difficulty arises when the first-order portal veins are occluded at the porta hepatis, whereas the portal trunk is patent. By definition it should not be diagnosed as EHO, but its pathophysiology is the same and should be treated as EHO.

EHO is a relatively uncommon disease in the Western countries. Webb and Sherlock documented 97 cases seen in 18 years up to 1970 at the Royal Free Hospital, London. Thus, a major liver center of the world sees several cases per year. By contrast, EHO is very common in India. At All India Institute for Medical Sciences, 87 cases of EHO and 83 cases of NCPF were treated in 6 years. In Chandigarh, 100 cases of EHO and 38 cases of NCPF were seen in an unspecified period. In Japan, EHO is less common than IPH. The incidence of EHO among 247,728 autopsies done in 1975 to 1982 was 0.055%. The IPH Study Group of Japan studied 184 surgically and angiographically confirmed cases of EHO in comparison with 469 cases of IPH. It was found that the epidemiology is clearly different, but both have similar clinicopathologic features. The age distribution demonstrated two peaks. There were more cases in the first decade, and another peak in the fifth decade. The number of patients younger than 20 years of age was about the same as the number older than age 20. There were slightly more men (male-to-female ratio of 1.2 : 1). In India, most patients with EHO are younger than 25 years of age, and only a few are older than 40 years of age.

There are many etiologic factors, and the cause of EHO varies with the patient. Studies in children with EHO have found frequent histories of umbilical sepsis and other infec-

tions. Catheterization for umbilical exchange transfusion does not seem to cause portal thrombosis frequently, however. In adults, the reported etiologies include intraabdominal sepsis, biliary tract disease, pancreatitis, appendicitis, pylephlebitis, duodenal ulcer, subacute bacterial endocarditis, postoperative infection, abdominal wound, hypercoagulable diseases such as polycythemia, and coagulation factor deficiency. Table 16–1 lists the past history elicited from the patients with EHO whom we studied. Although about half of young patients with EHO had no history that might cause portal thrombosis (so-called idiopathic), many of them could have had some infections not diagnosed at the time.

Liver pathology is not very characteristic. At operation for portal decompression or devascularization, the liver looks grossly normal. Histologically (wedge biopsy), there is portal fibrosis in about 40% of adult cases, but fibrosis is minimal or absent in children. If the intrahepatic portal branches are thrombosed, they are organized and recanalized, and the cut section looks like a sponge. It is not clear whether some of the adult cases of EHO with severe portal fibrosis in Japan are similar to the hepatoportal sclerosis cases in Mikkelsen's series who had portal thrombosis. The spleen is enlarged in EHO, but the weight is about two thirds that of the IPH spleen. In EHO, PVP is the pressure measured in the portal vein upstream from the obstruction. Little information is available regarding the difference in pressure between complete and incomplete obstructions. As shown in Table 16–2, WHVP is low in EHO, and clearly the portal obstruction or resistance is presinusoidal and most likely prehepatic. PVP in EHO is somewhat higher, but WHVP is lower compared with IPH, hence a greater difference (PVP-WHVP).

Clinical Features and Diagnosis. The presenting symptoms and signs are hematemesis, splenomegaly noted as an abdominal mass, anemia, abdominal distention due to ascites, and abdominal venous dilatation. Unlike IPH, hematologic changes are very mild if present. The averages in our study were: white blood cell count of 5000; red blood cell count of 3.7×10^6; hemoglobin level of 10.2 g/dL; and platelet count of 140×10^3. Liver function tests are only minimally abnormal and show average values: aspartate aminotransferase (AST), 38 IU/L; bilirubin, 1.5 mg/dL; γ-globulin, 20.8%; ICG clearance rate (k value), 0.132, a slight reduction; and normal albumin. Esophageal varices

Table 16–2 Portal Vein Pressure and Wedge Hepatic Vein Pressure in Extrahepatic Portal Vein Obstruction Compared with Idiopathic Portal Hypertension

| Pressure (mm H₂O) | EHO | | | |
	Age <20 (n = 93)	Age ≧20 (n = 91)	Average	IPH
PVP	389	352	371	334
WHVP	159	172	165	204
PVP—WHVP	229	180	205	132

EHO, extrahepatic portal vein obstruction; IPH, idiopathic portal hypertension; PVP, portal vein pressure; WHVP, wedged hepatic vein pressure.

were found in 90% of our patients, and gastric varices in 36%. Occlusion of the portal vein has to be demonstrated by ultrasound and more accurately by portography. In our survey, the portal vein, including the porta hepatis alone, was occluded in 71.5%; portal and superior mesenteric veins in 2.5%; portal and splenic veins in 13.6%; portal, superior mesenteric and splenic veins in 10.1%; and portal and other veins in 2.5%.

A fresh thrombus within the portal vein can be identified by ultrasound as an echogenic material within the lumen. Blood flow should then be studied by Doppler ultrasound in and around the thrombus. If it is a complete block, no flow signal will be obtained, and if incomplete or mural thrombosis, some flow signal will be obtained. A portogram is desirable for diagnosis, but nonsurgical direct portography is difficult technically. Figure 16–11 shows an uncommon finding in which a fresh portal thrombus was penetrated by a catheter that was passed percutaneously.

Cavernous Transformation. Portal obstruction is followed by formation of the so-called cavernous transformation. Cavernous or cavernomatous transformation was once thought to be a congenital malformation that mimics cavernomatous hemangioma. It is a hepatopetal collateral route consisting of many winding thin veins that can be readily identified by ultrasound as an irregular vascular structure near the hepatic hilum (Fig. 16–12). The mechanism of cavernous transformation remains an enigma. It is a venous neovascularization to compensate for the lack of portal venous flow into the liver. These thin veins enter the liver and then join patent intrahepatic portal branches at various levels, depending on the sizes of portal branches that were thrombosed. Clearly, some humoral mechanism is operative to form veins that carry blood from the mesenteric blood bed into the liver to make up for the reduction of nutrient rich portal blood flow. Cavernous transformation may be identified by superior mesenteric arterial portography and can also be indirectly suspected from a markedly widened

hilar portal area on CT. It develops even if the portal obstruction is incomplete whenever portal venous flow is reduced beyond a critical level. The time required to form cavernous transformation was estimated in patients with hepatocellular carcinoma in whom the cancer invaded the portal trunk; it was only several weeks.

Treatment and Prognosis. Management of variceal bleeding and encephalopathy is no different from that in cirrhosis and other portal hypertensive diseases. The most serious complication is thrombosis of the superior mesenteric vein, which may cause bowel infarction that requires an urgent surgery. Since the liver function is good, mortality from bleeding and encephalopathy is generally low, yet there are some fatalities from such complications. Incomplete portal obstruction or a web may be corrected by percutaneous transhepatic angioplasty. In the London series, 24 of 97 patients (25%) died between 3 weeks and 20 years, with an average survival of 10 years. Although disputed, prophylactic surgery for portal hypertension has been successful in Japan where the 10-year survival rate was 100% in 25 patients who underwent prophylactic surgery.

SCHISTOSOMIASIS (BILHARZIASIS)

Epidemiology. Of the three cardinal *Schistosoma* species, *S. japonicum, S. mansoni,* and *S. haematobium,* the first two are known to cause liver disease. *S. haematobium* mainly affects the urinary tract, but in an advanced stage, the liver also develops portal fibrosis. *S. japonicum* is capable of producing many more ova than *S. mansoni,* hence more severe liver disease. It is widely distributed in the world, particularly in China, Philippines, Laos, South Vietnam, Thailand, and Central Celebes. *Schistosomiasis japonica* was once called Katayama's disease because it was studied extensively in Japan, but since then it has been eradicated; no recent cases have been reported in this country. In China, it

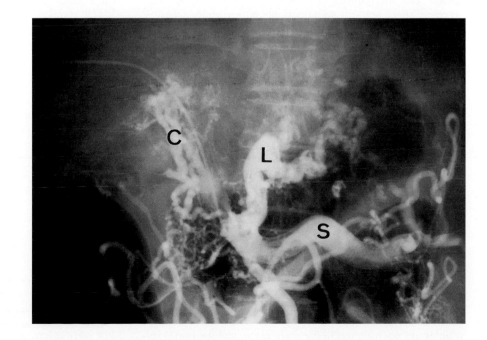

Figure 16–11
The catheter passed percutaneously through the liver penetrated a soft thrombus in the portal vein. Injected contrast medium opacified an enlarged left gastric (L); splenic vein (S); and cavernous transformation (C).

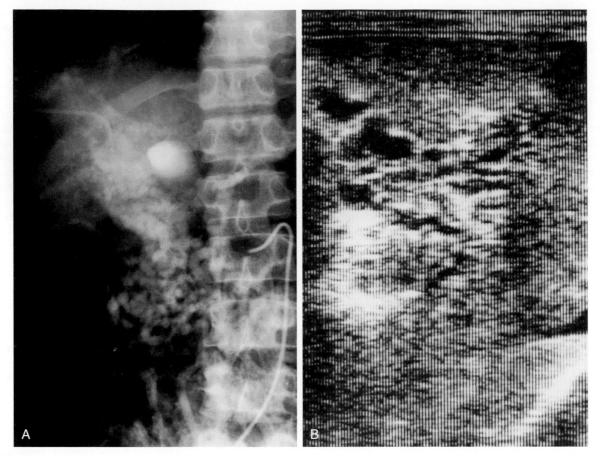

Figure 16–12
Cavernous transformation of the portal vein opacified by superior mesenteric arterial portography (A). The right panel (B) shows the ultrasound of the same, demonstrating an irregular vascular structure in the porta hepatis.

had been estimated that about 100 million people were infected. During the Mao regime, vigorous efforts were made to eradicate the disease. The campaign was partially successful, and the number of patients has clearly decreased; however, there are still some patients with chronic schistosomiasis. *S. mansoni* is endemic in lower Egypt, in most parts of Africa, Middle East, and South America. In Brazil alone, about 4.5 million people are infected.

The infection occurs when the cercariae enter the body through the skin, and adult worms eventually inhabit tributaries of the inferior *(mansoni)* or superior *(japonicum)* mesenteric veins. They lay several hundred to a thousand eggs per day for several years, then cease egg production. Their life span is 10 to 30 years. The ova that have flowed into portal venules and got stuck in the portal tract incite inflammation, which is followed by marked fibrosis.

Pathophysiology. The transition from acute to chronic schistosomiasis is insidious, and there is no clear definition of the time lapse to separate acute and chronic diseases. The major pathology is seen in the liver where inflammatory reactions occur due to the ova deposited in the portal venules. They are exudative, partially necrotizing, and granulomatous. Such reactions eventually lead to portal fibrosis, which increases with time. The reactions are incited by mechanical, chemical, and immunologic stimuli. The hepatic venules are not affected in the early stage, and the portal re-

sistance is mainly presinusoidal. However, changes are complicated and include the collapse of lobules by egg emboli and formation of wide fibrous bands. As the changes in the portal tracts advance, lobular distortion, destruction of portal venules, and intrahepatic collateral formation occur. Hepatic veins are affected due to circulatory disturbance as evident from WHVP in advanced cases (Table 16–3). Due to tissue collapse, the liver surface becomes grossly uneven

Table 16–3 Portal Vein Pressure and Wedged Hepatic Vein Pressure in Chronic *Schistosomiasis japonica* in Relation to Splenomegaly

Liver Histology	Splenomegaly	Average Pressure (mm H_2O)	
		PVP	WHVP
No fibrosis	No (n = 23)	161	138
	Yes (n = 5)	316	153
Portal fibrosis	No (n = 19)	188	141
	Yes (n = 13)	347	184
Cirrhosis*	No (n = 7)	267	294
	Yes (n = 8)	367	341

*Advanced schistosomiasis.
PVP, portal vein pressure; WHVP, wedged hepatic vein pressure.

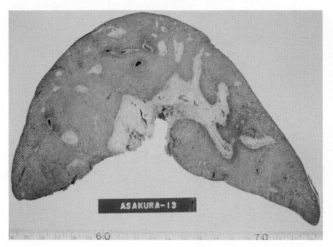

Figure 16–13
Schistosomiasis japonica showing a typical clay pipe-stem portal fibrosis in the cut section of the liver.

with bosselated areas and furrows, and the liver comes to look like a turtle shell in the case of schistosomiasis japonica. Kage and Nakashima grossly classified hepatic schistosomiasis japonica into the lobar, granular, mixed, and pipe stem types. With heavy deposition of eggs, and when they are calcified, plain x-ray film of the abdomen will demonstrate intrahepatic calcification. The portal vein may develop inflammation with a heavy egg load, and the vein wall may eventually calcify. A few patients with chronic schistosomiasis develop a huge splenomegaly. Again, splenomegaly does not reflect the degree of portal hypertension but is perhaps induced by an unknown diathesis of the person. During the clinical follow-up, splenomegaly develops within a relative short time as observed among the Japanese patients with schistosomiasis. The distribution of portal fibrosis is not homogeneous, and disfigurement of the liver seems to be related to the distribution of the worms within portal venules. More often, the lower anterolateral area of the right lobe undergoes severe atrophy, and on colloid scintigraphy, the liver assumes an inverted triangle configuration. In a strict sense, hepatic fibrosis is different from cirrhosis, and there will be no diffuse nodule formation in advanced schistosomiasis; however, the expression of "cirrhosis" has often been used for very disfigured livers. Severe gross change of the liver is uncommon in schistosomiasis mansoni, and rather the large portal tract expands with fibrosis to assume a picture called *clay pipe-stem fibrosis* (Fig. 16–13). Table 16–3 gives the PVP and WHPV measured in patients with schistosomiasis japonica. Again, the presence of large splenomegaly increased WHVP over that in nonsplenomegalic patients.

Clinical Features and Diagnosis.   In the acute stage, which mimics acute bacterial infection such as typhoid fever with fever and splenomegaly, there is no sign of portal hypertension. As the disease turns chronic and the liver develops portal fibrosis, esophageal varices, splenomegaly, and other signs of portal hypertension emerge. The degree of fibrotic changes is dependent mainly on the number of worms and ova deposited and on the duration of the disease. Many patients with mild fibrosis remain asymptomatic.

Even if the patient bleeds from esophageal varices, the liver function is usually good and the patient will survive if treated properly.

Laboratory study shows various grades of hypersplenism or reduced blood cells. Encephalopathy is uncommon without a precipitating factor, and so is ascites. If the disease is very severe, a decompensated state of the liver may develop with muscle wasting, hypoalbuminemia, and chronic ascites. Other coexisting factors, such as hepatitis B virus infection and alcoholism, may aggravate the clinical conditions and change the natural history. In the case of *S. mansoni,* extrahepatic manifestations have been described such as pneumonia caused by dead worms after chemotherapy and a mass formation along the colon.

Definitive diagnosis is made by the demonstration of schistosomal ova. It is done by biopsy of the rectal mucosa or the liver. Since the worms concentrate more densely in the distal colon, the rectal mucosa always has abundant ova. In patients with a very heavy egg deposition in the liver, the ova may be seen being released from the biopsy specimen when it is placed on the slide glass with a drop of saline and pressed by a coverglass; it clouds the saline.

Various immunologic diagnostic methods have been proposed and are in use, such as those based on complement fixation, hemagglutination, immunofluorescence, and immunoprecipitation. An enzyme-linked immunosorbent assay (ELISA) and enzyme-linked immunoelectrodiffusion assay (ELIEDA) have been used for schistosomiasis mansoni. For schistosomiasis japonica, the circumoval precipitin test (COPT) developed by Oliver-Gonzalez seems to be the most reliable. Radiologic examination using modern imaging techniques is also useful. A liver with advanced schistosomiasis is recognized by ultrasound from irregular hyperechoic bands, and calcified portal tracts are seen on plain CT (Fig. 16–14). The liver configuration may change to an inverted triangle on colloid scintigraphy, as already discussed. Liver histology shows numerous ova in the portal tract, and they are calcified if the disease is old (Fig. 16–15).

Treatment.   Currently used chemical agents for eradication of the worms in the acute stage of the disease are prazi-

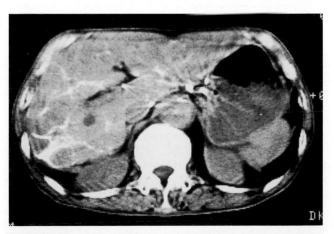

Figure 16–14
Computed tomography scan of the liver with schistosomiasis japonica. Irregular calcification of the portal areas is apparent.

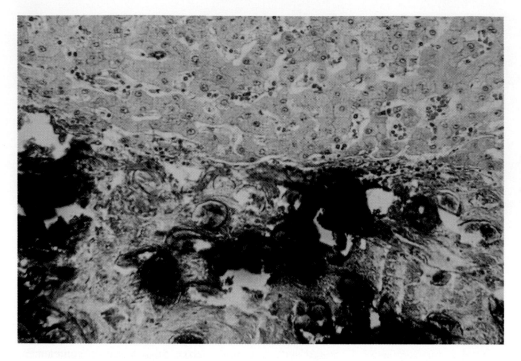

Figure 16–15
Calcified *Schistosoma japonicum* ova deposited in the portal tract.

quantel and oxamniquine. According to Caetano da Silva, the cure rate with oxamniquine is 80% in adults and 65% in children. Even if it does not kill all the worms, there will be a sharp reduction in egg laying. The side effects of this medication include dizziness, headache, and abdominal and muscle pains. However, in chronic patients, the worms no longer lay eggs and the patient may not require specific treatment. The adult worms lay eggs for several years after which egg production ceases. The eggs die within several weeks, and the interior of the egg is lost or undergoes calcification. Administration of toxic drugs may not benefit the patient. It is questionable whether prophylactic sclerotherapy or decompression surgery is indicated in patients who have not bled, but in patients who have bled, an elective measure for the prevention of rebleeding is indicated, as in liver cirrhosis.

OBSTRUCTION OF THE HEPATIC VEINS

Obstruction of the hepatic vein or a block to hepatic venous outflow is mainly caused by hepatic vein thrombosis and compression by a space-occupying, expanding lesion. It is generally called Budd-Chiari syndrome, but the definition is not well established and some hepatologists (notably Ludwig and Benhamou) suggest other names. In hepatic vein thrombosis, the ostia of the major hepatic veins are often involved and the disease may be confused with an idiopathic type of Budd-Chiari syndrome in which the hepatic portion of the inferior vena cava (IVC) is the primary site of thrombosis. Hepatic venule obstruction is generally called venoocclusive disease and is discussed separately. Therefore, in this chapter, an attempt is made to separate primary hepatic vein thrombosis or obstruction and primary IVC thrombosis.

Etiology and Epidemiology. Malignant tumors may cause incomplete or complete obstruction of major hepatic veins, but obstruction is relatively uncommon. They more often invade the IVC first then the hepatic vein. The reports include hepatocellular carcinoma, renal cell carcinoma, Wilms tumor, adrenal carcinoma, and leiomyosarcoma of the IVC. In an Indian series, it occurred in 11 (8.9%) of 123 cases of Budd-Chiari syndrome, excluding primary IVC obstruction. In the regions of the world where hydatid disease is endemic, hepatic vein obstruction by echinococcosis is not rare. An enlarging cyst caused by *Echinococcus granulosa* may compress upon the hepatic vein, and *E. multilocularis* may directly invade a large hepatic vein to cause obstruction. Liver abscess itself may not obstruct the hepatic vein, but extending pyogenic inflammation induces thrombosis within a large vein. Hepatocellular carcinoma is known to invade into the hepatic vein, sometimes further into the IVC and right atrium, but in such cases, typical clinical presentation is masked because the liver is already markedly invaded by the cancer with severe clinical manifestations. Thus, infectious and parasitic etiologies show a geographic distribution with a large difference between developing and developed countries.

Hepatic Vein Thrombosis. There are often underlying thrombogenic conditions of which primary myeloproliferative disorders are the most common in Western countries. According to Valla, there are just as many latent cases of myeloproliferative disorder as cases of full-blown polycythemia vera. The latent cases may be diagnosed by a bone-marrow culture and by demonstration of erythroid colony formation. Other hypercoagulable conditions as a cause of hepatic vein thrombosis include oral contraceptive use, paroxysmal nocturnal hemoglobinuria, lupus anticoagulant and anticardiolipin antibodies, and pregnancy and puerperium. Coagulation factor deficiencies cause thrombosis in the venous system of the whole body but seldom result in hepatic vein thrombosis. Low levels of coagulation factors may be caused by hepatic failure rather than by congenital deficiency. In India, pregnancy and puerperium-associated hepatic vein thrombosis are often fulminant and the major causes of fatality. The exact relationship between pregnancy and hepatic vein thrombosis is not very clear, but it may increase the thrombogenic potential of an underlying coexistent coagulation disorder. Vasculitis as a manifestation of collagen disease may cause hepatic vein thrombosis, such as Behçet's disease, sarcoidosis, and immunoallergic vasculitis. Certain drugs, such as dacarbazine, causes hepatic vein thrombosis by an immunoallergic mechanism, but it primarily affects small hepatic veins, and thrombosis extends into larger veins. In most studies, a considerable proportion of the cases were idiopathic, but in the French series, almost 90% of the patients had demonstrable underlying or etiologically associated disorders.

Pathophysiology.   A large part of the hepatic vein outflow tract must be occluded for clinical symptoms to develop. Patients with only one of the three major hepatic veins occluded may remain asymptomatic. Pressure increases in the sinusoids that drain into the affected vein and the flow within the upstream lobules decreases. Increased sinusoidal pressure causes sinusoidal dilatation and congestion, as reflected by hepatomegaly. Increased sinusoidal pressure increases hepatic lymph, and when the increase surpasses the capacity of the lymphatic drain, fluid of a high protein content leaks through the liver surface. A similar situation can be created in vitro in a liver perfusion system by raising the perfusion pressure. The liver surface acutely produces fluid like a sweating skin. It may mimic the state of the liver immediately after intraoperative ligation of the hepatic vein. A fluid with a protein content close to that of plasma comes out of the liver surface. However, in an actual patient with hepatic vein thrombosis, ascites does not have such a high protein level, perhaps due to changes in the permeability of the sinusoid wall and dilution by a low protein fluid coming from the mesentery.

Beside the three major hepatic veins, the liver has one vein caudal to them, namely the inferior right hepatic vein. In almost one half of the patients, this vein is not affected during the first attack. The flow within this vein greatly increases and compensates for the lack of flow in the other veins, resulting in a marked enlargement of the caudate lobe. A gross disfigurement is readily seen by ultrasound and CT, and upon injection of radiocolloid, the activity concentrates in the enlarged caudate lobe in a central concentration of radioactivity.

After thrombosis, the blood coming from the hepatic artery has to leave the liver, and small and large collateral channels develop between the obstructed areas and the areas of the liver where veins are patent, or the parietal and diaphragmatic veins. The pattern of collateral route formation varies greatly with each patient, with intra- and extrahepatic collaterals eventually going into the hemiazygos and azygos in retrograde flow within the portal vein. Centrilobular congestion and ischemia cause centrilobular necrosis. Hepatic failure may ensue depending on the extent of thrombosis and the acuteness of the obstruction. It could be fulminant. Centrilobular necrosis is soon followed by fibrosis, and within a relatively short period compensatory regeneration becomes recognizable as a nodule formation. The liver

eventually develops congestive cirrhosis in which the spatial relationship between the portal tract and central vein is reversed from that found in conventional cirrhosis. Hemodynamically, WHVP and intrahepatic sinusoidal pressure are elevated, and so is FHVP, making hepatic vein pressure gradient very low.

Clinical Features and Diagnosis.   The patient with acute hepatic thrombosis typically presents with ascites, abdominal pain, and liver enlargement. Other common signs include splenomegaly, edema, jaundice, and fever. Hepatic encephalopathy and gastrointestinal bleeding are less common. In a fulminant form, which is rare, hepatic failure sets in within a few days with marked aminotransferasemia and renal failure. The severity depends on the number of veins involved. Some patients present with chronic disease with less prominent signs, such as progressive ascites and low-grade aminotransferasemia; however, these patients, if left untreated, may develop slowly progressive hepatic failure or gastrointestinal bleeding. Ascites is resistant to therapy and is very annoying for the patient. In a recent French experience the 3-year survival rate was 50%.

Diagnosis.   The three cardinal signs, ascites, abdominal pain, and hepatomegaly, should arouse suspicion of hepatic vein thrombosis in patients who have hematologic disorders quoted earlier and other thrombogenic conditions. Abdominal ultrasound should be carried out immediately. It will readily demonstrate hepatic vein thrombosis as an echogenic material within the lumen of one or more of the hepatic veins (Fig. 16–16). An enlarged caudate lobe may also be recognized. CT is also useful because it confirms the findings obtained with ultrasound. Injection of contrast medium will show in the early phase its concentration in the center of the liver or over the caudate lobe (Fig. 16–17). Space-occupying lesions as the cause of hepatic vein obstruction are readily found by CT and ultrasound. MR imaging is about the same as CT in its diagnostic capability. If the inferior right hepatic vein is patent, radiocolloid scintigraphy will show central concentration as al-

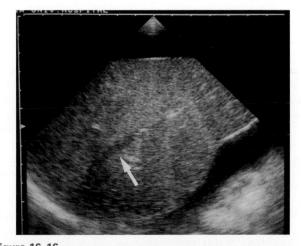

Figure 16–16
Ultrasound of the liver demonstrating a thrombosed middle hepatic vein *(arrow)* in Budd-Chiari syndrome.

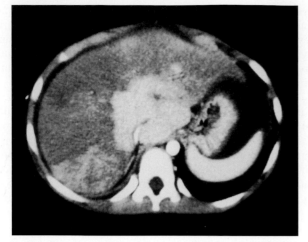

Figure 16–17
An enlarged caudate lobe is markedly enhanced by contrast medium on an enhanced computed tomography scan in Budd-Chiari syndrome. If the inferior right hepatic vein is occluded, no central concentration occurs.

ready described. A liver biopsy is not necessary to make the diagnosis, because imaging techniques suffice; however, in chronic cases, it may provide histologic information on the severity of hepatic fibrosis and cirrhosis. However, a diagnosis of hepatic vein obstruction may be difficult to make from biopsy alone in some of the chronic cases, because the liver shows only fibrosis without evidence for centrilobular congestion. In chronic cases, ultrasound will delineate collateral routes that have developed in and around the liver. With the aid of ultrasound, one can insert a thin needle into a patent portion of the hepatic vein and opacify the vein to demonstrate partial patency of the vein. Injection of contrast medium blindly into the hepatic parenchyma may show contrast flow into the portal vein when there is a retrograde portal flow. Catheterization of the hepatic vein through either the superior or the inferior vena cava may achieve opacification of a hepatic vein.

Treatment. In an acute case, further thrombosis must be prevented with heparin and a vitamin K antagonist. If the diagnosis was made in a very early stage of hepatic vein thrombosis, one can place a catheter in the affected hepatic vein through the vena cava and infuse a thrombolytic agent, such as tissue plasminogen activator (TPA), but its efficacy is uncertain. In a situation in which only the opening of the hepatic vein into the IVC is closed as a membrane of a short segment occlusion, transhepatic or surgical angioplasty is possible. Dorsocranial liver resection and direct hepatoatrial anastomosis have been attempted. The surgical approach depends on the status of the IVC and the portal vein. In the absence of obstruction in the IVC and portal vein, a side-to-side portacaval shunt or a mesocaval shunt is the choice in order to restore an outflow tract. Liver transplantation is indicated in fulminant patients and in those who have developed severe

cirrhosis. Otherwise, portacaval shunt is just as effective as liver transplantation.

INFERIOR VENA CAVA OBSTRUCTION (THROMBOSIS)

This disease corresponds to membranous obstruction of the inferior vena cava (MOVC), which was included in the Budd-Chiari syndrome and still is. However, the primary lesion in this disease occurs in the hepatic portion of the IVC, not in the hepatic vein within the liver. The etiology is unknown, but the disease is endemic in certain developing countries such as Nepal, China, India, and among South African blacks. The disease should be treated separately from classical Budd-Chiari syndrome. Thrombosis occurring at the level of the diaphragm frequently occludes the ostia of major hepatic veins and causes hepatic vein outflow obstruction. Thus, the pathophysiology of this disease is practically the same as that of classical Budd-Chiari syndrome. The thrombus organizes and turns into fibrous tissue that obstructs the IVC. It has been called membranous obstruction, but more often it is thicker than a membrane.

Epidemiology. This disease is common in developing countries judging from the literature. By contrast, only three reports of MOVC were made between 1960 and 1980, when Mitchell and associates analyzed 253 cases of Budd-Chiari syndrome in the English literature. MOVC was not too uncommon in Japan. In 1968, Nakamura and associates collected 90 autopsy cases of Budd-Chiari syndrome of which 71 were with no known etiology: 7 were classical type with hepatic vein thrombosis within the liver; 72% had obstructive lesions both in IVC and hepatic vein ostia; and 18% in IVC only. They also noted that 41% of these 71 cases had a complicating HCC. When our national group for the study of aberrant portal hemodynamics studied 157 authentic cases of Budd-Chiari syndrome, only 5.7% were of the classical type and the remainder had obstructive IVC disease, mainly with involvement of the hepatic vein ostia. At the liver center of Bir Hospital, Kathmandu, Nepal, there were 150 cases of IVC thrombosis, which constituted approximately one fifth of all patients with chronic liver disease, and all were idiopathic. In Beijing, Wang operated on 430 cases of Budd-Chiari syndrome, which included only seven cases of hepatic vein thrombosis. Thus, most cases of hepatic vein outflow block involve IVC thrombosis in these countries. A study in Chandigarh, India, analyzed 171 cases of Budd-Chiari syndrome of which 64% were idiopathic or MOVC. In 1982 in Pretoria, South Africa, Simson reported on the frequent complicating HCC (47%) among 101 black cases of MOVC. These primary IVC obstruction or thrombosis is much more prevalent in developing countries, whereas it is much less common in developed countries. The frequency of complicating HCC varies with the country. It is very high among African blacks but is much less elsewhere. It was 6.4% among 157 cases of Budd-Chiari syndrome in 10 years in Japan.

Pathophysiology, Clinical Features, and Diagnosis. The cause of MOVC was thought to be a congenital vascular malformation, and some people still believe in this theory.

However, this is an adult disease with the peak age in the 6th decade in Japan. If this were a congenital malformation, the patient should present with ascites, hepatomegaly, and venous dilatation shortly after birth. In our study of 17 autopsy cases of Budd-Chiari syndrome, there was only one case of classical Budd-Chiari syndrome with unobstructed IVC. The remainder had a thick or thin IVC obstruction with and without fresh thrombosis. Histologic examination of the membrane showed that it was an organized thrombus, with a normal IVC wall structure beneath it. Clearly, the vascular malformation theory has to be discarded. The etiology of IVC thrombosis is not known at the moment. For some reason, the hepatic portion of IVC is predisposed to thrombosis. Some investigators theorized that the diaphragmatic movements induce microscopic injuries to the endothelium of IVC that invite thrombosis. From my own experience in Nepal, where most patients have fever with occasional positive blood cultures, bacterial infection is one of the possible causes. Our national study in Japan failed to demonstrate a hypercoagulable state in these patients with MOVC.

The clinical presentation is virtually the same as that of classic Budd-Chiari syndrome but is generally less severe, because the three veins are seldom occluded simultaneously and completely. Abdominal pain, ascites, and hepatomegaly, particularly enlargement of the caudate lobe, are prominent, but most patients sustain the acute episode. They will subsequently have repeated episodes of varying severity at variable intervals and go into a chronic state. Liver histology shows centrilobular congestion and bleeding in the acute stage, but as the disease turns chronic, congestive findings become less prominent with increasing fibrosis. Signs of portal hypertension, such as esophageal varices, splenomegaly, and dilatation of abdominal collateral veins, become more evident (Fig. 16–18), and the liver will eventually turn into congestive cirrhosis. Repeated episodes of the symptoms are perhaps due to new thrombosis occurring at the same level of IVC. Hepatic veins, except for their orifices, are not involved.

Diagnosis is the demonstration of thrombosis or occlusion of IVC by ultrasound and perhaps by MR imaging. Such imaging diagnosis will delineate intrahepatic collaterals and collateral veins that originate in IVC and run cephalad along the vertebral column. The portal vein flow is usually antegrade.

Treatment. If the obstructive lesion is thin, angioplasty may be carried out. For the IVC membrane, several balloon catheters are passed from the femoral veins to perforate the membrane, and the hole is dilated. For a thin hepatic vein occlusion, transhepatic angioplasty may be performed. If these procedures are not applicable or have failed, surgical angioplasty may be carried out. Other options include shunting between the IVC and the right atrium, between the IVC and the right subclavian vein, and between the cranial hepatic resection and the hepatoatrial anastomosis.

VENO-OCCLUSIVE DISEASE

In Jamaica, approximately one third of cirrhosis seen at autopsy is a nonportal fibrosis with occlusion of centrilobular veins and centrilobular fibrosis. Most of these patients are young. The onset is often acute with jaundice, hepatomegaly, and ascites. Varices and variceal bleeding are the prominent clinical features. This is a toxic injury of the liver that is manifested histologically by centrilobular necrosis and congestion. It is believed that the disease in Jamaica is caused by pyrrolizidine alkaloids of *Senecio* and *Crotalania* plants contained in natural "bush-tea" drunk by some local residents. These alkaloids produce similar lesions in animals. This disease is extremely uncommon in Japan, where only one case has ever been reported. There was an outbreak of a similar disease in northwest India in 1974 in which one whole farming village was affected with a 10% mortality, and all dogs that were affected died of ascites. Although the investigators failed to identify the offending toxin, ingestion of moldy maize was thought to be related to this epidemic of toxic liver disease which mimicked VOD.

Similar lesions are seen after bone marrow transplantation in patients who received alkylating agents as preparation for transplantation. The incidence ranges from 7% to 50%. It also occurs after radiation to the liver. Clearly, VOD is caused not only by bush-tea alkaloids but also by several organic compounds. Centrilobular damage is followed by thrombotic occlusion, and thrombosis may extend toward larger hepatic vein branches, but portal hemodynamic changes that ensue are not well characterized. The diagnosis is made by liver biopsy. No specific imaging feature is known.

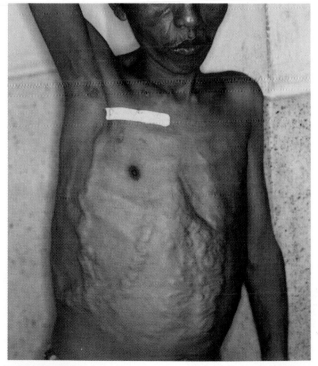

Figure 16–18
A patient with a chronic case of inferior vena cava obstruction. Marked dilatation of the subcutaneous veins, ascites, and emaciation are evident in this Nepalese man.

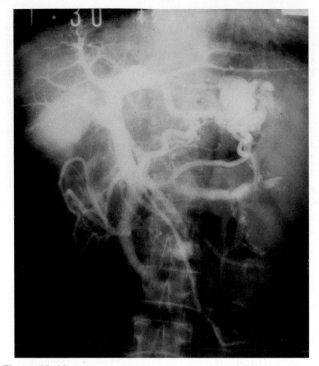

Figure 16–19
Portal hypertension in sarcoidosis. Percutaneous transhepatic portogram demonstrating splenomegaly, an enlarged hepatofugal left gastric vein, and splenorenal shunts.

SARCOIDOSIS

The liver is involved histologically in 17% to 90% of the cases of sarcoidosis depending on the reports, but clinical manifestations of the liver disease are uncommon. In a se-

ries of 300 cases, there was clinical or biochemical evidence of liver disease in 20. The granulomas occur in any area of the liver but are more frequent in the portal tracts causing injury to the portal veins. Portal hypertension, which is rather uncommon, is presinusoidal in the early phase of the disease and is caused by peripheral portal vein thrombosis; however, in advanced cases with marked fibrosis, there will be sinusoidal obstruction to portal blood flow as well. In some patients, signs of portal hypertension may be the presenting symptom, as shown in Figure 16–19. Portography demonstrated a marked splenomegaly and collateral left gastric and splenorenal shunts. The liver grossly showed furrows similar to those seen in a schistosomiasis liver in the patient. Portal hypertension is thought to be presinusoidal.

CONGENITAL HEPATIC FIBROSIS

This is a form of autosomal recessive polycystic kidney disease that is generally divided into several types according to the age of onset. Of these, the ones presenting in childhood and adolescence are frequently associated with portal hypertension besides kidney disease. Infants present with abdominal distention from enlarged organs, respiratory distress, and hypertension. Young adults seek medical attention because of variceal bleeding or hepatosplenomegaly. Liver function is good, but portal hypertension is prominent. The liver is enlarged and firm, with a fine reticular pattern of portal fibrosis. No cysts are grossly recognized. Microscopically, there is diffuse periportal fibrosis varying in thickness (Fig. 16–20). The fibrous bands encircle single lobules or a group of them. There are numerous uniform small bile ducts and an interrupted circular arrangement of the ducts (ductal plate malformation within the fibrous band). The portal hemodynamic changes vary with the report. One study in one

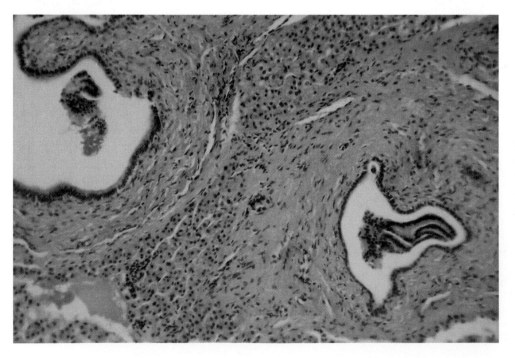

Figure 16–20
Congenital hepatic fibrosis containing dilated bile ducts. The liver parenchyma is sandwiched by thick fibrous bands in the portal tracts.

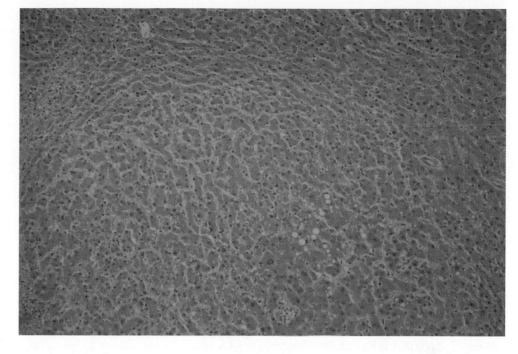

Figure 16–21
Nodular regenerative hyperplasia. A regenerative nodule is seen compressing the surrounding hepatocytes.

patient demonstrated a considerable gradient between PVP and WHVP, and another report in which six patients were investigated did not favor the increased presinusoidal resistance. The diagnosis depends mainly on liver histology, and no specific imaging feature is known.

HEMATOLOGIC DISORDERS

Myeloproliferative disease, agnogenic myeloid metaplasia, and certain other hematologic disorders are known to cause portal hypertension. They include leukemia, lymphoma, mastocytosis, Gaucher's disease, and osteopetrosis. It is mainly presinusoidal and partially sinusoidal. It has been generally thought that portal hypertension is caused by increased hepatic blood flow and infiltration of malignant and hemopoietic cells within the sinusoids. More recently, however, Wanless emphasized portal vascular changes and thrombosis as the cause of portal hypertension. More studies are needed for the exact cause of portal hypertension.

NODULAR REGENERATIVE HYPERPLASIA AND PARTIAL NODULAR TRANSFORMATION

Both nodular regenerative hyperplasia and partial nodular transformation are rare disorders of poorly understood etiologies. In the former, 1- to 2-mm nodules of regenerating hepatocytes occur rather diffusely, compressing the intervening liver parenchyma. There is no fibrosis surrounding the nodules (Fig. 16–21). Partial nodular transformation was originally described by Sherlock and associates in patients with portal hypertension in whom the liver had a large regenerative nodule near the hepatic hilum. Similar nodules are seen in IPH. According to Wanless, such nodules are a result of portal circulation

disturbances. Nodules form in the areas of the liver where there is adequate portal perfusion in compensation for the parenchymal atrophy caused by decreased portal perfusion as a result of vascular changes. Therefore, these nodules are compensatory histologic changes and do not represent disease entities.

CHEMICALLY INDUCED NONCIRRHOTIC PORTAL HYPERTENSION

A number of chemicals, drugs, and organic compounds are known to cause portal hypertension. Of these, arsenic-induced portal hypertension is perhaps the most frequently described followed by vinyl chloride monomer, vitamin A (hypervitaminosis), mercaptopurine, thioguanine, azathioprine, busulfan, and chlorambucil. Portal fibrosis, perisinusoidal fibrosis, portal venular injury, and other histologic changes are described.

ARTERIOPORTAL COMMUNICATIONS IN THE SPLANCHNIC BED

Communication between the artery and the portal vein system can occur under various conditions, leading to flow of arterial blood into the portal vein and producing portal hypertension. The most common cause of arterioportal fistula is trauma, and other causes include rupture of an aneurysm, diagnostic punctures of the liver (biopsy, catheterization), and congenital arteriovenous fistula. If the communication is small in diameter, no portal hypertension results. According to Reynolds, forcibly increased portal blood flow following a wound induces hepatoportal sclerosis, which subsequently reduces the once increased portal inflow. Thus, increased portal venous flow will induce portal hypertension and portal sclerosis. Figure 16–22 shows a congenital arte-

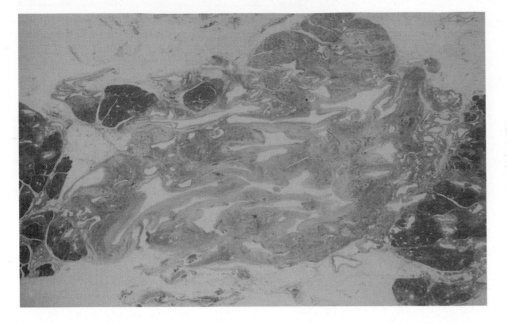

Figure 16–22
Congenital arteriovenous fistula found in the body of the pancreas. This caused marked portal hypertension.

riovenous shunt that is located in the pancreas and is causing severe portal hypertension.

SUGGESTED READINGS

Bolondi L, Gaiani S, Barbara L: Doppler flowmetery—clinical application in portal hypertensive patients. In Okuda K, Benhamou J-P (eds): Portal Hypertension: Clinical and Physiological Aspects. Tokyo: Springer, 1991, pp 161–182.

Burcharth F: Percutaneous transhepatic catheterization of the portal venous system. In Okuda K, Benhamou J-P (eds): Portal Hypertension: Clinical and Physiological Aspects. Tokyo: Springer, 1991, pp 127–137.

Caetano da Silva L: *Schistosomiasis mansoni*—clinical features. In Okuda K, Benhamou J-P (eds): Portal Hypertension: Clinical and Physiological Aspects. Tokyo: Springer, 1991, pp 309–318.

Dilawari JB, Bambery P, Chawla Y, et al: Hepatic outflow obstruction (Budd-Chiari syndrome): Experience with 177 patients and a review of the literature. Medicine 73:21–36, 1994.

Genecin P, Groszmann RJ: Portal hypertension. In Schif L, Schiff ER (eds): Diseases of the Liver. Philadelphia: JB Lippincott, 1993, pp 935–973.

Itai Y: CT and MRI in the diagnosis of portal hypertension. In Okuda K, Benhamou J-P (eds): Portal Hypertension: Clinical and Physiological Aspects. Tokyo: Springer, 1991, pp 207–217.

Kage M, Arakawa M, Kojiro M, Okuda K: Histopathology of membranous obstruction of the inferior vena cava in the Budd-Chiari syndrome. Gastroenterology 102:2081–2090, 1992.

Kage M, Nakashima T: The pathology of schistosomiasis. In Okuda K, Benhamou J-P (eds): Portal Hypertension: Clinical and Physiological Aspects. Tokyo: Springer, 1991, pp 289–300.

Kameda H, Yamazaki K, Imai F, et al: Obliterative portal venopathy: A comparative study of 184 cases of extrahepatic portal obstruction and 468 cases of idiopathic portal hypertension. J Gastroenterol Hepatol 1:139–149, 1986.

Kono K, Ohnishi K, Omata M, et al: Experimental portal fibrosis produced by intraportal injection of killed nonpathogenic *Escherichia coli* in rabbits. Gastroenterology 94:787–796, 1988.

Lebrec D: Hepatic vein catheterization. In Okuda K, Benhamou J-P (eds): Portal Hypertension: Clinical and Physiological Aspects. Tokyo: Springer, 1991, pp 117–125.

Matsutani S, Kimura K, Ohto M, Okuda K: Ultrasonography in the diagnosis of portal hypertension. In Okuda K, Benhamou J-P (eds): Portal Hypertension: Clinical and Physiological Aspects. Tokyo: Springer, 1991, pp 197–206.

Mitchell MC, Boitnott JK, Kaufman S, et al: Budd-Chiari syndrome: Etiology, diagnosis and management. Medicine 61:199–218, 1982.

Moriyasu F: The principle of Doppler ultrasound. In Okuda K, Benhamou J-P (eds): Portal Hypertension: Clinical and Physiological Aspects. Tokyo: Springer, 1991, pp 151–158.

Okuda K, Iuchi M: *Schistosomiasis japonica*—clinical features. In Okuda K, Benhamou J-P (eds): Portal Hypertension: Clinical and Physiological Aspects. Tokyo: Springer, 1991, pp 301–308.

Okuda K, Kono K, Ohnishi K, et al: Clinical study of eighty-six cases of idiopathic portal hypertension and comparison with cirrhosis with splenomegaly. Gastroenterology 86:600–610, 1984.

Okuda K, Nakashima T, Kameda H, et al: Idiopathic portal hypertension: A national study. In Brunner H, Thaler H (eds): Hepatology: A Festschrift for Hans Popper. New York: Raven Press, 1985, pp 95–108.

Okuda K, Shiomi S: Radionuclides in hemodynamic investigations. In Okuda K, Benhamou J-P (eds): Portal Hypertension: Clinical and Physiological Aspects. Tokyo: Springer, 1991, pp 183–194.

Okuda K, Suzuki K, Musha H, Arimizu N: Percutaneous transhepatic catheterization of the portal vein for the study of portal hemodynamics and shunts. Gastroenterology 73:279–284, 1977.

Okuda K, Takayasu K: Angiography in the study of portal hypertension. In Okuda K, Benhamou J-P (eds): Portal Hypertension: Clinical and Physiological Aspects. Tokyo: Springer, 1991, pp 219–237.

Reynolds TB: Portal hypertension. In Schiff L, Schiff ER (eds): Diseases of the Liver, 6th ed. Philadelphia: JB Lippincott, 1987, pp 875–901.

Sama SK, Bhargava S, Gopi Nath N, et al: Noncirrhotic portal fibrosis. Am J Med 51:160–169, 1971.

Valla D, Benhamou J-P: Obstruction of the hepatic veins or suprahepatic inferior vena cava. Dig Dis 14:99–118, 1996.

Wanless IR: On the pathogenesis of non-cirrhotic portal hypertension. In Boyer JL, Bianchi L (eds): Liver Cirrhosis: Proceedings of the VI International Congress of Liver Diseases. London: MTP Press, 1987, pp 293–311.

Wanless IR, Peterson P, Das A, et al: Hepatic vascular disease and portal hypertension in polycythemia vera and agnogenic myeloid metaplasia: A clinicopathological study of 145 patients examined at autopsy. Hepatology 12:1166–1174, 1990.

Chapter

17

Gastroesophageal Varices: Pathophysiology and Prevention of Bleeding

Arun J. Sanyal

Portal hypertension is defined as an increase in portal venous pressure over 5 mm Hg. Portal hypertension is responsible for the two major complications of cirrhosis (i.e., variceal hemorrhage and ascites). These two complications account for a large proportion of the 32,000 deaths and 20 million days of work loss related to cirrhosis annually. It is, therefore, important to prevent the development of these complications and to manage them aggressively when they do occur. Of these complications, variceal hemorrhage is more immediately life threatening and is associated with a 20% to 30% mortality with each episode of bleeding. Primary prevention of such hemorrhage is, therefore, an important goal of management in the patient with cirrhosis and gastroesophageal varices who has never bled.

The ideal treatment of portal hypertension and varices is one that is universally effective, safe, easy to administer, and inexpensive. Unfortunately, such treatment does not exist, and the physician is forced to choose from a menu of therapeutic options, none of which are ideal. The appropriate choice of therapy requires consideration of the following questions:

1. What is the natural history of the untreated disease or, in other words, is treatment necessary?
2. What is the relative efficacy and safety of one treatment vis-à-vis other available treatments?
3. How do you select patients for treatment to maximize the treatment benefit while minimizing the side effects of therapy?

Thus, the optimal management of varices requires an appreciation of their anatomy, hemodynamics, natural history, and the utility of specific therapies at specific stages in the natural history of portal hypertension. In this chapter, we re-view the anatomy and hemodynamics of varices and the primary prophylaxis of variceal hemorrhage.

GASTROESOPHAGEAL VARICES: ANATOMY AND CLASSIFICATION

The portal vein is formed by the confluence of the superior mesenteric vein and the splenic vein (Fig. 17–1). While the superior mesenteric vein drains deoxygenated blood from the small intestine, the head of the pancreas, the ascending colon, and part of the transverse colon, the splenic vein drains the spleen and the pancreas and is joined by the inferior mesenteric vein, which brings blood from the transverse and descending colon as well as the rectum. Thus, the portal vein normally receives blood from almost the entire intestine.

The tributaries of the portal vein also communicate with veins draining into the systemic venous circulation. Such portosystemic communications exist primarily in five locations: (1) at the cardia via the intrinsic and extrinsic veins of the region, (2) in the anal canal via anastomoses between the superior and middle hemorrhoidal veins, (3) in the falciform ligament via recanalization of the paraumbilical veins and direction of flow to the veins draining the abdominal wall, (4) the splenic venous bed and the left renal vein, and (5) the retroperitoneum. Of these, the gastroesophageal collaterals have the greatest clinical significance and allow portal blood to return to the heart when flow through the portal system is obstructed.

The veins draining the esophagus may be classified as intrinsic, extrinsic, and venae comitantes of the vagus nerve. The intrinsic veins are comprised of a subepithelial and submucosal plexus, which run along the length of the esophagus. These drain via perforating veins into an extrinsic

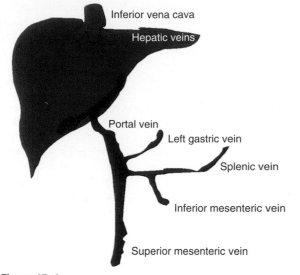

Figure 17–1
A schematic representation of the portal venous anatomy.

plexus of veins surrounding the esophagus. In the cervical region and superior mediastinum, they drain into the inferior thyroid and brachiocephalic veins, whereas in the posterior mediastinum they drain into the azygous vein. The extrinsic venous plexus around the abdominal part of the esophagus drains into the left gastric vein.

The intrinsic veins of the gastroesophageal junction are divided into four well-defined zones (Fig. 17–2): (1) the *gastric zone* is a 2- to 3-cm zone with its upper border at the gastroesophageal junction and consists of veins, arranged radially, in the submucosa and lamina propria; (2) the *palisade zone* commences at the gastroesophageal junction; it extends cranially for 2 to 3 cm and is a direct extension of the veins of the gastric zone, which runs in "palisades" or packs of longitudinally arrayed veins in the lamina propria. When portal pressures rise and impede drainage of the veins in the gastric zone into the left gastric vein, flow is directed via the veins of the palisade zone into the esophagus and eventually into the azygous vein. (3) The intrinsic veins drain into the extrinsic veins primarily in the *perforating zone* via valved perforating veins that normally allow only unidirectional flow. However, when flow through these veins increases in portal hypertensive subjects, the valves become incompetent and allow bidirectional flow. The perforating zone extends 2 to 3 cm cranially from the palisade zone, (4) The truncal zone is an 8- to 10-cm zone extending upward from the perforating zone. The intrinsic veins consist of three or four large venous trunks in the submucosa, which communicate with an irregular polygonal venous plexus in the submucosa. Blood in these veins flows from a cranial to a caudal direction and drains via the perforating veins into the extrinsic veins.

When portal hypertension occurs, the impediment to portal flow is partly compensated for by an increase in flow through portosystemic communications, thus allowing blood to return to the heart. These portosystemic communications, especially the intrinsic veins around the gastroesophageal junction, dilate and become varicose veins. Such gastroesophageal varices occur in four basic patterns: (1) varices in the fundus of the stomach, (2) gastric and palisade zone varices, (3) varices in the perforating zones, and (4) paraesophageal varices that involve the extrinsic esophageal veins.

Clinically, varices are classified by their location as esophageal or gastric varices. Esophageal varices are graded by their size (Fig. 17–3). A common system of classification is: F1: small straight varices; F2: enlarged, tortuous, occupy less than one third of lumen; F3: large, coil-shaped, occupy more than one third of lumen.

In contrast, gastric varices are classified primarily by

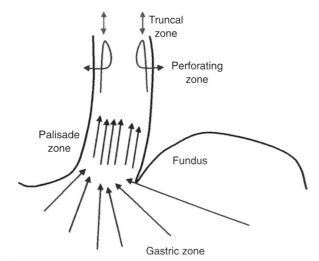

Figure 17–2
The intrinsic veins of the gastroesophageal junction. The venous anatomy allows subdivision of the region into four zones: the gastric, palisade, perforating, and truncal zones. (Redrawn from Vianna A: Anatomy of the portal venous system in portal hypertension. In McIntyre N, Benhamou J-P, Bircher J, et al (eds): Oxford Textbook of Clinical Hepatology. Oxford: Oxford University Press, 1991, pp 393–399.)

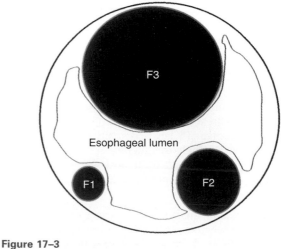

Figure 17–3
Gradation of esophageal varices.

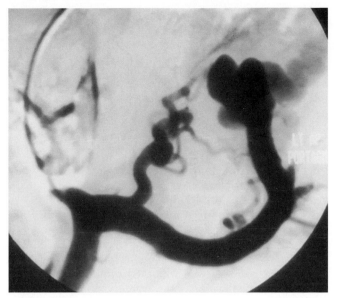

Figure 17–4
A spontaneous splenorenal shunt feeding a gastric varix.

their location. As agreed at the Baveno Consensus Conference, they are classified as follows:

A: Gastroesophageal varices (GOV): gastric varices in continuity with esophageal varices
Type I (GOV1): along the lesser curve (usually 2 to 5 cm in length)
Type II (GOV2): along the greater curve extending toward the fundus of the stomach

B: Isolated gastric varices (IGV):
Type I (IGV 1): isolated cluster of varices in the fundus of the stomach
Type II (IGV2): isolated gastric varices in other parts of the stomach

GOV1 are formed by a communication between the deep submucosal veins in the gastric zone with a branch of the left gastric vein. These varices allow blood from the left gastric vein to drain via palisade zone veins into the systemic circulation. GOV1 varices are invariably associated with large esophageal varices. In contrast, only 50% of GOV2 are associated with large esophageal varices. IGV1 are usually associated with either segmental portal hypertension (splenic vein thrombosis) or the presence of spontaneous collaterals from the splenic vein to the renal vein, which feed these varices (Fig. 17–4). Approximately 50% of cases of ectopic varices, including IGV2, are associated with portal vein thrombosis. The mechanisms underlying the predilection for varices to develop at sites away from the gastroesophageal junction when the portal vein is occluded remain unknown.

PATHOPHYSIOLOGY

The pressure in the portal vein is a direct product of portal inflow and outflow resistance:

$$\text{portal pressure} = \text{portal venous inflow} \times \text{outflow resistance} \qquad [1]$$

Portal pressure is determined by hepatic venous catheterization and measurement of the free hepatic venous (FHV) pressure and wedged hepatic venous pressure (WHVP) and calculation of the hepatic venous pressure gradient (HVPG):

$$\text{HVPG} = \text{WHVP} - \text{FHV} \qquad [2]$$

Wedged hepatic venous pressures reflect sinusoidal pressures and, in the absence of portal vein thrombosis, reflect portal venous pressures. The free hepatic venous pressure corrects for the effects of intra-abdominal pressures. Portal hypertension usually occurs when the resistance to flow through the portal venous bed is increased (Table 17–1). This may result from an obstruction to portal venous flow before it enters the hepatic sinusoids (presinusoidal portal hypertension, e.g., portal vein thrombosis), in the hepatic sinusoids (sinusoidal portal hypertension, e.g., cirrhosis), or beyond the hepatic sinusoids (postsinusoidal portal hypertension, e.g., hepatic vein thrombosis). In patients with cirrhosis, the increase in portal pressures is further compounded by a secondary increase in portal flow that results from splanchnic arteriolar dilatation.

A principal hemodynamic consequence of portal hypertension is diversion of portal flow to the systemic circulation via portosystemic communications that dilate to form varices. These varices, especially in the intrinsic veins around the GE junction, are likely to rupture bringing them to clinical attention. The likelihood of variceal rupture is determined by its wall tension, which may be defined as:

$$\text{wall tension} = (\text{transmural pressure gradient}) \times \text{radius of varix (r)/width of variceal wall (w)} \qquad [3]$$

Table 17–1 Causes of Portal Hypertension

Presinusoidal Portal Hypertension

Extrahepatic causes
  Portal vein thrombosis
  Cavernous transformation of the portal vein
  Extrinsic compression of the portal vein
  Arterioportal fistulas
Intrahepatic causes
  Schistosomiasis
  Sarcoidosis
  Primary biliary cirrhosis
  Idiopathic portal hypertension (noncirrhotic portal fibrosis)

Sinusoidal Portal Hypertension

Cirrhosis
Alcoholic hepatitis
Vitamin A and D toxicity

Postsinusoidal Portal Hypertension

Veno-occlusive disease
Budd-Chiari syndrome
Hepatic venous or inferior vena cava web
Restrictive heart disease
Constrictive pericarditis
Severe congestive heart failure

The transmural pressure gradient is the product of flow and resistance through the varix and is defined as:

$$P_1 - P_2 = Q \times R \qquad [4]$$

where P_1 and P_2 are the pressure within and outside the varix respectively, Q is the blood flow per unit time, and R is the resistance to flow through the varix. The resistance to flow may be calculated by Poiseuille's formula and expressed as:

$$R = 8nl/\pi r^4 \qquad [5]$$

where 1 is the length of the varix; n is related to blood viscosity (Reynolds number); and r is the radius of the vessel. Interposing equations 4 and 5 in equation 3, one may redefine the variceal wall tension as:

$$\text{Wall tension} = [Q \times (8nlk\pi r^4)] \times nw \qquad [6]$$

Thus, based on equation 6 above, long, large varices with high flow rates and a thin wall are most likely to rupture and bleed. Conversely, decreasing collateral flow, resistance to flow, or increasing wall thickness should decrease the risk of variceal rupture. Thus, in order to reduce the likelihood of variceal rupture, one must either decrease variceal flow or the radius of the varix since it is not feasible to increase the wall thickness of the varices. Variceal flow is decreased primarily by decreasing portal pressures. This is accomplished in most cases by inducing splanchnic arteriolar constriction, which reduces portal inflow (see equation 1) and forms the physiologic basis for most forms of pharmacologic treatment of portal hypertension. Whereas decreasing resistance to flow through the varices should decrease wall tension also, the results are less predictable due to an associated increase in collateral flow that negates the beneficial effects of decreased collateral resistance. This may explain some of the interindividual variability in hemodynamic response to pharmacologic treatment

MANAGEMENT OF THE CIRRHOTIC PATIENT WITH VARICES THAT HAVE NOT BLED

A key objective of management of the cirrhotic subject is the primary prevention of variceal hemorrhage. The steps involved in this process include identification of appropriate patients for treatment and an appreciation of the relative efficacy, side effects, and cost-effectiveness of the treatment modalities available. The first step in this process is to stratify patients according to their risk of bleeding so that only patients with a higher risk of bleeding may be selected for treatment with the potential for adverse effects. This requires an understanding of the natural history of gastroesophageal varices and the factors that predict variceal hemorrhage. A discussion of these factors follows.

Esophageal Varices (Natural History and Prediction of Bleeding)

Approximately 5% to 15% of patients with cirrhosis without varices develop varices de novo each year. It is estimated that most cirrhotic individuals will develop varices during their lifetime and that about a third of all patients with esophageal varices will even experience variceal hemorrhage. It, therefore, seems reasonable to treat portal hyper-

tension and esophageal varices before the onset of hemorrhage. It is, however, important to remember that, while on one hand each episode of hemorrhage is associated with a 20% to 30% risk of mortality, the beneficial effects of treatment may be diluted if a large number of patients (especially those not destined to bleed) experience adverse effects from treatment. These factors underscore the need to be able to identify those at greatest risk of bleeding and benefit from treatment. Several factors predict the risk of bleeding from esophageal varices.

Portal Pressures. It is both intuitively as well as clinically obvious that varices cannot bleed if they do not develop. Several studies have now shown that, at HVPG values less than 12 mm Hg, varices do not form and therefore do not bleed. Varix formation, as identified by endoscopy, is invariably associated with a HVPG greater than 12 mm Hg. However, the precise level of portal pressure above 12 mm Hg does not correlate well with the likelihood of bleeding. An important implication of these observations is that if the HVPG is maintained below 12 mm Hg, the risk of variceal hemorrhage can be minimized. Another corollary of these findings is that the occurrence of varices may be prevented by decreasing the portal pressures below 12 mm Hg before the development of varices; Clinical trials designed to test this hypothesis are currently under way.

Intravariceal Pressure. The portal pressure determines the degree of portosystemic shunting and is an indirect marker of variceal flow and transmural pressure gradient. Traditionally, intravariceal measurement necessitated puncture of the varices and, therefore, was not considered clinically useful. Recently, noninvasive measurement of variceal pressure has become technically feasible by attaching a pressure gauge to the distal end of an endoscope. The gauge is a small chamber covered by a latex membrane and perfused by N_2. When applied over a varix, the pressure needed to perfuse the gauge equals the pressure inside the varix. Using such a system (Table 17–2), it has been shown that more than 70% of patients with an intravariceal pressure higher than 16 mm Hg experienced hemorrhage within 1 year of measurement whereas only 9% of patients with pressures between 13 and 14 mm Hg bled during the same period. If these data are corroborated by other clinical trials, this is likely to be incorporated in clinical practice.

Table 17–2 Incidence of Variceal Bleeding Within 1 Year in Patients with Cirrhosis as a Function of the VP Level

VP (mm Hg)	Incidence of Bleeding (bleeders/total patients)
≤13	0/25 (9%)
>13 and ≤14	1/11 (9%)
>14 and ≤15	2/12 (17%)
>15 and ≤16	7/14 (50%)
>16	18/25 (72%)

From Nevens F, Bustami R, Scheys I, et al: Variceal pressure factor predicting the risk of a first variceal bleeding: A prospective cohort study in cirrhotic objects. Hepatology 27:15–19, 1998.

Varix Size and Location.   The likelihood of variceal rupture is also directly related to its diameter because the wall tension is directly related to its radius. Varices at the gastroesophageal junction and palisade zone are located more superficially within the wall of the esophagus. Consequently, they have a thinner coat and are most likely to bleed.

Variceal Features on Endoscopy.   Several endoscopic features of esophageal varices have been shown to predict the risk of hemorrhage. Together, these are often referred to as "red signs" due to their color. These findings include:

Red Wale Marks: These are longitudinal red streaks on varices that resemble red corduroy wales.

Cherry Red Spots: These are discrete red cherry-colored spots that are flat and overlie varices.

Hematocystic Spots: These are raised discrete red spots overlying varices and resemble "blood blisters."

Diffuse Erythema: This is self-evident and denotes a diffuse red color of the varix.

Degree of Liver Failure.   Patients with more advanced liver failure are more likely to experience variceal hemorrhage. Thus, with increasing bilirubin, and prothrombin time and decreasing albumin levels, the risk of bleeding increases.

Presence of Ascites.   Tense ascites is also an important risk factor for variceal hemorrhage.

All of these risk factors have been used to estimate the probability of variceal hemorrhage with relative precision (Table 17–3). Thus, in a patient with Child class C cirrhosis and large varices and red signs, the risk of hemorrhage is more than 76% within 1 year, whereas another patient with Child class A cirrhosis and small varices has a less than 10% likelihood of bleeding. The risk of bleeding also decreases over time following their identification, and most bleeding episodes occur within the first 2 years after identification of varices.

After the onset of active hemorrhage, bleeding stops spontaneously in approximately 50% of individuals. Patients with large spurting varices and those with Child class C cirrhosis are most likely to experience exsanguinating hemorrhage without specific intervention. The period following cessation of active bleeding is usually subdivided into two periods, based on the risk of rebleeding. The risk of rebleeding is extremely high in the period immediately after hemostasis is achieved and decreases over the next 6 weeks to baseline values. The risk factors for such early rebleeding include large varices, age older than 60 years, renal failure, and severe initial bleeding as defined by a hemoglobin less than 8 g/dL at admission. Also, overly aggressive volume replacement may cause rebound portal hypertension and precipitate early rebleeding. The long-term course after an index bleed is characterized by recurrent variceal hemorrhage, liver failure, and death. The risk of recurrent bleeding is related to the degree of liver failure, continued alcoholism, variceal size, renal failure, and the presence of a hepatoma. Overall, approximately 70% of untreated individuals rebleed as well as die within 1 year of their index bleed.

Gastric Varices (Natural History and Prediction of Hemorrhage)

The likelihood of bleeding from gastric varices depends on their location. Although GOV1 constitute more than 70% of gastric varices, only 11% of GOV1 ever bleed. In contrast, about 80% of IGV1 experience hemorrhage even though they comprise only 8% of all gastric varices. Bleeding from IGV1 occurs at lower portal pressures than those seen in nonbleeding subjects with esophageal varices. Furthermore, bleeding from such varices is more severe and the risk of encephalopathy is higher than in patients with bleeding esophageal varices. Overall, gastric varices bleed less frequently but more severely than do esophageal varices. Recently, the risk of bleeding from IGV1 was shown to correlate with the size of the varices (>10 mm), Child class and the presence of a red spot on the varices. Based on these findings, a prognostic index was calculated:

$$\text{Prognostic index} = 0.53*\text{Child class} + 0.78*\text{varix size} + 0.72*\text{red spot}$$

where Child class A = 0; B = 1; C = 2; the varix size scored as small (<5 mm) = 0, medium (5 to 10 mm) = 1, and large (>10 mm)= 2; and red spot scored as absent = 0

Table 17–3   Estimated 1-Year Percentage Probability of Bleeding as a Function of All Possible Combinations of the Endoscopic Variables Form (F) and Red Wale Markings in Child's Class A, B, and C Patients

	Child's Class								
	A			B			C		
	F1	F2	F3	F1	F2	F3	F1	F2	F3
Red wale markings									
	6	10	15	10	16	26	20	30	42
+	8	12	19	15	23	33	28	38	54
++	12	16	24	20	30	42	36	48	64
+++	16	23	34	28	40	52	44	60	76

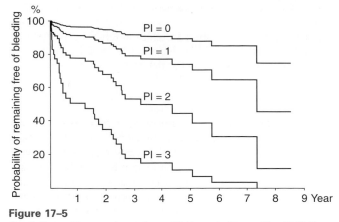

Figure 17–5
Prediction of hemorrhage from IGV type I. (From Kim T, Shijo H, Tokumitsu H, et al: Risk factors for hemorrhage from gastric fundal varices. Hepatology 25:307–312, 1997.)

and present = 1. The risk of bleeding correlated directly with the prognostic index (Fig. 17–5).

Esophageal variceal sclerotherapy causes spontaneous obliteration of 60% of GOV1. In those where GOV1 persists for more than 6 months after esophageal variceal obliteration, the risk for rebleeding is substantially greater than in those where varices disappear (28% versus 2%). GOV2 are not affected by esophageal sclerotherapy.

Treatment Modalities Available for Primary Prophylaxis of Variceal Hemorrhage

Currently, despite the multitude of available treatments, only pharmacologic treatment with nonselective β-blockers is currently recommended for primary prevention of variceal hemorrhage.

Pharmacologic Treatment

Nonselective β-Blockers:

An important determinant of portal pressure is the portal venous inflow, which is dependent on mesenteric arteriolar resistance. α-Adrenergic agonists constrict mesenteric arterioles and decrease portal blood flow, whereas β-adrenergic agonists cause splanchnic vasodilatation and increase portal venous inflow. β-Adrenergic antagonists block the β-receptor–mediated splanchnic vasodilatation and allow unopposed vasoconstriction mediated by α-adrenergic receptors. Propranolol and nadolol are the two most studied β-adrenergic antagonists.

Pharmacodynamic Effects. After either an oral or intravenous dose of propranolol, the hepatic venous pressure gradient decreases by 9% to 31%. This results primarily from a drop in portal pressures as measured by the wedged hepatic pressure with a smaller contribution from increased free hepatic venous pressure. This increment in FHP is caused by increased systemic venous pressure noted after β-blocker administration. At higher doses, a decrease in heart rate and cardiac output decrease the amount of blood delivered to the splanchnic bed and thus contribute to the decrease in portal pressures.

An important aspect of the pharmacodynamic effects of propranolol on portal pressures is the heterogeneity in response, and up to 50% of patients show a less than 10% decrease in portal pressures following acute administration. Several factors contribute to this heterogeneity: (1) a concomitant increase in collateral or hepatic sinusoidal resistance, which negates the hypotensive effects of decreased portal inflow, and (2) a compensatory increase in hepatic arterial flow that maintains sinusoidal perfusion and thus the increased wedge pressures. Also, the site of portal obstruction and etiology of cirrhosis, plasma propranolol levels, severity of liver failure or baseline hemodynamics and heart rate response to propranolol do not correlate with its portal hypotensive effects. In the long term, the portal hypotensive effects are maintained in most subjects. Tachyphylaxis does, however, occur in some patients and is clinically important, because only those with a sustained decrease in portal pressures may benefit from β-blockade.

Pharmacokinetic Considerations. Propranolol is highly lipophilic and is almost completely absorbed after oral administration. It undergoes first-pass elimination to a variable degree, causing plasma levels to vary by up to 20-fold. With increasing doses, the relative hepatic extraction decreases and allows plasma levels to rise. A sustained-release form of propranolol has also been developed. This form allows single daily dose administration. The clinical effects often do not correlate well with the plasma levels because of the formation of active metabolites, especially the (-) enantiomer, which are taken up by sympathetic nerve endings and subsequently released slowly over time.

In contrast, nadolol is water soluble and only incompletely absorbed orally. In contrast to propranolol, the interindividual pharmacokinetic variability is much less with nadolol. Nadolol does not cross the blood-brain barrier well and, theoretically, should have fewer side effects on the central nervous system (CNS). However, clinical trials have not shown a significant decrease in the incidence of CNS side effects compared to propranolol. It is excreted via the kidney, and its dose has to be modified in those with renal failure.

Adverse Effects. β-Blocker therapy is associated with a large number of side effects and, in clinical trials of β-blockers for portal hypertension, up to 20% of patients have had to discontinue treatment due to intolerable side effects.

The most clinically important side effects involve bronchoconstriction, development of heart failure, and impotence in cirrhotics. Many patients also complain of nonspecific deterioration in mental function. Despite the increase in renin activity and decrease in renal blood flow, renal dysfunction only occurs occasionally after propranolol administration. It is, however, worthy of note that the administration of β-blockers has not been shown to impair the hemodynamic response to acute blood loss.

Clinical Trials of β-Blockers for Primary Prevention of Variceal Hemorrhage. A total of 10 placebo-controlled clinical trials of propranolol or nadolol have been reported and reviewed extensively. The most common cause of cirrhosis was alcohol across all published trials, and all but one study enrolled patients with esophageal varices only. However, comparisons across trials are confounded by the differences in patient populations studied as well as treatment regimens used. Whereas one study excluded patients with Child class C cirrhosis, the others did not. Importantly, only those with large varices were enrolled in four studies, and only two studies specifically used a HVPG greater than 12 mm Hg as an entry criterion. Ten to 480 mg/day of short-acting propranolol or 40 to 320 mg/day of long-acting propranolol were used. Nadolol was used in two studies. The dose was titrated in these studies by measurement of heart rate with a 25% decrease in resting heart as the desired "endpoint." In addition, a resting heart rate of 55/mm was considered adequate in one trial.

Despite the heterogeneity between trials, several general observations can be made: (1) in the first year of follow-up (the period of greatest risk of bleeding), those treated with β-blockers had a lower risk of variceal hemorrhage than did those treated with placebo (0% to 18% versus 12% to 30%) (Fig. 17–6). These effects were even more pronounced after 2 years of follow-up. Also, there was a decrease in variceal hemorrhage-related mortality. However, these beneficial effects translated into an overall survival advantage in one study.

Meta-analyses of the data suggest that nonselective β-blockade reduce the risks of initial variceal hemorrhage by 45% and bleeding-related deaths by 50%. The factors associated with failure of treatment included younger age, large variceal size, advanced liver failure and lower doses of propranolol. On the other hand, compliance with treatment was an important predictor of a good outcome. It has also been shown that an important predictor of a favorable outcome is the degree of portal decompression achieved. Those patients who are able to sustain a drop in hepatic venous pressure gradient by 25% or to levels below 12 mm Hg over time did not bleed and had a significantly prolonged survival. It has been suggested, therefore, that repeated measurements of HVPG be used to guide pharmacologic

therapy of portal hypertension. However, the cost efficacy of such an approach remains to be demonstrated, and routine measurement of HVPG is not available at most community hospitals.

Nitrosovasodilators

Pharmacodynamics. An important mediator of the vasodilated state seen in patients with cirrhosis is nitric oxide (NO). The "nitrosovasodilator" group of drugs activate nitric oxide pathways and produce vasodilatation in their target vascular beds. At usual pharmacologic doses, these agents are primarily venodilators and decrease postsinusoidal resistance and thus a decrease in portal pressure. The cardiac output falls in patients with normal myocardial length-tension relationship due to a decrease in venous return. With increased doses, arterial dilatation and a decreased cardiac output produce hypotension and reflex splanchnic vasoconstriction. Finally, nitrate-mediated baroreceptor reflexes in the pulmonary capillary bed also trigger splanchnic vasoconstriction and contribute to their portal hypotensive action.

Effects on Portal Hemodynamics. Acute administration of either isosorbide mononitrate (ISMN) or dinitrate (ISDN) cause up to 40% decrease in HVPG, 30% decrease in portal flow, and 15% decrease in azygous flow. The effects of ISMN are more predictable than those of ISDN and ISMN is the nitrate of choice when this class of drugs is used for the treatment of portal hypertension. Tachyphylaxis does occur with repeated doses, and the long-term effects on portal pressure are variable. The portal hypotensive effects of nitrates are associated with an increase in plasma levels of sodium-retentive hormones due to the systemic vasodilatation produced by these drugs.

Clinical Trials of Nitrates for Primary Prevention of Variceal Hemorrhage. An important study prospectively randomized 118 patients to receive either ISMN (20 mg tid) or propranolol (to the maximum tolerated dose). Although no differences were noted during initial analysis 29 months after entry into the study, an increased mortality especially in those older than 51 years of age (72% versus 48%) was noted in those receiving ISMN after 7 years of follow-up (Fig. 17–7).

It is unclear whether the aforementioned findings reflect a beneficial effect of propranolol or an adverse effect of nitrates. The results of this study are further weakened because approximately 50% of patients enrolled in both arms withdrew from the study. Potential explanations for the increased mortality in those receiving nitrates include worsening of the hyperdynamic circulatory state and decrease in effective circulating volume, increased sodium retention, and tissue hypoxia with increased lactate levels in cirrhotic individuals. At this time, the data do not support a role for nitrates as monotherapy for the primary prophylaxis of variceal hemorrhage. Similarly, the role of combination therapy (β-blockers plus nitrates) for primary prophylaxis of variceal hemorrhage have not been validated in clinical trials and their use is considered experimental.

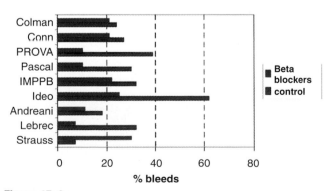

Figure 17–6
The effects of nonselective β-blockers on rates of variceal hemorrhage in clinical trials of β-blockers for primary prophylaxis of variceal hemorrhage. (From Sanyal AJ, Shiffman ML: The pharmacologic treatment of portal hypertension. Curr Clin Topics Gastrointest Pharmacol 1:242–275, 1997.)

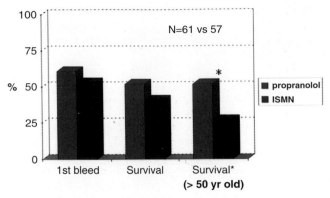

Figure 17–7
The relative effects of propranolol and isosorbide mononitrate on bleeding rates and mortality when used for primary prophylaxis of variceal hemorrhage. (Data redrawn from Angelico M, Carli L, Piat C, et al: Effects of isosorbide 5 mononitrate compared to propranolol on bleeding and long-term survival in cirrhosis. Gastroenterology 113:1632–1639, 1997.)

Surgical Portal Decompression

Four prospective randomized trials comparing surgical portacaval shunts to medical therapy were carried out more than 25 years ago. Although surgery effectively prevented variceal hemorrhage, the benefit was offset by severe encephalopathy, which developed in 30% to 60% of patients. Moreover, medically treated patients survived longer. Thus, this modality has been eliminated as an option for the primary prevention of variceal hemorrhage

Transjugular Intrahepatic Portosystemic Shunts (TIPS)

This procedure involves the creation of a tract between the hepatic vein and the intrahepatic portion of the portal vein using angiographic techniques. This tract is then dilated and kept patent by deployment of an expandable metal stent, thus creating a low-resistance pathway for blood from the hypertensive portal vein to return to the heart. Currently, no data exist to support a role for TIPS for primary prevention of variceal hemorrhage. Moreover, TIPS does not improve the outcome of liver transplant and, in some cases, may render the operation technically more difficult. TIPS is thus not recommended for primary prevention of variceal hemorrhage.

Endoscopic Sclerotherapy

Several studies have examined the utility of endoscopic sclerotherapy for the primary prevention of variceal hemorrhage. The data are difficult to compare owing to variability in patient populations and the use of sclerotherapy during episodes of active bleeding. Although three studies found sclerotherapy to be beneficial, a large multicenter study found a significantly higher mortality in those treated with sclerotherapy despite a decrease in variceal hemorrhage in these patients. When directly compared with β-blockers, sclerotherapy was found to be inferior for primary prophylaxis of variceal hemorrhage. Sclerotherapy should not be

used either alone or with β-blockers for the primary prevention of variceal hemorrhage.

Endoscopic Band Ligation

A recent study evaluated the role of endoscopic band ligation for the primary prevention of variceal hemorrhage. It demonstrated a decrease in rates of variceal hemorrhage and also demonstrated a survival advantage for treated patients. These exciting data now await validation in cirrhotic populations in the U.S.

Clinical Guidelines for Primary Prevention of Variceal Hemorrhage

Nonselective β-blockers are the only recommended treatment for the primary prevention of variceal hemorrhage in cirrhotic patients. They are both clinically effective and also cost effective. However, the potential for clinical benefit must be weighed against the risk of side effects, and only those at greatest risk of bleeding should be targeted for therapy.

All patients with cirrhosis should undergo an endoscopic examination as part of their evaluation. Patients with Child class B or C cirrhosis with esophageal varices of any grade and those with Child class A cirrhosis and large varices (especially with red signs) should be targeted for treatment. In those where varices are not present, endoscopy should be repeated at 2- to 3-year intervals. No evaluable data currently exist for the clinical utility of β-blockers for the various types of gastric varices, although it appears to make intuitive sense to treat those especially at high risk for bleeding.

It has been shown that those who experience a 25% or greater drop in HVPG or HVPG to values less than 12 mm Hg and maintain these changes over time are most likely to remain free of bleeding. It has, therefore, been recommended that the HVPG be measured before the initiation of therapy and after 1 to 3 months of treatment and also that the dosage of the drug be changed appropriately to achieve the desired endpoints. However, the cost-effectiveness of this approach remains to be demonstrated. Moreover, HVPG measurement is not possible at many medical centers. Where such facilities are unavailable, the dose should be titrated to achieve a decrease in resting heart rate to values of 55 to 60 beats/min.

SUGGESTED READINGS

Angelico M, Carli L, Piat C, et al: Effects of isosorbide 5 mononitrate compared to propranolol on first bleeding and long-term survival in cirrhosis. Gastroenterology 113:1632–1639, 1997.

Beppu K, Inokuchi K, Koyanagi N, Doe J: Prediction of variceal hemorrhage by esophageal endoscopy. Gastrointest Endosc 27:213–218, 1981.

Butler H: The veins of the esophagus. Thorax 6:276–296, 1951.

Cales P, Desmorat H, Vinel JP, et al: Incidence of large oesophageal varices in patients with cirrhosis: Application to prophylaxis of first variceal bleeding. Gut 31:1298–1302, 1990.

Conn HO, Grace ND, Bosch J, et al: Propranolol in the prevention of the first hemorrhage from esophagogastric varices: A multicenter, randomized clinical trial. Hepatology 13:902–912, 1991.

DeFranchis R: Prediction of the first variceal hemorrhage in patients with cirrhosis of the liver and esophageal varices. N Engl J Med 3(19):983–989, 1988.

DeFranchis R, Primignani M: Why do varices bleed? Gastroenterol Clin North Am 21:85–101, 1992.

Frishman WH: Nadolol: A new β-adrenoreceptor antagonist. N Engl J Med 305:678–682, 1982.

Grace ND: Prevention of initial variceal hemorrhage. Gastroenterol Clin North Am 21:149–161, 1992.

Graham DY, Smith JL: The course of patients after variceal hemorrhage. Gastroenterology 80:800–809, 1981.

Groszmann RJ, Bosch J, Grace ND, et al: Hemodynamic events in a prospective randomized trial of propranolol versus placebo in the prevention of a first variceal hemorrhage. Gastroenterology 99:1401–1407, 1990.

Hoffman BB, Lefkowitz RJ: Adrenergic receptor antagonists. In Goodman-Gilman A, Rall TW, Nies AS, Taylor P (eds): The Pharmacological Basis of Therapeutics, 8th ed. New York: Pergamon Press, 1990, pp 221–243.

Ideo G, Bellati G, Fesce E, Grimoldi D: Nadolol can prevent the first gastrointestinal bleeding in cirrhotics: A prospective randomized study. Hepatology 8:6–9, 1988.

Kim T, Shijo H, Tokumitsu H, Kubara K, et al: Risk factors for hemorrhage from gastric fundal varices. Hepatology 25:307–312, 1997.

Lay CS, Tsai YT, Teg CY, Doe J: Endoscopic variceal ligation in prophylaxis of first variceal bleeding in cirrhotic patients with high-risk esophageal varices. Hepatology 25:1347–1352, 1997.

Lebrec D, Poynard T, Capron JP, et al: Nadolol for prophylaxis of gastrointestinal bleeding in patients with cirrhosis: A randomized trial. J Hepatol 7:118–125, 1988.

Nevens F, Bustami R, Scheys I, et al: Variceal pressure is a factor predicting the risk of a first variceal bleeding: A prospective cohort study in cirrhotic subjects. Hepatology 27:15–19, 1998.

Polio J, Groszmann RJ: Hemodynamic factors involved in the development and rupture of esophageal varices: A pathophysiologic approach to treatment. Semin Liver Dis 6:318–331, 1986.

Poynard T, Cales P, Pasta L, et al: Beta-adrenergic antagonist drugs in the prevention of gastrointestinal bleeding in patients with cirrhosis and esophageal varices: An analysis of data and prognostic factors in 589 patients from four randomized clinical trials. N Engl J Med 324:1532–1538, 1991.

Prandi D, Rueff B, Roche-Sicot J, et al: Life-threatening hemorrhage of the digestive tract in cirrhotic patients. Am J Surg 131:204–209, 1976.

Rodes J: The evolution of knowledge on the pathophysiology of portal hypertension. In DeFranchis R (ed): Portal hypertension II: Proceedings of the Second Baveno Consensus Workshop on Definitions, Methodology and Therapeutic Strategies. Oxford: U.K. Blackwell Science, 1996, pp 18–29.

Sanyal AJ, Shiffman ML: The pharmacologic treatment of portal hypertension. Curr Clin Top Gastrointestinal Pharmacol 1:242–275, 1997.

Sarin SK: Diagnostic issues: Portal hypertensive gastropathy and gastric varices. In DeFranchis R (ed): Portal hypertension II. Proceedings of the Second Baveno International Consensus Workshop on Definitions, Methodology and Therapeutic Strategies. Oxford: Blackwell Science, 1996, pp 30–55.

Sarin SK, Lahoti D, Saxena SP, et al: Prevalence, classification and natural history of gastric varices: Long-term follow-up study in 568 patients with portal hypertension. Hepatology 95:434–440, 1992.

Shand DG: Propranolol. N Engl J Med 293:280–284, 1975.

Smith JL, Graham DY: Variceal hemorrhage: A critical evaluation of survival analysis. Gastroenterology 82:968–973, 1982.

Veterans Affairs Cooperative Variceal Sclerotherapy Group: Prophylactic sclerotherapy for esophageal varices in men with alcoholic liver disease: A randomized single-blind, multicenter clinical trial. N Engl J Med 324:1779–1784, 1991.

Vianna A, Hayes PC, Moscoso G: Normal venous circulation of the gastroesophageal junction: A route to understanding varices. Gastroenterology 93:876–889, 1987.

Waldman SA, Murad F: Cyclic GMP synthesis and function. Pharmacol Rev 39:163–196, 1987.

18

Complications of Cirrhosis: Ascites, Hyponatremia, Hepatorenal Syndrome, and Spontaneous Bacterial Peritonitis

Pere Ginès
Vicente Arroyo
Juan Rodés

The natural course of patients with cirrhosis is frequently complicated by the excessive accumulation of fluid in the peritoneal or pleural cavities and interstitial tissue. This is caused by an abnormal regulation of extracellular fluid volume, which is commonly associated with alterations in renal function (especially sodium retention) and, less commonly, water retention and reduced renal perfusion. Other than these abnormalities in renal function, cirrhotic patients with ascites may develop spontaneous bacterial peritonitis, an infection of ascitic fluid without any intra-abdominal source of infection. The present chapter reviews the pathogenesis, clinical findings, diagnosis, and treatment of these complications of cirrhosis.

ASCITES

Definition

Ascites is defined as the presence of fluid in the peritoneal cavity. Although the presence of ascites is highly suggestive of cirrhosis (or other chronic liver diseases associated with portal hypertension), the definitive diagnosis should always be established by clinical or exploratory findings or, preferably, by liver biopsy.

Pathogenesis of Ascites

The formation of ascites in cirrhosis is the consequence of a combination of abnormalities in renal function, which cause sodium retention with subsequent expansion of extracellular fluid volume, and alterations in portal and splanchnic circulation, which facilitate the accumulation of fluid in the peritoneal cavity by increasing lymph formation. Chrono-logically, sodium retention is the earliest alteration of kidney function observed in patients with cirrhosis. As sodium is retained iso-osmotically in the kidney, the retention of sodium causes fluid retention and expansion of the extracellular fluid volume, which results in ascites or edema formation. Sodium retention in cirrhosis is mainly caused by an abnormally increased tubular reabsorption of sodium that probably takes place both in the proximal and distal tubules. The main effectors of this increased sodium reabsorption are hyperaldosteronism and enhanced renal sympathetic nerve activity, although other intrarenal and extrarenal sodium-retaining mechanisms may also be involved (Table 18-1). Although many patients with ascites have an impaired ability to excrete water, this disorder is not required for the development of ascites. The only renal excretory function abnormality needed for the development of ascites is sodium retention.

Portal hypertension is another key pathogenic factor in the development of ascites in cirrhosis. The increased intra-hepatic vascular resistance causes not only a rise in hydrostatic pressure in the portal venous system but also a marked vasodilatation of the splanchnic arteries, which results in an increased portal venous inflow. Both abnormalities cause marked changes in the splanchnic microcirculation that result in an enhanced splanchnic lymph production. These alterations of splanchnic hemodynamics in patients with cirrhosis and portal hypertension are associated with changes in systemic hemodynamics, which are characterized by a hyperdynamic circulatory state with reduced systemic vascular resistance and a high cardiac index (Table 18-2). These hemodynamic changes play an important role in sodium retention by causing a baroreceptor-dependent activation of vasoconstrictor and antinatriuretic systems, mainly the renin-angiotensin-aldosterone system and the sympathetic nervous system.

Table 18–1   Factors Involved in Sodium Retention in Cirrhosis

Hyperaldosteronism
Increased renal sympathetic nerve activity
Reduced renal perfusion
Renal resistance to natriuretic peptides
Increased tubular sensitivity to aldosterone

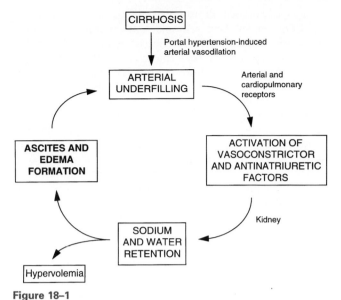

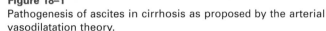

Figure 18–1
Pathogenesis of ascites in cirrhosis as proposed by the arterial vasodilatation theory.

The theory that best explains the pathogenesis of sodium retention and ascites formation in cirrhosis is the Arterial Vasodilatation Theory (Fig. 18-1). According to this hypothesis, sodium retention is the consequence of a homeostatic response raised by an underfilling of the arterial circulation secondary to arterial vasodilatation in the splanchnic vascular bed. The underfilling of the arterial circulation is sensed by arterial and cardiopulmonary receptors and results in hypervolemia by activating antinatriuretic factors. The retained fluid compensates initially the disturbance in the arterial circulation and suppresses the activation of sodium-retaining mechanisms. However, as the vasodilatation in the splanchnic circulation causes more marked arterial underfilling, the retained fluid does not fill adequately the intravascular compartment, mainly because fluid is leaking continuously into the peritoneal cavity and the sodium-retaining mechanisms become permanently activated. This theory also provides an explanation for the pathogenesis of dilutional hyponatremia and hepatorenal syndrome (see later).

Clinical Features

The main clinical symptom of patients with ascites and edema is discomfort caused by abdominal and leg swelling. In some cases, the accumulation of fluid is so important that respiratory function and physical activity may be impaired. Pleural effusion is common in patients with ascites. The effusion is usually mild or moderate and more frequent on the right side. In some cases, pleural effusions are large, recur after therapy, and constitute the main manifestation of the disease. These cases are usually caused by the existence of anatomic defects in the diaphragm that create a communication between the peritoneal and pleural cavities. Other com-

mon manifestations of patients with ascites include anorexia, malaise, and weight loss.

Diagnostic Approach to the Patient with Ascites (Table 18-3)

General Evaluation

The evaluation of a cirrhotic patient with ascites should include an assessment of liver function by standard biochemi-

Table 18-2   Hemodynamic Abnormalities in Splanchnic and Systemic Circulation in Patients with Cirrhosis and Ascites

Splanchnic Circulation	Systemic Circulation
Increased pressure in the portal venous system	Increased cardiac output
Vasodilatation of splanchnic arteries	Reduced systemic vascular resistance
Increased portal venous inflow	Reduced arterial pressure
Increased intestinal capillary pressure	Increased plasma volume
Increased splanchnic lymph flow	Overactivity of vasoconstrictor systems
Development of portocollateral circulation	

Table 18-3   Diagnostic Approach to the Patient with Cirrhosis and Ascites

General Evaluation

Standard liver tests
Abdominal ultrasonography (including the kidneys)
Upper gastrointestinal endoscopy
Liver biopsy (see text)

Evaluation of Ascitic Fluid

Protein measurement
Cell count
Culture

Evaluation of Renal Function

24-hour urine sodium
Diuresis after water load (IV 5% dextrose, 20 mL/kg)
Serum electrolytes and serum creatinine
Urine sediment and protein excretion

Evaluation of Circulatory Function

Arterial pressure
Plasma renin activity and plasma norepinephrine concentration

cal tests, abdominal ultrasonography, to rule out the existence of hepatocellular carcinoma, and upper gastrointestinal endoscopy, to assess the presence of esophageal or gastric varices or hypertensive gastropathy. In patients with previously unknown liver disease, the diagnosis of cirrhosis should be confirmed either histologically or by a combination of exploratory (cutaneous stigmata), ultrasonographic (diffuse parenchymal heterogeneity, nodular liver edge or signs of portal hypertension), and endoscopic findings (presence of gastroesophageal varices). Percutaneous liver biopsy should be performed preferably after resolution of ascites, because ascites increases the risk of complications. In patients with coagulation disturbances, a biopsy may be performed using a transjugular approach.

Evaluation of Ascitic Fluid

A diagnostic paracentesis should be performed in every cirrhotic patient with ascites for protein measurement, cell count, and culture. The protein concentration of ascitic fluid is usually low in cirrhotic patients, with 60% of patients having an ascitic fluid protein concentration lower than 10 g/L. However, values above 30 g/L are not uncommon. The difference between serum and ascites albumin is greater than 1.1 g/dL. The protein concentration of ascitic fluid is an important predictive factor in cirrhosis, because patients with ascites protein lower than 10 g/L have a higher prob-

ability of developing spontaneous bacterial peritonitis and shorter survival expectancy than do patients with protein concentrations higher than 10 g/L (Fig. 18-2). The ascitic fluid red blood cell count is usually low (<1000 cells/mm³), although bloody ascites (>50,000 red blood cells/mm³) may be seen in some patients. A superimposed hepatocellular carcinoma should be excluded in these latter patients. The ascitic fluid white blood cell count is less than 500 per mm³ in most patients, and mononuclear cells predominate (>75%). As discussed later, a high number of polymorphonuclear cells in the ascitic fluid is indicative of peritoneal infection. The result of the ascitic fluid culture is negative unless a peritoneal infection is present. However, a few patients may have a positive ascitic fluid culture without an increased polymorphonuclear cell count. This condition is known as bacterascites.

Evaluation of Renal Function

The evaluation of renal function in patients with cirrhosis and ascites is important in the prognosis and patient's response to therapy. The evaluation should be performed in conditions of low-sodium diet and after at least 4 days without the administration of diuretics. Parameters to be measured include 24-hour urine volume and sodium excretion, urine volume after a water load of 5% dextrose (20 mL/kg), serum electrolytes, and serum creatinine. In patients with renal failure (serum creatinine >1.5 mg/dL), tests of urine sediment, 24-hour urine protein, and a renal ultrasound should also be performed.

Evaluation of Circulatory Function

The evaluation of circulatory function should include the measurement of arterial pressure in conditions of bed rest, low-sodium diet, and without diuretic therapy. The measurement of the activity of vasoconstrictor systems (plasma renin activity and plasma norepinephrine concentration), which estimate the degree of disturbance in systemic hemodynamics, is also valuable.

Treatment

The objective of the treatment of ascites or edema in cirrhosis is to reduce the patient's discomfort due to abdominal or leg swelling. Besides, the decrease in the amount of fluid in the peritoneal cavity reduces the risk of complications related to abdominal hernias, such as incarceration or rupture. With this in mind, the therapeutic measures in these patients should be oriented to reduce the amount of ascites and edema and to prevent their reaccumulation after therapy (Table 18-4).

The initial step in the management of cirrhotic patients with ascites or edema is sodium restriction, because the amount of extracellular fluid retained within the body depends on the balance between the sodium ingested in the diet and the sodium excreted in the urine. As long as the sodium excreted is lower than that ingested, patients will accumulate ascites or edema. Conversely, when sodium excretion is greater than intake, ascites or edema will decrease. The reduction of sodium content in the diet to 40 to 60 mEq/day (1 to 1.5 g of salt) causes a negative sodium balance and

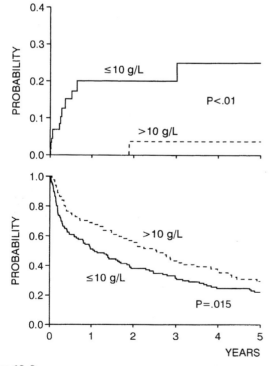

Figure 18–2
Probability of developing spontaneous bacterial peritonitis *(top)* and survival *(bottom)* in cirrhotic patients with ascites according to the protein concentration in ascitic fluid. (Reproduced in part from Llach J, et al: Incidence and predictive factors of first episode of spontaneous bacterial peritonitis in cirrhosis with ascites: Relevance of ascitic fluid protein concentration. Hepatology 16:742–747, 1992.)

Table 18–4 Therapeutic Approach to the Patient with Ascites

Mild or Moderate Ascites

Sodium restriction (40–60 mEq/day)
Spironolactone alone or associated with loop diuretics

Large Ascites

Sodium restriction (40–60 mEq/day)
Therapeutic paracentesis plus IV albumin (8 g/L of ascites) followed by diuretic therapy
Consider liver transplantation

Refractory Ascites

Repeated therapeutic paracentesis plus IV albumin (8 g/L of ascites) or peritoneovenous shunt
Consider liver transplantation

loss of ascites and edema in patients with mild sodium retention (5% to 20% of the whole population of patients with ascites). In patients with moderate or marked sodium retention, such dietary sodium restriction is not sufficient by itself to achieve a negative sodium balance, but it may slow the accumulation of fluid. These patients would require theoretically a more severe restriction of sodium (<20 mEq/day). However, such intense sodium restriction is difficult to accomplish and may impair nutritional status.

Patients with mild or moderate accumulation of ascitic fluid should be treated initially with bed rest and sodium restriction. If this fails to result in diuresis and weight loss, patients should be started on diuretics (Table 18-5). As plasma aldosterone concentration is usually increased in patients with ascites and plays an important role in the increased tubular sodium reabsorption, spironolactone, a drug that competes with aldosterone for the binding to the mineralocorticoid receptor in the collecting tubular epithelial cells, is the diuretic of choice in these patients. Other diuretics acting in the distal tubules, such as amiloride or triamterene, are less effective. Spironolactone is initially given at a dose of 100 mg/day and increased as needed every 4 to 5 days up to a maximum dose of 400 mg/day. Loop diuretics, especially furosemide (20 mg/day initially and increased up to 160 mg/day) or bumetanide or torasemide, which act by inhibiting the Na^+-K^+-$2Cl^-$ cotransporter in the loop of Henle, are commonly given in combination with spironolactone to increase the natriuretic efficacy. Loop diuretics should not be used as single therapy in patients with cirrhosis, because they are less effective than spironolactone, particularly in patients with marked sodium retention. The response to diuretic therapy in cirrhotic patients should be evaluated by measuring body weight, urine volume, and sodium excretion regularly. Diuretics should be given at the minimum effective dose to achieve a weight loss of approximately 300 to 500 g/day in patients with ascites without edema and 800 to 1000 g/day in patients with ascites and edema. An inadequate sodium restriction is a common cause of failure to diuretic therapy, especially in nonhospitalized patients. This situation should be suspected when body weight and ascites do not decrease, despite a high urine volume and natriuresis. Complications of diuretic therapy in patients with cirrhosis are common and include electrolyte disturbances (hyponatremia and hypo/hyperkalemia), renal impairment, hepatic encephalopathy, gynecomastia, and muscle cramps. Hyponatremia occurs more frequently in patients with marked renal dysfunction and during treatment with high doses of loop diuretics. A rise in serum potassium levels is observed in most patients treated with spironolactone but only rarely is important enough to warrant a reduc-

Table 18–5 Diuretics for the Treatment of Ascites or Edema in Cirrhosis

Generic Name	Mechanism	Dose	Site of Action	Comments
Potassium-Sparing Diuretics				
Spironolactone	Antagonist of the mineralocorticoid receptor	25–400 mg/day	Collecting duct	Diuretic of choice Serum potassium must be monitored carefully when renal failure is present. Gynecomastia is a common side effect.
Amiloride	Inhibitor of Na^+ channel	5–10 mg/day	Collecting duct	Less effective than spironolactone
Triamterene	Inhibitor of Na^+ channel	100–300 mg/day	Collecting duct	Similar potency to amiloride
Loop Diuretics				
Furosemide	Inhibitor of Na^+-$2Cl$-K^+ cotransporter	20–160 mg/day	Thick ascending limb of Henle's loop	Use in combination with spironolactone
Bumetanide	Inhibitor of Na^+-$2Cl$-K^+ cotransporter	1–4 mg/day	Thick ascending limb of Henle's loop	Use in combination with spironolactone
Torasemide	Inhibitor of Na^+-$2Cl^-$-K^+ cotransporter	10–40 mg/day	Thick ascending limb of Henle's loop	Use in combination with spironolactone Longer half-life than furosemide

tion or suppression of the medication. However, special attention should be paid to patients with renal failure in whom spironolactone may cause marked hyperkalemia. Hypokalemia usually does not develop, unless patients are treated with loop diuretics alone. The impairment of renal function during diuretic therapy is due to intravascular volume depletion and is usually rapidly reversible after therapy is discontinued. Although aggressive diuretic therapy has been described as a precipitating factor to hepatorenal syndrome, there is no convincing evidence to support this relationship.

In patients with a large accumulation of ascitic fluid (either tense ascites or otherwise), particularly those requiring hospitalization, therapeutic paracentesis has proved to be an effective and less costly approach to initial management than prolonged bed rest and conventional diuretic therapy. In this approach, either all or part (4 to 6 L) of fluid is removed by a specially designed peritoneal needle using strict aseptic techniques. Albumin should be infused intravenously, at a dose of 8 grams per liter of ascitic fluid removed, to avoid circulatory dysfunction caused by a decrease in effective intravascular volume after paracentesis. This circulatory disorder develops almost constantly when patients are treated with paracentesis without plasma volume expansion and is of clinical relevance, because it is associated with a greater risk of a recurrence of ascites and impaired survival. Synthetic plasma expanders (e.g., dextran-70 or hemaccel) are less effective than albumin in the prevention of this disorder. Because paracentesis does not modify the pre-existing sodium retention, maintenance diuretic therapy in conjunction with sodium restriction should be instituted to avoid a recurrence of ascites.

A few cirrhotic patients (10% to 20%) have refractory ascites, a condition defined as ascites that either does not respond or the reaccumulation of which after paracentesis cannot be prevented by diuretics or cannot be treated with maximal doses of diuretics because of the development of diuretic-induced complications (Table 18-6). The best therapeutic option in these patients is repeated therapeutic paracentesis with albumin. An alternative option is the use of peritoneovenous shunt, a prosthesis that has a pressure-sensitive, one-way valve allowing ascitic fluid to flow from the peritoneal cavity to the superior vena cava. The use of the shunt in patients with refractory ascites has declined greatly in recent years because of important side effects that cannot be prevented (e.g., obstruction, superior vena cava thrombosis, peritoneal fibrosis) and the introduction of therapeutic paracentesis. Preliminary studies suggest that transjugular intrahepatic portosystemic shunt (TIPS), which consists of the placement of a self-expandable metal stent between a hepatic vein and the intrahepatic portion of the portal vein using a transjugular approach, may be valuable in the management of patients with refractory ascites. Nevertheless, their use cannot be recommended at present because of insufficient information.

Prognosis

The prognosis of patients with cirrhosis and ascites is poor, with less than 50% of patients surviving 2 years after the onset of ascites (Fig. 18-3). Long-term survivors (>10 years) are very uncommon. Factors known to be associated with a poor prognosis are those that estimate the abnormalities in renal function and systemic hemodynamics (Table 18-7). In patients with ascites, these parameters are better predictors of prognosis than are liver function tests or the Child-Pugh score. The prognosis can also be estimated by observing the patient's response to therapy. When a satisfactory response is observed with only dietary sodium restriction and small doses of diuretics, then the outlook is much better than if intensive diuretic therapy or frequent paracentesis are needed. Owing to this poor prognosis, all patients with ascites should be considered as potential candidates for liver transplantation, and the existence of factors indicative of poor prognosis should be assessed. The decision to perform a liver transplantation should not be delayed until patients are in very poor condition (i.e., refractory ascites or hepatorenal syndrome).

Table 18–6 Definition and Diagnostic Criteria of Refractory Ascites in Cirrhosis

Diuretic-Resistant Ascites. Ascites that cannot be mobilized or the early recurrence of which cannot be prevented due to a lack of response to sodium restriction (50 mEq/day sodium diet) and diuretic treatment (mean loss of weight less than 200 g/day during the last 4 days of intensive diuretic therapy—spironolactone 400 mg/day and furosemide 160 mg/day—and urinary sodium excretion less than 50 mEq/day).

Diuretic-Intractable Ascites. Ascites that cannot be mobilized or the early recurrence of which cannot be prevented due to the development of diuretic-induced complications(**) that preclude the use of an effective diuretic dosage.

**Diuretic-induced complications: Diuretic-induced hepatic encephalopathy: development of hepatic encephalopathy in the absence of other precipitating factors. Diuretic-induced renal failure: increase in serum creatinine by greater than 100% to a value above 2 mg/dL in patients with ascites responding to diuretic treatment. Diuretic-induced hyponatremia: decrease in serum sodium concentration by greater than 10 mEq/L to a level lower than 125 mEq/L. Diuretic-induced hypokalemia or hyperkalemia: decrease of serum potassium concentration to less than 3 mEq/L or increase to more than 6 mEq/L despite appropriate measures to normalize potassium levels.

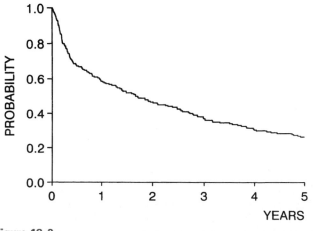

Figure 18–3
Survival of cirrhotic patients with ascites.

Table 18–7 Adverse Prognostic Factors in Cirrhosis with Ascites

Previous ascites	Hyponatremia
Absence of hepatomegaly	Low urine sodium
Poor nutritional status	High plasma renin activity
Low serum albumin	High plasma aldosterone
High serum bilirubin	High plasma norepinephrine
Increased serum creatinine	Low arterial pressure
Reduced water excretion after water load	Esophageal varices

Measurements of renal and hormonal function should be obtained after a minimum of 4 days on a low-sodium diet and without diuretics.

HYPONATREMIA

Definition

Hyponatremia in cirrhotic patients with ascites is usually caused by an inability of the kidneys to excrete water, which results in increased total body water and dilution of extracellular fluid volume. Therefore, hyponatremia is not equivalent to sodium depletion because total sodium content is increased owing to sodium retention.

Pathophysiology

The pathogenesis of water retention in cirrhosis involves several mechanisms, including a reduced delivery of filtrate to the ascending limb of the loop of Henle, the diluting site of the nephron, reduced renal synthesis of prostaglandins (particularly prostaglandin E_2), and increased secretion of arginine-vasopressin (AVP). The latter is probably the most important factor in the disturbed renal water handling in cirrhosis because: (1) plasma AVP levels are commonly increased in cirrhotic patients and correlate closely with the reduction in free water excretion; (2) in experimental animals there is a close chronologic relationship between the appearance of water retention and AVP hypersecretion; (3) Brattleboro rats (rats with a congenital deficiency of AVP) with cirrhosis do not develop water retention; (4) kidneys from cirrhotic rats with ascites show increased gene expression of aquaporin-2, the AVP-regulated water channel; and (5) the administration of specific antagonists of the tubular effect of AVP (V_2 antagonists) restores the impaired water excretion in experimental and human cirrhosis.

The increased plasma AVP levels in cirrhosis are secondary to an enhanced hypothalamic release owing to a nonosmotic stimulus. The mechanism of this nonosmotic hypersecretion is probably hemodynamic, because plasma AVP levels are suppressed by maneuvers that increase effective arterial blood volume and the administration of antagonists of the vascular effect of AVP (V_1 antagonists) is followed by arterial hypotension (Fig. 18-4).

Prevalence and Clinical Features

The prevalence of hyponatremia in hospitalized cirrhotic patients with ascites is approximately 30%. As discussed previously, hyponatremia indicates the existence of a marked disturbance in water excretion. Besides water reten-

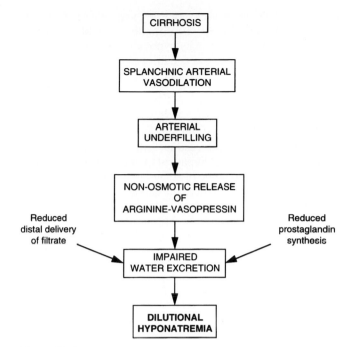

Figure 18–4
Proposed pathogenic mechanisms of dilutional hyponatremia in cirrhosis.

tion, most patients with hyponatremia have avid sodium retention and renal vasoconstriction with reduced renal blood flow and glomerular filtration rate and also marked activation of vasoconstrictor systems.

It should be noted that a normal serum sodium concentration in a cirrhotic patient with ascites should not be interpreted as indicative of a normal renal capacity to excrete water, because a large proportion of patients with ascites have moderate impairment in their capacity to excrete water. These patients are able to maintain a normal serum sodium concentration when their water intake is kept within normal limits, but they may develop hyponatremia when water intake is increased. A common example is hyponatremia observed in hospitalized cirrhotic patients who are maintained with intravenous (IV) 5% dextrose in an amount that exceeds their urine output. Other causes of hyponatremia are shown in Table 18-8.

In some patients, hyponatremia is asymptomatic, but in others it may be associated with clinical symptoms similar to those found in dilutional hyponatremia of other etiologies, including anorexia, headache, difficulty in mental con-

Table 18–8 Major Causes of Hyponatremia in Cirrhotic Patients with Ascites

Spontaneous
Induced
    Excessive administration of IV fluids
    Diuretics
    Nonsteroidal anti-inflammatory drugs
    Vasopressin analogues
    Therapeutic paracentesis without plasma expansion

centration, lethargy, nausea, vomiting and, occasionally, seizures. In most cases it may be difficult to establish whether these symptoms are caused by hyponatremia, the underlying liver disease, or associated conditions.

Treatment

No pharmacologic therapy exists for dilutional hyponatremia, and the only therapeutic measure that may improve or stop the progressive decrease in serum sodium concentration is water restriction. In patients with marked hyponatremia, fluid intake should be restricted to 500 to 1000 mL/day. The administration of hypertonic saline solutions is not recommended, because it invariably leads to further expansion of extracellular fluid volume and accumulation of ascites and edema. A number of drugs that increase selectively renal water excretion (aquaretic agents), including antagonists of the V_2 receptor of AVP and kappa-opioid agonists, are currently under investigation for their potential use in the treatment of hyponatremia in cirrhosis.

Prognosis

Spontaneous dilutional hyponatremia is usually a late event in the natural history of cirrhosis with ascites. The median survival time of patients with hyponatremia is 15 months, compared with 24 months for patients who do not have hyponatremia (Fig. 18-5). In patients without overt renal failure, the presence of hyponatremia is a predictive factor for the development of hepatorenal syndrome.

HEPATORENAL SYNDROME

Definition

Hepatorenal syndrome (HRS) is a common and serious complication of cirrhosis that is characterized by impaired renal function and marked disturbances in the arterial circu-

lation and activity of vasoactive systems. In the renal circulation there is a marked increase in vascular resistance, whereas total systemic vascular resistance is reduced, which results in arterial hypotension. This reduction in systemic vascular resistance is mainly caused by an arterial vasodilatation of the splanchnic circulation, because nonsplanchnic vascular beds appear to be also vasoconstricted.

Pathophysiology

The pathophysiologic hallmark of HRS is a vasoconstriction of the renal circulation. The kidneys are structurally intact. The mechanism of this vasoconstriction is poorly understood and possibly multifactorial, involving increased vasoconstrictor and reduced vasodilator factors that act on the renal circulation. The most accepted theory on the pathogenesis of HRS (Arterial Vasodilation Theory) proposes that renal hypoperfusion represents the extreme manifestation of an underfilling of the arterial circulation secondary to a marked vasodilatation of the splanchnic area (Fig. 18-6). This arterial underfilling would result in a progressive baroreceptor-mediated activation of vasoconstrictor systems (i.e., renin-angiotensin and sympathetic nervous systems) that would cause vasoconstriction not only in the renal circulation but also in other vascular beds (lower and upper extremities). The splanchnic area would escape to the effect of vasoconstrictors and a marked vasodilation would persist, probably because of the existence of very potent local vasodilator stimuli. In early phases following the development of ascites, renal perfusion would be maintained within normal or near-normal levels despite the overactivity of vasoconstrictor systems by an increased synthesis/activity of renal vasodilator factors. The development of renal hypoperfusion leading to HRS would occur either as a result of a maximal activation of vasoconstrictor systems that could

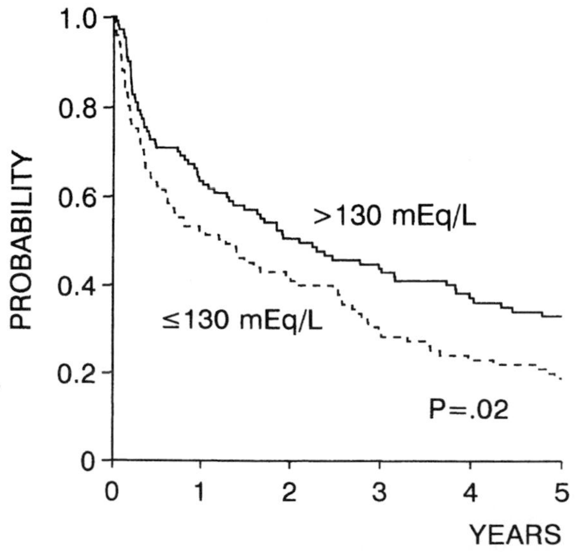

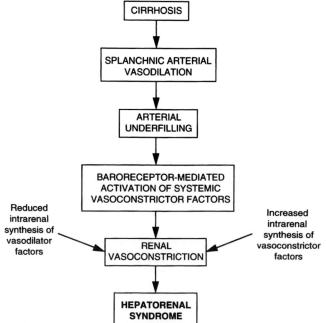

Figure 18–5
Survival of cirrhotic patients with ascites with and without hyponatremia.

Figure 18–6
Proposed pathogenic mechanisms of hepatorenal syndrome in cirrhosis.

Table 18–9   Common Causes of Renal Failure in Cirrhosis Other than Hepatorenal Syndrome

Prerenal failure due to volume depletion (diuretics, vomiting, diarrhea)
Acute tubular necrosis
Glomerulonephritis
Nephrotoxicity (nonsteroidal anti-inflammatory drugs, aminoglycosides)

Table 18–10   Diagnostic Criteria of Hepatorenal Syndrome*

Major Criteria

1. Low glomerular filtration rate, as indicated by serum creatinine greater than 1.5 mg/dL or 24-hour creatinine clearance lower than 40 ml/min
2. Absence of shock, ongoing bacterial infection, fluid losses, and current treatment with nephrotoxic drugs
3. No sustained improvement in renal function (decrease in serum creatinine to 1.5 mg/dL or less or increase in creatinine clearance to 40 mL/min or more) following diuretic withdrawal and expansion of plasma volume with 1.5 L of a plasma expander
4. Proteinuria lower than 500 mg/day and no ultrasonographic evidence of obstructive uropathy or parenchymal renal disease

Additional Criteria

1. Urine volume lower than 500 mL/day
2. Urine sodium lower than 10 mEq/L
3. Urine osmolality greater than plasma osmolality
4. Urine red blood cells less than 50 per high-power field
5. Serum sodium concentration lower than 130 mEq/L

*All major criteria must be present for the diagnosis of hepatorenal syndrome. Additional criteria are not necessary for the diagnosis but provide supportive evidence. From Arroyo V, Ginès P, Gerbes A, et al: Definition and diagnostic criteria of refractory ascites and hepatorenal syndrome in cirrhosis. Hepatology 23:164, 1996.

not be counteracted by vasodilator factors, decreased activity of vasodilator factors, and/or increased production of intrarenal vasoconstrictor factors. An alternative theory proposes that renal vasoconstriction is the result of a direct relationship between the liver and the kidney, without any relationship with disturbances in systemic hemodynamics. The link between the liver and the kidney would be either a liver vasodilator factor, the synthesis of which would be reduced as a consequence of liver failure, or a hepatorenal reflex causing renal vasoconstriction.

Clinical Features and Diagnosis

HRS is a common complication of cirrhotic patients with ascites. The incidence of HRS in patients with cirrhosis hospitalized for the treatment of ascites is approximately 10%. Two different types of HRS, which represent distinct expressions of the same pathogenic mechanism, exist. *Type I HRS* is characterized by rapid and progressive impairment of renal function as defined by a doubling of the initial serum creatinine to a level higher than 2.5 mg/dL or a 50% reduction of the initial 24-hour creatinine clearance to a level lower than 20 mL/min in less than 2 weeks. Renal failure in these patients is often associated with progressive oliguria, marked sodium retention, and hyponatremia. Patients with type I HRS are usually in a very severe clinical condition and show signs of advanced liver failure. In approximately half of the cases, this type of HRS develops spontaneously without any identifiable precipitating factor, whereas in the remaining patients it occurs in close chronologic relationship with some complications or therapeutic interventions (e.g., bacterial infection, particularly spontaneous bacterial peritonitis, paracentesis without plasma expansion). *Type II HRS* is characterized by moderate and stable reduction of GFR that does not meet the criteria proposed for type I. Unlike type I HRS, type II HRS usually occurs in patients with relatively preserved hepatic function. The main clinical consequence of this type of HRS is diuretic-resistant ascites.

There is no specific test for the diagnosis of HRS. The diagnosis of HRS is based on the exclusion of other common causes of renal failure that may occur in patients with cirrhosis (Table 18-9) and demonstration of a low GFR. Criteria for the diagnosis of HRS are shown in Table 18-10. Although a cut-off value of serum creatinine of 1.5 mg/dL may seem low, cirrhotic patients with ascites with serum creatinine above 1.5 mg/dL have a GFR below 30 mL/min, which represents only one fourth of the normal GFR for healthy subjects of the same age. The low serum creatinine values relative to the reduction in GFR are probably related to a reduced endogenous production of creatinine caused by the poor nutritional status of cirrhotic patients. Most cases of

HRS have urine sodium below 10 mEq/L and urine osmolality above plasma osmolality because of the preservation of tubular function. Nevertheless, some patients may have high urine sodium and low urine osmolality, similar to what occurs in acute tubular necrosis. Conversely, cirrhotic patients with acute tubular necrosis may have low urine sodium and high osmolality. For these reasons, urinary indices are not considered major criteria for the diagnosis of HRS.

Treatment

Various therapeutic modalities have been used in patients with HRS, with only minor or no beneficial effects. Recent reports suggest that the administration of systemic vasoconstrictors, particularly ornipressin, or the insertion of TIPS may be useful. However, the efficacy of these methods should be evaluated in controlled investigations. The only effective treatment for HRS at present is liver transplantation. However, a significant proportion of patients die before transplantation can be done because of their extremely short survival rate. Therefore, liver transplantation should be indicated before the development of HRS. Patients with ascites who are more likely to develop HRS are those with very reduced urine sodium, dilutional hyponatremia, arterial hypotension, and marked activation of renin-angiotensin and sympathetic nervous systems.

Prognosis

The prognosis of patients with HRS is very poor. Type I HRS is the complication with the worst prognosis for cirrhotic patients. The median survival time of these patients is less than 2 weeks, which is a survival time shorter than that

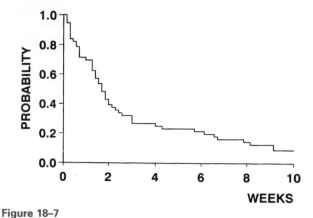

Figure 18–7
Survival after the development of hepatorenal syndrome.
(From Ginès A, Escorsell A, Ginès P, et al: Incidence, predictive
factors, and prognosis of the hepatorenal syndrome in
cirrhosis with ascites. Gastroenterology 105:229–236, 1993.)

of patients with acute renal failure of other etiologies (Fig.
18-7). The combination of several factors, including renal
failure, liver failure, and, in some cases, associated conditions, accounts probably for this extremely poor outcome.
The median survival of patients with type II HRS is usually
several months, which is a longer survival time than those
with type I but shorter than patients with ascites without renal failure.

SPONTANEOUS BACTERIAL PERITONITIS

Definition

Spontaneous bacterial peritonitis (SBP) is a common and
severe complication of cirrhotic patients with ascites, which
is characterized by spontaneous infection of ascitic fluid
without an intra-abdominal source of infection. The prevalence of SBP in hospitalized patients with ascites ranges
from 10% to 30%. Cirrhotic patients with hydrothorax may
also develop a spontaneous infection of pleural fluid.

Pathophysiology

The isolation of aerobic gram-negative bacteria in most episodes of SBP suggests that the gastrointestinal tract is the
source of bacteria. Although the pathogenesis of SBP is not
completely understood, it is generally accepted that it involves three major steps: (1) passage of bacteria from the
intestinal lumen to the systemic circulation; (2) bacteremia
secondary to the impairment of the reticuloendothelial system (RES) phagocytic activity, and (3) infection of ascites
caused by defective antimicrobial activity of ascitic fluid.
Studies in experimental animals with cirrhosis suggest that
bacterial translocation (i.e., passage of bacteria from the intestinal lumen to mesenteric lymph nodes) is the mechanism
by which bacteria from the intestinal lumen reach the systemic circulation. Bacterial translocation may increase under several circumstances, such as hemorrhagic shock. This
may explain, at least in part, the high incidence of infections
caused by enteric bacteria in cirrhotic patients with gastro-

intestinal hemorrhage. The reduced phagocytic activity of
the RES (a system that removes bacteria from the circulation) is another important pathogenic factor in the development of SBP. Cirrhotic patients with reduced activity of the
RES are highly predisposed to develop SBP, whereas this
infection is rarely seen in patients with normal activity of
the RES. Finally, a reduced antimicrobial activity of the ascitic fluid also plays a very important role in the development of SBP. Patients with reduced antimicrobial activity of
ascitic fluid have a greater risk of developing ascitic fluid
infection than those with normal antimicrobial activity of
the ascitic fluid. As the antimicrobial activity of ascites correlates with total ascitic fluid protein concentration, patients
with low ascites protein content (<10 g/L) have a greater
risk of developing SBP compared with patients with higher
ascites protein concentration (see Fig. 18-2).

The most accepted theory on the pathogenesis of SBP is
shown in Figure 18-8. The initial step involves translocation
of bacteria from the gut flora to mesenteric lymph nodes.
This translocation would occur either spontaneously or as a
consequence of some precipitating events (i.e., gastrointestinal hemorrhage). An increased permeability of the gut related to histologic changes in the gut mucosa or intestinal
bacterial overgrowth may facilitate bacterial translocation.
The bacteria then reach the systemic circulation through the
lymphatic system. In cases of SBP that are not caused by
bacteria from enteric origin, the bacteria would reach the
systemic circulation from other areas (i.e., respiratory or urinary tracts or skin). In patients with normal activity of the
RES, bacteria are efficiently removed from the circulation,
but persistent bacteremia develops in patients with impaired
activity of the RES. Subsequently, bacteria may reach the
ascitic fluid through an hematogenous route. The development of SBP depends on the antimicrobial activity of the ascitic fluid. Infection of ascites does not occur in patients
with good antimicrobial activity of the ascitic fluid. By contrast, patients with reduced antimicrobial activity of the ascitic fluid develop SBP. A similar mechanism may explain
the development of spontaneous bacterial empyema.

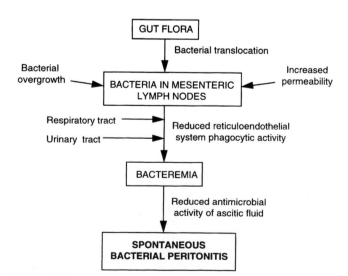

Figure 18–8
Proposed pathogenic mechanisms of spontaneous bacterial
peritonitis in cirrhosis.

Table 18–11   Clinical Signs or Symptoms at Presentation in a Series of 161 Cirrhotic Patients with Spontaneous Bacterial Peritonitis

Clinical Signs or Symptoms	% of Patients
Abdominal pain	80
Fever	70
Hepatic encephalopathy	58
Hypoperistalsis	32
Diarrhea	19
Septic shock	16
Gastrointestinal bleeding	15
Vomiting	13
No symptoms	10

Clinical Features and Diagnosis

The clinical spectrum of SBP is very variable (Table 18-11). A very high degree of clinical suspicion is required to make a diagnosis, because only a relatively low percentage of patients show the typical features of an acute peritoneal infection with fever, chills, diffuse abdominal pain, rebound tenderness, and reduced bowel sounds. Fever may be the only clinical sign in a large proportion of patients. In other cases, the infection is manifested by hepatic encephalopathy or septic shock. In 10% of cases, SBP may be totally asymptomatic. Renal failure develops in one third of patients with SBP. The development of renal failure may occur despite the resolution of the infection and is associated with a poor prognosis. Mechanisms responsible for renal failure during SBP are currently unknown. Patients who survive an episode of SBP are at high risk of developing recurrent episodes of SBP during follow-up. As many as 70% of patients who survive 1 year after the first episode of SBP will develop a new episode of infection within this period. Gram-negative bacteria are the most common isolates in recurrent episodes of SBP, regardless of the type of bacteria responsible for the first episode. Factors associated with a greater risk of a recurrence of SBP are impaired liver function and low protein concentration in ascitic fluid.

The diagnosis of SBP is based on examination of ascitic fluid. A diagnostic paracentesis should be performed routinely in all cirrhotic patient admitted to hospital with ascites and in those hospitalized patients in whom a peritoneal infection is suspected because of fever, abdominal pain, shock, hepatic encephalopathy, or renal impairment. It is commonly accepted that the presence of a polymorphonuclear leukocyte count greater than 250 mm^3 in the ab-

sence of an intra-abdominal source of infection is indicative of SBP and should prompt the administration of broad-spectrum antibiotics. The determination of pH or lactate levels in ascitic fluid is not useful in the diagnosis of SBP. The concentration of bacteria in ascitic fluid of patients with SBP is usually very low (1 microorganism/mL or less). This low concentration accounts for the high frequency of culture-negative SBP when using conventional culture methods. The inoculation of 10 mL of ascitic fluid into blood culture bottles immediately after paracentesis improves the rate of positive ascitic fluid cultures. The most common isolates are gram-negative bacilli from intestinal origin, especially *Escherichia coli*. Pneumoccci and other gram-positive bacteria are less common. Anaerobic and microaerophilic organisms, although very abundant in gut flora, rarely cause SBP.

Despite the use of sensitive methods of ascitic fluid culture, between 20% and 40% of episodes of SBP diagnosed by high polymorphonuclear count are culture-negative. This condition, known as culture-negative SBP, or culture-negative neutrocytic ascites, should be considered as SBP and patients should be managed with antibiotics (Table 18-12). Bacterascites is a different condition that consists of a positive ascitic fluid culture with a normal polymorphonuclear count and represents probably an early colonization of ascitic fluid by bacteria without inflammatory response. Because some patients with bacterascites may develop SBP, a follow-up paracentesis is advisable in these patients to rule out progression of the infection.

The main condition to be considered in the differential diagnosis of SBP is peritonitis secondary to gut perforation or peritoneal abscess, because the latter is also associated with an increased polymorphonuclear count in ascitic fluid. Although secondary peritonitis is less common than SBP, the differentiation between the two conditions is very important, because surgical treatment is required for secondary peritonitis. The ascitic fluid in cirrhotic patients with secondary peritonitis is usually characterized by markedly high polymorphonuclear count, protein levels over 10 g/L, increased LDH, and multiple organisms in the Gram stain or culture. Nevertheless, the existence of perforation or abscesses causing secondary peritonitis should be confirmed by appropriate methods, such as abdominal x-ray, ultrasound, computed tomography (CT) scan, or radioisotope scintigraphy.

Treatment

Empirical antibiotic therapy should be initiated in patients with a polymorphonuclear count in ascitic fluid greater than

Table 18–12   Diagnosis of Spontaneous Bacterial Peritonitis and Related Conditions

Condition	PMN Count in Ascites	Ascitic Fluid	Comments
Culture-positive SBP	>250/mm^3	Positive	Requires antibiotic therapy
Culture-negative SBP	>250/mm^3	Negative	Requires antibiotic therapy Better prognosis than culture-positive SBP
Bacterascites	<250/mm^3	Positive	May progress to SBP

PMN, polymorphonuclear; SBP, spontaneous bacterial peritonitis.

Table 18–13 Antibiotics Used in the Treatment of Spontaneous Bacterial Peritonitis

Antibiotic	Dose	SBP Resolution	Comments
Cefotaxime (or other third-generation cephalosporins)	2 g/12hr IV	75–90%	Antibiotic of choice
Ofloxacin	400 mg/12hr PO	84%	Advantage of oral administration May substitute cefotaxime in patients without GI hemorrhage, ileus, or septic shock
Amoxicillin-clavulanic acid	1 g–200 mg/6hr IV	85%	No comparison with cefotaxime in randomized studies

GI, gastrointestinal; SBP, spontaneous bacterial peritonitis.

250 mm³ before the detection of the causative organisms by ascitic fluid culture. The antibiotics of choice as initial empirical treatment for cirrhotic patients with SBP are third-generation cephalosporins, owing to their broad antibacterial spectrum, high efficacy, and few side effects (Table 18-13). Although cefotaxime has been the drug more commonly used, other cephalosporins, such as ceftriaxone, have similar efficacy. In randomized comparative studies, cefotaxime has been shown to be more effective than other types of antibiotics, such as aztreonam or aminoglycosides plus ampicillin. Amoxicillin-clavulanic acid seems also effective, but comparative studies between this antibiotic and third-generation cephalosporins are lacking. Ofloxacin is as effective as IV cefotaxime in terms of resolution of infection and survival and has the additional advantage of oral administration and low cost. Nevertheless, patients in severe condition (i.e., septic shock) or with complications that may impair oral absorption of drugs (gastrointestinal hemorrhage or ileus) should be treated with IV antibiotics. Treatment with antibiotics should be maintained until all signs of infection (e.g., fever, abdominal pain, normalization of blood polymorphonuclear count) completely disappear and the polymorphonuclear count in ascitic fluid is reduced to below 250 mm³.

Prognosis

The resolution of SBP in patients treated with third-generation cephalosporins is obtained in 75% to 90% of cases. Factors associated with a lack of response to therapy are renal impairment, high blood polymorphonuclear count,

hospital acquired SBP, and high AST levels. Despite the high rate of resolution of the infection, the mortality rate of patients with SBP during hospitalization remains very high, between 20% and 40%. The most important predictor of survival in patients with SBP is the development of renal impairment during the infection. Other prognostic factors are shown in Table 18-14.

The long-term prognosis of cirrhotic patients who have recovered from an episode of SBP is poor. The 1-year survival probability is only 40% (Fig. 18-9). Because of this short survival, patients recovering from an episode of SBP should be considered for liver transplantation. The main causes of death in these patients are recurrent episodes of SBP, liver failure, and gastrointestinal hemorrhage.

Prevention

The administration of antibiotics is a useful method in the prevention of SBP in specific subsets of cirrhotic patients with a high risk of developing this complication (Table 18-15). Antibiotic prophylaxis is effective in patients with gastrointestinal hemorrhage and in patients who have recovered from the first SBP episode. In patients with gastrointestinal hemorrhage, the administration of norfloxacin or ofloxacin during and shortly after the bleeding episode re-

Table 18–14 Adverse Predictive Factors of Spontaneous Bacterial Peritonitis in Cirrhosis

Response to Therapy	Survival
Renal impairment	Renal impairment
High blood PMN count	Older age
Hospital-acquired	Positive ascitic fluid culture
High AST levels	High Child-Pugh score
	GI bleeding
	High PMN count in ascites
	Ileus

AST, aspartate transaminase; GI, gastrointestinal; PMN, polymorphonuclear.

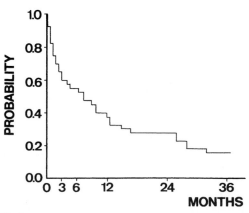

Figure 18–9
Survival of patients with cirrhosis after resolution of the first episode of spontaneous bacterial peritonitis. (From Tító LL, et al: Recurrence of spontaneous bacterial peritonitis in cirrhosis: Frequency and predictive factors. Hepatology 8:27–31, 1988.)

Table 18–15   Effective Antibiotic Prophylaxis of Spontaneous Bacterial Peritonitis (SBP) in Cirrhotic Patients with Ascites

Condition	Antibiotic Regimen	Duration	Comments
Gastrointestinal hemorrhage	Norfloxacin 400 mg bid (PO or gastric tube)	7 days	Reduce the incidence of SBP and other bacterial infections compared with the placebo
	Ofloxacin 400 mg/day (IV or PO)	10 days	Reduce the incidence of SBP and other bacterial infections compared with the placebo
	Ciprofloxacin 200 mg/day plus amoxicillin-clavulanic acid 1 g–200 mg/8hr IV	10 days	Reduce the incidence of SBP and other bacterial infections compared with the placebo
Prevention of SBP recurrence (secondary prophylaxis)	Norfloxacin 400 mg/day PO	Indefinitely	Prevents recurrence due to gram-negative bacilli Does not increase the incidence of SBP due to gram-positive bacteria or gram-negative-resistant bacteria
Prevention of first SBP in patients with low ascites protein (<10–15 g/L) (primary prophylaxis)	Norfloxacin 400 mg/day PO, or Ciprofloxacin 750 mg/wk PO, or Trimethoprim (160 mg) Sulfamethoxazole (800 mg)/5 times a week PO		No experience in therapy longer than 6 months

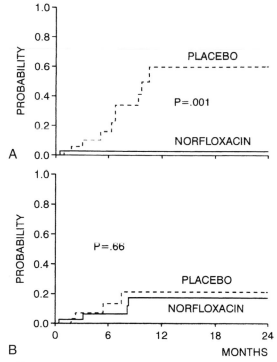

Figure 18–10
Probability of the recurrence of spontaneous bacterial peritonitis in patients treated chronically with norfloxacin (400 mg/day) as secondary prophylaxis and patients treated with a placebo. **A,** Episodes caused by gram-negative bacteria. **B,** Episodes caused by gram-positive bacteria or culture-negative bacteria. (From Ginès P, et al: Norfloxacin prevents spontaneous bacterial peritonitis recurrence in cirrhosis: Results of a double-blind, placebo-controlled trial. Hepatology 12:716–724, 1990.)

duces greatly the incidence of SBP or bacteremia. Long-term norfloxacin is also very effective in the prevention of a recurrence of SBP in cirrhotic patients. The probability of a recurrence of SBP at 1 year of follow-up is reduced from 70% to 20%, and is attributed to gram-negative bacilli (60% versus 3% at 1 year) (Fig. 18-10). The antibiotic prophylaxis does not increase the probability of developing SBP or other infections caused by gram-positive bacteria or gram-negative resistant organisms. Bacteriologic studies of the fecal flora in patients treated with norfloxacin show a marked reduction or disappearance of gram-negative bacilli from the fecal flora a few days after the initiation of treatment. By contrast, no significant changes in gram-positive cocci, anaerobic bacteria, and *Candida* species occur during treatment. Antibiotic prophylaxis after resolution of SBP should be given to all patients with SBP, regardless of the type of bacteria responsible for the index episode, because gram-negative bacteria are the most common isolates in recurrent SBP. Antibiotic prophylaxis (e.g., with norfloxacin, ciprofloxacin, and trimethoprim-sulfamethoxazole) may be also effective in the prevention of the first episode of SBP (primary prophylaxis) in patients with low (<10 to 15 g/L) ascitic fluid protein, but this indication requires further evaluation in controlled studies.

SUGGESTED READINGS

Ascites

Benoit JN, Granger DN: Splanchnic hemodynamics in chronic portal hypertension. Semin Liver Dis 6:287–298, 1986.

Clària J, Jiménez W, Ros J, et al: Pathogenesis of arterial hypotension in cirrhotic rats with ascites: role of endogenous nitric oxide. Hepatology 5:343–349, 1992.

Ginès A, Arroyo V, Monescillo A, et al: Randomized trial comparing albumin, dextran-70 and polygeline in cirrhotic patients with ascites treated by paracentesis. Gastroenterology 111:1002–1010, 1996.

Ginès P, Arroyo V, Quintero E, et al: Comparison of paracentesis and diuretics in the treatment of cirrhotics with tense ascites. Results of a randomized study. Gastroenterology 93:234–241, 1987.

Ginès P, Arroyo V, Vargas V, et al: Paracentesis with intravenous infusion of albumin as compared with peritoneovenous shunting in cirrhosis with refractory ascites. N Engl J Med 325:829–835, 1991.

Ginès P, Titó L, Arroyo V, et al: Randomized comparative study of therapeutic paracentesis with and without intravenous albumin in cirrhosis. Gastroenterology 94:1493–1502, 1988.

Groszmann RJ: Hyperdynamic circulation of liver disease 40 years later: Pathophysiology and clinical consequences. Hepatology 20:1359–1363, 1994.

Llach J, Ginès P, Arroyo V, et al: Prognostic value of arterial pressure, endogenous vasoactive systems, and renal function in cirrhotic patients admitted to the hospital for the treatment of ascites. Gastroenterology 94:482–487, 1988.

Ochs A, Rössle M, Haag K, et al: The transjugular intrahepatic portosystemic stent-shunt procedure for refractory ascites. N Engl J Med 332:1192–1197, 1995.

Schrier RW, Arroyo V, Bernardi M, et al: Peripheral arterial vasodilation hypothesis: A proposal for the initiation of renal sodium and water retention in cirrhosis. Hepatology 8:1151–1157, 1988.

Hyponatremia

Gines P, Berl T, Bernardi M, et al: Hyponatremia in cirrhosis: From pathogenesis to treatment. Hepatology 28:851–864, 1998.

Ginès P, Jiménez W: Aquaretic agents: A new potential treatment of dilutional hyponatremia in cirrhosis. J Hepatol 24:506–512, 1996.

Hepatorenal Syndrome

Arroyo V, Ginès P, Gerbes A, et al: Definition and diagnostic criteria of refractory ascites and hepatorenal syndrome in cirrhosis. Hepatology 23:164–176, 1996.

Ginès A, Escorsell A, Ginès P, et al: Incidence, predictive factors, and prognosis of the hepatorenal syndrome in cirrhosis with ascites. Gastroenterology 105:229–236, 1993.

Gonwa TA, Morris CA, Goldstein RM, et al: Long-term survival and renal function following liver transplantation in patients with and without hepatorenal syndrome experience in 300 patients. Transplantation 51:428–430, 1991.

Spontaneous Bacterial Peritonitis

Andreu M, Solà R, Sitges-Serra A, et al: Risk factors for spontaneous bacterial peritonitis in cirrhotic patients with ascites. Gastroenterology 104:1133–1138, 1993.

Felisart J, Rimola A, Arroyo V, et al: Cefotaxime is more effective than is ampicillin-tobramycin in cirrhotics with severe infections. Hepatology 5:457–462, 1985.

Follo A, Llovet JM, Navasa M, et al: Renal impairment after spontaneous bacterial peritonitis in cirrhosis: Incidence, clinical course, predictive factors and prognosis. Hepatology 20:1495–1501, 1994.

García-Tsao G, Lee FY, Barden G, et al: Bacterial translocation to mesenteric lymph nodes is increased in cirrhotic rats with ascites. Gastroenterology 108:1835–1841, 1995.

Ginés P, Rimola A, Planas R, et al: Norfloxacin prevents spontaneous bacterial peritonitis recurrence in cirrhosis: Results of a double blind, placebo-controlled trial. Hepatology 12:716–724, 1990.

Navasa M, Follo A, Llovet JM, et al: Randomized, comparative study of oral ofloxacin versus intravenous cefotaxime in spontaneous bacterial peritonitis. Gastroenterology 111:1011–1017, 1996.

Rolachon A, Cordier L, Bacq Y, et al: Ciprofloxacin and long-term prevention of spontaneous bacterial peritonitis: results of a prospective controlled trial. Hepatology 22:1171–1174, 1995.

Runyon B. Low-protein-concentration ascitic fluid is predisposed to spontaneous bacterial peritonitis. Gastroenterology 91:1343–1346, 1986.

Singh N, Gayowski T, Yu VL, et al: Trimethoprim-sulfamethoxazole for the prevention of spontaneous bacterial peritonitis in cirrhosis: A randomized trial. Ann Intern Med 122:595–598, 1995.

Soriano G, Guarner C, Tomás A, et al: Norfloxacin prevents bacterial infection in cirrhotics with gastrointestinal hemorrhage. Gastroenterology 103:1267–1272, 1992.

Toledo C, Salmerón JM, Rimola A, et al: Spontaneous bacterial peritonitis in cirrhosis: Predictive factors of infection resolution and survival in patients treated with cefotaxime. Hepatology 17:251–257, 1993.

Xiol X, Castellví JM, Guardiola J, et al: Spontaneous bacterial empyema in cirrhotic patients: a prospective study. Hepatology 23:719–723, 1996.

19

Portosystemic Encephalopathy

Kevin D. Mullen
Steedman A. Sarbah
Annette Kyprianou

Portosystemic (or portal-systemic) encephalopathy (PSE) is a term used to describe a wide spectrum of neuropsychiatric abnormalities in patients with chronic liver disease or well-established portosystemic shunting of splanchnic venous blood. In its clinically overt form, most patients not only have portosystemic shunting of blood but also clear evidence of reduction in hepatic parenchymal function. The relative importance of loss of hepatic function versus portosystemic shunting of blood in the genesis of the syndrome is debated.

It is widely accepted that PSE occurs because gut-derived "toxins" escape hepatic detoxification and accumulate in the systemic circulation. Whether accumulation of these gut derived "toxins" leads to PSE by a direct mechanism or by inducing secondary changes in brain neurochemistry is uncertain. Progress in our understanding of the pathogenesis of this syndrome has been slow for three main reasons: (1) ethical constraints in obtaining appropriate sample sites for measuring "toxin" levels (e.g., cerebrospinal fluid); (2) poor understanding of the mechanisms responsible for maintenance of consciousness; and (3) lack of an animal model for this syndrome. Despite these limitations, quite effective empirical therapy has been developed to treat PSE.

NOMENCLATURE AND TERMINOLOGY ISSUES

PSE is close to being replaced by the term hepatic encephalopathy (HE). Already in widespread use, HE is being adopted by a working group appointed to standardize terminology in this field. However, until a consensus is reached, the terms PSE and HE will be used, sometimes interchangeably. It is anticipated that a final recommendation on this issue will have been made at the World Congress of Gastroenterology in Vienna in 1998. Meanwhile, in the literal absence of any agreed upon nomenclature, terminology, and diagnostic criteria for this syndrome, the literature in this field is confusing. In particular, terms such as acute and chronic HE have different meanings for clinicians. A mnemonic type of classification may become the accepted terminology (Table 19–1).

PATTERNS OF CLINICAL PRESENTATION

Even with a lack of consensus on some key issues, a discrete number of patterns of presentation of PSE are recognized (Table 19–2). One of the drawbacks for the term PSE is that it is not readily applicable to encephalopathy seen in acute liver failure. This may be reasonable because there are many differences in the encephalopathy seen in acute liver failure and that observed in patients with chronic liver disease (Table 19–3). Nonetheless, there are some common links, including the presence of some evidence of portosystemic shunting and portal hypertension in acute liver failure (Table 19–4).

Little else will be said about encephalopathy in acute liver failure (see Chapter 22), except to emphasize the new term *a*cute *l*iver *f*ailure *a*ssociated *h*epatic *e*ncephalopathy, or ALFA-HE. This is likely to be endorsed by the working groups mentioned earlier.

Returning to the patterns of clinical presentation in chronic liver disease, one important point bears emphasis. The term episode or episodic implies an event that is self-limited; that is, the patient returns to a normal neurologic state after recovery as implied by Adams and Foley almost 50 years ago. However, in a provocative article, Kreiger and associates have raised the possibility that recovery from overt episodes of PSE may not be complete.

Table 19–1 Classification of Hepatic Encephalopathy

Type A—*Acute liver failure associated hepatic encephalopathy* (ALFA-HE)
Type B*—Classic PSE in patients with "normal" liver function and portosystemic *bypass*
Type C—HE in patients with chronic liver disease/*cirrhosis*

*This type is retained because it is very well described in historical articles in the literature. It is relatively uncommon.
PSE, portosystemic encephalopathy.

Table 19–2 Presentation Patterns of Portosystemic Encephalopathy

- Subclinical
- Acute episode—spontaneous
- Acute episode—precipitated
- Recurrent episodes—spontaneous
- Recurrent episodes—precipitated
- Chronic mild
- Chronic severe ⇄ hepatocerebral degeneration

Acute, onset within hours to days; episode, clinically evident but full recovery within 1 month; spontaneous, no precipitating factor evident; precipitated, defined precipitating event present; chronic, present for 1 month or longer; mild, neurologic deficit present but capable of daily functions; severe, neurologic deficit sufficient to affect daily living.

EPIDEMIOLOGY

Unlike some of the other complications of liver disease, PSE is not easy to define, diagnose, or quantify in terms of severity. Hence, unlike ascites, variceal bleeding, and the hepatorenal syndrome, the epidemiology of PSE is difficult to discern from the literature.

Based on ICD-9 discharge coding (572.2), there were ap-proximately 50,000 episodes of PSE in the United States in 1994 to 1995. No doubt this does not include all cases of clinically significant PSE that occurred, but little other data are available. Based on data from MetroHealth Medical Center and Cleveland Clinic Foundation (1996 to 1997), the incidences of PSE by ICD-9 coding were 2.5/1000 and 3.6/1000 discharges, respectively. Considering that both of these hospitals treat a fairly large population of patients with liver disease (MetroHealth Medical Center is a county hospital; Cleveland Clinic Foundation is a liver transplant center), estimates of 50,000 to 100,000 cases of PSE for the entire United States may be reasonable.

It is not possible to accurately predict the lifetime incidence of PSE in a cirrhotic patient based on the existing literature. In a recently published large series of cirrhotic patients with hepatitis C, who were followed from the time of diagnosis, 5 of 384 developed PSE as the first sign of hepatic decompensation (mean period of follow-up was 61 months). Incidences of 10% to 13% of PSE are encountered in sclerotherapy populations, which may reflect a figure with some validity. Postsurgical shunt patients and patients with transjugular intrahepatic portosystemic shunt (TIPS) have widely varying incidences of PSE. However, in almost all studies, methods to evaluate PSE are poorly described or simply are invalid. Furthermore, follow-up periods were radically different because of the study design or factors such as liver transplantation. In the best of hands, postsurgical shunt PSE is in the 5% to 15% range, a figure remarkably similar to that found in patients undergoing TIPS procedures. PSE that is intractable or difficult to manage is much less common, and this problem should be of most concern to physicians. A distinction between PSE responsive to medical management and PSE refractory to medical management is not always evident in the published literature.

Much better data are needed on the epidemiology and natural history of PSE in patients with chronic liver disease. It is likely that as the etiology of the majority of liver dis-

Table 19–3 Difference in Clinical Pattern

	PSE	vs.	ALFA-HE
Precipitating factor	Common		Rarely easily identified
Response to treatment	Usually good		Frequently poor
Short-term mortality	Low to moderate		Very high
Cerebral edema	Rare		Common
Seizures	Uncommon		20–30% of cases
Hypoglycemia	Uncommon		Common

ALFA-HE, acute liver failure associated hepatic encephalopathy; PSE, portosystemic encephalopathy.

Table 19–4 Common Links Between PSE and ALFA-HE

	PSE	ALFA-HE
Evidence of portosystemic shunts	Prominent in most cases	Varices seen in some cases
Splenomegaly	Often	Seen in 30% ? of cases
Elevated blood ammonia	Very often	Less prominent but present
Response to flumazenil	10–30% ?	Reported
Detection of benzodiazepines	70–80% ?	70–80%

ALFA-HE, acute liver failure associated hepatic encephalopathy; PSE, portosystemic encephalopathy.

ease in the United States changes, we will see an alteration in the incidence and natural history of PSE. Formerly, the bulk of patients had exclusively alcohol as a cause for cirrhosis. These patients generally presented with PSE at a time when both florid evidence of portosystemic shunt and liver function failure (as represented by reduced serum albumin and prolongation of the prothrombin time) was evident. As more patients with chronic hepatitis C progress over decades to cirrhosis, PSE is being seen in patients with better preserved liver function and yet evidence of major portosystemic shunting of blood. Only longitudinal studies of these types of patients will be able to establish whether this will have a major impact on our approach to management of PSE. Certainly, it is of concern that we may be facing for the first time a large group of patients with cirrhosis surviving into their 60s and 70s, because age in some studies predicts susceptibility to the development of PSE.

PATHOGENESIS

Reflecting the difficulty of this area, hypotheses of the pathogenesis of PSE abound (Table 19-5). Considering our lack of understanding of the fundamental molecular mechanisms involved in the maintenance of consciousness, sleep, or induction of anesthesia, perhaps it is not surprising we have had such difficulty in defining the cause of PSE. Nonetheless some excellent concepts have been proposed that can be tested to a variable extent. A discussion of every facet of each hypothesis would be too lengthy for this chapter, thus selected comments will be made. Interested readers might want to peruse the more detailed articles that have been published.

Approach to Studies in Pathogenesis

As will be discussed further in the section on diagnosis and management, there are some important clinical features of PSE. Some of these may offer important clues to the pathogenesis of PSE. Despite the occasional suggestion that the liver may synthesize a "brain preservative substance," there is really no evidence that supports this concept. Instead, an inescapable conclusion is that PSE is in some way related to the failure of the liver to clear one or more "toxins" that originate in the intestine. Every clinician who has observed the emergence of patients from severe PSE after gut cleansing or lactulose or oral antibiotic therapy knows that the gut is the key. Most but not all the precipitating factors that in-

Table 19–5 Hypothesis of Pathogenesis of PSE

- Direct ammonia neurotoxicity
- Multiply synergist neurotoxins
- False neurotransmitter/plasma amino acid imbalance
- Tryptophan and its metabolites
- γ-Amino-butyric acid (GABA)
- Endogenous benzodiazepines
- Astrocyte dysfunction
- Endogenous opiates
- Manganese

PSE, portosystemic encephalopathy.

duce clinical episodes of PSE can be explained by enhanced generation, absorption, or failure to clear gut-derived "toxins." It has been largely assumed that this putative gut-derived "toxin" or "toxins" directly affect brain function. Although this is the most parsimonious hypothesis (e.g., direct ammonia neurotoxicity), other considerations should not be excluded. As proposed many years ago, toxins could alter brain function or structure leading to sensitization of the brain to other toxins. Another concept best illustrated by the tryptophan hypothesis is that excessive gut-derived entry of tryptophan into the brain can lead to radical alterations in brain neurochemistry.

Before addressing the specific hypothesis, it is interesting to examine another largely unexplored concept. It has been assumed that the putative toxins involved in PSE may be present in all individuals. Only, it has been proposed, in the presence of liver disease or portosystemic shunting do these toxins gain access to the systemic circulation. Largely ignored is the possibility that alterations in gut motility in portal hypertension or other factors could lead to a situation peculiar to this syndrome, that is, production of toxins which do not occur in normal individuals. An interesting example of this is the production of D-lactate in patients with jejuno-ileal bypass operations.

Ammonia Hypothesis

There is no question that this hypothesis has a vast amount of circumstantial evidence in its favor. Ammonia is clearly derived from the gut and is usually efficiently cleared by the liver. If one chooses selected studies, there is an excellent correlation between ammonia levels in arterial blood and the severity of PSE. Moreover, almost every effective therapy in the management of PSE can be explained on the basis of reduced generation, absorption, or enhanced clearance of ammonia. In addition, there is excellent evidence that chronic elevation of blood ammonia levels leads to the characteristic astrocyte changes seen at brain autopsy in cirrhotic patients. As a great deal of new information on the role of astrocyte in maintenance of brain function has become available, the possibility that ammonia-induced astrocyte changes may be a key factor in PSE is becoming more attractive.

One of the major negative features of the ammonia hypothesis was the insistence of many of its proponents that no other compound should be ever considered as a possible contributing factor to the pathogenesis of PSE. This led to the suppression or rejection of many interesting manuscripts that reported new findings. This era has ended, but it cost our specialty a number of promising new investigators. Just as disturbing as this publication blockade was the fact that the scientific community (neurologists in particular) was led to believe that the problem of the pathogenesis of PSE was solved. To date, there still appears to be no publication (in English) that shows a correlation of arterial ammonia levels using a reliable ammonia assay with the severity of PSE. The otherwise excellent studies of Stahl used outdated methods. However, even if there is a lack of correlation of arterial blood levels of ammonia and the severity of PSE, this does not rule out a major role of ammonia in the genesis of this syndrome. Rather than direct neurotoxicity, it is more likely that ammonia induces secondary changes in brain neurochemistry and structure (e.g., astrocyte changes) in concert with other compounds.

Synergistic Neurotoxin Hypothesis

This hypothesis is associated primarily with the work of Zieve, who championed the idea of multiple toxins. Choosing from a plethora of potential gut-derived neurotoxins, he focused on ammonia, mercaptans (metabolites of the amino acid methionine), and the fatty acid, octanoic acid. The concept of multiple toxins causing PSE is certainly realistic. One problem is that the hypothesis is difficult to prove. Originally, it was claimed that doses of these compounds administered individually did not induce encephalopathy but when injected together into experimental animals, they *synergistically* caused coma. One major problem with this work was the subsequent realization that the mercaptan assays used were probably invalid. In addition, it was never proved that levels of these compounds in blood sufficient to cause coma were present in either animal models or humans with PSE. The concept that multiple toxins may well be involved in the pathogenesis of PSE is still appropriately widely believed. However, rather than focus on octanoic acid and mercaptans attention has been given to other gut-derived compounds, such as tryptophan and γ-aminobutyric acid (GABA) in combination with ammonia.

False Neurotransmitter/Plasma Amino Acid Imbalance Hypothesis

This rather complicated hypothesis was developed by Fischer and colleagues. The basic premise was that true neurotransmitters (e.g., dopamine) were replaced in brain by false (weak) neurotransmitters, such as octopamine. This was proposed to arise from the abnormal plasma amino acid profile seen in most patients with cirrhosis (not only in those with PSE as originally suggested). Reduced branched chain amino acids (valine, isoleucine, leucine) and increases in aromatic amino acids (phenylalanine, tyrosine) in plasma promoted excessive entry of aromatic amino acids across the blood-brain barrier. Increased efflux of glutamine from the brain, arising from the detoxification of ammonia was proposed to further augment this process. An excess of aromatic amino acid was thought to inhibit tyrosine-3-hydroxylose (the key enzyme controlling the synthesis of dopamine and norepinephrine), leading to a depletion of the true or normal neurotransmitters. In addition, false neurotransmitters, like octopamine and β-phenylethanolamine were generated from aromatic amino acids and were postulated to compete with dopamine. The net result was marked impairment in dopaminergic neurotransmission in PSE.

This particular hypothesis is difficult to summarize succinctly and as such proves difficult to incorporate in any lecture on the hypothesis of the pathogenesis of PSE. Autopsy studies of patients dying of PSE have indicated no evidence of either increased false neurotransmitters or depletion in dopamine or noradrenaline. It has largely been discredited but has one lasting legacy. This is the so-called hepatic formulations of amino acid products for nutritional support of patients with advanced liver disease and PSE. Some evidence still exists that the "hepatic formulation" is less encephalopathogenic than similar standard amino acid formulations, especially with regard to oral administration. However, these formulations did not simply increase branched-chain amino acid and reduce aromatic amino acid content in the intravenous line of products. Debate continues as to whether a higher calorie nitrogen ratio or a lower glycine content was responsible for better tolerance. Proving better tolerance has been more convincing for oral formulations. Isolated reports of dramatic improvement in intractable PSE still appear with intravenous hepatic formulations. However, careful attention to empirical treatment (see later section) seems to be more important in arousing patients with PSE in most situations.

Tryptophan Hypothesis

Unlike many hypotheses, where marked disparity is noted between findings in animal models and humans with PSE has occurred, relatively consistently excess entry of tryptophan in brain has been demonstrated. Serotonin, the main but not exclusive product of tryptophan in brain tissue, is known to modulate a variety of central nervous system (CNS) processes. Despite strong evidence that serotonin turnover is increased in PSE, based on measurement of its main metabolite, 5-hydroxyindole acetic acid, it is not apparent that excessive serotonin neurotransmission occurs in the syndrome. Indeed, there is evidence for a "synaptic deficit" of serotonin in PSE. What this implies is that despite undoubted overproduction of serotonin in presynaptic nerves, there are mechanisms preventing this serotonin from reaching postsynaptic receptors. Post mortem studies of patients with HE at death display upregulation of some serotonin receptor subtypes. This can be interpreted to reflect an adaptive response to lack of serotonin stimulation. Evidence exists for overactivity of monoamine oxidase activity in presynaptic nerves and leaking of synaptic vesicles of serotonin, possibly caused by ammonia. Finally, two observations in humans with cirrhosis suggest a synaptic deficit rather than an excess as a factor in PSE. The first is precipitation of PSE by ketanserin, a serotonin antagonist, in patients with portal hypertension. Also, serotonin uptake inhibition does not aggravate mild PSE.

Alternative pathways for excess CNS tryptophan could lead to neurotoxic metabolites. The most investigated type has been quinolinic acid, but correlation with the severity of HE has not been demonstrated. Other compounds generated from tryptophan have periodically been investigated as possible contributions to PSE. In light of the clear origin of tryptophan from the gut and consistent findings of excess entry of tryptophan into the CNS in advanced liver disease, this particular area of investigation should continue to be the subject of some attention.

γ-Amino Butyric Acid/Benzodiazepine Hypotheses

Many investigators consider that these two hypotheses are distinct, which is inappropriate. Currently, the only widely accepted mechanism of action of benzodiazepines (BZs) is modulation of CNS GABA transmission. Originally, it was proposed based on studies in an experimental animal model of acute liver failure (galactosamine-induced liver failure in the rabbit) that excess GABAergic neurotransmission was a significant mediation of PSE. Subsequent realization that GABA was produced by enteric flora and cleared by the liver further supported the concept. Enormous blood levels of GABA were noted with radioreceptor assays in humans with PSE. Because GABA penetrates the blood-brain barrier poorly, an important issue early in these studies was whether blood-borne GABA could penetrate into the CNS. This was shown to be true in several acute liver failure models. Gut production of GABA was reported in one study to be reduced by neomycin therapy. Enthusiasm for this hypothesis was reduced considerably when it was realized that several amino acids (especially glutamine) interfered with the radioreceptor assay for GABA. A weakness of the GABA hypothesis from the outset was failure to ever show downregulation of GABA receptors, which should have been evident, if excess GABAergic neurotransmission was present in PSE.

The GABA hypothesis lives on in a modified form. Direct pharmacologic testing of rabbits with "PSE" using relatively specific GABA antagonists like bicuculline revealed a response compatible with increased GABAergic "tone" being present. However, rather than excess GABA being responsible, the notion that BZ augmentation of GABAergic neurotransmission was responsible was raised. This was postulated on the basis of amelioration of HE with the specific BZ antagonist, Ro 15-1788, now known as flumazenil. Although there has by no means been a consistent reporting of this phenomenon, the only acceptable interpretation of the effect is that it arises from "antagonism" of "endogenous" BZ augmentation of GABAergic neurotransmission. The nature of these BZs and their origin is still an area of active research today.

Current animal models of PSE are actually animal models of encephalopathy in acute liver failure. Many extraneous complications occur in these models, which makes it difficult to be sure whether encephalopathy is due to "hepatic" or other causes (Table 19–6). Failure to arouse animals with acute liver failure using BZ antagonists may be relevant if the comatose state is actually caused by HE. Our research team abandoned these acute liver failure models because of this issue, but investigators continue to use these models for most, if not all, experimental investigations. One major problem is the lack of an animal model of chronic liver disease (with maybe one exception) with overt HE/PSE. Because of this, we turned our studies to humans about a decade ago which resulted in some other problems.

Unlike animal models of liver failure in whom raised blood or CNS (or cerebrospinal fluid) levels of BZs are accepted as an interesting if unexplained phenomenon there is an additional issue in humans. When, and if, increased BZ levels are found the inclination is to suggest (not inappropriately) that these findings could be due to occult or surreptitious prescription intake of BZs. In our studies, which included measures to avoid taking blood samples from patients with any possibility of BZ intake in the 3 months prior to study inclusion, we found increased BZ levels in 70% to 80% of patients. If these findings occurred from undetected BZ drug intake, then every study done since the release of chlordiazepoxide in 1960 has to be questioned. One simply cannot propose widespread BZ drug intake in cirrhotic patients as a cause for PSE in the case of studies, which had measures to prevent this from happening, without declaring all other clinical studies of the pathogenesis of PSE to be potentially invalid.

The continuing weakness of the BZ hypothesis is still the lack of clear identification of the compounds responsible for BZ activity in blood. In addition, the source for these compounds remained obscure. Recently, using what may be a valid model of human PSE, a positive gradient of BZ levels was found between portal and systemic blood in dogs with congenital portacaval shunts (C-PCS). Combined with the finding of substantial quantities of BZs in stool in a number of species, this hypothesis has now perhaps found its gut connection. There is a lot more work needed, not the least of which is the development of reliable reproducible assays to allow all laboratories to measure and detect these compounds. Table 19–7 and Table 19-8 outline the the advantages and advantages for this hypothesis at present.

Table 19–6   Causes of "Coma" in Acute Liver Failure Animal Models

- Dehydration
- Acidosis
- Hypothermia
- Cerebral edema
- Hepatic encephalopathy
- Hypoglycemia
- Electrolyte disturbances
- Endotoxemia
- Renal failure
- Inanition

Table 19–7   Evidence in Support of the Benzodiazepine Hypothesis

- Presence of elevated BZ levels in animal models and human PSE
  Cerebrospinal fluid, blood, brain tissue, urine, stool
- Correlation of "BZ" level with the severity of PSE
- In vitro evidence of isolated Purkinje neuron BZ-mediated events in an animal model
- Autoradiographic evidence of BZs on brain BZ receptors in an animal model
- Response of PSE to BZ receptor antagonists

BZ, benzodiazepine; PSE, portosystemic encephalopathy.

Table 19–8   Problems with Benzodiazepine Hypothesis

- Detection of BZs not universal (laboratory-dependent)
- Source of BZs uncertain
- Identity of full profile of BZs still unresolved
- Only 20–30% of patients with severe PSE respond to BZ antagonists
- Widespread occult use of prescription BZs

BZ, benzodiazepine; PSE, portosystemic encephalopathy.

Astrocyte Dysfunction Hypothesis

As mentioned earlier, complex molecular interactions between brain neurons and astrocytes have been described. Alterations in neurotransmitter glutamate synthesis and regulation have been noted in animal models of liver disease and in various in vitro systems mimicking the syndrome of PSE. Neurosteroid production by the abnormal astrocytes seen in liver disease, the interrelationship of astrocytes swelling, cerebral edema, and PSE are all being explored at present. Out of this area may well arise some important new advances in our understanding of the pathogenesis of PSE.

Endogenous Opiates Hypothesis

An important, but often overlooked, paper by Yurdaydin and associates reports a significant increase in selected areas of brain and plasma opiate peptide levels in the thioacetamide-induced acute liver failure model. This very detailed paper also describes improvement in neurobehavioral status after administration of various opioid antagonists. Isolated reports of reversal of severe PSE in patients not receiving narcotics supports the concept that some patients with PSE may have endogenous opioid-induced encephalopathy. Unlike the parallel situation in the endogenous BZ area, long-acting oral opiate antagonists are available. Surprisingly no clinical trials in human PSE have yet appeared. The role of endogenous opiates in liver disease–associated pruritus is receiving increased attention these days.

Manganese Hypothesis

The latest hypothesis of the pathogenesis of PSE implicates excess deposition of manganese in brain (especially the basal ganglia) as a cause of this syndrome. Early reports of hyperintensity of the basal ganglia on T_1 weighted magnetic resonance imaging (MRI) in patients with advanced liver disease were reminiscent of that seen with industrial manganese poisoning. Despite the fact that a number of metals can be deposited in the basal ganglia and other brain regions in chronic liver disease, the paramagnetic properties of manganese made it an attractive possibility as the cause of these MRI findings. Post mortem studies have now indicated excess manganese in brain tissue of patients dying with PSE. Moreover, after many years of neglect the art of neurologic examination has been once again applied to patients with PSE. Not only have all sorts of neurologic signs compatible with basal ganglia dysfunction been identified in patients with PSE (not a major surprise), but one provocative report suggests that they do not resolve completely with PSE treatment. It has been proposed that PSE may actually be a slowly progressive neurodegenerative disorder. This interesting concept is difficult to reconcile with the usual course of treated PSE but raises all types of implications that need to be examined further.

DIAGNOSIS

The diagnosis of clinically evident PSE depends on two elements, The first element involves recognition that the patient has underlying significant liver dysfunction is

critical. Quite literally the diagnosis of PSE will not be entertained at all if liver disease is not suspected. The second element is that one has to recognize that the patient has the cardinal features of PSE: alterations in consciousness or behavior or varying degrees of a generalized motor disturbance.

Recognition of Underlying Significant Liver Dysfunction

There is a widespread belief that all patients with PSE of the clinically obvious variety will also have obvious liver disease. This, like many things in medicine, is not true. The term dysfunction rather than disease was used earlier to deliberately include a group of patients who have PSE not on the basis of intrinsic parenchymal liver disease (e.g., cirrhosis) but due to major portosystemic shunting of blood (Table 19-9). In many parts of the world, splanchnic venous thrombosis, schistosomiasis, and idiopathic portal hypertension are common situations where portosystemic shunting of blood is well developed in the absence of significant liver disease. Some of these patients develop PSE, particularly after major variceal bleeding. Unless a previous diagnosis of these conditions is known, the diagnosis of PSE can be easily missed. However, what is perhaps even more interesting is that even though patients with major portosystemic shunts and normal liver function can develop PSE, it is relatively infrequent. It seems that portosystemic shunting on its own, even if total, is often not sufficient to induce PSE, hence the concern for the use of the term PSE in the first place.

In the United States, common causes for major portosystemic shunting and apparently normal liver function are quiescent chronic hepatitis C–induced cirrhosis, cirrhosis in reformed alcoholics, nonalcoholic steatohepatitis–associated cirrhosis, and in the occasional patient with a congenital shunt. In any or all of these situations, PSE may occur which can baffle the clinician, especially if there is no biochemical suggestion of liver dysfunction. Perhaps reflecting our practice interest, we see a lot of these patients. Interestingly, one also sees PSE in a minority of patients following successful liver transplant. Presumably, this occurs because portosystemic shunts take some time to close after orthotopic liver transplantation.

Most patients do not pose such great difficulty in diagnosis of significant underlying dysfunction. Aspects of the history, physical diagnosis, and laboratory findings in "occult" liver dysfunction are listed in Table 19–10. Once the diagnosis of significant liver disease/dysfunction is made, then

Table 19–9 Causes of Noncirrhotic Portosystemic Shunts

- Idiopathic portal hypertension
- Noncirrhotic portal fibrosis
- Schistosomiasis
- Congenital hepatic fibrosis
- Splanchnic venous thrombosis
- Partial nodular transformation
- Nodular regenerative hyperplasia
- Congenital cause
- Postsurgical shunt

Table 19–10 Some Clues to Underlying "Occult" Liver Dysfunction*

History

Risk factors for hepatitis B and C
Past history alcohol abuse
Native of endemic area of schistosomiasis
Family history of liver disease

Physical Examination

Spider nevi
Fetor hepaticus
Splenomegaly
Gynecomastia

Laboratory Test

Thrombocytopenia
Hyperammonemia
Elevated globulins
Pancytopenia

*Generally liver disease and portosystemic shunting are obvious but faced with an obscure "encephalopathy" any of the above may provide helpful clues in considering PSE.

one is ready to attribute any neurologic changes seen to possible PSE. The common neurologic symptoms found in patients with PSE are listed in Table 19–11. The patients presenting with psychiatric syndromes can be a challenge, since in our observation these patients often have well preserved liver function (i.e., the underlying liver disorder may be missed). The constipating effects of the older antidepressants often aggravated mild PSE presenting as depression. Listed in Table 19–12 are some clinical features that are not typical of PSE. Some used to be listed as features of PSE, but we suspect that this arose from intermingling of cases of ALFA-HE with PSE. Alcohol withdrawal syndrome can be difficult at times to distinguish from PSE, especially in patients with delirium tremors associated with sepsis.

MANAGEMENT

The diagnosis of PSE is essentially clinical. Once one suspects that it is present, then empirical treatment is initiated.

Table 19–11 Clinical Signs of Portosystemic Encephalopathy

• Varying degrees of loss of consciousness
• Asterixis
• Hyperreflexia*
• Positive Babinski*
• Increased tone
• Dysarthria
• Parkinsonian features
• Fine motor hand dysfunction
• Monotonous speech
• Decorticate posturing
• Hyperventilation

*Can be transiently asymmetric.

Table 19–12 Atypical Features of Portosystemic Encephalopathy

• Vivid visual hallucinations*
• Seizures*
• Prolonged asymmetry of motor findings†
• Hypoventilation
• Diaphoresis*

*More suggestive of delirium tremens.
†Concomitant neuropathy can be confusing.

First-Line Treatment of PSE

Empirical or first-line treatment consists of the following:

• Gut cleansing with gastric lavage, laxatives, and enemas.
• Low-protein (zero protein if totally comatose) high-carbohydrate diet.
• Delivery of lactulose into the intestine.

Concurrently, other causes of encephalopathy are sought and treated (Table 19–13) and finally also concurrent precipitating factors for the development of PSE are sought and treated (Table 19–14).

Patients in severe PSE (stages III to IV) should be managed initially in intensive care units, unless the patient is known to frequently be admitted with severe, but treatment responsive PSE. Ruling out or treating other causes of encephalopathy, identifying and correcting precipitating factors, and instigating empirical therapy are labor intensive. Current staffing on medical wards makes management of severe PSE difficult to accomplish.

It is not widely appreciated that correction of precipitating factors can return most patients to their baseline mental

Table 19–13 Other Causes of Encephalopathy in Patients with Portosystemic Encephalopathy

• Hypoxia	• Intracranial bleed
• Hypercapnia	• CNS sepsis
• Hypoglycemia	• Acidosis
• Hyperglycemia	• Hypovolemia
• Electrolyte disturbances	• Renal failure
• Sepsis	• Post-ictal
• Delirium tremens	• Intra-ictal

CNS, central nervous system.

Table 19–14 Precipitating Factors for Portosystemic Encephalopathy

• Gastrointestinal hemorrhage	• Cessation of lactulose*
• Sedative and analgesics	• Dehydration
• Constipation/ileus	• Superimposed hepatic injury
• Hypokalemia/alkalosis	• Postoperative
• Sepsis	• Ketanserin/propranolol
• Uremia	• Zinc deficiency ?
• Excessive oral protein	• Post portosystemic shunt

*Not strictly a precipitating factor, but commonly seen.

and neurologic state. Herewithin lies the problem of designing clinical treatment trials in PSE. Since correction of precipitating factors can take 48 to 72 hours to have an effect the benefit of additional therapy introduced during this time period is difficult to gauge. It is possible for some ineffective therapy to be given the credit for improvement that is due to correction of precipitating factors.

Blood Ammonia Testing

We discourage blood ammonia testing for the diagnosis and monitoring of patients with PSE for the following reasons: (1) Unless a proper handling technique is used, many ammonia assays will give artefactually elevated ammonia levels. After venipuncture, ammonia concentrations rise in blood due to the enzyme adenylic deaminase present in erythrocytes. Hemolysis is also a major issue, because 75% of the whole blood content of ammonia resides in erythrocytes. Unless measures are in place to reduce deaminase activity (i.e., prompt placement of blood onto ice or prompt assay, such as within 20 to 30 minutes), then the assay should not be done at all. (2) Correlation of blood ammonia (usually sera) with the severity of PSE or merely with its presence or absence is uncertain, especially with venous blood sampling. (3) The absence of hyperammonemia does not rule out PSE. (4) The presence of real hyperammonemia does not per se make a diagnosis of PSE.

The clear role of an accurate and properly assayed blood ammonia determination is for obscure cases of encephalopathy. The finding of significant hyperammonemia may indicate an acquired or congenital urea cycle enzyme defect. More commonly, in adult practice, it may be the first indication that a patient without clinical or laboratory evidence of liver disease has established portosystemic shunting. However, in most cases, PSE is diagnosed clinically on the basis of known or strongly suspected underlying chronic liver disease and a neurologic picture compatible with this syndrome. Knowledge of the serum ammonia level does not alter management.

General Points About Empirical Therapy

The guiding principle of the management of patients with suspected severe HE is to clear the gut out as much as possible. This is true whether or not the episode is precipitated by a major gastrointestinal hemorrhage. Two extremes of approach to this are seen.

The first approach is literally that no attempt is made to clear the gut, because of fear of inserting a nasogastric tube in patients with probable esophageal varices. This is associated with enthusiastic irrigation of the rectum with enemas. The role of the rectum in generation of the toxins involved in PSE is unknown, but in our experience, giving enemas alone is usually ineffective. This may be in part caused by a loss of enema delivery skills in modern nursing.

The second and potentially even more harmful approach is the induction of a near-cholera state with grossly overenthusiastic use of lactulose. Making the rectal fluid effluent similar in appearance (except for bile staining) to that infused via a nasogastric tube certainly qualifies as aggressive therapy. However, it can easily induce dehydration or gross hypernatremia and will retard the improvement in PSE gen-

erally seen in most patients. As has been stated often, the best regimen is that which induces two loose bowel movements a day. One can be forgiven for overshooting this mark initially, especially in the grossly comatose patient, but profuse diarrhea should never be the goal of treatment.

Returning to the fear of nasogastric tube insertion, one as usual finds no published studies to encourage the timid in this regard. Simply put, it is believed that these tubes do not cause variceal bleeding. However, there may be significant reasons for caution in placing them after an initial bout of variceal band ligation.

Lactulose is the preferred laxative for the treatment of PSE in the United States. In patients without concomitant renal failure and a low serum magnesium, magnesium citrate may be an ideal laxative to commence gut cleansing. Most nasogastric tubes are very inefficient in removing clots and blood from the stomach. In the United States, only gastroenterologists seem inclined to use large-bore tube irrigation of the stomach. This is done prior to therapeutic endoscopy to allow visualization of entire upper gastrointestinal tract. In Europe, there are devices that pulverize and rapidly suction clots from the stomach.

Large amounts of blood in the intestines are a major precipitant for PSE. If one cannot clear blood from the stomach, then accelerating its exit from the lower intestine is warranted. Luckily, blood itself is a laxative, which results in relatively quick evacuation. Nonetheless, prompt delivery of lactulose is required to shorten the subsequent course of PSE.

The zero or low-protein diet is always part of the empirical treatment regimen for PSE. This simply arises from the common practice of not feeding patients for days after admission. One of the virtues it was said of branched chain enriched intravenous formulations was the fact that nutritional support was maintained while severe PSE was treated. As a general rule, we try and restart an adequate protein intake as soon as possible. If, despite all measures, HE is not improved in 72 hours, then other second liver treatments for HE need to be instituted (see next section).

Second-Line Treatment of PSE

Listed in Table 19–15 are almost all of the therapies available for the treatment of PSE. If first-line measures have not been effective, our first choice for second-line therapy is metronidazole. This is very effective, but care has to be taken to avoid accumulation of metronidazole, which is cleared by the liver. After a few days of 250 mg PO qid, the dose is titrated downward as PSE improves. Our impression is that efficacy may be reduced with repeated courses. Metronidazole is not recommended for long-term treatment. Neomycin is thought to be equivalent in efficacy, but concerns regarding systemic absorption have tended to limit its use. There is a widespread opinion that the 6 g/day in divided doses is too high for routine clinical use. We only give 2 g/day which is tolerated well by patients. However, the only placebo-controlled trial using neomycin at this dose failed to show any benefit. Other trials indicating efficacy of oral neomycin at varying doses are actually comparison trials of neomycin versus other agents. Interestingly, clear-cut reversal of neurobehavioral changes in an animal model of HE have been reported with neomycin.

Table 19–15 Therapies Used to Treat Hepatic Encephalopathy

Reduction of gut toxin production and absorption
  Lactulose
  Lactitol
  Lactose
  Neomycin
  Kanamycin
  Sorbitol
  Paromomycin
  Metronidazole
  Vancomycin
  Ribostamycin
  Rifaximine
  Nicotinohydroxamic (urease inhibitor)
Elimination of ammonia
  Sodium benzoate
  Branched-chain keto acids
  Ornithine aspartate
  Arginine
  Glutamate
  Sodium phenylacetate
Dietary manipulation
  Branched-chain amino acids
  Vegetable supplementation
  Zinc supplementation
  Benzodiazepine receptor antagonist administration
Repletion of brain dopamine levels
  L-Dopa
  Bromocriptine
Alteration of intestinal flora
Modification of portosystemic shunts

Oral vancomycin has been reported to be effective in one trial of lactulose-resistant patients. Paromomycin and rifaximine are not available for routine clinical use, even though both appear to be effective.

The sequence that we generally follow is to rigorously ensure that we have succeeded in accomplishing first-line measures (most often we have not done this in an optimum fashion). Then we proceed to use oral metronidazole therapy for 3 to 4 days, followed by vancomycin substitution. This line of approach is followed in the severe cases (grades III and IV) and usually works well, except in cases of protracted ileus or true end-stage liver disease. Even though more suited to milder severity of HE, if we still have a patient in severe HE after first- and second-line measures, we will then go on to third-line treatment. This is usually started about 3 to 4 days after the patient's admission to the hospital.

Third-Line Treatment of PSE

Based on one very well conducted study, sodium benzoate 5 g PO bid probably should be used more frequently to treat resistant HE. Even though it is not an approved treatment (no therapy is actually approved by the Food and Drug Administration for HE), sodium benzoate is widely available in hospitals because of its use by pediatricians to treat urea cycle enzyme–deficient children. A parenteral form of this drug would be particularly helpful to have available in some cases.

Infusion of branched-chain amino acid–enriched formulations, either intravenously or by the nasoenteric route, has a role to play in treatment of some resistant cases of HE. Its role is more often found in the recurrent cases of HE, where the normal oral protein intake is not tolerated. Vegetable-based protein diets in theory could also be applied if they could be delivered. The occasional resistant HE case is due to concomitant zinc deficiency. Zinc repletion in these cases clearly can be beneficial, even though oral zinc supplementation trials have had variable results.

Based on recent reports, ornithine aspartate infusion could be helpful. Treatment of severe HE has not been reported yet with this formulation, which is only available in Europe. Bromocriptine in isolated cases can correct truly intractable HE, but not with any consistency. Administration of flumenazil can be associated with dramatic improvement in 20% to 40% of cases, but the effect is short-lived and a long-acting BZ antagonist is not yet available.

Severe Treatment Unresponsive PSE

One assumes that liver transplant assessment has already begun long before intractable PSE has occurred. Sometimes, patients come late in their course and PSE is so bad that a great deal of the transplant work-up cannot be completed. In particular, requirements for alcohol abstinence programs may be impossible. Other individuals are simply not liver transplant candidates or are refused on the basis of concerns about irreversible hepatocerebral degeneration. Whatever the reason for liver transplantation not being an option, one has to look to some rather heroic measures to treat individual cases of truly intractable PSE. Colonic exclusion or resection is not done very often these days, and evidence for its benefit has been limited. A more successful approach for selected cases has been attempts to nonsurgically reduce the amount of portosystemic shunting of blood. Embolization, reduction in the diameter of existing TIPS stents, and other techniques are now performed by some expert interventional radiologists (or gastroenterologists in Europe).

When confronted with intractable PSE cases, liver transplant surgeons often express concern regarding the potential for recovery from the neurologic perspective. Brain atrophy, abnormally hyperintense basal ganglia, tend to further reduce enthusiasm for transplant acceptance. One must emphasize that these findings are frequently seen in patients with cirrhosis and relatively normal mental status. Even in rare patients with true hepatocerebral degeneration, considerable improvement in CNS status can be seen after successful orthotopic liver transplantation. Transient awakening with flumazenil can help transplant teams in deciding whether to proceed, but this idea has not been tested systematically. Artificial liver support devices may play a role in these relatively rare intractable PSE cases in that if temporary awakening can be induced, liver transplantation can be offered. No studies have been done to establish whether this type of approach can distinguish irretrievable cases from those capable of normal neurologic status after liver transplantation. Even though these patients are relatively rare, artificial liver support devices may accomplish more in reversing PSE in these patients than trying to stabilize patients with fulminant liver failure.

SUGGESTED READINGS

Adams RD, Foley JM: The neurological disorder associated with liver disease. Res Publ Ass Res RCS Nerv Ment Dis 32:198–237, 1953.

Aronson L, Gacad R, Kaminsky-Russ K, et al: Detection of "endogenous" benzodiazepines in dogs with congenital portacaval shunts. Vet Surg 26:189–194, 1997.

Basile AS, Jones EA, Skolnick P: The pathogenesis and treatment of hepatic encephalopathy: Evidence for the involvement of benzodiazepine receptor ligands. Pharmacol Rev 43:27–71, 1991.

Butterworth RF: The neurobiology of hepatic encephalopathy. Semin Liver Dis 16:235–244, 1996.

Cordoba J, Blei AT: Treatment of hepatic encephalopathy. Am J Gastroenterol 92:1429–1439, 1997.

Fattovich G, Giustina G, Degos F, et al: Morbidity and mortality in compensated cirrhosis type C: A retrospective follow up study of 384 patients. Gastroenterology 112:463–472, 1997.

Ferenci P, Puspök, Steindl P: Current concepts in the pathophysiology of hepatic encephalopathy. Eur J Clin Invest 22:573–581, 1992.

Ferenci P: Treatment of hepatic encephalopathy in patients with cirrhosis of the liver. Dig Dis 14 (Suppl 1):40–52, 1996.

James JH, Zipparo V, Jeppson B, et al: Hyperammonemia, plasma amino acid imbalance and blood brain amino acid transport: A unified theory of portal systemic encephalopathy. Lancet 2:772–775, 1979.

Jones EA, Weissenborn K: Neurology and the liver. J Neurol Neurosurg Psychiatry 63:279–293, 1997.

Kreiger S, Jaub M, Jansen O, et al: Neuropsychiatric profile and hypertensive globus pallidus on T_1-weighted magnetic resonance images in liver cirrhosis. Gastroenterology 111:147–155, 1996.

Langer B, Taylor BR, Greig PD: Selective or total shunts for variceal bleeding. Am J Surg 160:75–79, 1990.

Marchesini G, Dioguardi FJ, Bianchi GP, et al: Long term oral branched-chain amino acid treatment in chronic hepatic encephalopathy. J Hepatol 11:92–101, 1990.

Mullen KD, Szauter KM, Kaminsky-Russ K: Endogenous benzodiazepine activity in physiological fluids of patients with hepatic encephalopathy. Lancet 336:81–83, 1990.

Mullen KD, McCullough AJ: Problems with animal models of chronic liver disease. Suggestions for improvement in standardization. Hepatology 9:500–503, 1989.

Mullen KD, Gacad R: Hepatic encephalopathy. Gastroenterologist 4:188–202, 1996.

Norenberg MD: Astrocyte ammonia interactions in hepatic encephalopathy. Semin Liver Dis 16:245–253, 1996.

Riordan SM, Williams R: Treatment of hepatic encephalopathy. N Engl J Med 337:473–479, 1997.

Rössle M, Haag K, Blum HE: The transjugular intrahepatic portosystemic stent-shunt: A review of the literature and our experiences. J Gastroenterol Hepatol 11:293–298, 1996.

Sherlock S, Summerskill WHJ, White LP, Phear EA: Portal-systemic encephalopathy: Neurological complications of liver disease. Lancet 2:453–457, 1954.

Stahl J. Studies of the blood ammonia in liver disease: Its diagnostic, prognostic and therapeutic significance. Ann Intern Med 58:1–24, 1963.

Thurn JR, Pierpont GL, Ludvigsen CW, Eckfeldt JH: D-Lactate encephalopathy. Am J Med 79:717–721, 1985.

Walker CO, Schenker S: Pathogenesis of hepatic encephalopathy with special reference to the role of ammonia. Am J Clin Nutr 23:619–632, 1970.

Yurdaydin C, Li Y, Ha JK, et al: Brain and plasma levels of opioid peptides are altered in rats with thioacetamide-induced fulminant hepatic failure: Implications for the treatment of hepatic encephalopathy with opioid antagonists. J Pharmacol Exp Ther 273:185–192, 1995.

Zieve L, Doizaki WM, Zieve FJ: Synergism between mercaptans and ammonia and fatty acids in the production of coma: A possible role for mercaptans in the pathogenesis of hepatic coma. J Lab Clin Med 83:16–28, 1974.

20

Complications of Cirrhosis: Hemostatic Failure

J. Heinrich Joist
Charles S. Eby

Abnormal bleeding, predominantly epistaxis, gingival bleeding, ecchymoses, and bleeding from the gastrointestinal tract, is common in patients with advanced cirrhosis. This is not surprising, because the liver plays a central and complex role in hemostasis. It is the sole or major site of synthesis of all of the recognized procoagulant blood coagulation factors (except tissue factor [TF]), several important regulatory anticoagulant proteins of the coagulation system (antithrombin III [AT], protein C [PC], protein S [PS], C_1 inhibitor), and components of the fibrinolytic system (plasminogen, α_2-antiplasmin). The liver also functions as an important site for clearance from the circulation of activated coagulation factors and plasminogen activators.

In addition, the diverse spectrum of hemostatic abnormalities in cirrhosis includes synthesis of abnormal fibrinogen and functionally impaired vitamin K–dependent clotting factors, vitamin K deficiency caused by intrahepatic cholestasis, thrombocytopenia, impaired platelet function, consumption coagulopathy (CC), disseminated intravascular coagulation (DIC), or accelerated fibrinolysis.

Although the levels of both prohemostatic and antihemostatic factors may be decreased in advanced liver disease, severe liver disease may lead to a shift in the delicately controlled hemostatic system toward defective primary hemostasis (hemostatic platelet plug formation) and secondary hemostasis (reduced fibrin formation and enhanced clot dissolution), predisposing to abnormal bleeding (Fig. 20–1).

Although the focus of this chapter is on hemostatic abnormalities in cirrhosis, it should be noted that there is substantial overlap in the hemostatic abnormalities observed in patients with severe acute infectious or toxic hepatitis, advanced chronic hepatitis, and acute or chronic biliary obstruction.

PATHOPHYSIOLOGY AND CLINICAL FEATURES

Thrombocytopenia

Mild to moderate thrombocytopenia may be observed in one third or more of patients with cirrhosis. The number of megakaryocytes in the bone marrow is usually normal or increased, indicating that decreased platelet production is not a major component of liver disease associated thrombocytopenia. However, it has been shown that the liver is the major site of production of thrombopoietin (TPO), a glycoprotein that binds to megakaryocyte-committed progenitor cells in the bone marrow and stimulates platelet production. Furthermore, in preliminary investigations, no TPO was detected in plasma of thrombocytopenic cirrhotic patients immediately before liver transplantation, and TPO levels rapidly increased post-transplantation followed by an increase in platelet counts 4 to 6 days later. Thus, the relationships between advanced liver disease, thrombopoietin synthesis, platelet production, and liver disease–associated thrombocytopenia require further evaluation.

The major mechanism involved in thrombocytopenia in chronic liver disease appears to be increased platelet pooling in the spleen caused by congestive splenomegaly. Thus, whereas in normal subjects, the spleen contains about one third of the total platelet mass, in the cirrhotic patient with congestive splenomegaly, up to 90% of the total platelet mass may be sequestered in the spleen with the liver playing a minor role. Interestingly, in one study, shortened fibrinogen survival could be increased toward normal with the administration of heparin, whereas no such effect of heparin on shortened platelet survival could be demonstrated. This indicates that mechanisms for shortened plate-

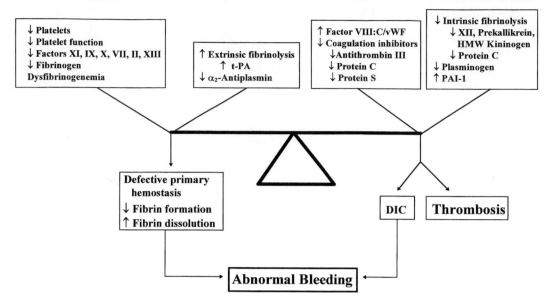

Figure 20–1
Hemostatic abnormalities that may cause hemostatic system imbalance and contribute to abnormal bleeding and thrombosis in cirrhosis.

let survival other than thrombin-mediated platelet consumption (i.e., DIC) may be operative, such as increased splenic sequestration and perhaps accelerated destruction of platelets by immune mechanisms. Increased amounts of platelet-associated IgG, as well as increased concentrations of immune complexes in serum, have been demonstrated in patients with cirrhosis. Furthermore, complete and sustained resolution of thrombocytopenia and a decrease in platelet-associated IgG have been reported in some patients with chronic liver disease and increased platelet-associated IgG following partial splenic embolization. However, direct evidence for immune-mediated platelet destruction in cirrhotic patients is lacking as is clear evidence for efficacy of immunomodulating agents (e.g., high-dose intravenous [IV] immunoglobulin) or immunosuppressive agents such as glucocorticoids in ameliorating thrombocytopenia.

Two other readily correctable causes of thrombocytopenia to be considered in patients with alcoholic cirrhosis are folic acid deficiency, caused by inadequate dietary intake, and direct toxic effects of ethanol on megakaryocytes or circulating platelets.

Platelet Dysfunction

Various in vitro platelet functional abnormalities have been described in patients with chronic liver disease, including reduced platelet adhesiveness, impaired primary and secondary platelet aggregation to adenosine diphosphate (ADP), and impaired platelet aggregation to epinephrine, thrombin, and ristocetin in citrated platelet-rich plasma. In some studies, a mild to moderate prolongation of the bleeding time in the absence of thrombocytopenia, or out of proportion to the extent of thrombocytopenia, was observed and appeared to correlate with the presence of abnormal platelet aggregation and the severity of the liver disease. However, others have reported bleeding times that were

generally appropriate for blood platelet concentrations, as well as normal platelet adhesiveness and normal platelet aggregation to ADP, epinephrine, and collagen in patients with stable liver cirrhosis.

The platelet functional abnormalities in chronic liver disease have been attributed to extrinsic factors such as the inhibitory effect of elevated plasma fibrinogen/fibrin degradation products (FDP) on platelet aggregation, acquired dyslipidemia, or ethanol. There are also data indicating that the platelet functional defect may be intrinsic, that is, demonstrable in washed platelets from patients with liver disease and not inducible by short-term incubation of normal platelets in plasma from cirrhotic patients. Possible mechanisms are a decrease in arachidonic acid available for formation of the proaggregatory and platelet release–potentiating prostaglandin metabolite, thromboxane A_2, a decrease in total platelet adenine nucleotides associated with an increased ATP/ADP ratio (findings suggestive of acquired platelet-dense granule storage pool deficiency), increased platelet cholesterol, a decrease in platelet surface GP1b expression, the primary receptor for von Willebrand factor (vWF), and impairment of platelet transmembrane signaling mechanisms.

Coagulation Factor Abnormalities

Progressive loss of liver parenchymal cells in chronic liver disease is associated with a progressive decrease in the plasma levels of all procoagulant coagulation factors, except factor VIII, primarily as a result of impaired synthesis. Of the vitamin K–dependent clotting factors, factors VII, X, and II are usually decreased proportionately, whereas the reduction in factor IX is frequently less pronounced. The extent of the reduction in the levels of factors VII, II, and X correlates with the severity of the disease as assessed by other laboratory tests and clinical signs and symptoms. Hypocarboxylated forms of prothrombin and a decreased ratio of factor II activity over factor II antigen have been demonstrated in some studies, consistent with impaired utilization of vitamin K. Low levels of factor V are frequently observed in patients with chronic liver disease and are thought by some to be more accurate predictors of the extent of liver damage than the levels of vitamin K–dependent factors.

Factor VIII:C is almost always mildly to moderately increased in patients with cirrhosis, as are vWF antigen and ristocetin cofactor (R:CoF). In some patients with advanced cirrhosis, factor VIII:C may be lower than vWF antigen, and vWF may be qualitatively abnormal (lack of larger multimers as observed in patients with type 2 von Willebrand disease), possibly because of proteolytic degradation by thrombin, plasmin, or other cellular or plasma proteases.

Fibrinogen is normal or increased in most patients with stable cirrhosis. However, mild to moderate hypofibrinogenemia may be seen with advanced cirrhosis. This may result from impaired synthesis; loss into extravascular spaces (ascites, edema); accelerated, thrombin-mediated consumption; increased fibrinogen catabolism by plasmin or other proteases; uncompensated, massive hemorrhage; or a combination thereof. Dysfibrinogenemia, characterized by abnormal fibrin polymerization, is common in cirrhosis. The functional defect appears to be related mainly to an excessive content of sialic acid. Dysfibrinogenemia may be responsible in some patients for the common finding of a prolonged thrombin time in the presence of normal or only minimally reduced fibrinogen concentration and normal or minimally elevated serum FDP. Whether dysfibrinogenemia may contribute to abnormal bleeding is unclear.

The levels of the contact system coagulation factors, factors XII, XI, prekallikrein, and HMW kininogen, are mildly to moderately decreased in advanced chronic liver disease, probably as a result of decreased synthesis. The clinical significance of these abnormalities is unknown.

Consumption Coagulopathy

Accelerated activation of coagulation and thrombin formation resulting in consumption coagulopathy (CC), also frequently called disseminated intravascular coagulation (DIC), has been postulated to occur commonly in patients with cirrhosis. This concept is supported by several findings, such as thrombocytopenia; hypofibrinogenemia (rare); shortened fibrinogen survival, which may be prolonged toward normal by the administration of heparin; increased levels of prothrombin fragment 1 (reflecting increased generation and action of factor Xa); fibrinopeptide A (FPA) (indicating increased generation of thrombin), increased thrombin/AT complexes, soluble fibrin; and increased plasma levels of plasma degradation products of cross-linked fibrin (D-dimer). However, in other studies, only infrequent and then only marginal elevations of FPA were found in cirrhotic patients; fibrinogen survival was normal; and there was poor correlation between increases in plasma FPA, hypofibrinogenemia, thrombocytopenia, and extent of liver disease. Furthermore, thrombocytopenia may be caused by hypersplenism; shortened survival of fibrinogen could be due to a loss of fibrinogen into extravascular spaces (ascites, edema) or accelerated clearance of abnor

mal fibrinogen; and elevated FPA could result from impaired clearance by the diseased liver or fibrinogen degradation by plasmin or other proteases.

Release of procoagulant substances into the bloodstream from necrotic hepatocytes and liberation of clot-promoting, intestine-derived endotoxins into the congested portal system have been invoked as possible triggering mechanisms for CC. In addition, there are major alterations of hemostatic control mechanisms and factors that could shift the hemostatic balance toward regional (portal system) or systemic, accelerated intravascular fibrin formation and accumulation, and thrombosis (see Fig. 20–1). Among these are impaired clearance of tissue factor and activated clotting factors by the reticuloendothelial system and the diseased liver, compounded by excessive accumulation of activated clotting factors caused by stasis in the expanded portal system and also by reduced plasma levels of important inhibitors of blood coagulation. Thus, decreases in AT correlating with the extent of hepatic dysfunction have been reported. Interestingly, although a moderate reduction of AT as seen in inherited AT deficiency is a major risk factor for venous thromboembolism, similar reductions in procoagulant coagulation factors generally do not increase the risk of abnormal bleeding. It has been suggested that CC, as reflected by increased plasma-soluble fibrin, is likely to occur if AT activity falls below 30% of normal. AT deficiency in cirrhosis is thought to be caused predominantly by impaired synthesis. However, IV administration of AT concentrates in cirrhotic patients with marked deficiency of the inhibitor has been shown to be associated with an increase in fibrinogen or fibrinogen survival and decreases in thrombin AT complexes and prothrombin fragment 1. This supports the concept that AT deficiency with impaired neutralization of thrombin, factor Xa, and other coagulation proteases may indeed contribute to accelerated fibrinogen catabolism in cirrhotic patients. The plasma concentration of another major regulatory protein of the coagulation system, PC, is also decreased in patients with cirrhosis, usually in proportion to the degree of clinical and laboratory liver function abnormalities, along with its cofactor in plasma, PS. In contrast, tissue factor pathway inhibitor (TFPI) is generally normal. DIC in cirrhotic patients is often difficult to ascertain because of the numerous other hemostatic system alterations associated with liver disease. Furthermore, the issue of the importance of DIC in regard to abnormal bleeding in patients with chronic liver disease remains controversial.

Abnormal Fibrinolysis

Accelerated fibrinolysis has long been recognized in patients with cirrhosis. This hyperfibrinolytic state, indicated by a shortened whole blood or euglobulin clot lysis time and an increase in serum FDP, has been attributed mainly to increased concentrations of plasminogen activators in plasma, in particular, tissue plasminogen activator (TPA), secondary to impaired hepatic clearance and lack of appropriate increases in TPA inhibitors (PAIs), especially PAI-1. Decreased levels of α_2-antiplasmin and histidine-rich glycoprotein have also been reported. This combination of abnormalities could contribute to the observed shortened survival and decreased levels of plasminogen, elevated levels of plasma D-dimer, and plasmin/α_2-antiplasmin complexes. Endogenous activation of fibrinolysis is mediated through activation of the contact system factors, factor XII, prekallikrein, and HMW kininogen, which may be decreased in chronic liver disease, and, indirectly, through activation of the PC system, which may also be impaired. This impairment of endogenous fibrinolysis may conceivably compensate for the accelerated stimulation of extrinsic (t-PA-mediated) fibrinolysis. DIC may also contribute to enhanced fibrinolysis in liver cirrhosis as suggested by the partial correction of shortened plasminogen survival by the administration of heparin. A relation between accelerated fibrinolysis and mucous membrane bleeding in patients with chronic liver disease and between hyperfibrinolysis and fatal hemorrhagic episodes in patients with decompensated cirrhosis has been suggested. However, whether and to what extent accelerated fibrinolysis contributes to abnormal bleeding in cirrhosis remains uncertain.

ASSESSMENT AND MANAGEMENT

Laboratory Evaluation

In patients with suspected cirrhosis, particularly when they present with abnormal bleeding or are about to undergo surgery or other invasive procedures, a hemostatic screening profile, consisting of a platelet count, activated partial thromboplastin time (APTT), and prothrombin time (PT), is commonly used to provide information with regard to the nature and extent of the hemostatic impairment. Some clinicians also use the bleeding time to assess platelet function. However, the bleeding time is not a specific test of platelet function but reflects the overall function of many factors involved in primary hemostasis, such as platelet-injured vessel wall interaction (hemostatic platelet plug formation), that is, the platelet number, platelet function, subendothelial vessel wall connective tissue structure/function, and vWF level and function. Furthermore, the bleeding time is highly operator-dependent, because it is affected by many analytic variables. At present, there is inadequate evidence that the bleeding time is sufficiently predictive of the risk of abnormal bleeding in individual patients with cirrhosis to be clinically useful.

Because the coagulation disorder of cirrhosis commonly involves a reduction in the levels of all coagulation factors (except factor VIII), both APTT and PT may be prolonged, particularly with more advanced cirrhosis. However, dependent on the reagents used, the extent of the PT prolongation usually exceeds that of the APTT (Table 20–1). Further-

more, even with moderate to severe cirrhosis, the PT may be prolonged whereas the APTT may be normal, presumably because the APTT is unaffected by factor VII deficiency and is insensitive to mild reductions of factor V or vitamin K–dependent coagulation factors X and II. This combination of prolonged PT and minimal or no prolongation of APTT is similar to that found in patients with other common, acquired coagulopathies such as vitamin K deficiency, warfarin anticoagulation, and DIC. This combination also contrasts with that found usually in plasma containing heparin or in patients with the lupus anticoagulant (usually selective prolongation of APTT, or APTT prolonged to a much greater extent than PT). Fibrinogen, commonly measured with the Clauss method, is frequently normal but may be decreased with severe cirrhosis. In this test, a standard amount of thrombin is added to a plasma sample, and the rate of fibrin clot formation is proportional to the concentration of fibrinogen. The thrombin time (TT), using more dilute thrombin, is particularly sensitive to impaired fibrin polymerization and may be prolonged in patients with hypofibrinogenemia, dysfibrinogenemia, or high levels of FDP and sometimes in patients without such abnormalities. In patients with a prolonged PT, the TT and fibrinogen assay may be useful in differentiating liver disease, which may lower fibrinogen (severe cirrhosis) and prolong the TT, from vitamin K deficiency or warfarin anticoagulation in which fibrinogen and TT are normal (see Table 20–1).

The PT is now commonly reported in seconds, along with the normal reference interval as well as an international normalized ratio (INR), which was developed specifically to improve standardization of reporting of PT ratios for patients taking warfarin. The INR minimizes the considerable variability in PT results obtained with the same plasma specimen among different laboratories, owing mainly to the use of different tissue thromboplastin reagents with different sensitivities to reductions in the vitamin K–dependent coagulation factors and, to a lesser extent, use of different coagulation instruments. With the INR system, the patient's PT (in seconds) is divided by the mean of the PT normal reference interval, and this ratio value is raised to the power of the international sensitivity index (ISI) of the PT reagent used (INR = PT ratio^{ISI}). The ISI value is obtained by calibrating a given PT reagent against a World Health Organization reference thromboplastin reagent using a series of plasmas from patients on warfarin therapy and normal controls. However, the findings of several recent studies indicate that the INR system does not reliably reduce interlaboratory variation when the PT is performed on plasmas from patients with acquired coagulopathies caused by liver dis-

Table 20–1 Hemostatic Abnormalities in Liver Disease and Vitamin K Deficiency

Condition	Platelets	APTT	PT	Factor V	Factor VII	TT	Fibrinogen	FDP D-Dimer
Cirrhosis (stable)	N or ↓	N or ↑	↑	↓ or N	↓	↑ or N	N or ↓	N or ↑
Cirrhosis (decompensated)	↓	↑ or N	↑↑	↓	↓↓	↑ or N	↓ or N	N or ↑
Vitamin K deficiency	N	↑ or N	↑↑	N	↓↓	N	N	N

APTT, activated partial thromboplastin time; PT, prothrombin time; TT, thrombin time; FDP, fibrinogen/fibrin degradation products; N, normal; ↑ increased; ↓ decreased.

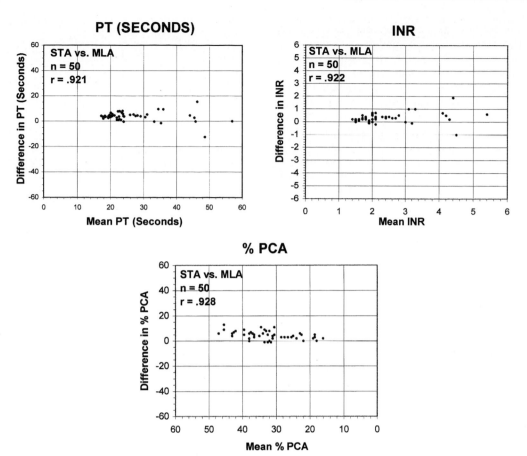

Figure 20–2

Comparison of different methods of expression of prothrombin time results in patients with advanced liver disease. Prothrombin times (PT) were performed on 50 plasma specimens from patients with prolonged PT and known liver disease (bilirubin ≥2.0 mg/dL), not taking warfarin, using two coagulation instrument/reagent systems (STA/Neoplastine Ci+, Diagnostica Stago, France; MLA 1600, Hemoliance, U.S.A./Innovin, Dade International, Inc., U.S.A.). PT results are given in seconds and expressed as international normalized ratio (INR) and percentage prothrombin complex activity (%PCA) based on a standard curve using dilutions of normal pool plasma (NPP) and saline. Differences between two reagent/instrument systems are plotted on the ordinate against means of the respective PT expressions on the abscissa. (From Joist JH, Jagadeesan K, Chance D, et al: Unpublished data.)

ease. This is demonstrated in Figure 20–2, which shows unpublished data from our own laboratory. The INR variability increases considerably and progressively with INR levels higher than 3. In contrast, expression of PT results in percentage prothrombin complex activity (PCA) using a standard dilution curve prepared with mixtures of normal pool plasma and saline, yields improved comparability of results among different PT reagent/instrument systems with increasing prolongation of PT results. However, at present in the US, PT results are generally reported in seconds and in INR values (but not in % PCA) and the correlation coefficient of INR values at INR less than 3 seems to be no worse than that of the PT in seconds.

TREATMENT

Management of Abnormal Bleeding

Because a number of factors and mechanisms, including systemic hemostatic and local vascular abnormalities, may contribute to abnormal bleeding with liver disease, it may be difficult to determine which is most important in a particular clinical situation. The therapeutic approach should be tailored to the nature, site, and extent of bleeding. Epistaxis, gastrointestinal bleeding, bleeding from biopsy sites, or major bleeding following portacaval shunt or surgery, may require different strategies. In addition, attempts at correction of the hemostatic disorder must be closely linked to and coordinated with other measures, such as mechanical compression or sclerotherapy or band ligation of esophageal varices, administration of drugs to reduce production of or neutralize gastric acid, or intervention by surgical procedures or drugs to reduce portal pressure.

Platelet transfusions may be helpful in patients with marked thrombocytopenia and serious abnormal bleeding. The platelet increment after transfusion may, however, be much less than expected (8000 to 10,000/μL per random donor unit or 40,000 to 50,000/μL per pheresis unit infused) because of sequestration of transfused platelets in the enlarged spleen. Portal decompression by portacaval anastomosis or intrahepatic portosystemic shunt (TIPS) may partially correct the thrombocytopenia in some but not all patients. Splenectomy may be associated with improvement of the platelet count but carries considerable risks, such as sepsis and portal vein thrombosis, and is considered by some to be contraindicated in patients with portal hypertension and hypersplenism. Partial splenic embolization (to reduce splenic blood flow by 40% to 80%) may be effective in yielding a prompt and durable, clinically significant increase in platelet concentrations. However, there can be significant complications associated with this procedure, such as transient pain, ileus, fever, nausea, ascites, splenic abscess, and pleural effusion. In preparation for major surgery, platelet concentrates should be given to maintain platelet counts of more than $100,000/\mu L$ perioperatively. It appears that other invasive procedures such as endoscopy, thoracentesis, paracentesis, and lumbar puncture may be carried out safely with platelet counts of more than $50,000/\mu L$. Whether recombinant TPO is effective in temporary correction of thrombocytopenia in patients with cirrhosis prior to surgery or invasive procedures remains to be investigated.

Heparin therapy has been proposed in patients with acute and chronic liver disease because of laboratory evidence of DIC and reports of improvement of hemostasis abnormalities—in particular, prolongation of shortened fibrinogen and plasminogen survival with heparin administration; however, clinical benefit of this approach remains to be demonstrated. Because the contribution of DIC to the bleeding diathesis in patients with liver disease is frequently difficult to determine by laboratory tests, and because heparin may worsen abnormal bleeding, its use cannot be recommended.

Antithrombin III concentrates have been shown to improve hemostatic alterations in cirrhosis. However, these concentrates carry the risks of transmission of viral diseases; they are expensive; and their safety and clinical benefit have yet to be established by controlled studies.

1-Deamino-8-D-arginine vasopressin (DDAVP) administration to patients with stable cirrhosis has been reported to be associated with significant improvement in global coagulation tests and levels of coagulation factors VIII, IX, XI, and XII, as well as shortening of bleeding time and appearance in plasma of vWF multimers larger than those present in a patient's plasma before treatment or in normal plasma. Clinical benefit could not be evaluated, because none of the patients was apparently bleeding at the time of infusion. Furthermore, because the levels of factor VIII:C, vWF antigen, and R:CoF are commonly increased in patients with chronic liver disease, the potential risk of thromboembolic complications with the use of DDAVP must be considered. In another recent prospective study, DDAVP combined with a potent vasoconstricting agent (Terlipressin) yielded less effective control of variceal bleeding than Terlipressin alone.

The use of synthetic *fibrinolytic inhibitors* such as ϵ-aminocaproic acid (Amicar) and tranexamic acid has been proposed in view of laboratory evidence of a hyperfibrinolytic state, and preliminary data have suggested usefulness in the control of bleeding in cirrhotic patients undergoing portacaval shunt surgery and liver transplantation and in controlling abnormal bleeding after tooth extraction. However, because of reports of post-liver transplant thrombosis associated with the administration of Amicar, routine use of fibrinolytic inhibitors is not recommended.

A trial with vitamin K_1 (5 to 10 mg IV or SC) is appropriate if the PT is not excessively prolonged (INR <5) and the patient is not bleeding acutely or at increased risk for bleeding (e.g., status after surgery, before surgery, or pre- or postinvasive procedures). Patients with vitamin K deficiency uncomplicated by liver disease show a substantial or complete correction of the PT within 12 to 24 hours. In patients with serious bleeding, factor VII and V activities may be determined on a blood specimen collected before administration of vitamin K_1 to arrive at a diagnosis more rapidly and to assess the need for administration of fresh frozen plasma. Because both factors V and VII are synthesized by the liver but only one (factor VII) is vitamin K dependent, a reduction in both factors is consistent with liver disease, whereas a reduction in factor VII alone is consistent with vitamin K deficiency. A selective reduction in factor V would be consistent with DIC.

Fresh frozen plasma (FFP) contains all of the coagulation factors and inhibitors present in circulating blood and is, therefore, theoretically the most suitable agent for correction of the multiple defects found in liver disease. In practice, however, effective replacement is difficult because the large amounts of FFP required to correct a markedly prolonged PT to an INR of ≤1.5 (6 to 8 units, 1200 to 1600 mL, in an average-size adult patient, or 20 mL/kg) are frequently not well tolerated by patients with an already expanded plasma volume, particularly with pre-existing cardiovascular or pulmonary compromise. Furthermore, because of the relatively short biologic half-life of factors VII and V, additional continued or intermittent infusions of FFP may be required to maintain adequate plasma concentrations and sustain PT/INR improvement. Because FFP in general is not treated with heat or vapor or other viral inactivation measures, the risks of transmission of viruses (albeit very small) as well as yet unknown pathogens must be considered. However, solvent/detergent–treated FFP is now commercially available but derived from large pools of donors and is appreciably more costly.

When frozen plasma is slowly thawed at 4°C, an insoluble precipitate remains. This precipitate is rich in fibrinogen, vWF, and factor VIII. Following separation from plasma and further warming, these *cryoprecipitate proteins* become soluble and may be infused as a concentrated source of fibrinogen in an actively bleeding cirrhotic patient with marked hypofibrinogenemia or dysfibrinogenemia.

Prothrombin-complex concentrates (PCC) contain high concentrations of factors IX, X, and II and also variable concentrations of factor VII. Because other coagulation factors that are decreased in liver disease, such as factor V, are not present in significant amounts in PCC, administration of PCC may fail to correct adequately the abnormal PT and to control bleeding unless accompanied by the infusion of FFP.

Although the risk of transmitting hepatitis viruses and HIV has been largely eliminated with the introduction of effective donor screening and heat-treated and solvent/detergent-treated PCC, some of these concentrates contain variable amounts of activated coagulation factors (IX_a, X_a, VII_a, II_a) that may not be adequately neutralized in patients with advanced liver disease because of impaired hepatic clearance as well as reduced plasma concentrations of antithrombin III, PC, and PS. Thus, the administration of some

Table 20–2 Minimal Hemostasis Test Guidelines and Abnormal Bleeding with Percutaneous Liver Biopsy

Reference (No. of Cases)	PT (Seconds Prolonged)	Platelets ($\times 10^3/\mu$L)	Bleeding Time (Minutes)	Bleeding Complications (%)
Sherlock et al (50)	$\leq$3	$\geq$80	—	0
Westaby et al (200)	<4	>80	—	1.5
Garcia-Tsao and Boyer (346)	$\leq$3	$\geq$60	$\leq$10	0
Janes and Lindon (405)	<2	>50	—	2

PCC has been reported to be associated with thromboembolic complications, including deep vein thrombosis, pulmonary embolism, and DIC in patients with liver disease and hemophilia. Although the concomitant administration of FFP (to increase the levels of ATIII, PC, and PS) or ATIII concentrate or heparin may diminish the risk of thromboembolic complications, PCC cannot be generally recommended in patients with liver disease, and they are considered contraindicated for procedures such as portacaval shunt surgery.

Recombinant factor VIIa (rVIIa) has been shown to be effective in fully correcting mildly to moderately prolonged PT levels in nonbleeding cirrhotic patients. The rVIIa effect is dose-dependent and at the highest dosage (80 μg/kg) lasts approximately 12 hours. Highly variable, but generally small increases in prothrombin F1.2, indicating accelerated intravascular coagulation, were observed but no decreases in AT, fibrinogen, or platelets, and none of the patients exhibited clinical signs or symptoms of CC. These interesting and promising findings need to be confirmed, and the efficacy of rVIIa in controlling abnormal bleeding in cirrhotic patients with coagulopathy and safety must be established in controlled studies.

Prevention of Abnormal Bleeding with Liver Biopsy and Other Invasive Procedures

Percutaneous liver biopsy frequently provides important information on the exact nature of the liver disorder and the extent of hepatocellular damage and may have prognostic and, with the emergence of α-interferon and other antiviral agents, therapeutic implications. Clinically significant bleeding after outpatient percutaneous liver biopsy is an uncommon complication in patients with liver disease with mildly prolonged ($\leq$4 sec) PT as long as the platelet count is more than 60,000/μL. Important variables that affect the incidence of abnormal bleeding include the diameter and type of biopsy needle used, the number of passes made, the severity of hemostasis defects, liver pathology, operator experience, and sensitivity of post-procedure criteria to detect bleeding (direct observation of liver capsule puncture site, ultrasound evidence of hepatic hematoma, tachycardia and hypotension, and red blood cell transfusion required). Guidelines based on retrospective, single institution experiences have been published for determining safety of percutaneous liver biopsy (Table 20–2). However, differences in patient population, biopsy technique, post-procedure monitoring, and laboratory methods make general acceptance of such guidelines difficult. A recent survey of academic hepatologists from different countries has highlighted the diversity of use of hemostatic tests and practice guidelines (Table 20–3). Responses from 85 American gastroenterology training centers indicated that PT prolongations no greater than 2 or 4 seconds were acceptable to 59% and 7% of respondents, respectively. Congenital deficiencies of single coagulation factors with levels 40 U/dL or higher and mild, combined deficiencies of vitamin K–dependent coagulation factors with levels 40 U/dL or higher are generally not associated with abnormal bleeding. Since levels of vitamin K–dependent coagulation factors of 40 U/dL or higher correspond approximately to a PT-INR of 1.5 or lower, this may be a reasonable, arbitrary safety limit, pending data from controlled clinical outcome studies.

When hemostasis test results are thought to exceed particular guidelines or practice limits, treatment options include vitamin K_1, FFP or platelets, or DDAVP. Another alternative is to obtain liver tissue by a different and, perhaps, safer approach such as laparoscopic liver biopsy, computer tomography (CT)–guided biopsy with Gelfoam packing of the biopsy core, or transjugular intrahepatic biopsy. The management recommendations outlined here for percutaneous liver biopsy, in general, also apply to other invasive procedures, such as paracentesis, thoracentesis, placement of central venous and arterial catheters, and lumbar puncture.

Table 20–3 International Survey of Hemostasis Test Usage with Percutaneous Liver Biopsy

Country and No. of Centers Responding	Minimal Platelet Count ($\times 10^3/\mu$L)			Bleeding Time Performed
	30–50	*50–80*	*>80*	
Canada (10)	40%	40%	20%	0%
US (83)	11%	41%	48%	36%
Europe (73)	7%	59%	34%	23%
Asia (50)	16%	68%	16%	54%

Peritoneovenous Shunt Related Coagulopathy

The LeVeen shunt, introduced in 1974, directs ascitic fluid from the peritoneal cavity to the superior vena cava via a subcutaneous tube that contains a one-way valve. Potential benefits of diversion include reduction of abdominal distention, improved renal function, and improved quality of life. However, rapid reinfusion of large amounts of ascitic fluid may acutely precipitate life-threatening DIC, and chronically, thrombosis of the venous limb and tip of the shunt or of the superior vena cava. Procoagulant (tissue factor, activated coagulation factors) and fibrinolytic (elevated FDP) substances have been described in ascitic fluid, as have endotoxins. The development and extent of LeVeen shunting–associated DIC appears to be dependent on the rate of infusion and volume of reinfused ascites, the degree of liver dysfunction, and a pre-existing hypercoagulable state or CC. Initial reports of 20% to 100% of patients developing post-LeVeen shunt DIC, causing severe bleeding and death in some cases, as well as high rates of recurrent ascites due to thrombosis of shunts or superior vena cava have led to several modifications of the procedure. Most important, patients with clinical or laboratory evidence of appreciable, ongoing CC and accelerated fibrinolysis are at highest risk of acute complications and should not undergo LeVeen shunting. Removal of ascites fluid before initiation of shunting and perioperative antibiotics appears to reduce postoperative morbidity and mortality. Introduction of a titanium tip on the venous return limb of the LeVeen shunt may further reduce the incidence of shunt thrombosis. With the advent of TIPS for management of refractory ascites, fewer (if any) LeVeen shunts are being performed.

PROGNOSIS

Patients with cirrhosis are clearly at increased risk for major bleeding complications and death. The Child-Turcotte classification (encephalopathy, ascites, total bilirubin, albumin, nutritional status) was originally developed to stratify the severity of liver disease and to predict short-term risk of death before portosystemic shunting. Subsequently, nutritional status was replaced by PT, and application of the Child-Turcotte classification as modified by Pugh (Child-Pugh) was expanded to predict the likelihood of death in cirrhotic patients managed medically. Data from recent prospective studies seem to indicate that the extent of decrease of factor VII activity may be a useful predictor of patient survival, whereas platelet concentration is not. Neither platelet count nor bleeding time appears to be a useful predictor of gastrointestinal bleeding. Hyperfibrinolysis (elevated D-dimer, increased TPA activity) may be associated with an increased risk of first variceal hemorrhage, but this finding requires confirmation.

SUGGESTED READINGS

Agnelli G, Parise P, Levi M, et al: Effects of desmopressin on hemostasis in patients with liver cirrhosis. Haemostasis 25:241–247, 1995.
Alvarez OA, Lopera GA, Patel V, et al: Improvement of thrombocytopenia due to hypersplenism after transjugular intrahepatic portosystemic shunt placement in cirrhotic patients. Am J Gastroenterol 91:134–137, 1996.
Aoki Y, Hira K, Tanikawa K: Mechanism of thrombocytopenia in liver cirrhosis: Kinetics of indium-111 tropolone labeled platelets. Eur J Nucl Med 20:123–129, 1993.
Basili S, Ferro D, Leo R, et al: Bleeding time does not predict gastrointestinal bleeding in patients with cirrhosis. J Hepatol 24:574–580, 1996.
Bernstein DE, Jeffers L, Erhardtsen E, et al: Recombinant factor VIIa corrects prothrombin time in cirrhotic patients: A preliminary study. Gastroenterology 113:1930–1937, 1997.
Carmassi F, De Negri F, Morale M, Ferrini L: Antithrombotic and antifibrinolytic effects of antithrombin III replacement in liver cirrhosis. Lancet 349:1069, 1997.
Garcia-Tsao G, Boyer JL: Outpatient liver biopsy: How safe is it? Ann Intern Med 118:150–153, 1993.
Hillaire S, Labianca M, Borgonovo G, et al: Peritoneovenous shunting of intractable ascites in patients with cirrhosis: Improving results and predictive factors of failure. Surgery 113:373–379, 1993.
Janes CH, Lindon KD: Outcome of patients hospitalized for complications after outpatient liver biopsy. Ann Intern Med 118:96–98, 1993.
Joist JH: Hemostatic abnormalities in liver disease. In Coleman RW, Hirsh J, Marder VJ, Salzman EW (eds): Hemostasis and Thrombosis: Basic Principles and Clinical Practice. Philadelphia: JB Lippincott, 1994, p 906.
Kajiwara E, Akagi K, Azuma K, et al: Evidence for an immunological pathogenesis of thrombocytopenia in chronic liver disease. Am J Gastroenterol 90:962–966, 1995.
Laffi G, Cinotti S, Filimberti E, et al: Defective aggregation in cirrhosis is independent of in vivo platelet activation. J Hepatol 24:436–443, 1996.
Moller S, Bendtsen F, Christensen E, Henriksen JH: Prognostic variables in patients with cirrhosis and oesophageal varices without prior bleeding. J Hepatol 21:940–946, 1994.
Peck-Radosavljevic M, Zacherl J, Meng YG, et al: Is inadequate thrombopoietin production a major cause of thrombocytopenia in cirrhosis of the liver? J Hepatol 27:127–131, 1997.
Robert A, Chazouilleres O: Prothrombin time in liver failure: Time, ratio, activity percentage, or International Normalized Ratio? Hepatology 24:1392–1394, 1996.
Sangro B, Bilbao I, Herrero I, et al: Partial splenic embolization for the treatment of hypersplenism in cirrhosis. Hepatology 18:309–314, 1993.
Sanyal AJ, Freedman AM, Purdum PP, et al: The hematologic consequences of transjugular intrahepatic portosystemic shunts. Hepatology 23:32–39, 1996.
Scherer R, Kabatnik M, Erhard J, Peters J: The influence of antithrombin III (AT III) substitution to supranormal activities on systemic procoagulant turnover in patients with end-stage chronic liver disease. Intensive Care Med 23:1150–1158, 1997.
Sherlock S, Dick R, Von Leeuwen DJ: Liver biopsy today: The Royal Free Hospital Conference. J Hepatol 1:75–85, 1984.
Sue M, Caldwell SH, Dickson RC, et al: Variation between centers in technique and guidelines for liver biopsy. Liver 16:267–270, 1996.
Violi F, Basili S, Ferro D, et al: Association between high values of D-dimer and tissue-plasminogen activator activity and first gastrointestinal bleeding in cirrhotic patients. Thromb Haemost 76:177–183, 1996.
Violi F, Ferro D, Basili S, et al: Association between low-grade disseminated intravascular coagulation and endotoxemia in patients with liver cirrhosis. Gastroenterology 109:531–539, 1995.
Violi F, Ferro D, Basili S, et al: Prognostic value of clotting and fibrinolytic systems in a follow-up of 165 liver cirrhotic patients. Hepatology 22:96–100, 1995.
von Flue M, Rothembuhler JM, Bianchi L, et al: Portal venous thrombosis following splenectomy in portal hypertension: Risks and management. J Suisse Med 123:2309–2317, 1993.
Westaby D, MacDougall BRD, Williams R: Liver biopsy as a day-case procedure: Selection and complications in 200 consecutive patients. BMJ 281:1331–1332, 1980.
White GC, Marder VJ, Colman RW, et al: Approach to the bleeding patient. In Coleman RW, Hirsh J, Marder VJ, Salzman EW (eds): Hemostasis and Thrombosis: Basic Principles and Clinical Practice. Philadelphia: JB Lippincott, 1994, pp 1134–1147.
Younger HM, Hadoke PW, Dillon JF, Hayes PC: Platelet function in cirrhosis and the role of humoral factors. Eur J Gastroenterol Hepatol 9:989–992, 1997.

21

Malnutrition in Cirrhosis

Arthur J. McCullough

The nutritional management of patients with liver disease remains a much discussed but controversial area of clinical hepatology. At a strategic level, there can be little doubt that adequate nutritional sustenance is a fundamental component to the survival and sense of well-being in these patients. However, the logistics of identifying patients in need of nutritional therapy as well as choosing the type, duration, and quantity of nutritional supplements remain elusive and ill defined. In addition, questions persist regarding the cost-effectiveness of nutritional therapy, its effect on quality of life, and the definition of the appropriate goals and outcomes to be achieved from such therapy in patients with liver disease.

Nonetheless, the importance of nutrition in the management of these patients is emphasized by the following nutritional axioms relevant to chronic liver disease.

1. Malnutrition is common but underdiagnosed.
2. Alterations in energy metabolism and nutritional status are similar to those observed in starvation.
3. The occasional need for sodium and protein restriction conflicts directly with nutritional requirements in these patients.
4. Complications of cirrhosis such as encephalopathy and sepsis usually occur in conjunction with muscle wasting and negative nitrogen balance.
5. Correction of malnutrition may improve the clinical outcome of these patients.

Most clinicians employ a common sense approach to feeding patients with liver disease, whereas many investigators advocate the aggressive use of nutritional supplements and specialized formulations. The aim of this more aggressive approach is to correct pre-existing protein-calorie malnutrition (PCM) and to stimulate hepatic regeneration. Nascent clinical studies suggest that more aggressive nutritional therapy may, in fact, benefit certain types of patients with liver disease. These studies are encouraging and emphasize the need for a greater understanding of the etiologic factors responsible for PCM so that the specific role of nutrition in the diagnosis, prognosis, and therapy of chronic liver disease can be improved and better defined.

PREVALENCE

Early data focusing on alcoholic liver disease reported weight loss, nausea, and vomiting to occur in 60%, 55%, and 87% of such patients, respectively. The results of these symptoms are shown in Table 21–1, which is a compilation of studies and displays the frequency of PCM in alcoholics with or without structural liver disease. There are quantitative differences among these studies, which may have been due, in part, to the presence of structural liver disease, the proportion of calories derived from alcohol, and nonuniformity in the precision with which nutritional status was assessed. Nonetheless, several facts seem apparent.

1. In hospitalized patients with alcoholic hepatitis, the prevalence of PCM is significant but varies according to disease severity and the extent of nutritional assessment performed. The Veterans' Administration (VA) cooperative study, which is the largest and most comprehensive study performed in patients with severe alcoholic hepatitis, reported a prevalence of almost 100% for PCM. The prevalence of PCM in that study correlated with the severity of liver dysfunction (shown in Table 21–2) but not with the histologic alterations. In hospitalized patients with less severe alcoholic hepatitis, the prevalence of PCM ranges between 30% and 40%.

Table 21–1 Malnutrition in Alcoholic Patients

	Structural Disease Present	Structural Disease Absent
Number of studies	5	8
Prevalence (%) of malnutrition	10–100%	0–40%
% of dietary calories from alcohol	35–65%	24–41%

Table 21–3 Prevalence of Protein-Calorie Malnutrition

	Alcoholic Liver Disease	Nonalcoholic Liver Disease
Sarin (1997)	54–82%	50–80%
Caregaro (1997)	34%	34%
Thuluvath (1994)	37%	33%
IMCP (1992)*	40%	27%

*Italian Multicenter Cooperative Project in liver cirrhosis.

PROGNOSIS

It has been difficult to demonstrate a causal relationship between malnutrition and survival in patients with cirrhosis, because multiple pathophysiologic processes are occurring simultaneously. However, a growing number of reports now confirm this association (Table 21–4). Nutritional status was first used as a prognostic factor in the Child-Turcotte classification for estimating mortality in patients undergoing portacaval shunt surgery. Many studies have now reported its value in predicting operative mortality and long-term survival in patients with chronic liver disease. PCM also has prognostic value in patients undergoing liver transplantation or other abdominal operations. The disappearance of ascites following the placement of a peritoneal venous shunt improved nutrition and immunity. PCM also predicted altered immunity and susceptibility to infection and mortality in patients hospitalized for cirrhosis and ascites. In addition, the VA cooperative study mentioned earlier demonstrated that improved food intake and survival correlated with improved nutritional status. These data indicate that the recognition and treatment of malnutrition are important considerations in the management of patients with liver disease, especially for those types of patients listed in Table 21–4.

ASSESSMENT OF NUTRITIONAL STATUS

Because the presence of PCM has prognostic value and influences clinical decisions regarding nutritional therapy in patients with liver disease, accurate methods of assessing nutritional status are vital. The measurement parameters most commonly used in clinical practice to diagnose PCM are shown in Table 21–5. Unfortunately, assessment of nutritional status (especially protein deficiency) in patients with liver disease is difficult to accomplish. Fluid excess is universal in end-stage liver disease and is common even in earlier stages of disease. This fluid excess causes weight to height parameters (e.g., the percentage of ideal body weight) to underestimate both the prevalence and the degree of malnutrition. In addition, alcohol and chronic liver disease itself may cause alterations in visceral protein synthesis, cellular immunity, and total lymphocyte count independently from PCM. In fact, visceral proteins appear to correlate better with the degree of liver damage than the degree of PCM. In contrast, markers of lean body mass and fat stores are less dependent on either alcoholism or structural liver disease.

Despite the limitations of these standard methodologies, more sophisticated measurements of body cell mass (BCM) also provide evidence for PCM in chronic liver disease. The

2. Patients hospitalized for alcoholic liver disease have the worst nutritional status compared with other types of hospitalized patients.
3. Although the data are more limited in patients with alcoholic liver disease who are not admitted to a medical facility, the available information suggests that approximately 30% of such patients are malnourished.
4. In alcoholics without liver disease, the prevalence of PCM is also variable and is dependent on the amount of alcohol intake. In those patients who derive less than 30% of the caloric intake from alcohol, PCM is uncommon. In contrast, the prevalence of PCM increases to above 50% in patients who derive more than 50% of their calories from alcohol.

Despite the large amount of data on alcoholic liver disease, there have been only a few studies regarding PCM in nonalcoholic liver disease. Early studies suggested that the prevalence of PCM was low in nonalcoholic liver disease and less severe than in alcoholic liver disease. However, recent data indicate that PCM is prevalent in both these forms of liver disease. Table 21–3 displays the only four studies that measured PCM in both alcoholic and nonalcoholic liver disease. These studies demonstrate that the prevalence of PCM is almost identical in these two types of liver disease. Although the prevalence is similar, the pattern of PCM is different. Nonalcoholic cirrhosis is associated with a decrease in both fat and muscle mass, whereas alcoholic cirrhosis is associated with a decrease in muscle mass but a relative sparing of fat stores. Disease-specific patterns of PCM have also been demonstrated in cirrhotic patients awaiting liver transplantation.

Therefore, clinicians need to be aware that PCM is common in both alcoholic and nonalcoholic liver disease, especially because it has prognostic significance.

Table 21–2 Protein-Calorie Malnutrition in Alcoholic Hepatitis*

Disease Severity†	Prevalence of Malnutrition (%)
Mild	4.7
Moderate	47
Severe	72.2

*Adapted from Mendenhall CL, Anderson S, Weesner RE, et al: Protein-calorie malnutrition associated with alcoholic hepatitis. Am J Med 76:211–222, 1984. Copyright© 1984, with permission from Excerpta Medica Inc.
†Grading based on prothrombin time and serum bilirubin.

Table 21–4   Protein-Calorie Malnutrition as a Poor Prognostic Factor in Cirrhosis

Condition or Procedure	Clinical Outcome Measured	Study Author (year)
Cirrhosis	Survival	Caregaro (1996)
		Merli (1996)
	Immunodeficiency	Qiao (1988)
		O'Keefe (1980)
Cirrhotic patients having abdominal surgery	Survival	Garrison (1984)
	Postoperative complications	Ouchi (1988)
Hospitalized patients with ascites/cirrhosis	Survival	Llach (1988)
		Blendis (1986)
		Franco (1987)
Alcoholic hepatitis	Survival	Mendenhall (1984, 1986)
	Liver function	
Liver transplantation	Patient/graft survival	Shaw (1985, 1986)
		Lautz (1992)
		Moukarzel (1990)
		Selberg (1997)
Hepatectomy	Postoperative complications	Fan (1995)

BCM, which comprises the central energy-expending mass of working tissue, has been found to be decreased in both alcoholic and nonalcoholic cirrhosis by three different measurements: (1) total body potassium; (2) intracellular water; and (3) total body protein. Therefore, it is important for the clinician to remember that all the methods commonly used for nutritional assessment in cirrhotic patients are influenced or potentially influenced by the presence of liver disease alone or in combination with renal failure, alcohol ingestion, and expansion of the extracellular water compartment. Nonetheless, nutritional assessment is useful in patients with liver disease, especially when a composite score emphasizing anthropometry and creatinine height index is performed and combined with overall clinical judgment.

ETIOLOGY OF PROTEIN-CALORIE MALNUTRITION

Table 21–6 lists the major potential causes of malnutrition in these patients. In addition to the well described factors of maldigestion, malabsorption, and decreased hepatic storage, the importance of poor dietary intake cannot be overemphasized. This poor intake occurs before, during, and after hospitalization. It is important to emphasize that poor dietary intake is an extremely relevant factor in both hospitalized

and ambulatory patients with liver disease. Furthermore, it is now recognized that the liver may play an important role in controlling food intake. Factors 1 and 2 listed in Table 21–6 can at least potentially be treated by a clinician who institutes prompt and aggressive nutritional therapy. However, a number of studies have now demonstrated that PCM may exist in cirrhosis despite adequate dietary intake and nutrient absorption. This suggests that factors 3 through 6 in Table 21–6 are also important in the altered PCM in chronic liver disease.

ENERGY METABOLISM

Energy Expenditure

Quantitative disturbances in energy expenditure in cirrhosis are variable as shown in Table 21–7. Most studies using indirect calorimetry find no difference in absolute energy expenditure between cirrhotic and control patients. The exceptions to this observation are two studies that demonstrated an increased absolute energy expenditure: one in children with cirrhosis and extrahepatic portal vein obstruction and the other in patients with primary biliary cirrhosis. However, four of the studies also demonstrated increased energy expenditure when caloric consumption is expressed per unit

Table 21–5   Nutritional Assessment Parameters of Factors Influencing Their Accuracy*

| Measurements | Malnutrition | | Alcohol Toxicity | Liver Disease | Renal Function |
	Protein	Protein-Calorie			
Visceral proteins	X		X	X	
Lymphocyte count	X		X	X	X
Cellular immunity	X		X	X	X
% Ideal body weight		X		X	X
Anthropometry		X		(?)	(?)
Creatinine height index		X		(?)	X

*Modified from McCullough AJ, Tavill AS: Disordered energy and protein metabolism in liver disease. Semin Liver Dis 11:265–277, 1991.

Table 21–6 Potential Causes of Malnutrition in Liver Disease*

1. Decreased quality and quantity of food
   Disease related
      Anorexia, nausea, and vomiting
   Iatrogenic
      Unpalatable diets
      Purgation and neomycin enteropathy
2. Impaired nutrient digestion and absorption
   Pancreatic and bile salt deficiency
   Stressful complications
3. Increased energy requirements
   Energy cost of alcohol metabolism
   Stressful complications
4. Accelerated protein breakdown
5. Protein oxidation*
6. Inefficient protein synthesis

*Factors 1 and 2 can be altered currently by nutritional therapy.
†Protein oxidation is a term used to describe irreversible amino-nitrogen loss occurring at the amino acid level but extrapolated to precursor tissue protein.

of lean body mass (estimated from urinary creatinine excretion). Furthermore, energy expenditure correlates directly with lean body mass in cirrhosis. However, patterns of energy expenditure may be dependent on the type of liver disease. In primary biliary cirrhosis and alcoholic hepatitis, energy expenditure increases with worsening liver function. In contrast, energy expenditure decreases with the worsening function in alcoholic and posthepatitic cirrhosis. Therefore, if urinary creatinine excretion reflects total lean body mass,

it appears that cirrhotic patients have increased resting energy expenditure that correlates with the severity of liver disease and that may be dependent on the type of liver disease.

However, it should be emphasized that there are inherent difficulties in the measurement of both lean body mass and energy expenditure. Furthermore, these difficulties are compounded by differences among patient populations, such as gender, genetics, type and stage of liver disease, and variability within individual organs and total body expenditures. These difficulties have also been emphasized in a large study of patients awaiting liver transplantation. In this heterogeneous group of patients, a wide range of energy expenditure exists with 18% of patients being hypermetabolic, 51% normal metabolic, and 31% hypometabolic. Energy expenditure correlated with lean body mass rather than the type, duration, or severity of liver disease. This suggests that hypermetabolism (although present in a proportion of patients) is not a constant feature of cirrhosis and may be influenced more by extrahepatic than hepatic factors. Prediction of resting energy expenditure by means of standard equations (e.g., the Harris-Benedict equation) gives reliable results in patients when applying actual body weight. However, the variance in measured resting energy expenditure among cirrhotic patients is larger than the variance observed in healthy individuals, because more than 50% of the cirrhotic patients have measured energy expenditure outside the 95% predicted range. Therefore, although it is preferable to directly measure energy expenditure in these patients, the Harris-Benedict equation can be used to calculate energy expenditure, but the error in this calculation is larger than in healthy controls. When increased energy expenditure is

Table 21–7 Resting Energy Expenditure in Chronic Liver Disease Based on Indirect Calorimetry

Study	Cirrhotic Patients	Control Group	Data Expressed as
Owen (1983)	1.05 ± 0.17 (n = 8)	1.00 ± 0.16 (n = 10)	kcal/min/1.73 m^2
Jhangiani* (1986)	1507.8 ± 255.2 (n = 8)	1470.3 ± 191.2 (n = 7)	kcal/day/m^2
John (1989)†	1566 ± 306.7‡ (n = 10)	1923 ± 246 (n = 20)	kcal/day
Moderate disease			
Severe disease	1878 ± 211.9		
Shanbhogue† 1987	1730 ± 300 (n = 10)	1800 ± 330 (n = 10)	kcal/day
Merli et al (1990)	21.9 ± 2.0 (n = 25)	21.4 ± 1.0 (n = 10)	kcal/kg/day
Schneeweiss et al† (1990)	1.06 ± 0.14 (n = 22)	0.98 ± 0.09 (n = 20)	kcal/min/1.73/m^2
Green (1991)	4.46 ± 0.81‡ (n = 7)	3.65 ± .23 (n = 7)	kj/hr/kg
Müller† (1991)	27.1 ± 4.1 (n = 10)	25.6 ± 2.5 (n = 10)	kcal/kg/day
Vermeij (1991)	1645 ± 315 (n = 10)	1530 ± 235 (n = 50)	kcal/day
Ksiazyk§ (1996)	143.7 ± 29.5 (n = 25)	116.1 ± 5.9 (n = 14)	kj/kg

Results are expressed as mean ± SD.
*Measurements performed 2 hours postprandial. All other studies performed measurements after an overnight fast.
†Cirrhotic patients had increased energy expenditure when expressed per gram of urinary creatinine excretion.
‡$P < .01$ vs. severe disease and controls.
§Patient group included children with cirrhosis (n = 11) and extrahepatic portal vein obstruction (n = 14).

present in patients with liver disease, the cause or causes remain unknown and proposals are speculative. Ascites increases energy expenditure by approximately 10%.

Diet-induced thermogenesis is also not quantitatively different in patients with cirrhosis. Energy expenditure measured by treadmill or bicycle exercise experiments is reported to be normal, at least in clinically stable patients with cirrhosis. Therefore, in most patients, the correction factors for activity can be applied when calculating total energy requirements in patients with cirrhosis. However, the maximum workload and the anaerobic threshold are both reduced and plasma lactic acid concentrations are increased proportionally to workload in patients with cirrhosis. These data suggest a reduced anaerobic capacity to oxidize energy in response to increased energy needs or a reduced physical fitness in these patients.

The stressful complications associated with the cytokine response, which often occur in advanced liver disease, may also increase energy expenditure on an intermittent or continuous basis. In addition, cirrhotic patients may not have the normal metabolic or hormonally adapted decrease in energy expenditure, which occurs in response to insufficient nutrient intake and decreased lean body mass.

Fuel Substrate

Regardless of the rate of energy expenditure, it is now clear that the preferred fuel substrate is altered in most patients with cirrhosis. All except two of the available studies shown in Table 21–8 reported decrease in respiratory quotient after an overnight fast in cirrhotic patients. This indicates that cirrhotic patients obtain approximately 75% of their calories from fat after an overnight fast compared with 35% for controls who would take approximately 48 to 72 hours of starvation to obtain the low RQ levels obtained in cirrhosis after only 12 to 18 hours. Consequently, food should not be withheld from cirrhotic patients for any extended period, but rather frequent interval feedings with a nighttime snack should be given. The potential clinical advantage of this approach has been confirmed with studies that evaluated nitrogen balance in cirrhotic patients who are fed the same amount of calories distributed over different time intervals. Those patients who received an evening snack to supply energy during the sleeping hours were able to maintain a greater positive nitrogen balance than did patients who were

given less frequent interval feeding. In addition, the habitual dietary intake in these patients indicates that they prefer the breakfast meal, thus indirectly confirming this need for energy after periods of fasting.

Carbohydrate Metabolism

Most experts conclude that approximately 80% of patients with cirrhosis are glucose intolerant, but only 10% will develop frank diabetes mellitus. It should be emphasized that although there is a high prevalence of glucose intolerance, most cirrhotic patients have fasting plasma levels of less than 140 mg/dL, and the 2-hour postprandial glucose concentration is usually about 200 mg/dL during a glucose tolerance test. Therefore, there is little risk for the development of the microvascular complications of diabetes in most cirrhotic patients despite this glucose intolerance.

Consequently, the glucose intolerance and insulin resistance in cirrhotic patients have often been considered an interesting observation without important clinical consequences. However, with the pathophysiology of carbohydrate intolerance being increasingly understood, the role of altered glucose metabolism in determining substrate fuel metabolism and protein balance is assuming greater importance. The major abnormalities of glucose metabolism in cirrhosis are provided in Table 21–9 along with their likely etiologies. This area has been reviewed extensively by Petrides and DeFronzo.

Altered Glucose Metabolism in Cirrhosis

Insulin Resistance

Insulin resistance is a ubiquitous finding in all types and stages of cirrhosis. Using the euglycemic insulin clamp technique, the average affinity constant for insulin is threefold higher in cirrhotic patients than in controls. Furthermore, the insulin dose response curve in cirrhosis is shifted to the right, an abnormality that correlates with the increased insulin response to an oral glucose tolerance test and indicates a decrease in insulin sensitivity. Collectively, these studies demonstrate that insulin's action upon glucose metabolism is decreased by approximately 40% to 50%. This insulin resistance occurs even in the early stages of cirrhosis and with physiologic concentrations of insulin. Al-

Table 21–8 Respiratory Quotients in Cirrhosis*

Author (Year)	Cirrhotic Patients (No.)	Control Group (No.)
Owen (1983)	0.74 ± 0.02 (9)†	0.85 ± 0.02 (10)
Mullen (1986)	0.75 ± 0.01 (6)†	0.85 ± 0.03
Jhangiani (1986)	0.84 ± 0 (8)	0.83 ± 0.04 (7)
Merli (1990)	0.78 ± 0.04 (25)†	0.87 ± 0.05 (10)
Schneeweiss (1990)	0.72 ± 0.01 (22)†	0.84 ± 0.01 (20)
Petrides (1991)	0.82 ± 0.5 (8)	0.84 ± 0.10 (12)
Müller (1992)‡	0.73 ± 0.02 (123)†	0.83 ± 0.03 (30)

*All respiratory quotients are corrected for urinary nitrogen excretion except for the data of Jhangiani.
†Significantly less than controls.
‡Results estimated from Figure 21–2 in article.
The numbers in parentheses indicate the number of patients studied.

Table 21–9 Glucose Metabolism in Liver Disease

Abnormality	Etiology of Abnormality
Hyperinsulinemia	Decreased hepatic extraction
	Portosystemic shunting
	Increased insulin secretion (?)*
Insulin resistance	Decreased receptor binding (?)
	Post receptor defect
	Increased levels of insulin antago- nists
	Hyperinsulinemia
Glucose intolerance	Decreased glucose uptake and glyco- gen formation in muscle
	Decreased hepatic glycogen forma- tion (?)
Altered energy metabolism	Decreased hepatic sensitivity to glu- cagon
State of accelerated starvation	Increased metabolic rate (?)
	Decreased glycogen stores
Increased use of fats as a fuel source	Increased lipolysis
	Hormonal and metabolic milieu favors early use of alternative fuel

*(?) Indicates an etiology which has either not been investigated or for which conflicting data exist.

though the presence of insulin resistance in cirrhosis is gen- erally accepted, its etiology (and the sequelae of this insulin resistance) is multifactorial and remains a much discussed but not completely understood area of clinical investigation. The etiology of hyperinsulinemia is also multifactorial; pos- sible factors include increased insulin secretion, diminished hepatic extraction, and portosystemic shunting.

Based on indirect calorimetry as well as euglycemic in- sulin clamp studies, glucose oxidation is normal in cirrhosis, but nonoxidized glucose disposal is reduced by 50%. Be- cause nonoxidative glucose disposal predominantly repre- sents glycogen formation, impaired glycogen synthesis is the primary defect responsible for peripheral insulin resis- tance. This has been confirmed both in human cirrhosis and in animal models of liver disease and is consistent with other insulin resistance states that have diminished muscle glycogen synthesis (Table 21–10).

Fat Metabolism

Consistent with this state of insulin resistance and acceler- ated starvation, cirrhotic patients have a number of distur- bances in fat metabolism, which are shown in Table 21–11.

Fatty Acid Turnover

As shown in Table 21–12, all four studies that have inves- tigated fatty acid turnover in cirrhosis demonstrated in- creased lipolysis (or the appearance of fatty acids into se- rum). Furthermore, this increase in lipolysis is resistant to the usual suppressive effect of insulin, particularly at low physiologic insulin levels, and appears directly related to the concentration of free fatty acids in serum.

Although total free fatty acids are increased in serum, the abnormalities are not uniform across the range of individual free fatty acids. Monounsaturated free fatty acids (18:1 and

Table 21–10 Abnormal Glucose Metabolism in Different Insulin Resistance States*

	Cirrhosis	Obesity	NIDDM
Total body glucose uptake	†	†	†
Glucose oxidation	NL	†	†
Nonoxidative glucose disposal	†	†	†
Suppression of hepatic glucose production	NL	†	†

*Modified from Petrides AS, Groop LC, Riely CA, DeFranzo RA: Effect of physiologic hyperinsulinemia on glucose and lipid metabolism in cirrhosis. J Clin Invest 88:561–570, 1991.
†, Decreased activity; NL, normal activity; NIDDM, non–insulin- dependent diabetes mellitus.

16:1) are profoundly elevated, whereas there is a reduction in the saturated and polyunsaturated fatty acids (PUFA). Perhaps most important, arachidonic acid (one of the PUFA) is decreased. This has potential importance because it is the major long chain PUFA in tissue and serum phospholipids and may adversely affect cell membrane function. In addi- tion, arachidonic acid and the other 20 carbon PUFA are the precursors in the biosynthesis of prostaglandins and related eicosanoids, which have important roles in regulating kid- ney function and the immune system. These observations have led some others to suggest dietary supplements with PUFA in cirrhotic patients.

Lipid Oxidation and Synthesis

As has been mentioned earlier, most studies indicate that in the postabsorptive state and during short-term starvation, fat constitutes a significantly larger proportion of total caloric expenditure in cirrhotic patients than was observed in nor-

Table 21–11 Abnormalities in Fat Metabolism

Abnormality	Clinical and Biochemical Consequences
Elevated serum free fatty acid and glycerol levels	Low respiratory quotient
	High lipid turnover
	Increased fat oxidation
	Increased production of ketone bodies (?)
Deficiency of certain fatty acids (particu- larly arachidonic acid)	Abnormal prostaglandin synthesis (cyclooxygenase)
	Abnormal leukotriene synthesis (lipoxygenase)
Increased cholesterol- phospholipid ratio	Decreased RBC life span (?)
	Abnormal platelets aggregation
	Abnormal phagocytosis by macro- phages
Decreased membrane fluidity	Abnormal transport of ions and nutrients across membranes (?)
	Target cell formation
	Spur cell anemia

Table 21–12   Fatty Acid Turnover and Serum Levels in Cirrhosis*

Study (Year)	FFA Levels		FFA Turnover†	
	Cirrhotic Patients	*Control Patients*	*Cirrhotic Patients*	*Control Patients*
Owen (1983)	948 ± 192*	578 ± 162	7.2 ± 1.7*	4.7 ± 1.3
Merli (1986)	893 ± 95*	340 ± 140	5.2 ± 0.4*	1.8 ± 0.4
Petrides et al (1991)	933 ± 43*	711 ± 44	9.1 ± 1.2*	6.0 ± 0.5
Romijn (1991)	634 ± 90*	400 ± 38	7.1 ± 1.2	4.5 ± 0.5‡
			11.2 ± 1.1*	6.8 ± 0.6§

*Results expressed as mean ± SD.
†All studies used 1-^{14}C palmitate, except Merli and associates who used 1-^{14}C oleate, and are expressed as μmol/kg body weight/min except for Romijn and Owen who normalized data for lean body mass and 1.73 m^2, respectively.
‡Study performed after a 16-hour fast.
§Study performed after a 22-hour fast.

mal controls. Consequently, it was not surprising when two different studies obtained results that indicated that fatty acid oxidation was increased in cirrhosis. However, the rate of total lipid oxidation (measured by indirect calorimetry) exceeds the rate of plasma free fatty acid oxidation (measured by labeled CO_2 in the breath doing a labeled fatty acid infusion) by 40% to 50%. Therefore, there may be a disassociation between the rate of free fatty acid turnover and fatty acid oxidation in cirrhosis.

Recent information suggests that cirrhotic patients have decreased lipid synthesis and an impaired formation of triglyceride lipoproteins following both carbohydrates and fat feeding. This may indicate a problem with storage of dietary energy and may contribute to the loss of adipose tissue.

Energy Overview

Based on this information, cirrhosis should be considered a state of accelerated starvation. The inability of cirrhotic patients to normally store energy precursors results in an early conversion to alternative fuels with resultant loss of lean and fat mass.

Protein Metabolism

Cirrhosis continues to be considered a catabolic disease associated with increased rates of protein breakdown and negative nitrogen balance. However, as shown in Table 21–13, the available data based on different methodologies are conflicting and responsible for the current controversies regarding protein kinetics in cirrhotic patients. Of the various methodologies shown in Table 21–13, the most extensively used method is the measurement of protein kinetics, which is based on labeled amino acid turnover. Table 21–14 shows the results of the studies using this methodology. Although a consensus opinion has not currently been reached, the majority of the data indicate that protein breakdown is increased in cirrhosis. In addition, recent studies utilizing long-term refeeding experiments support the concept of increased protein degradation.

According to recommended dietary allowance (RDA) recommendations, healthy individuals have an average requirement of 0.6 g/kg/day. Allowing for 2 standard deviations and suboptimal composition of dietary protein in a mixed diet, the RDA recommendation is for 0.8 g/kg/day. In

refeeding experiments, cirrhotic patients have an average requirement of 0.8 g/kg on a mixed diet. When adding the 2 standard deviations, this recommendation is increased to 1.2 to 1.3 g/kg/day. Therefore, the average requirement of cirrhotic patients equals the recommendation of the RDA for healthy people. Techniques using the urinary excretion of the end products of nitrogen metabolism have repeatedly suggested increased protein breakdown, whereas leucine tracer methodology has consistently found normal protein degradation rates. With the realization that lean body mass is decreased in cirrhosis, protein degradation per unit of metabolically active tissue is increased regardless of the methodology. In addition, it should be stressed that most protein kinetic studies performed on cirrhotic patients have been performed during stable periods of the patients' clinical course. Therefore, patients with chronic disease may exhibit abnormalities in protein metabolism, particularly during periods of diminished nutritional intake, daily activity, and intercurrent illness. Acute episodes of liver injury associated with monocyte-derived cytokines such as alcoholic hepatitis also may have profound effects on protein metabolism. In the refeeding studies mentioned previously, cirrhotic patients, even when clinically stable, have a spontaneous intake that is very close to the requirement for protein balance and, therefore, are susceptible to rapid protein wasting during periods associated with decreased dietary intake

Table 21–13   Measurement of Protein Breakdown in Cirrhosis

Experimental Technique	Protein Degradation*	
	Increased	*Normal*
Amino acid studied		
Tracer kinetics		
^{14}C-tyrosine†	(X)	
^{13}C-leucine	X	X
^{13}C-keto-isocaproic acid	X	X
^{15}N-glycine	X	X
Nitrogen balance	X	X
3-CH$_3$ histidine	X	X

*X represents studies that indicate increased or normal rates of protein degradation.
†In the ^{14}C-tyrosine study, historical controls were used without normalization for body weights.

Table 21–14 Protein Kinetics* in Cirrhosis Using [1-^{13}C] or 1-^{14}C] Leucine

	Protein	
Study	*Degradation*	*Oxidation*
Millikan (1985)†		
Controls (n = 5)	3.57 ± 0.48	0.45 ± 0.05
Cirrhotics		
Compensated (n = 4)	3.53 ± 1.0	0.49 ± 0.08
Decompensated (n = 4)	3.05 ± 0.25	0.32 ± 0.05
Mullen (1986)		
Controls (n = 6)	3.61 ± 0.7	0.53 ± 0.11
Cirrhotics (n = 6)	3.64 ± 0.8	0,33 ± 0.10‡
Shanbhogue (1987)§		
Control (n = 7)	5.86 ± 1.75	1.49 ± 1.18
Cirrhotics (n = 20)	6.97 ± 2.16	1.36 ± 1.41
Morrison (1990)‖¶		
Controls (n = 8)	5.53 (3.5–8.4)	1.55 (1.1–2.7)
Cirrhotics (n = 11)	5.69 (3.9–6.3)	1.87 (1.5–2.0)‡
Petrides (1991)**		
Controls (n = 9)	2.20 ± 0.20	0.33 ± 0.11
Cirrhotics (n = 8)	2.70 ± 0.20	0.37 ± 0.10
McCullough (1992)¶		
Controls (n = 7)	4.19 ± 0.9	0.83 ± 0.13
Cirrhotics (n = 7)	6.56 ± 1.6‡	1.06 ± 0.24‡
McCullough (1992a)††		
Controls (n = 6)	5.82 ± 0.76	1.13 ± 0.16
Cirrhotics (n = 6)	6.96 ± 0.82‡	0.99 ± 0.22
Tessari (1993)		
Controls (n = 26)¶	4.35 ± 1.50	ND
Cirrhotics (n = 15)	3.96 ± 1.14	ND
Tessari		
Controls (n = 26)¶	5.75 ± 1.50	ND
Cirrhotics (n = 15)	4.85 ± 0.95‡	ND

*All study results are calculated in g/kg/day and expressed as mean ± SD, except for the study of Morrison and associates, in which only median values with ranges are provided.
†Values represent the mean values of the two postabsorptive studies.
‡$P < .05$ versus controls.
§Values represent the absolute flux and oxidation rates as provided in the article divided by the mean weights of each group in order to standardize kinetic rates for body weight. Kinetics were determined during a 43.6% branched-chain amino acid solution at a rate of 14.7 g/hr of amino acids. These patients had end-stage liver disease and were awaiting hepatic transplantation.
‖These patients were severely wasted with decreased body weight, fat stores, and muscle mass. Kinetics were based on the plasma enrichment of leucine's ketoacid-α-ketoisocaproic acid, rather than leucine itself, and the results are expressed as medians with ranges.
¶Kinetics based on leucine's ketoacid-α-ketoisocaproic acid.
**Values represents means converted from data expressed per m^2 to per kg body weight from the mean weight and surface area values provided in the article.
††Data normalized to body cell mass rather than body weight.

such as ascites, sepsis, and gastrointestinal bleeding. In the absence of other parameters that can identify patients with an increased protein requirement, it has been suggested that patients who have an increased protein requirement can be identified by the measurement of urinary nitrogen excretion at an intake of 1 g/kg/day. Patients in a positive balance on this intake can be considered not to have an increased requirement. The other patients who were not in positive nitrogen balance on this amount of dietary protein require larger amounts of protein to achieve nitrogen balance. Therefore, dietary or hormonal manipulation aimed at reducing protein degradation may be more successful in these patients.

NUTRITIONAL REQUIREMENTS

Nitrogen

Based on studies using isotopic tracer methodology and perioperative balance studies, protein requirements did not appear to be increased in stable cirrhosis. Dietary intakes of 0.8 to 1 g/kg/day have been shown to achieve positive nitrogen balance in both compensated and decompensated patients. It should be emphasized that in stress situations like alcoholic hepatitis or decompensated liver disease, these requirements may increase to 1.5 to 2 g/kg/day. However, these methodologies are limited to a brief period of obser-

Table 21–15   Nutritional Requirements in Cirrhosis

	Liver Disease		Energy Substrate	
	Protein (g/kg/day)	Energy (kcal/kg/day)	% CHO	% Fat
Cirrhosis (uncomplicated)	1–1.5	30–40	67–80%	20–33%
Cirrhosis (complicated)				
a. Malnutrition	1–1.8	40–50	72%	28%
b. Cholestasis	1–1.5	30–40	73–80%	20–27%
c. Encephalopathy				
Grade 1 or 2	0.4–1.2	25–40	75%	25%
Grade 3 or 4	0.4	20–35	75–86%	14–25%
Liver transplant				
a. Peri-transplant	1.2–1.75	30–50	70–80%	20–30%
b. Post-transplant	1.0	30–35	>70%	≤30%

vation that may not reflect the entire metabolic status of an individual. As such, these methodologies may reflect a failure of metabolic adaptation rather than true nutritional requirements. Consistent with this possibility are the results from recent long-term refeeding studies in cirrhosis, which concluded that protein requirements are actually higher in these patients than was previously suggested. Consolidation of these various observations have been made and are provided in Table 21–15 as nutritional guidelines for cirrhotic patients. Apart from any specific numeric recommendation for an amount of protein required in cirrhosis, perhaps the most important information for the clinician is provided by long-term studies (which used up to 1.8 g/kg/day of mixed protein) that demonstrate that patients with cirrhosis can tolerate large protein loads. Therefore, there is no need for routine protein restriction used as prophylaxis to prevent the development of hepatic encephalopathy.

In addition to the observation that routine protein restriction is not required in these patients, two important factors pertinent to protein metabolism are germane to the treatment of these patients. First, it is now generally accepted that a low-protein diet reduces renal plasma flow and the glomerular filtration intake rate. Recent information indicates that levels of protein intake influence renal function in cirrhosis. A moderately high-protein diet and intravenous amino acids increase plasma flow and the glomerular filtration rate in cirrhosis, whereas protein restriction may produce the converse effects. Second, the therapeutic use of β-blockers for the management of portal hypertension is gaining acceptance, and wider use of these agents in cirrhotic patients can be expected. However, it has been observed that β-adrenergic blockade accelerates protein oxidation, possibly by decreasing plasma catecholamines and increasing protein requirements as well as adversely affecting glucagon metabolism and hepatic metabolic activity.

Energy

As already discussed, absolute resting energy requirements in stable cirrhosis as well as in alcoholic hepatitis are similar to control groups. However, energy expenditure appears to be increased per unit of lean body mass. Therefore, with the information currently available, it seems logical to base energy requirements on urinary creatinine excretion or some

other marker of lean body mass. Consideration for maintenance or repletion therapy must be considered. For the present, 30 to 40 kcal/kg body weight seems appropriate for maintenance of most patients with stable cirrhosis, whereas malnourished patients or patients undergoing liver transplantation may require as much as 50 kcal. These increased caloric needs should be coordinated with frequent interval feedings and a nighttime snack.

The suggested proportions of carbohydrate and fat are also provided in Table 21–15 based on the assimilation of a large number of metabolic studies in cirrhosis. Although insulin resistance and carbohydrate intolerance are common in cirrhosis, carbohydrate is the preferred energy substrate in cirrhosis after a mixed meal. The metabolism of absorbed lipids seems to be normal in cirrhosis. Administration of lipid emulsion produced normal increments in plasma triglyceride, free fatty acids, and ketone bodies in cirrhosis. In addition, whole body lipid oxidation rate was normal, and lipid oxidation became saturated at a fat intake of approximately 1 g/kg/day with amounts above 1 g/kg/day utilized for lipid synthesis.

NUTRITIONAL THERAPY

The collective data discussed to date indicate that the recognition and treatment of malnutrition are important considerations in the management of patients with chronic liver disease. Guidelines have been developed for the overall nutritional management of patients with liver disease, and Table 21–16 provides a general approach to the daily feeding of patients with cirrhosis. However, only recently has nutritional therapy been demonstrated to have clinical value in terms of altering the morbidity and mortality of these patients. Table 21–17 shows several studies suggesting that nutritional intervention with both standard and branched-chain amino acid (BCAA) formulations can be beneficial when used in carefully selected patients. Severely malnourished hospitalized cirrhotic patients with decompensated alcoholic liver disease and patients following liver transplantation benefit from short-term nutritional therapy as specified in Table 21–17. With longer nutritional therapy (6 to 12 months), patients with chronic encephalopathy and low BCAAs to aromatic amino (AA) acid ratios and symptomatic cirrhotic outpatients show more substantial improvement. In addition to these general guidelines for stable

Table 21–16 General Guidelines for a Daily Diet in Patients with Cirrhosis*

- Protein = 1.0 − 1.5 g/kg body weight
- Total calories = 1.2–1.4 × REE with a minimum of 30 kcal/kg body weight
  50–55% as carbohydrate (preferably as complex carbohydrates)
  30–35% as fat; preferably high in unsaturated fat and with adequate essential fatty acids
  15% of total calories given as a nighttime snack
- Nutrition should be given enterally by voluntary oral intake or by small-bore feeding tube; PPN is the second choice; TPN is the last choice.
- Salt and water intake should be adjusted for the patient's fluid volume and electrolyte status.
- Liberal multivitamins and minerals
- Specialized BCAA enriched supplements not usually necessary
  Most patients tolerate standard AA supplements.
  Reserve BCAA formulations for patients who cannot tolerate the necessary amount of standard AA (which maintain nitrogen balance) without precipitating encephalopathy.
  Avoid supplements providing only BCAA; they do not maintain nitrogen balance.

*Modified from Normpleggi DJ, Bonkovsky HL: Nutritional supplementation in chronic liver disease: An analytical review. Hepatology 19:518–533, 1994.
AA, amino acids; BCAA, branched-chain amino acid; PPN, peripheral parenteral nutrition; REE, resting energy expenditure; TPN, total parenteral nutrition.

and decompensated cirrhotic patients, several specific types of patients should be addressed.

Alcoholic Hepatitis

The goal of nutritional therapy in alcoholic hepatitis is to supply optimal nutritional replacement to correct preexisting PCM while providing sufficient amino acids to encourage hepatic regeneration and normalization without precipitating encephalopathy. It is important for the clinician to recognize and understand the significance of the degree of malnutrition in these patients. There have been eight published controlled trials on the use of standard intravenous amino acids as primary therapy for alcoholic hepatitis (Table 21–18). The results are conflicting, but six of the eight studies showed improvement in histology or liver function. Two of the studies concluded that supplemental amino acids were not beneficial; however, one of these studies treated patients with cirrhosis as opposed to alcoholic hepatitis, and the other study failed to achieve nutritional supplementation in the treatment group. These combined data indicate that protein feeding is well tolerated, and there is no reason to routinely restrict protein in patients with alcoholic hepatitis. Furthermore, the benefit of achieving positive nitrogen balance as well as improving liver function emphasizes the fact that nutritional support is helpful. Other manipulations have also been attempted to improve nutritional status in these patients. In a VA Cooperative Study, 30 days of oxandrolone was compared with prednisolone or placebo in patients with moderate or severe alcoholic hepatitis. Although short-term survival did not differ among the groups, when dietary intake was analyzed retrospectively, oxandrolone had a beneficial affect on long-term survival, but only in moderately malnourished patients who ingested significant calories. However, because of its potential hepatotoxicity and nonuniform efficacy in these patients, the use of oxandrolone cannot be recommended until more data are available.

Perioperative State

Several studies indicate that parenteral nutrition with standard amino acid formulations are well tolerated and equally effective as branched-chain–enriched formulations when used as perioperative nutritional therapy in cirrhotic patients. However, only one study shows any clinical or financial benefits of perioperative nutrition in cirrhotic patients

Table 21–17 Nutritional Therapy in Liver Disease

Author (Year)	Patient Profile	Therapy	Benefit
Short-Term			
Cabre (1990)	Severely malnourished cirrhotics	Enteral feeding (2115 kcal)	Child's score mortality ($P = .065$)
Reilly (1990)	Hypoalbuminemic after liver transplant	Total parenteral nutrition (1.5 g/kg amino acids and 35 kcal/kg/day)	Nitrogen balance Length in intensive care unit Hospital cost
Kearns (1992)	Decompensated alcoholic liver disease	Enteral feeding (1.5 g protein/kg)	Encephalopathy, bilirubin Antipyrine clearance
Long-Term			
Marchesini (1990)	Chronic encephalopathy	BCAA vs. casein supplements (0.24 g/kg)	Encephalopathy Nitrogen balance Bilirubin
Yoshida (1989)	BCAA/AAA < 1.0	BCAA supplements (16 g)	Delayed death (2–4 yr)
Hirsch (1993)	Symptomatic alcoholic cirrhotics	Enteral supplement (1000 kcal)	Less frequent hospitalizations for infections

BCAA, branched-chain amino acid; AAA, aromatic amino acid.

Table 21–18 Studies Investigating Standard Amino Acid Supplements in Alcoholic Hepatitis

Positive Results	No. of Patients	Comments
Nasrallah (1980)	35	Improved mortality and LFTs
Diehl (1980)	15	Improved hepatic steatosis
Achord (1987)	28	Improved histology and LFTs
Simon (1988)	34	Improved LFTs in severe disease
Mezey (1991)	54	Improved biochemical, metabolic, and nutritional parameters
Bonkovsky (1991)	39	Improved Child-Pugh score when combined with oxandrolone
Negative Results		
Calvey (1985)	64	Nutritional supplementation not achieved
Naveau (1866)	40	60% had inactive cirrhosis

LFT, liver function test.

when compared with no nutritional therapy. In this study, the perioperative nutrition decreased postoperative septic complications, weight loss, and the need for diuretics while improving hepatic function in patients undergoing major resection for hepatocellular carcinoma.

Liver Transplantation

Malnutrition is reported to be an independent risk factor for both adults and children undergoing liver transplantation. In addition to the usual postoperative nutritional concerns, protein catabolism is greatly increased during the first 2 weeks after liver transplantation; protein requirements increase up to 1.8 g/kg/day. Despite this informa-

tion, there have only been two randomized studies that have demonstrated the benefits of nutritional therapy in the transplant patient. During the first 7 postoperative days in adult patients, isotonic glucose (500 kcal/day) was compared with total parenteral nutrition (TPN) containing 35 kcal/kg/day nonprotein calories with 1.5 g/kg/day of either a standard or BCAA–enriched solution. Both TPN groups had significantly better nitrogen balance with beneficial trends for shorter length of stay in the intensive care unit and lower hospital costs. Another study in pediatric patients awaiting liver transplantation showed that a formulation enriched with BCAAs was more effective than standard amino acids. Based on this information, liver transplant patients should receive at least 1.5 g/kg protein per day and 40 kcal/kg perioperatively. BCAAs may be more effective in the pediatric patient, but this awaits further study.

Hepatic Encephalopathy

Nutritional therapy in conjunction with other management of hepatic encephalopathy have been extensively reviewed by Marchesini and associates. The readers are referred to this source for further reading. However, the most controversial area in the field of nutrition for hepatic encephalopathy involves the use of BCAAs. As a nutritional therapy, BCAAs are attractive because they stimulate protein synthesis, decrease protein degradation, may be used as an energy source in peripheral tissues, and are ketogenic, thus supplying another source of energy. Based on these nutritional attributes as well as potential therapy for hepatic encephalopathy, BCAAs have been used in both acute and chronic encephalopathy.

Acute Hepatic Encephalopathy

Table 21–19 summarizes the seven randomized controlled trials of intravenous BCAA therapies in acute hepatic encephalopathy, but only one study compared BCAA with standard amino acids. In summary, although the evidence indicates that intravenous BCAAs may play some role in

Table 21–19 Randomized Controlled Trials of Intravenous Branched-Chain Amino Acid Therapy

Author	Type of Treatment	Duration of Treatment	Total IV AA kg/day	BCAA (kg/day)	Observation Period
Rossi-Fanelli (1982)	C	2 Days	0	0	4 Days
	T		57	57	
Wahren (1983)	C	5 Days	0	0	5 Days
	T		40	40	
Michel (1985)	C	5 Days	78	15	5 Days
	T		78	28	
Cerra (1985)	C	3 Days	0	0	10 Days
	T		77	28	
Fiaccadori (1985)	C	7 Days	0	0	7 Days
	T		53	22	
Strauss (1986)	C	5 Days	0	0	5 Days
	T		60	≤21	
Vilstrup (1990)	C	6 Days	0	0	16 Days
	T		70	29	

C, control; T, treatment; IV, intravenous.

Table 21–20 Controlled Trials on Oral BCAA Treatment

Author	Period of Study	BCAA (g/day)	Alternative Treamtent	Outcome	Results
Eriksson (1982)	2 weeks	30	CHO	Encephalopathy	ND
Sieg (1983)	3 months	15	CHO	Latent encephalopathy	ND
Sinko (1983)	3 months	7–21	?	Encephalopathy	ND
McGhee (1983)	11 days	15	Casein	Encephalopathy	ND
				Nitrogen balance	ND
Horst (1984)	3 weeks	20–60	Proteins	Encephalopathy	Favorable to BCAA
				Nitrogen balance	ND
Guarnieri (1984)	3–4 months	0.45/kg	CHO/lipid	Encephalopathy	ND
				Nitrogen balance	Favorable to BCAA
Christie (1985)	3 days	30	Casein	Encephalopathy	ND
				Antropometry	ND
				Nitrogen balance	ND
Egberts (1985)	1 week	0.25/kg	Casein	Latent encephalopathy	ND
				Nitrogen balance	Favorable to BCAA
Fiaccadori (1988)	4 weeks	25	Casein	Encephalopathy	ND
				Nitrogen balance	ND
Swart (1989)	5 days	12–28	Proteins	Latent encephalopathy	ND
				Nitrogen balance	ND
Marchesini (1991)	3 months	0.24/kg	Casein	Encephalopathy	Favorable to BCAA
				Nitrogen balance	Favorable to BCAA

ND, no difference among treatment groups; BCAA, branched-chain amino acid.

accelerating arousal from coma, there is no significant benefit on survival or nutritional parameters

Chronic Encephalopathy

Table 21–20 summarizes 11 controlled trials that have been used in a meta-analysis of the use of oral BCAAs in chronic hepatic encephalopathy. This meta-analysis was unable to support any benefit of oral BCAAs in this state. There are methodologic problems in many of the studies published, but there is no evidence that encephalopathy is improved. However, two of the larger studies do show some improvement, and future clinical trials are needed to investigate potential of nutritional benefits of these specialized formulations when used for long periods.

Nonetheless, there is clear evidence that specialized formulations enriched in BCAAs are better tolerated than standard amino acids in a small subset of patients with cirrhosis. These patients cannot ingest an adequate amount of protein with standard amino acids without precipitating encephalopathy. Therefore, it seems appropriate to use branched-chain–enriched formulations only in patients who cannot tolerate adequate nitrogen intake in the form of dietary proteins without precipitating encephalopathy. If the amounts of protein (stated in Table 21–15) cannot be provided without precipitating hepatic encephalopathy, formulations with BCAAs should be substituted for standard formulations. There are two oral enteral feedings (Nutrihep, which is 50% BCAA enriched, and Hepatic Aid II, which is 46% BCAA enriched) and two intravenous formulations (Hepatamine and Hepatasol—both of which are 36% BCAA enriched). The cost of these specialized formulations is approximately 14 times that of standard amino acids or casein, and therefore their use must be judiciously employed.

SUMMARY

Although more investigation is needed to study the effect of nutritional intervention in liver disease, clinicians need to recognize that malnutrition is virtually ubiquitous in all types of cirrhosis. It has prognostic significance, and its treatment has been shown to provide beneficial clinical outcomes. Therefore, it is important to identify malnutrition and treat it with increased amounts of conventional feedings while maintaining specialized formulations in only those patients who cannot tolerate standard dietary needs without precipitating encephalopathy (Table 21–21).

Table 21–21 Nutritional Therapy in Liver Disease: General Guidelines

1. Nutritional regimens (see Tables 21-15 and 21-16)
   Trace metals/vitamins that influence nutrition
2. Treat complications that influence nutrition
   Sepsis (hypoglycemia)
   Ascites (↑ energy needs)
3. No need for routine protein restriction
   As prophylaxis against hepatic encephalopathy
   Patient selection for branched-chain amino acids
      Protein intolerance (HE)
      BCAA/AA <1.0
      Pediatric transplant patients
      Oral better than IV (?)
4. Enteral preferred over intravenous feeding
   Varices not a contraindication for feeding tubes
5. Long-term treatment most important
   Nighttime snack (frequent feedings)

SUGGESTED READINGS

Cabrè E, Gassull MA: Nutritional support in liver disease. Eur J Gastroenterol Hepatol 7:528–532, 1995.

Campillo B, Bories PN, Leluan M, et al: Short-term changes in energy metabolism after 1 month of a regular oral diet in severely malnourished cirrhotic patients. Metabolism 44:765–770, 1995.

Chang WK, Chao YC, Tang HS, et al: Effects of extra carbohydrate supplementation in the late evening on energy expenditure and substrate oxidation in patients with liver cirrhosis. J Parenter Enteral Nutr 21:96–99, 1997.

Fan ST, Lo CM, Lai ECS, et al: Peri-operative nutritional support in patients undergoing hepatectomy for hepatocellular carcinoma. N Engl J Med 331:1547–1552, 1994.

Heymsfield SB, Waki M, Reinus J: Are patients with chronic liver disease hypermetabolic? Hepatology 11:502–505, 1990.

Kondrup J, Nielsen K, Juul A: Effect of long-term refeeding on protein metabolism in patients with cirrhosis of the liver. Br J Nutr 77:197–212, 1997.

Kondrup J, Müller MJ: Energy and protein requirements of patients with chronic liver disease. J Hepatol 27:239–249, 1997.

Kondrup J, Nielsen K: Protein requirement and utilization in patients with cirrhosis of the liver. Z Gastroenterol (Suppl 5) 34:26–31, 1996.

Kruszynska Y, Williams N, Perry M, Home R: The relationship between insulin sensitivity and skeletal muscle enzyme activities in hepatic cirrhosis. Hepatology 8:1615–1619, 1988.

Lamont LS, Patel DG, Kalhan SC: β-Adrenergic blockade alters whole body leucine metabolism in humans. J Appl Physiol 67:221–225, 1989.

Levine JA, Morgan MY: Weighed dietary intakes in patients with chronic liver disease. Nutrition 12:430–435, 1996.

Marchesini G, Fabbri A, Bianchi G, Bugianesi E: Branched-chain amino acids in liver disease. In Cynober LA (ed): Amino Acid Metabolism and Therapy in Health and Nutritional Disease. Boca Raton: CRC Press, 1995, pp 337–347.

McCullough AJ, Mullen KD, Smanik EJ, et al: Nutritional therapy and liver disease. Gastroenterol Clin North Am 18:619–643, 1989.

McCullough AJ, Glamour T: Differences in amino acid kinetics in cirrhosis. Gastroenterology 104:1858–1865, 1993.

McCullough AJ, Tavill AS: Disordered energy and protein metabolism in liver disease. Semin Liver Dis 11:265–277, 1991.

McCullough AJ, Bugianesi E: Protein-calorie malnutrition and the etiology of cirrhosis. Am J Gastroenterol 92:734–738, 1997.

Mendenhall CL, Moritz TE, Roselle GA, et al: The study of oral nutritional support with oxandrolone in malnourished patients with alcoholic hepatitis results of a Department of Veterans Affair Cooperative Study. Hepatology 17:564–573, 1993.

Mullen KD, Weber FL: Role of nutrition in hepatic encephalopathy. Semin Liver Dis 11:292–304, 1991.

Muller MJ: Malnutrition in cirrhosis. J Hepatol 23 (Suppl):31–35, 1995.

Müller MJ, Lautz HU, Plogmann B, et al: Energy expenditure and substrate oxidation in patients with cirrhosis: The impact of cause, clinical staging and nutritional state. Hepatology 15:782–794, 1992.

Müller MJ, Rieger A, Willmann O, et al: Metabolic responses to lipid infusions in patients with liver cirrhosis. Clin Nutr 11:193–206, 1992.

Normpleggi DJ, Bonkovsky HL: Nutritional supplementation in chronic liver disease: An analytical review. Hepatology 19:518–533, 1994.

Petrides AS, Groop LC, Riely CA, DeFronzo RA: Effect of physiologic hyperinsulinemia on glucose and lipid metabolism in cirrhosis. J Clin Invest 88:561–570, 1991.

Petrides AS, DeFronzo RA: Glucose metabolism in cirrhosis: A review with some perspectives for the future. Diabetes Metab Rev 5:691–709, 1989.

Plauth M, Merli M, Kondrup J, et al: ESPEN Guidelines for Nutrition in Liver Disease and Transplantation. Clin Nutr 16:43–55, 1997.

Tavill AS, McCullough AJ (eds): Nutrition and the liver. Semin Liver Dis 11:265–348, 1991.

Teran JC, Mullen KD, McCullough AJ: Glutamine—a conditionally essential amino acid in cirrhosis. Am J Clin Nutr 62:897–900, 1995.

Verboeket–Van DeVenne WPHG, Westerterp KR, et al: Habitual pattern of food intake in patients with liver cirrhosis. Clin Nutr 12:293–297, 1993.

22

Fulminant Hepatic Failure

Andres T. Blei

Fulminant hepatic failure (FHF) is a rare clinical entity. In the United States (US), it has been estimated that 2000 cases/yr present with this syndrome. Nonetheless, the dramatic onset of illness, the rapidity at which clinical progression may occur, and its high mortality make FHF a true medical emergency.

The nomenclature of this syndrome has been controversial. Two critical issues in its definition are the appearance of changes in mental state and the time span during which symptoms evolve. In 1970, the term fulminant hepatic failure was coined to describe the onset of encephalopathy within 8 weeks of the first evidence of illness, without indication of any pre-existing liver disease. In the mid-80s, French investigators divided FHF into fulminant (encephalopathy within 2 weeks) and subfulminant (encephalopathy between 2 and 12 weeks). More recently, a further division into hyperacute (encephalopathy within a week), acute (1 to 4 weeks), and subacute (5 to 26 weeks) has been proposed. The rationale for subdividing the disease is based on different clinical characteristics (e.g., a greater prevalence of cerebral edema with a short interval between onset and encephalopathy) as well as on different prognoses. A longer interval between jaundice and encephalopathy is associated with a poor spontaneous survival rate.

ETIOLOGY

Geographic differences will result in variations of the etiology of the syndrome. Table 22–1 lists a series from the US. However, this may not be the experience in different areas of the world, underlining the existence of regional variations. In one specialized referral center in Great Britain, almost 75% of 342 cases were related to acetaminophen toxicity, in most cases of a suicidal nature. The American data

reflect the experience of 12 centers, which are also geographically dispersed. In India, hepatitis E plays an important pathogenic role in cases of non-A, non-B hepatitis. In Japan, hepatitis B is a relatively more frequent cause of FHF. Several entities deserve comment.

Viral hepatitis is a major etiologic category (Table 22–2), although the incidence of FHF within the broader group of patients with viral hepatitis is very low (0.35% of hepatitis A and up to 1% of hepatitis B). Hepatitis A is a rare cause of FHF and carries a better prognosis; in the West, the shift toward the acquisition of this infection at a later age may result in a more virulent course. Hepatitis B is the most common cause of FHF worldwide, especially in the Far East. Special virologic factors may predispose to FHF in hepatitis B. These factors include a role for mutant strains, for coinfection or superinfection with the delta (hepatitis D) virus, and for spontaneous or chemotherapy-related reactivation of hepatitis B virus. In the case of hepatitis C, most studies indicate that this virus does not result in a fulminant course. But the role of hepatitis C may be more complex: Two reports, from France and Japan, noted coinfection with hepatitis C in up to one half of patients with fulminant hepatitis B. With regard to hepatitis E, the virus has a propensity in India for a fulminant course in pregnant women; it plays a minor role in the West, mainly related to travelers to endemic areas.

In all series of FHF, a sizable number of cases (10% to 45% in the West) are defined as non-A, non-B, non-C, non-D, non-E (non-A–E) hepatitis and in whom no etiology can be discerned. It is still unclear whether this entity represents the effects of an undiscovered infectious agent; the epidemiology of this entity has not been fully defined. Parvovirus B19 has been proposed as the cause of some pediatric cases of non-A–E FHF associated with aplastic ane-

Table 22–1 Etiology and Prognosis in Patients with Fulminant Hepatic Failure

	No.	OLT	Spontaneous Survival
Acetaminophen	60	7	34
Drugs	34	17	7
Hepatitis B	30	19	4
Indeterminate	43	26	11
Hepatitis A	20	7	8
Wilson's disease	18	17	0
Autoimmune hepatitis	17	5	4
Miscellaneous	73	24	6
TOTAL	295	122 (41%)	74 (25%)

This table depicts a recent experience with orthotopic liver transplantation (OLT) from 12 centers in the United States. The miscellaneous group includes a wide variety of etiologies (see text). From Schiodt FV, Atillasoy E, Shakil AO, et al: Etiology and outcome for 295 patients with acute liver failure in the United States. Liver Transpl Surg 5:29–34, 1999.

mia. Togavirus-like particles have been reported in some patients with non-A–E FHF. Using polymerase chain reaction in blood or tissues, some of these non-A–E cases have been shown to exhibit hepatitis B. It is likely that this problematic group may consist of more than one pathogenic agent.

In the immunosuppressed population, fulminant hepatitis has been associated with herpes simplex and Coxsackie B infections. Other causes of viral hepatitis, such as Epstein-Barr and cytomegalovirus, seldom develop a fulminant presentation.

The ingestion of acetaminophen for suicidal intentions is increasing throughout the Western world. However, hepatotoxicity does not arise only from suicidal attempts. Drug doses that are not considered toxic (<4 g/day in adults, <80 mg/kg in infants) have been associated with severe liver injury. An accelerated production of toxic metabolites of acetaminophen may occur in alcoholics, in whom cytochrome P-450 activity is chronically induced (related to the production of the toxic intermediates). In the case of infants, short periods of fasting may result in depletion of glutathione, an intracellular scavenger of the toxic metabolite, which may then account for the drug's hepatotoxicity. The early administration of N-acetylcysteine, a sulfhydryl donor that replenishes glutathione, can prevent the development of hepatic injury. In the US, an intravenous preparation of N-acetylcysteine is not yet available and requires oral administration, which is frequently associated with gastric intolerance.

Idiosyncratic drug reactions may result in acute liver failure. A prominent example is isoniazid, which is used increasingly with the re-emergence of tuberculosis worldwide. Coadministration of rifampin has been noted as an additional risk factor, because the latter may induce the formation of toxic metabolites from isoniazid. Halothane injury is less frequently seen after the substitution of this halogenated anesthetic with similar but less toxic compounds. Ketoconazole, diphenylhydantoin and sodium valproate can also induce severe hepatotoxicity. In fact, the rate of introduction of new pharmaceutical agents is such that a full evaluation of their potential hepatotoxicity only arises after more widespread clinical use. For drugs that cause an idiosyncratic injury, it is not surprising that a "pre-marketing" evaluation fails to detect their potential for liver toxicity.

An acute presentation of chronic liver disease does not fit the definition of FHF but shares many clinical features. Reactivation of hepatitis B may occur as the initial clinical presentation of infection with this virus. In patients with Wilson's disease, the liver is usually cirrhotic, and liver cell necrosis is associated with massive copper release; this, in turn, results in hemolysis and variable degrees of renal failure. The diagnosis can be difficult to make because low ceruloplasmin levels are seen in all forms of FHF due to massive hepatic necrosis; an elevated serum copper may be a laboratory clue. Autoimmune hepatitis has also been reported to present with a fulminant picture.

A group of rare etiologies is important to list because specific therapies may be administered. Acute fatty liver of pregnancy, commonly seen in the third trimester, responds to fetal delivery. Massive infiltration of the liver by lymphoma requires urgent chemotherapy. Intoxication with *Amanita phalloides* (Fig. 22–1) is seen in mushroom gatherers and is associated with prominent muscarinic effects, such as sweating and diarrhea; it may respond to specific measures, including penicillin and cholestyramine. Ische-

Table 22–2 Acute Viral Hepatitis and Fulminant Hepatic Failure in the USA

Type	Case Fatality (%)	No. of Estimated Icteric Cases	No. of Deaths
Hepatitis A	0.2–0.4	75,000	120–304
Hepatitis B	1.0–1.2	100,000	950–1220
NANB	1.5–2.5	37,500	570–950
TOTAL		212,500	1640–2474

Data compiled by the Viral Hepatitis Surveillance Program (operated by the Center for Disease Control) and the Sentinel Counties Study. Data from Hoofnagle JH, Carithers RL Jr., Shapiro C, Ascher N: Fulminant hepatic failure: Summary of a workshop. Hepatology 21:240–252, 1995.

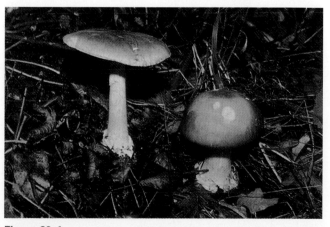

Figure 22–1
A classical view of the poisonous *Amanita phalloides*.

mia of the liver may be a manifestation of left ventricular dysfunction even without the presence of congestive heart failure. An acute Budd-Chiari syndrome, with hepatic venous outflow block, may be amenable to thrombolytic therapy. Intoxication with carbon tetrachloride or phosphorus requires prompt recognition of exposure.

PATHOLOGY OF ACUTE LIVER FAILURE

Different etiologies of acute liver failure result in different pathologic presentations of hepatic injury. Three main patterns can be discerned.

Centrilobular Necrosis: Zone 3 of the hepatic acinus is more susceptible to ischemic injury as the lobular gradient of oxygen decreases from the portal venule to the central vein. Hepatocytes in zone 3 possess cytochrome P-450 activity and are more prone to injury from toxic metabolites generated through this pathway, as is the case of acetaminophen and with organic solvent poisoning such as carbon tetrachloride. In acute venous outflow block, marked centrilobular congestion accompanies necrosis of centrilobular hepatocytes.

Bridging/Multilobular Necrosis: Necrotic "bridges" that link portal-to-portal or portal-to-central areas can coalesce and result in areas of multilobular necrosis. Varying degrees of necrosis are present in such cases, also called "submassive" hepatic necrosis. Inflammation of portal tracts can be prominent, and intralobular changes include swollen hepatocytes, giant cell transformation, features of pseudoacinar changes, and cholestasis. Acute yellow atrophy is an older term that describes a shrunken, massively necrotic liver. With "massive" necrosis, inflammation is sparse, and hemorrhage can be detected within the parenchyma together with varying degrees of bile ductular proliferation (Fig. 22–2).

Liver biopsy, performed using the jugular venous approach, can determine the extent of necrosis and has been used by some groups to determine prognosis. Although this

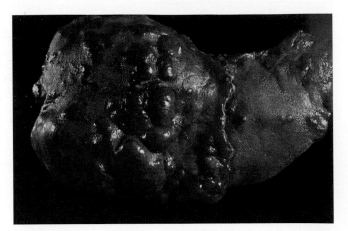

Figure 22–3
Macroscopic appearance of a liver from a patient with indeterminate etiology of fulminant hepatic failure. The apparent nodular areas in the right lobe represent islands of preserved parenchyma. The smooth appearance of the left lobe reflects massive collapse. (Courtesy of Sambasiva Rao, MD, Department of Pathology, Northwestern University.)

approach may be more useful when the extent of injury is diffuse, as is the case of acetaminophen toxicity, it may be less helpful in viral, drug, or idiopathic etiologies, where not all lobes experience the same degree of necrosis (Fig. 22–3).

Microvesicular Steatosis: Certain etiologies of FHF exhibit small droplets of fat in hepatocytes that otherwise do not displace the nucleus and are not associated with patterns of necrosis (Fig. 22–4). Examples include acute fatty liver of pregnancy, valproate-induced hepatotoxicity, FHF associated with intravenous tetracycline, and Reye's syndrome. Recent conditions include intoxication with *Bacillus ceruleus* and the nucleoside analogue, fialurudine, which was discontinued as a potential therapy for hepatitis B because of toxicity and death. Many of these agents and etiologies share as a common link the presence of mitochondrial injury

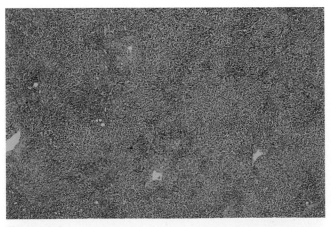

Figure 22–2
An example of liver histology in massive hepatic necrosis from acetaminophen toxicity. (Courtesy of Sambasiva Rao, MD, Department of Pathology, Northwestern University.)

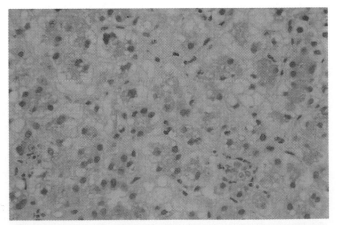

Figure 22–4
An example of liver histology in a patient with acute fatty liver of pregnancy. Note the presence of microvesicular steatosis. (Courtesy of Sambasiva Rao, MD, Department of Pathology, Northwestern University.)

with subsequent "energy failure." This has been well delineated in the case of fialuridine, which is directly toxic to mitochondrial DNA and results in decreased activity of the electron transport chain within this organelle.

MECHANISMS OF INJURY

Numerous mechanisms may account for the development of FHF, as illustrated in the following etiologies.

Both host and viral factors may account for the rarity of FHF in the context of all cases of viral hepatitis. However, it is unlikely that such massive injury arises from direct cytotoxicity to liver cells. Infected hepatocytes are injured by cytotoxic T lymphocytes, which are directed against viral antigens with subsequent cell necrosis; recent reports have noted that such lymphocytes can also induce apoptosis (the disappearance of single hepatocytes as a result of DNA fragmentation by endonucleases) in the case of viral hepatitis B and C. Release of cytokines (especially tumor necrosis factor [TNF]-α and nitric oxide) may mediate the inflammatory response, whereas some of these cytokines can be generated within the liver itself, as is the case of TNF-α synthesized in Kupffer cells as a result of endotoxin activation. Whatever the pathway, the excessive nature of this reaction may account for the massive hepatic destruction seen in FHF. In the case of hepatitis B mutants that lack expression of core antigen, it has been proposed that the lack of tolerance to this viral component may explain the reports of FHF with such mutants. Direct cytotoxicity to hepatocytes may arise from herpesviruses, but such a course for this infection is still more likely in the immunosuppressed population.

Drug hepatotoxicity can also be direct or can involve an immunoallergic mechanism. In the case of direct toxicity, it is the formation of intermediate toxic metabolites that cause injury. These metabolites are produced during detoxification steps, generally cytochrome P-450 mediated, that are characterized as either phase I (the introduction of polar groups) or phase II (conjugation with glucuronic acid, sulfate, or glutathione). When the ability to neutralize these metabolites is lost (the case of glutathione depletion in the face of acetaminophen intoxication), cell injury may arise. These intermediate compounds are reactive metabolites that will result in protein covalent binding or cause lipid peroxidation, with injury to different cellular elements or metabolic pathways. In the case of immunoallergic drug injury, the drug's metabolite binds to cellular proteins and forms a hapten, which will act as a neoantigen. Halothane hepatotoxicity is a good example of this process, where circulating antibodies can be detected to the new modified proteins and whose binding to hepatocytes initiates injury to the liver. This sequence explains the usual clinical scenario for this rare lesion, with previous febrile reactions upon first exposure and a short time elapsed between the second exposure to this anesthetic agent and hepatotoxicity.

Ischemia may injure the liver via a decrease in oxygen supply and is well documented in the setting of liver transplantation via changes associated with reperfusion. Numerous cellular events are disrupted with hypoxia, but impairment of the mitochondrial respiratory chain function is critical for injury to occur. Reperfusion injury may be related to the generation of reactive oxygen species with subsequent cellular damage via lipid peroxidation or complement-mediated cell lysis. Damage to the organ's endothelium may also promote adherence of neutrophils with subsequent obstruction to sinusoidal flow.

Endotoxinemia may be a common additional factor that amplifies the initial mechanism of injury. Kupffer cell uptake results in the generation of TNF-α and nitric oxide. Hepatic circulatory disturbances as well as increased adhesiveness of leukocytes and platelets may all contribute to the original injury.

CLINICAL FEATURES

Physical Signs

A typical patient with FHF is a previously healthy individual who presents with nonspecific symptoms of malaise and nausea and then develops jaundice and changes in mental state over a variable period. Some etiologies of FHF are not associated with prominent jaundice, such as acetaminophen toxicity (where the injury is mainly centered in zone 3 of the acinus) and herpetic hepatitis (where the course is extremely rapid). Hence, the diagnosis of FHF may not be obvious clinically and requires laboratory evidence of liver failure. Physical findings consistent with chronic liver disease are generally absent, such as the presence of hepatomegaly, spider angioma, or ascites. Some of the etiologies in the spectrum of FHF are exceptions to this rule, such as hepatomegaly caused by massive infiltration by lymphoma or stigmata of cirrhosis in patients with fulminant Wilson's disease. For most patients, the liver is not palpable and may actually decrease in size as changes occur over several days. Splenomegaly is not a feature of FHF. Changes in mental state may not be present in subjects with a more protracted (subacute) course, and it is important to differentiate this latter entity from an icteric presentation of chronic liver disease, because ascites and renal failure may also develop in the subacute setting.

Laboratory Abnormalities

Laboratory testing is critical for diagnosis as well as for providing clues of etiology. A very prolonged prothrombin time can be the first suggestion of the diagnosis. In the standard liver chemistry panel, serum aminotransferases (aspartate aminotransferase [AST], alanine aminotransferase [ALT]) are very elevated (generally >1000 IU/mL); extreme levels (20,000 to 30,000 IU/mL) suggest acetaminophen toxicity. Aminotransferases may decrease as the liver parenchyma is destroyed; a very prompt decrease (within 1 to 2 days) suggests hepatic ischemia. Alternatively, a mild to moderate elevation in aminotransferases (5- to 10-fold) and marked jaundice in the clinical setting of FHF can provide a clinical clue for fulminant Wilson's disease. Bilirubin values are also elevated in FHF, although a few etiologies (see the previous paragraph) can present with values less than 10 mg/dL; fractionation is seldom helpful. Alkaline phosphatase is either normal or modestly increased; in fulminant Wilson's disease, it can be characteristically subnormal (see Chapter 12). A marked rise in lactate dehydrogenase can be a clue to hepatic infiltration by lymphoma.

Laboratory testing for viral etiologies needs to consider several unique aspects. Liver destruction can be so massive that hepatitis B surface antigen (HBsAg) may not be detected, and exclusion of hepatitis B requires determination of IgM-anti-HBc. If hepatitis C must be ruled out, the time lag before development of an antibody response requires assays that measure circulating HCV RNA. If hepatitis E is suspected, few laboratories can accurately measure the appropriate antibody (in the US, the Centers for Disease Control and Prevention [CDC] [800-545-6783] will assay). Anti-HAV-IgM and delta antibody are more straightforward in their interpretation.

Multiorgan Failure

Multiple organ systems are affected in FHF, and a sequence of events that leads to multiorgan failure may account for this marked clinical diversity. However, there are unique features to the syndrome, such as the development of cerebral edema, that distinguishes FHF from the multiorgan failure of other conditions such as sepsis. We will review several organ systems that are affected and provide an integrated view as a summary.

Liver Failure

Two major complications that arise from the rapid onset of liver failure are hypoglycemia and coagulation disturbances; they occur as a consequence of the liver's synthetic failure. Hypoglycemia can be extreme (<30 mg/dL of plasma glucose) and result in marked symptomatology (e.g., tachycardia and sweating) as well as add to the disturbance of consciousness. It requires constant provision of intravenous glucose, starting at 10% concentrations.

The *coagulopathy of FHF* is complex, because the liver is the site of synthesis of most coagulation and fibrinolysis factors. Clinically, a bleeding diathesis is manifested by an increased propensity to gastrointestinal hemorrhage and complications from invasive procedures.

The impairment of the γ-carboxylation of coagulation factors II, VII, IX, and X is a vitamin K–dependent posttranslational deficit that results in a prolongation of the prothrombin time in chronic liver disease. In FHF, massive necrosis results in complete synthetic failure. An international normalized ratio (INR) standardizes the activity of thromboplastins used in the prothrombin time assay. Other nonvitamin K–dependent factors are also synthesized in the liver; factor V has a half-life of 12 to 16 hours, and its activity has been used as a prognostic parameter in FHF.

Other coagulation factors may be increased, such as factor VIII and von Willebrand factor, a likely manifestation of endothelial cell activation in the liver. The synthesis of inhibitors of coagulation (e.g., antithrombin III, protein C, and protein S) is decreased. Very low fibrinogen levels may reflect increased peripheral destruction in addition to decreased synthesis; abnormal fibrinogen molecules, rich in sialic acid, have also been described in FHF. Components of the fibrinolytic system are synthesized in the liver, and reduced levels of plasminogen and α_2-antiplasmin have been reported in FHF.

Thrombocytopenia is common in FHF, and the platelet count is lower in nonsurvivors than in survivors (mean of 58,000 versus 97,000 platelets/mL). This reduction may be partly related to decreased production of hepatic factors necessary for platelet synthesis; studies of the activity of the newly described thrombopoietin have not yet been reported in this disease. Increased platelet adhesiveness may reflect the activity of an increased von Willebrand factor; it poses difficulties with extracorporeal support systems, where the tubing may be a stimulus for further platelet adhesion. On the other hand, platelet aggregation is decreased, with a resultant marked prolongation of the bleeding time.

Systemic Hemodynamics and Its Consequences

Patients with FHF exhibit a hyperdynamic circulatory state, manifested by a decreased systemic vascular resistance, a high cardiac output, and a lower mean arterial pressure. The cause of this circulatory phenomenon is unclear. Endothelial factors may result in an increased synthesis of nitric oxide, which is a powerful vasodilator, and increased levels of circulating cyclic GMP, nitrates and nitrites have supported this concept. The stimulus for nitric oxide formation via the activation of endothelial nitric oxide synthase may be proinflammatory cytokines and especially TNF-α, whose levels are increased in FHF.

Several clinical consequences arise from this circulatory disturbance. It is associated with arteriovenous shunting of blood within the microcirculation, thus decreasing oxygen delivery to tissues. This oxygen debt contributes to the presence of lactic acidosis in FHF and may underlie the manifestations of multiorgan failure that are present in the fully developed syndrome. Acidosis is a poor prognostic sign in acetaminophen toxicity, and lactate levels higher than 4 ng/mL are associated with decreased survival.

The abnormal arterial vasodilatation underlies the pathogenesis of renal failure in FHF, a functional abnormality caused by excessive renal arterial vasoconstriction. Homeostatic mechanisms, including the sympathetic nervous system, endothelins, and the renin-angiotensin-aldosterone system, are activated to restore the lowered arterial pressure; these renal vasoconstrictive stimuli are unopposed by a decreased production of renal vasodilators, such as prostaglandins of the E family. As a result, more than half of patients with FHF develop renal failure, with avid sodium renal retention manifested by a low U_{Na} (<10 mEq) and $U_{osm}>P_{osm}$. This can progress to overt acute tubular necrosis. Acetaminophen toxicity includes direct effects of metabolites on kidney structure, including distal tubular damage that increases urinary phosphate loss. Hypophosphatemia in FHF can be severe, resulting in muscle weakness and respiratory depression.

Infections

In large series of patients, bacteriologically proved infections occurred in up to 80% of individuals with FHF and were suspected in another 10%. Bacterial or fungal infections can occur as early as 2 to 5 days after the onset of the disease. Several mechanisms account for the high frequency of infections in patients with FHF. These include defects in intracellular killing by polymorphonuclear leukocytes, the decreased function of the hepatic reticuloendothelial system, and the hypocomplementemia that arises from its decreased hepatic synthesis. The latter may be especially important in reducing the capacity to opsonize bacteria and yeasts. Experimental models of FHF have shown the presence of intestinal bacterial translocation, and this may be an important route for acquisition of gram-negative infections. Endotoxinemia is common in FHF, and the release of pro-inflammatory cytokines, such as TNF-α and interleukin (IL)-6, may add to the picture of multiorgan failure, similar in some respects to that seen in septic conditions.

The clinical diagnosis of infection can be difficult to establish. Fever and leukocytosis are absent in up to 30% of patients; hemodynamic instability can be a clue to its presence and can be confused with the hyperdynamic state previously discussed. Pneumonia is the most common type, with urinary tract infections, bacteremias, and intravenous catheter–related infections comprising the rest. The latter category emphasizes the need for rigorous care of intravenous lines and urinary catheters in the intensive care unit. Predominant organisms are *Staphylococcus aureus,* *Escherichia coli,* and coagulase-negative staphylococcal species. Fungal infections pose special problems in diagnosis; in one prospective series, these infections were found in 30% of cases. It is suspected when the clinical picture or laboratory tests deteriorate after a period of improvement, and tends to be present in the second week of the course of FHF. Leukocytosis can be severe (>20,000 WBC/mm^3), and renal failure may develop. When detected, *Candida albicans* is the most common species and is isolated from either the bloodstream or the lung.

Hepatic Encephalopathy

The presence of an abnormal mental state defines the syndrome of FHF. The cause of hepatic encephalopathy is the subject of a long-standing controversy. It is most likely a multifactorial event in which hyperammonemia is a major factor in the development of an abnormal mental state. The entry of ammonia into the brain may be facilitated by changes in the permeability of the blood-brain barrier and, once in the brain tissue, results in a cascade of neurochemical events that end in neurotransmitter failure. Among them, alterations in glutamatergic neurotransmission have been described in animal models of FHF, and an increased extracellular glutamate level is a robust finding in several species. The latter observation may explain the recent reports of subclinical seizures that have been reported in patients with FHF and deep encephalopathy. Ammonia may also result in abnormalities of GABAergic, serotoninergic, and dopaminergic neurotransmission. Other proposed neurotoxins include "endogenous" benzodiazepines, whose levels have been found to be increased in the plasma and brain of patients with FHF, subjects in whom exogenous benzodiazepines were not administered. Once in brain tissue, these substances may bind to the GABA$_A$ receptor in the brain and result in neuroinhibition. The concomitant presence of hypoxemia, hypokalemia, and hypoglycemia may all contribute to the varied neurologic symptomatology.

Early symptoms can include excitation and mania, which can be erroneously treated with sedatives in the outpatient setting. Patients can progress quickly from stage I (confusion) and II (obtundation) to stage III (stupor) and IV coma (unresponsiveness), and traditional signs of hepatic encephalopathy, such as asterixis and fetor hepaticus, may be absent. Decerebrate posturing and myoclonic seizures may be present in more advanced stages. A sudden respiratory arrest may occur in stages III and IV encephalopathy. Infection should be ruled out as a precipitating cause of encephalopathy, but in most patients no other reason for the abnormal mental state can be found beyond the presence of liver failure.

Brain Edema

This unique complication of FHF is observed in patients in stages III and IV coma. Neuropathologically, the brain at autopsy is heavy and may show temporal lobe or uncal herniation, unequivocal evidence of brain edema as a cause of death. Pathologic examination after perfusion fixation of the brain of animal models and in human brain biopsies at the time of death indicates the presence of astrocyte swelling and intact tight intracellular junctions of the capillary endothelial cells. Alzheimer's type II astrocytes are seen in human brains examined after immersion fixation.

The mechanisms that lead to brain swelling are still being explored (Fig. 22–5). It is unlikely that a breakdown of the blood-brain barrier, as seen in other causes of vasogenic

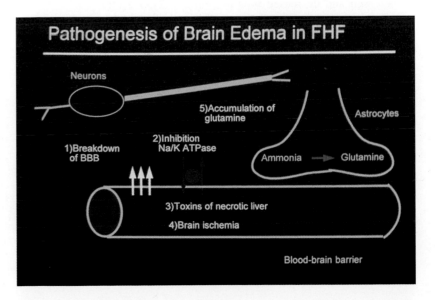

Figure 22–5
Several possible mechanisms may account for brain edema in fulminant hepatic failure.

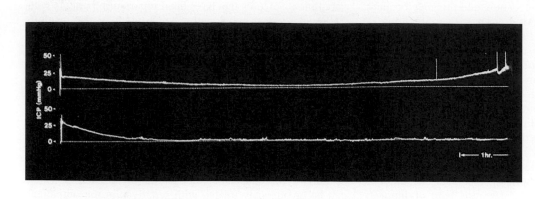

Figure 22–6
In an animal model of fulminant hepatic failure *(top)*, intracranial pressure rises in the last 2 hours of the clinical course, culminating in the development of intracranial pressure waves. The initial reduction in pressure reflects a stabilization step. The *bottom panel* reflects tracings in a normal animal. (From Webster S, Gottstein J, Levy R, Blei AT: Intracranial pressure waves and intracranial hypertension in rats with ischemic acute hepatic failure. Hepatology 14:715–720, 1991.)

edema, is present. Corticosteroids are ineffective in the therapy of this condition; protein levels in the cerebrospinal fluid are normal; and computed tomography (CT) scans of the brain seldom show patchy involvement with edema; in fact, the results of most CT scans are negative. A cellular (or cytotoxic) etiology may be present and the accumulation of glutamine (the product of ammonia detoxification) in astrocytes has been proposed to act as an intracellular osmole that attracts water into brain tissue. Cerebral hyperemia, absolute or relative, has been proposed as the initial factor that facilitates entry of water into the brain. Loss of cerebral vascular autoregulation has been described in these patients, and this abnormality places patients at risk of a reduction of cerebral perfusion when a decrease of arterial pressure is present, resulting in brain ischemia.

Most of the clinical signs of brain edema arise from the elevation of intracranial pressure, with displacement of brain structures accounting for the presence of pupillary abnormalities, alteration of caloric reflexes, and decerebrate or decorticate posturing (Fig. 22–6). However, elevations of intracranial pressure of up to 60 mm Hg can remain clinically silent, and the clinical detection of elevated intracranial pressure is difficult. Conflicting evidence exists as to the nature of cerebral perfusion in this setting, with reports of increased and decreased flow as well as "relative" hyperemia (higher flows for the cerebral metabolic requirements, an entity also called "luxury" perfusion). It is clear, however, that persistent elevations of intracranial pressure that result in a prolonged reduction of cerebral perfusion pressure [(mean arterial pressure) − (intracranial pressure)] to less than 40 mm Hg will result in a high likelihood of development of cerebral ischemia and secondary neurologic damage.

Other Disturbances

Respiratory alterations are common. Patients may require intubation at the time of deep encephalopathy, but hypoxemia is common as pulmonary arteriolar vasodilatation (part of the hyperdynamic state) may result in functional arteriovenous shunting in the lung. Pulmonary edema may occur as a result of "leaky" capillaries, with normal left heart pressures; intracranial hypertension may also contribute to this phenomenon. Adult respiratory distress syndrome may even be present after a successful liver transplant.

Gastrointestinal hemorrhage is the result of superficial gastric erosions. Portal hypertension is present in many patients as a result of the increased portal vascular resistance that results from the collapse of the liver parenchyma (Fig. 22–7). However, complications from portal hypertension are seldom detected. Another unique gastrointestinal complication is the development of acute pancreatitis, whose etiology is unclear. Acute pancreatitis may be detected in up to 5% of cases. When present, it may contraindicate the performance of a liver transplantation.

Protein catabolism is increased and, in cases of subacute liver failure with a more protracted course, protein-calorie malnutrition may develop. Parenteral alimentation is especially difficult in view of the potential for fluid overload.

PROGNOSIS

Few centers have developed a large experience in the management of this devastating illness, and FHF has been traditionally associated with up to a 90% mortality. The concentration of patients in specialized units, the improvements in

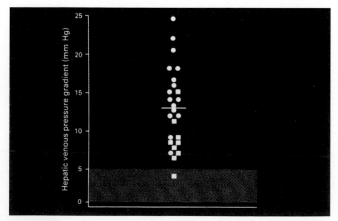

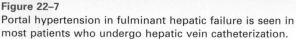

Figure 22–7
Portal hypertension in fulminant hepatic failure is seen in most patients who undergo hepatic vein catheterization.

Figure 22–8
Prognostic factors in fulminant hepatic failure.
Survival is related to etiology of the syndrome as
well as to the development of complications.
(Adapted from O'Grady JG, Alexander GJM,
Hayllar KM, Williams R: Early indicators of
prognosis in fulminant hepatic failure.
Gastroenterology 97:439–445, 1989.)

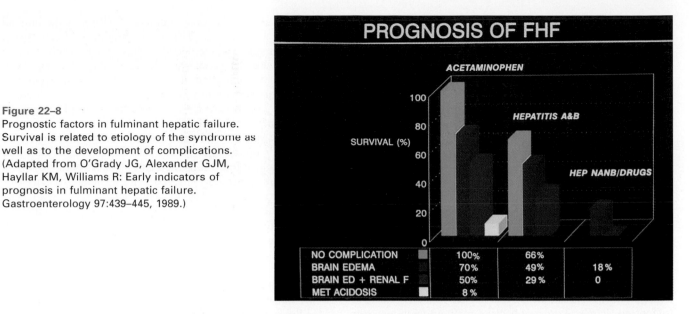

critical care, together with earlier recognition and management of the multiple complications of FHF, has led to an improved survival. Still, a considerable number of patients succumb to this disease, with spontaneous survival varying between 20% and 50%, with better prognosis for patients with FHF related to acetaminophen intoxication or hepatitis A. Prediction of survival has acquired a new urgency in the era of liver transplantation, when the decision to proceed with the transplant needs to take into account the rapidity with which deterioration can occur as well as the current shortage of organ donors.

Prognostic criteria based on clinical parameters on admission to the hospital have been proposed by the Liver Unit at Kings' College Hospital in London, based on a multivariate analysis of 588 subjects (Fig. 22–8). Patients are divided according to etiology, acetaminophen versus nonacetaminophen, whereas encephalopathy is not a criterion for prognosis (Table 22–3). These criteria have been examined at other centers and have acceptable positive predictive value (~80%) in predicting death. In Clichy, France, the combination of factor V deficiency (<20% in patients younger than 30 years of age; <30% in patients older than 30 years of age) and any grade of encephalopathy was associated with a poor prognosis, independent of the etiology of FHF.

The role of liver biopsy in determining the number of viable hepatocytes, as already discussed, is controversial. Other proposed tools to determine prognosis include the liver volume measured with CT scanning, the amount of fresh frozen plasma used to correct the coagulopathy, and the determination of somatosensory evoked potentials. Their prognostic use awaits confirmation. Circulating levels of group-specific component (Gc) protein are decreased in FHF and as an actin scavenger (released from dead hepatocytes) has been postulated to provide prognostic information; low levels would allow circulating actin to polymerize in the peripheral microcirculation.

A particularly vexing problem is the patient with a subacute (or subfulminant) course, in whom no neurologic symptoms may have developed but in whom evidence of liver failure does not improve over time. These patients have a poor prognosis, and they can succumb quickly to a devastating infection.

MANAGEMENT AND THERAPY

Prompt recognition of the presence of FHF is critical. During the early stages, when the patient is not overtly jaundiced, the clinical picture can be confused with gastrointestinal disturbances, flu-like symptomatology, or a psychiatric picture if excitation or mania are present. In an emergency room, a prolonged prothrombin time may be the critical laboratory clue, particularly on weekends when liver chemistry panels may not be available. Early referral to specialized centers is recommended, especially in subjects in

Table 22–3   Indicators of Poor Prognosis in Fulminant Hepatic Failure

Patients with Acetaminophen Toxicity
- pH <7.30 (regardless of grade of encephalopathy and after correction of volume status)

        or

- Prothrombin time >100 sec and serum creatinine >300 μmol/L in patients with grade III or IV encephalopathy

Patients with Non-Acetaminophen Toxicity
- Prothrombin time >100 sec (regardless of grade of encephalopathy) or three of the following:
  - Age <10 or >40 years
  - Etiology: Non-A-non-B hepatitis, drug reactions
  - Interval jaundice-encephalopathy >7 days
  - Prothrombin time >50 sec
  - Serum bilirubin >300 μmol/L (>17mg/dL)

From O'Grady JG, Alexander GJ, Hayllar KM, Williams R: Early indicators of prognosis in fulminant hepatic failure. Gastroenterology 97:439–445, 1989.

whom emergency liver transplantation is a therapeutic option. Comatose patients pose special challenges for transfer. Long ambulance rides may increase the risk of worsening the patient's neurologic condition. For air transport, acceleration and deceleration forces during takeoff and landing may prove deleterious to a swollen brain; such patients may be best transferred via a helicopter. There are four aspects to consider in the management of these patients.

Recognition of the Cause of FHF

There is an urgent need to recognize the etiology in view of the availability of specific disease-related measures. A history obtained from the patient or his or her relatives and a careful physical examination may provide important clues, because specific laboratory testing may not become available for 24 to 48 hours. These include the complete set of blood counts and liver-related chemistries, testing for hepatitis viruses, immunologic markers (antinuclear antibody, antismooth muscle antibody), and copper-related studies. A toxicology screen is ordered because methamphetamine use ("Ecstasy") by adolescents has been associated with FHF. Antidotes for poisoning with acetaminophen or mushrooms are available, although they are most efficacious when administered before overt hepatic injury is present. Ultrasound imaging may provide critical information on the possible existence of chronic liver disease and the patency of the hepatic veins.

Management of the Complications of FHF

Survival of patients is in many cases related to the quality of care provided in the intensive care setting. Patients require the insertion of a urinary catheter, intravenous catheters, cardiac monitoring and in most cases, an arterial line. Constant surveillance of clinical status, meticulous care to avoid hospital-acquired infections, and prompt recognition of changes in mental state are critical.

Metabolic Disturbances: Intravenous glucose therapy is routine, and 10% dextrose is required in many cases, because hepatic gluconeogenesis is absent. Blood glucose controls are needed every 2 hours, and hypoglycemia should be excluded when alterations of mental state occur. Hypophosphatemia may be made worse by glucose infusion and requires parenteral correction. The presence of renal failure may give rise to difficulties in the management of potassium and magnesium, which should be monitored. Hyponatremia is common in these individuals and should be corrected cautiously, especially in patients who will undergo emergency transplantation, in order to avoid additional neurologic complications. Metabolic acidosis may reflect disturbances in the peripheral microcirculation and is difficult to treat; in the case of renal failure, correction may be possible with dialytic procedures.

Coagulopathy: The prothrombin time and factor V levels are prognostic parameters on the patient's admission to the hospital. The evolution of these parameters may be especially useful to show improvement of the laboratory picture. Thus, administration of fresh frozen plasma (2 to 4 units every 4 to 6 hours) may be necessary when bleeding occurs, but the ability to use coagulation tests to assess the clinical evolution is then lost. The administration of fresh frozen plasma in cases where bleeding has not occurred is more controversial. Its prophylactic effectiveness has not been proved, and its administration can be problematic in cases of renal failure, where they can contribute to fluid overload. In this setting, some groups advocate the use of plasmapheresis, a maneuver that also permits the performance of invasive tests, such as the placement of intracranial pressure monitors. Low platelet counts may predispose to bleeding from the gastrointestinal tract, and platelet counts less than 30,000 are commonly treated with platelet transfusions. Prophylaxis of gastrointestinal hemorrhage with H_2-receptor antagonists is instituted; a proton pump inhibitor may be preferable to avoid effects on mental state seen with the former drugs, but an intravenous formulation is not yet available.

Hemodynamic and Renal Problems: The peripheral vasodilatation that these patients exhibit poses difficulties for fluid therapy; monitoring of central pressures facilitates patient management. When hyperdynamic features are present, with a high cardiac output and a low peripheral resistance, sepsis needs to be ruled out. The latter can be superimposed on the hyperdynamic circulatory state and arterial hypotension may supervene. The use of pressor agents, however, may adversely affect oxygen delivery and tissue microcirculation. Availability of drugs to enhance oxygen exchange in the periphery is desirable; N-acetylcysteine has been reported to produce such an effect via the formation of nitrosothiols, resulting in microvascular vasodilatation. This has led to the use of N-acetylcysteine not merely as an antidote to acetaminophen but also as a general support measure for patients with FHF. This experience needs to be confirmed in other centers. It should be remembered that an elevation of arterial pressure and bradycardia may indicate the presence of intracranial hypertension.

Management of functional renal failure requires adequate fluid management and exclusion of sepsis, a common aggravating factor. Low doses of dopamine (2 to 4 μg/kg/hr) are commonly instituted but its efficacy is questionable. When renal failure is progressive or when acute tubular necrosis is present, dialytic methods are needed. Hemodialysis may be problematic in patients with encephalopathy, because rapid fluid shifts may aggravate osmotic disequilibria between plasma and the brain. Slower methods, such as continuous venovenous hemofiltration, are preferable.

Infections: The predominance of gram-positive bacteria, especially *S. aureus,* points at the skin as the source of entry of organisms. As mentioned, maximal efforts should be made to avoid contamination of intravenous line sites. Microbial surveillance is done regularly in many centers on a daily basis, because clinical markers of infection are often not helpful. The administration of a prophylactic selective parenteral and enteral regimen (colistin, tobramycin, amphotericin B, cephalosporin for 5 days, vaginal clotrimazole) was not superior to the administration of antibiotics when infection was suspected or proved. More limited antibiotic prophylaxis with a third-generation cephalosporin and flucloxacillin reduces the incidence of infection with *S.*

aureus but favors the appearance of resistant organisms. The role of prophylactic antibiotics is still questionable (Fig. 22–9), but in our center, therapy is started against *S. aureus, E. coli,* and fungal species (fluconazole, amphotericin B) when the patient is listed for liver transplantation. Fungemia can be a devastating infectious complication and may preclude the performance of the transplant procedure. Aminoglycosides are avoided because of the susceptibility to renal damage in the setting of liver disease.

Hepatic Encephalopathy and Brain Edema: For patients with an abnormal mental state, protein is restricted to 40 g/day; branched-chain amino acid solutions have no proven value in this setting. Infection, gastrointestinal hemorrhage and renal failure can contribute to the development of hepatic encephalopathy. Hypoglycemia, hypoxemia, and electrolyte alterations may also affect the patient's mental state. Drugs with potential neuroactive effects are avoided. A particular problem in management is the young patient who develops an excitatory state, where injury to self can occur. Sedation in this setting is unavoidable, generally with intravenous benzodiazepines; propofol is a short-acting alternative. Most patients receive treatment of encephalopathy with lactulose, administered via a nasogastric tube; its efficacy in this setting has not been tested in clinical trials. Neomycin, a poorly absorbable antibiotic active against urease-containing bacteria, should be avoided because of its potential renal toxicity. Flumazenil, 1 mg intravenously, may be useful if ingestion of benzodiazepines is suspected; its role in the management of the encephalopathy of FHF is still under investigation.

Management of brain edema is difficult, because the clinical signs of intracranial hypertension may be absent. CT may be useful to exclude other neurologic conditions, such as intracerebral hemorrhage, but is seldom helpful for the diagnosis of brain swelling. Furthermore, transportation of the patient to a radiology suite is complicated and the lack of rigorous nursing supervision may pose unacceptable risks. As brain herniation may suddenly develop, with concomitant respiratory arrest, patients in grade III and IV encephalopathy should undergo endotracheal intubation prophylactically. Monitoring of intracranial pressure is reserved for patients awaiting liver transplantation, because placement of such a device is not associated with prolongation of survival; it may also be very important for intraoperative management. There is concern that intracranial pressure monitors may result in additional morbidity and mortality. In a survey of the experience with such monitors in the US, piercing of the dura mater with subdural bolts, intraventricular catheters, or thin monitors placed on the brain surface was associated with fatal intracranial hemorrhage. Epidural transducers are less precise but provide a better margin of safety and are preferred by most centers.

The elevation of intracranial pressure can be progressive and culminates in the development of intracranial pressure waves, which are the basis for brain displacement and herniation (Fig. 22–10). The patient's head is kept at a 20-degree angle to reduce venous pressure. Mannitol, 0.5 g/kg, is administered intravenously as a bolus over 30 minutes. In patients with renal failure, repeated boluses will require dialysis to avoid hyperosmolarity. Hyperventilation as a measure to reduce intracranial pressure is seldom effective. Barbiturate coma may be used as a last resort, but the decrease in arterial pressure associated with this therapy may pose additional problems. The decision to proceed with a liver transplant when the cerebral perfusion pressure is less than 40 mm Hg for more than 2 hours is a difficult one, because patients in this setting may exhibit some elements of irreversible neurologic damage.

Support of the Failing Liver

Corticosteroids have been shown to be ineffective in FHF. Measures to favor hepatic regeneration, such as prostaglandin E and insulin/glucagon infusions, have not been shown to be beneficial in clinical trials. Methods that replace some aspects of the hepatic clearance function will remove toxins

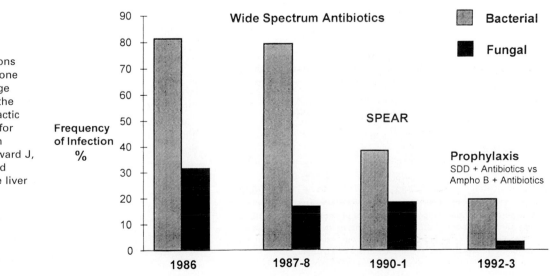

Figure 22–9
The incidence of infections decreased over time in one institution (King's College Hospital, London) with the introduction of prophylactic measures. See the text for additional details. (From Rolando N, Philpott-Howard J, Williams R: Bacterial and fungal infection in acute liver failure. Semin Liver Dis 16:389–402, 1996.)

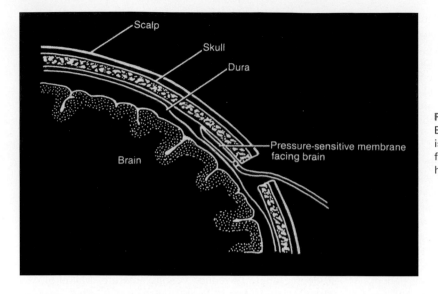

Figure 22–10
Epidural monitor to measure intracranial pressure is the favored approach in fulminant hepatic failure in order to decrease the risk of hemorrhage.

from the blood, via dialytic methods or via plasmapheresis but do not trigger hepatic regeneration.

The search for an "artificial liver" has spanned close to 4 decades of research. Dialysis and plasmapheresis may play a limited role. The proposed benefits of charcoal hemoperfusion have not been substantiated in clinical trials. Although an improvement in mental state was observed in the 1960s with the use of extracorporeal perfusion of pig livers, no effect on ultimate survival was seen. The possibility of using such an approach as a "bridge" to liver transplant has renewed interest in this therapeutic modality. This has included bioartificial devices, where the patient's blood is perfused through a dialysis-type cartridge that contains porcine or modified human hepatocytes (Table 22–4). The ultimate role of these technologic developments, which are expensive and complex, awaits testing in controlled clinical trials.

Emergency Liver Transplantation

Knowledge of the patient's prognosis upon admission to the hospital facilitates the initial decision to place the patient on a liver transplant list. Infection with the human immunodeficiency virus is excluded, and noninvasive tests of cardiac

function are obtained. The urgency in obtaining an organ donation results in the acceptance of marginal livers, and in desperate circumstances ABO incompatible livers have been used. Overall survival of patients with FHF after transplantation is lower than with other conditions, averaging 60% to 65% at 1 year; this percentage also reflects the difficulties that arise in the management of the patient during the postoperative period.

The current criteria used to proceed with emergency transplantation are not infallible; it would appear that a small percentage of currently transplanted patients could have spontaneously survived. In the absence of a perfect predictive tool, this error may be unavoidable, because the alternative, the patient's death while awaiting the reversibility of the condition, is unacceptable. Uncontrolled infection, pancreatitis, and intractable intracranial hypertension with brain ischemia are contraindications to the transplant procedure.

Orthotopic liver transplantation has been the usual surgical procedure. Auxiliary liver transplantation, in which a portion of normal liver is placed in either a heterotopic or orthotopic position, has been evaluated with the hope of providing transient support while the injured liver undergoes full regeneration. At that time, immunosuppression is discontinued and the patients would be able to avoid the need for lifelong medication. Unfortunately, this sequence does not occur in all patients, but preliminary studies suggest that patients with hyperacute failure (short interval between the onset of jaundice and encephalopathy) may be the most likely to benefit from this approach. Living donor liver transplantation for FHF has been done in Japan, where organ donation confronts different societal rules on the definition of death than in the West.

Issues of cost and accessibility make liver transplantation a nonuniversal mode of therapy for FHF. The development of this devastating illness could be thwarted in many cases with efforts directed toward universal vaccination for hepatitis B, the avoidance of the combination of acetaminophen and alcohol, and elucidation of the pathogenesis of non-A–E hepatitis.

Table 22–4 Bioartificial Liver for Fulminant Hepatic Failure

	No.	Pre-BAL	Post-BAL	P Value
Glasgow	9	7.2 ± 0.8	7.3 ± 0.7	NS
ICP (mm Hg)	9	19.1 ± 2.2	9.0 ± 1.2	0.005
CLOCS	10	25.2 ± 2.6	29.8 ± 2.1	0.01
Lactate	9	4.5 ± 0.5	4.1 ± 0.4	NS
NH_3	9	152 ± 15	119 ± 10	0.05

BAL, bioartificial liver–Glasgow Coma Scale (0 [worst] to 15 [best]); ICP, intracranial pressure; CLOCS, comprehensive level of consciousness score; NH_3, ammonia. From Blei AT: Pathogenesis of brain edema in fulminant hepatic failure. Progr Liver Dis 13:331, 1995.

SUGGESTED READINGS

Acharya SK, Dasarathy S, Kumer TL, et al: Fulminant hepatitis in a tropical population: Clinical course, cause, and early predictors of outcome. Hepatology 23:1448–1455, 1996.

Berk PD, Popper H: Fulminant hepatic failure. Am J Gastroenterol 69:349–400, 1978.

Bernuau J, Goudeau A, Poynard T, et al: Multivariate analysis of prognostic factors in fulminant hepatitis B. Hepatology 6:648–651, 1986.

Bernuau J, Rueff B, Benhamou JP: Fulminant and subfulminant liver failure: Definitions and causes. Semin Liver Dis 6:97–106, 1986.

Bhaduri BR, Mieli-Vergani G. Fulminant hepatic failure: Pediatric aspects. Semin Liver Dis 16:349–55, 1996.

Bismuth H, Samuel D, Castaing D, et al: Liver transplantation in Europe in patients with acute liver failure. Semin Liver Dis 16:415–25, 1996.

Blei AT, Olafsson S, Webster S, Levy R: Complications of intracranial pressure monitoring in fulminant hepatic failure. Lancet 341:157–158, 1993.

Ellis A, Wendon J: Circulatory, respiratory, cerebral, and renal derangements in acute liver failure: pathophysiology and management. Semin Liver Dis 16:379–388, 1996.

Gazzard BG, Portmann B, Iain M, et al: Causes of death in fulminant hepatic failure and relationship to quantitative histological assessment of parenchymal damage. Q J Med 94:615–626, 1975.

Harrison PM, Wendon JA, Gimson AES, et al: Improvement by acetylcysteine of hemodynamics and oxygen transport in fulminant hepatic failure. N Engl J Med 324:1852–1857, 1991.

Hoofnagle JH, Carithers RL Jr, Shapiro C, Ascher N: Fulminant hepatic failure: Summary of a workshop. Hepatology 21:240–252, 1995.

Hughes RD, Williams R. Use of bioartificial and artificial liver support devices. Semin Liver Dis 16:435–444, 1996.

Lee WM: Management of acute liver failure. Semin Liver Dis 16:369–378, 1996.

Losser MR, Payen D: Mechanisms of liver damage. Semin Liver Dis 16:357–367, 1996.

McCashland TM, Shaw BW Jr, Tape E: The American experience with transplantation for acute liver failure. Semin Liver Dis 16:427–433, 1996.

Muñoz SJ: Difficult management problems in fulminant hepatic failure. Semin Liver Dis 13:395–413, 1993.

Navasa M, Gatcia-Pagan JC, Bosch J, et al: Portal hypertension in acute liver failure. Gut 33:965–968, 1992.

O'Grady JG, Schalm S, Williams R: Acute liver failure: Redefining the syndromes. Lancet 342:273–275, 1993.

O'Grady JG, Alexander GJM, Hayllar KM, Williams R: Early indicators of prognosis in fulminant hepatic failure. Gastroenterology 97:439–445, 1989.

Pereira SP, Langley PG, Williams R: The management of abnormalities of hemostasis in acute liver failure. Semin Liver Dis 16:403–414, 1996.

Rolando N, Gimson A, Wack J, et al: Prospective controlled trial of selective and enteral antimicrobial regimen in fulminant liver failure. Hepatology 17:196–201, 1993.

Rolando N, Philpott-Howard J, Williams R: Bacterial and fungal infection in acute liver failure. Semin Liver Dis 16:389–402, 1996.

Wendon JA, Harrison PM, Keays R, Williams R: Cerebral blood flow and metabolism in fulminant hepatic failure. Hepatology 19:1407–1413, 1994.

Williams R: Classification, etiology, and considerations of outcome in acute liver failure. Semin Liver Dis 16:343–348, 1996.

23

Drug Hepatotoxicity

Stephan Krähenbühl
Jürg Reichen

SIGNIFICANCE OF DRUG-INDUCED LIVER INJURY

Drug-induced liver disease represents an important clinical problem for several reasons. Because the liver is the major site of drug metabolism, reactive metabolites with the potential to damage hepatocytes or other liver cells are generated; this toxicity can occur by direct effects or by immunologic mechanisms. Between 500 and 1000 drugs have been listed that can cause abnormalities of liver function tests or liver injury. Drug-induced hepatic injury is a frequent cause of fulminant hepatic failure and has a particularly bad prognosis. Drug-induced liver injury accounts for approximately 0.1% to 0.2% of all hospital admissions and for 2% to 3% of the hospital admissions caused by adverse drug reactions. Finally, drug-induced liver disease can mimic virtually every other form of hepatobiliary disease and must therefore always be included in the differential diagnosis of liver disease of unknown etiology.

EPIDEMIOLOGY

Reliable data on the risk and frequency of drug-induced liver injury are rare. Most of the drug-induced liver injuries are idiosyncratic and have a low incidence. In order to be able to estimate the frequency for a rare event, a large population must be studied; thus, to detect a relative risk of 2 for a given event in a cohort study and assuming a level of significance of 0.05, a power of 0.9, and a background incidence in the control group of 0.001, a total of 63,000 patients would have to be studied in both the exposed group and the nonexposed group. A possible solution to this problem are record linkage studies, in which prescriptions for a particular drug are linked with hospital discharge diagnoses

or disease registries, with nonexposed patients serving as a control group. Using this technique, the relative risk for acute liver failure associated with the use of nonsteroidal anti-inflammatory drugs (NSAIDs) has been estimated to be 2.3 with an absolute risk of 9 cases per 100,000 person years.

Comprehensive hospital drug monitoring is a way to determine frequencies of adverse drug reactions in hospitalized patients. Using this type of epidemiologic study, 20 patients with drug-induced hepatitis were diagnosed among 66,995 patients monitored, indicating a frequency of 1:3350 in hospitalized patients. This figure is clearly higher than that observed for hepatotoxicity in general practice where a prevalence of 0.3 per 100,000 patients has been reported.

In several studies, the frequency of drug-induced liver disease was determined prospectively in patients admitted to the hospital. Halls and associates reported that 157 of 1999 consecutive admissions were drug related; among them three involved injury to the liver. Of 320 consecutive patients with hyperbilirubinemia, 2% were identified to be related to drugs. Similarly, Bjorneboe and associates identified 640 patients with jaundice among 23,600 consecutive admissions. Among these patients, 15 had a drug-related cause, amounting to 2.3% of the jaundiced patients. Thus, epidemiologic studies indicate that 1 of 600 to 3500 hospitalizations are caused by drug-induced liver injury, amounting to 2% to 3% of all admissions due to adverse drug reactions.

The collection of spontaneous reports of drug-induced liver injuries is not suitable for the estimation of their frequency. However, most of the available knowledge about the existence and possible mechanisms of drug-induced liver disease is derived from case reports in medical journals or reports to national drug surveillance centers or drug companies.

DIAGNOSIS AND CAUSALITY ASSESSMENT

Because almost all types of hepatobiliary disease can be mimicked by an adverse drug reaction and since there is no specific diagnostic test for drug-induced hepatic disease, the assessment of a causal relationship between the administration of a drug and liver injury is a very difficult task, demanding a considerable amount of expertise and experience. There are numerous methods to assess causality, most of them incorporate factors such as:

1. The chronology of the administration of the drug, in particular the intervals between the beginning or the end of treatment and the onset of the adverse reaction
2. The course of the reaction after stopping the drug or during continued treatment
3. The respective roles of drugs and diseases in this particular type of liver injury
4. The response to readministration of the drug
5. The results of laboratory tests
6. Knowledge that the drug can cause this particular type of liver disease

During several international consensus meetings in France, systems for causality assessment of drug-induced liver injuries were discussed. The system finally proposed comprises three chronologic criteria (time to onset of the reaction, course of the reaction after withdrawing or during continuation of the drug, and response to drug readministration) and clinical information about the patient. In the absence of other causes, a reaction appearing 5 to 90 days after the beginning of the treatment is suggestive of a drug reaction. After stopping the drug, an event is still compatible with a drug reaction when it occurs before 15 days for hepatocellular injuries or before 1 month for mixed or cholestatic reactions. The course is suggestive for a drug effect when the alanine aminotransferase (ALT) levels decrease to less than 50% within 8 days after stopping the drug or when alkaline phosphatase activity or bilirubin concentration decreases more than 50% within 6 months. Important clinical information about the patient includes the nature of the underlying disease, use of alcohol, and a detailed drug history. Non–drug-related causes of liver injury should be assessed and excluded as well as possible. Based on this information, the probability that liver injury may be caused by a drug can be estimated as illustrated in Table 23–1.

CLASSIFICATION

Clinical Picture

The diagnosis of drug-induced hepatic injury is usually made by circumstantial evidence, after exclusion of other causes. A positive rechallenge would, in most cases, provide the definitive answer regarding the etiology but should be performed extremely cautiously because of the potential severity of the drug reaction. Typically, drug hepatotoxicity begins 1 to 2 months after initiating a drug, but latency may also be longer. The clinical picture is highly variable, reflecting the whole spectrum of hepatobiliary disease. Most often drug-induced liver disease manifests itself as acute or chronic hepatitis or as a cholestatic syndrome with jaundice and pruritus. If the patient is rechallenged with the same

Table 23–1   Assessment of the Probability that Liver Injury is Caused by a Drug

Probability	Criteria
Very probable	Reintroduction of the drug causes the same reaction. Intentional reintroduction is ethically unacceptable in most cases because of the potential severity of the reactions.
Probable	Other principal causes were ruled out; the drug is known to cause this type of liver injury.
Possible	The appearance of the reaction is timely and compatible with the administration of the drug; other causes are not excluded with certainty.
Excluded	The time is incompatible (the drug is administered after the reaction or the reaction appears more than 2 weeks [hepatocellular injury] or more than 4 weeks [cholestatic injury] after stopping the drug). A non–drug-related cause has been proved with certainty.

drug, liver injury usually reappears after one or two doses in allergic drug reactions but after a longer period of time in metabolic toxicity. After stopping the drug, the symptoms improve rapidly (within days) in patients with hepatocellular injury but only slowly (weeks to months) in patients presenting with a cholestatic syndrome.

In order to be able to compare reports about drug-induced injuries, it is important to use a common language. Based on the report of the consensus conference in France, the terms liver injury and abnormality of liver tests should be preferred when no liver biopsy is available. Liver injury is defined by an increase in ALT or conjugated bilirubin higher than 2N (N = upper limit of normal) or a combined increase in aspartate aminotransferase (AST), alkaline phosphatase (ALP), and total bilirubin with one of these values higher than 2N. Liver injury is considered to be hepatocellular, when ALT alone is increased or when $R > 5$ (R = ALT/alkaline phosphatase, both expressed as a multiple of N). Liver injury is cholestatic when ALP alone is increased or $R < 2$, and mixed when $2 < R < 5$. Liver injury that lasts for longer than 3 months is called chronic. Liver injury is severe when the patient is jaundiced, has a prothrombin ratio of less than 50% or develops hepatic encephalopathy. Fulminant liver failure is defined as for non–drug-related causes by the appearance of severe acute liver disease with hepatic encephalopathy in a previously healthy person. If the determination of the liver tests or the clinical picture does not meet the criteria for liver injury but is abnormal, the term abnormality of liver tests should be used.

Mechanisms of Drug-Induced Liver Disease

Type A Versus Type B Reactions

Type A reactions occur in a predictable, dose-dependent fashion and are usually well known from clinical trials or from toxicity in experimental animals. Type A reactions develop, therefore, mainly because of inadequate usage of these agents and usually produce a specific histologic picture. Examples of agents from this type are carbon tetrachloride and acetaminophen (centrilobular lesions), yellow phosphorus (midzonal lesions), and allylalcohol (periportal lesions).

Type B reactions are unpredictable and typically occur at therapeutic doses. This type of toxicity has a low frequency and is, therefore, most often not known from clinical trials or from toxicity studies in animals. The histologic pattern is not uniform, and liver injury can be accompanied by systemic features such as fever, rash, eosinophilia, and sometimes by the appearance of autoantibodies in serum. Possible mechanisms for this type of adverse drug reaction includes drug allergy with the immune response directed against hepatocytes, cholangiocytes, or other structures in the liver and genetic abnormalities or environmental influences on metabolite production and detoxification.

Molecular Mechanisms of Hepatotoxicity

The mechanism of toxicity is well established only for a few hepatotoxins. As discussed earlier, most drug-induced liver diseases are rare, idiosyncratic reactions that are mediated by abnormal production or detoxification of toxic metabolites or an abnormal immune response that is mostly not characterized in detail (Fig. 23–1).

In the case of toxin-induced cell death, electrophilic metabolites deplete the cellular glutathione pool and bind covalently to macromolecules. An example of this mechanism is paracetamol (acetaminophen), whose hepatotoxic metabolite N-acetyl-p-benzoquinone imine (NAPQI) is normally detoxified by covalent binding to glutathione. When high doses of paracetamol are ingested, sulfation and glucuronidation—normally the predominant metabolic pathways—are saturated and the hepatic glutathione pool is rapidly exhausted. After depletion of the hepatic glutathione stores, NAPQI binds to hepatocellular proteins, including enzymes and transport proteins, impairs their function, and finally leads to cell death. The predominantly centrilobular localization of paracetamol-induced liver injury is caused by the perivenular localization of cytochrome P-450 (CYP) 2E1, the most important enzyme for the formation of NAPQI.

Oxidative processes are also considered to be important in the pathogenesis of paracetamol-induced hepatic cell damage. NAPQI is an oxidant, leading to the oxidation of thiol groups of hepatocellular proteins. The formation of free radical metabolites or reactive oxygen species may initiate the chain reaction of lipid peroxidation, which is an important phenomenon in several types of liver injuries, in-

DRUG

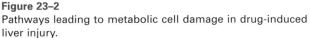

Figure 23–1
General mechanisms leading to drug-induced liver injury.

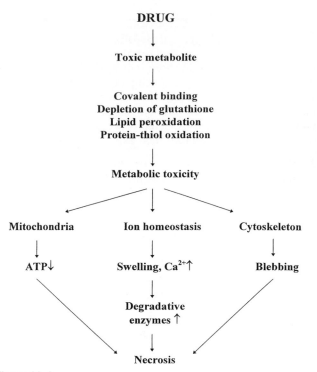

Figure 23–2
Pathways leading to metabolic cell damage in drug-induced liver injury.

cluding also carbon tetrachloride-induced (CCl_4) liver necrosis. Thus, glutathione depletion, covalent binding, protein-thiol oxidation, and lipid peroxidation are the chemical consequences of excess reactive metabolites, compromising specific cell functions (mitochondria, ion homeostasis, cytoskeleton) and eventually leading to cell death (Fig. 23–2).

Nonparenchymal cells such as Kupffer cells and neutrophils as well as endotoxin and cytokines can contribute to the extent of the cell damage initiated by biochemical events in hepatocytes (Fig. 23–3). For instance, blockage of Kupffer cell activation reduces the extent of liver injury by CCl_4 in experimental animals. Similarly, neutrophil depletion decreases the extent of liver damage from CCl_4 or paracetamol. Thus, toxic metabolites generated in hepatocytes lead to the release of radicals, aldehydes derived from lipid peroxidation, and interleukin (IL)-8. These factors can activate Kupffer cells, leading to the release of cytokines such as IL-1, tumor necrosis factor (TNF), and IL-8 as well as reactive oxygen intermediates. These factors can lead to further injury to hepatocytes and also to endothelial and stellate cells. IL-8 and endothelial damage promote neutrophil adherence and induce further damage by the release of proteases and reactive oxygen intermediates by the neutrophils. Thus, not only the initial formation of toxic metabolites determines the ultimate extent of liver disease, but also the interplay among hepatocytes, nonparenchymal cells, and neutrophils.

Immune mechanisms are involved in some cases of drug-induced liver disease. As illustrated in Figure 23–4 in immunologic liver injury, exposure to toxic metabolites strongly influences or may even be a prerequisite for the development of liver injury. Metabolites generated by CYP or

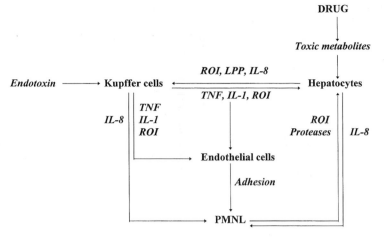

Figure 23–3

Interaction between hepatocytes, nonparenchymal liver cells, polymorphonuclear leukocytes, and cytokines in drug-induced liver injury. (LPP, lipid peroxidation products; ROI, reactive oxygen intermediates; PMNL, polymorphonuclear leukocytes.)

UDP-glucuronyltransferases may react with microsomal proteins, from where they can be transported to the plasma membrane by microtubular-dependent vesicular transport. The antigen may be the drug itself acting as a hapten, or the protein to which the drug or the metabolite is bound. The immune response can be directed either against the modified protein (reaction against the modified self: immunoallergic hepatitis) or against unmodified proteins (reaction against the self: autoimmune hepatitis). Hepatocytes are then destroyed by antibody or T lymphocyte-mediated mechanisms.

Histologic Picture According to Primary Target of Liver Injury

Histologically, drug-induced liver injuries can be classified in five major categories that span the whole spectrum of hepatobiliary diseases and include hepatitis, cholestasis, fibrosis, vascular injury, and hepatic neoplasm (Table 23–2).

Acute Hepatitis

Hepatocellular injury presents histologically with liver cell necrosis. Some hepatotoxins affect predominantly the cells of a specific region of the lobule, leading to zonal necrosis. Normally, there is no inflammatory response, and damaged hepatocytes in the periphery of the lesion may accumulate lipid. This kind of liver injury ends either fatally or with complete recovery, but chronic liver disease does not develop. The basis for the zonal preference of certain hepatotoxins is the production of toxic metabolites in this particular lobular location; for example, many CYP isoenzymes are located in the central zone of the liver lobules, explaining the centrilobular toxicity of paracetamol and carbon tetrachloride.

Hepatocellular injury can also present histologically as diffuse, spotty necrosis or as a viral hepatitis-like reaction with patterns of bridging, submassive or massive necrosis. Although diffuse spotty necrosis has a good prognosis, the fatality rate is high for viral hepatitis-like reactions. In the absence of repeated exposure, the development of chronic liver disease is unusual for both types of liver injury.

Granulomas consist typically of aggregates of epithelioid histiocytes, which may be accompanied by inflammatory cells, in particular eosinophils in the case of drug-induced granulomas. It is estimated that up to one third of hepatic granulomatous lesions are induced by drugs.

Chronic Hepatitis

The histologic picture of drug-induced chronic hepatitis is heterogeneous, presenting with an autoimmune-like or a chronic hepatitis-like picture with features of bridging necrosis, fibrosis, and cirrhosis. These forms of drug-induced liver injury occur mainly with prolonged use of agents that cause acute hepatitis, entering a self-perpetuated process

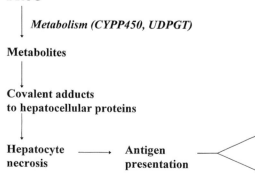

Figure 23–4

Immunopathogenesis of drug-induced liver injury.

Table 23–2 Pathologic Classification of Drug-Induced Liver Disease

Hepatocellular Injury

Acute hepatitis
  Zonal necrosis: CCl_4, paracetamol, yellow phosphorus
  Diffuse, spotty necrosis: aspirin and many others
  Viral hepatitis-like injury: diclofenac, halothane, isoniazid, sulfonamides
  Granuloma: allopurinol, carbamazepine, phenytoin, quinidine, etc.
Chronic Hepatitis
  Autoimmune like injury: α-methyldopa, dantrolene, diclofenac, nitrofurantoin
  Chronic viral hepatitis-like: amineptin, amiodarone, aspirin, etretinate, isoniazid
Microvesicular steatosis: aspirin, didanosine, fialuridine, tetracycline, valproate
Nonalcoholic steatohepatitis: amiodarone, calcium channel blockers, perhexiline
Phospholipidosis: amiodarone

Cholestasis

Acute cholestasis
  Bland cholestasis: estrogens, 17-alkylated steroids
  With inflammation: amoxicillin/clavulanate, erythromycin estolate, piroxicam
Chronic cholestasis
  Ductopenia and secondary biliary cirrhosis: ajmaline, carbamazepine, chlorpromazine, chlorpropamide, haloperidol, penicillins, thiobendazole, tricyclic antidepressants, tolbutamide
Macroscopic duct sclerosis: intra-arterial floxuridine

Fibrosis

Perisinusoidal: methotrexate, vitamin A

Vascular Alterations

Veno-occlusive disease: pyrrolizidine alkaloids, azathioprine, alkylating agents
Hepatic vein thrombosis: estrogens
Noncirrhotic portal hypertension: azathioprine, 6-thioguanidine
Peliosis hepatis: azathioprine, estrogens, anabolic steroids
Nodular regenerative hyperplasia: azathioprine, 6-thioguanidine

Neoplasms

Adenoma: estrogens
Hepatocellular carcinoma: estrogens, anabolic steroids, cyproterone
Angiosarcoma: vinyl chloride, thorotrast

with continued administration of this drug. Resolution can be prompt and complete after stopping the implicated drug (e.g., aspirin); delayed or liver injury may even progress after the drug (e.g., etretinate) is discontinued.

Microvesicular Steatosis

In this form of liver injury, fat is deposited in the form of small lipid droplets that are dispersed throughout the cyto-

plasm, leaving the nucleus in the center of the hepatocyte. Accumulation of fat in these cases is caused by inhibition of mitochondrial fatty acid oxidation by impairment of mitochondrial β-oxidation or of the respiratory chain. Clinically, these patients often present as a Reye-like syndrome that may progress to acute liver failure and carries a bad prognosis.

Nonalcoholic Steatohepatitis

Triglycerides are stored in the form of large droplets, which displace the nucleus to the periphery of the cell and give hepatocytes an adipocyte-like appearance. Normally, liver function is maintained in this type of liver injury. However, when the liver lesion resembles alcoholic hepatitis with infiltrates of polymorphonuclear leukocytes, Mallory bodies, hepatocellular necrosis, and fibrosis, it may progress to cirrhosis and end fatally.

Acute Cholestasis

Bland cholestasis is characterized by the accumulation of bile in canaliculi and hepatocytes, predominantly in the center of the liver lobe and in the absence of features of inflammation. Systemic symptoms are usually mild with the exception of pruritus, which may be severe.

Accumulation of bile in the presence of portal or lobular infiltrates represents another type of acute cholestasis that usually presents as mixed (hepatocellular and cholestatic) liver injury. This type of liver injury is frequently accompanied by systemic features such as rash, fever, and arthralgias, suggesting an immunologic mechanism. Normally, patients recover after cessation of the drug, but recovery is typically slower than for hepatocellular injuries, which often require several months.

Chronic Cholestasis

Ductopenic cholestasis, also called vanishing bile duct syndrome, is characterized by the destruction of more than 50% of the portal bile ducts. Initially, cholangitis with neutrophilic or eosinophilic infiltration of lobular and septal bile ducts is an important histologic feature, before loss of bile ducts occurs. Cholestasis may persist for years and may finally resolve or progress to secondary biliary cirrhosis. As shown in Table 23–2, an increased number of drugs is causing this condition.

Intra-arterial infusion of 5-fluorodeoxyuridine (floxuridine) induces diffuse strictures of large bile ducts, which resemble the histologic lesions of primary sclerosing cholangitis. The pathogenesis of this bile duct damage is drug-induced arteritis, which leads to ischemic bile duct damage.

Other Lesions

A primary fibrogenic reaction may be caused by selective stimulation of fibrogenesis by stellate cells, whereas vascular lesions appear to result from injury to endothelial cells of the sinusoids or terminal venule or from venous thrombosis. Hepatic tumors can develop owing to the proliferative effects of sex steroids on hepatocytes or vinyl chloride on vascular cells.

RISK FACTORS AND PREVENTION

As shown in Table 23–3, several factors influence suscepti-bility for drug-induced liver injury. Factors predisposing older patients to increased drug toxicity include altered drug disposition, in particular decreased renal function, changes in drug metabolism, and pre-existing diseases of the liver. A study from Denmark suggests a linear increase in hepatic drug toxicity from less than 10 cases per million persons/yr in the first 2 decades to approximately 40 cases in the eighth decade of life. Typical examples for drugs exhibi-ting increased toxicity in older patients include isoniazid, chlorpromazine, penicillins, methotrexate, and halothane, whereas the frequency of hepatic injury is higher in children or young adults for valproate, erythromycin, and aspirin.

The frequency of acute hepatitis caused by halothane,

Table 23–3   Risk Factors for Drug-Induced Liver Injury

Risk Factor	Drugs with Increased Risk for Hepatotoxicity
Age	
Geriatric patients	Halogenated hydrocarbons, isoniazid, methotrexate, non-steroidal anti-inflammatory drugs, paracetamol, penicil-lins
Pediatric patients	Erythromycin, valproate
Gender	
Women	Diclofenac, isoniazid, penicil-lins, sulindac
Men	Azathioprine
Enzyme Polymorphisms	
Thiopurine methyltrans-lerase	Azathioprine
Slow acetylators	Dihydralazine, isoniazid, sul-fonamides
Slow sulfoxidation	Estrogens
Interaction with Other Drugs or Toxins	
Induction of CYP	Halothane, isoniazid, valproate
Alcohol	Halothane, isoniazid, metho-trexate, paracetamol
Disease States	
Pre-existing liver disease	Isoniazid, methotrexate, parac-etamol
Juvenile rheumatoid arthri-tis, Still's disease	Aspirin
Decreased mitochondrial β-oxidation	Aspirin, valproate
Renal insufficiency	Allopurinol, methotrexate
Obesity	Methotrexate, paracetamol
AIDS	Penicillins, sulfonamides
Repetitive exposure	Halothane
Racial Background	
African	Isoniazid
Asian	Isoniazid

α-methyldopa, sulindac and diclofenac and for chronic hepatitis by α-methyldopa and oxyphenisatin is higher in women than in men. In contrast, vascular toxicity of aza-thioprine is found predominantly in men. Because immune mechanisms are involved in most forms of drug-induced hepatitis, the female predominance in certain types of drug toxicity may reflect the higher risk of developing autoim-mune disease in women.

Genetic factors determine the activity of pathways of drug metabolism such as the CYP isoenzymes and the con-jugation reactions and the effectiveness of the protective factors such as glutathione metabolism and the regulation of immune responses. These factors are, therefore, important determinants for individual susceptibility to hepatic toxicity of drugs. For instance, the incidence of isoniazid-induced hepatic injury is increased in slow acetylators with con-comitant intake of enzyme inducers such as rifampicin. In slow acetylators, more of the toxic hydrazine is formed from isoniazid by CYP isoenzymes and is only slowly detoxified by acetylation. Slow acetylation is also a risk factor for the hepatotoxicity of sulfonamides. For chlorpromazine and other neuroleptics, poor sulfoxidation in combination with extensive debrisoquine hydroxylation may be a risk factor. The formation of 4-en-valproic acid, a strong inhibitor of mitochondrial β-oxidation formed by microsomal metabo-lism, may explain the increased frequency of valproate-induced hepatotoxicity in patients receiving antiepileptic polytherapy, which usually includes the CYP-inducers phenytoin or carbamazepine. Microvesicular steatosis, which is associated with the administration of valproic acid, aspirin or tetracycline and results from inhibition of mito-chondrial β-oxidation, is considered to be more frequent in patients with preexisting mitochondrial disorders such as decreased β-oxidation, urea cycle defects or mitochondrial cytopathies. Other diseases predisposing to hepatic injury include juvenile rheumatoid arthritis and Still's disease in patients receiving aspirin, AIDS in patients treated with sul-fonamides and preexisting liver disease in patients treated with methotrexate. Induction of CYP 2E1 by alcohol and obesity may explain the known increase in susceptibility to paracetamol and isoniazid in alcoholics and obese patients. A positive family history may predict hepatotoxicity of halothane.

TREATMENT

Recognition that a particular liver injury may be induced by drugs and cessation of offending agents is crucial. In general, the longer the patient continues to ingest a toxic agent after the onset of symptoms, the worse will be the prognosis. There is no specific treatment for acute or chronic drug-induced hepatitis; in particular, there are no controlled trials proving that the use of steroids is beneficial in any drug-induced liver injury. Case reports or uncontrolled trials suggest that they may be helpful to control the systemic symptoms of hypersensitivity associated with the use of allo-purinol, carbamazepine, diclofenac, or phenytoin, but they have no effect on liver injury or survival. N-acetyl-cysteine following paracetamol overdose is currently the only spe-cific antidote available. For patients with drug-induced ful-minant liver failure, liver transplantation is associated with a better survival rate than conservative treatment.

Drug-induced cholestasis is treated symptomatically similar to other types of cholestatic liver disease. Pruritus is treated by administration of cholestyramine or ursodeoxycholic acid and fat-soluble vitamins are provided as necessary.

HEPATOTOXICITY OF INDIVIDUAL DRUGS

Since there are several recent, comprehensive reviews about this subject, we will discuss only the most important adverse drug reactions that affect the liver.

Anesthetics

Halothane

Two forms of liver injury can occur after the administration of halothane. One is a mild, self-limiting form of hepatotoxicity, which affects up to 30% of the patients and manifests itself with elevated serum aminotransferases and in some patients with fever. It is unclear whether these patients have a higher frequency of severe liver damage when re-exposed to halothane. Nevertheless, it is recommended that halothane should not be reused in patients with mild halothane-associated liver injury.

The second form is severe halothane-associated liver injury, which leads to fulminant liver failure in approximately 80% of the affected patients and has, therefore, a bad prognosis. Symptoms include fever, nausea, myalgias, and jaundice. These symptoms usually develop 5 to 9 days after exposure but can appear at any time between 1 and 26 days. Typically, this interval is reduced after re-exposure, suggesting an immunologic mechanism. The frequency of the severe form is approximately 1 case per 35,000 anesthesias but reaches $1:10,000$ after repeated exposure. The susceptibility is increased in adults, women, and obese patients. Although the development of chronic liver disease has been reported, liver damage is normally completely reversible in surviving patients.

Histologically, the lesions range from spotty to zonal centrilobular necrosis and may be difficult to differentiate from viral hepatitis. Occasionally, there is an eosinophilic infiltrate or formation of granulomas, both of which are compatible with an immunologic mechanism. Increased incidence after repeated exposure, shortened period between exposure and the onset of symptoms, and clinical and histologic findings suggest an immunologic mechanism, but centrilobular location of hepatocyte necrosis suggests a toxic mechanism. The main metabolites of halothane are trifluoroacetic acid and bromide, neither of which is hepatotoxic. In a perfused rat liver, hepatotoxicity can be demonstrated after the induction of CYP and under low oxygen tension. These conditions favor reductive metabolism of halothane, which leads to the formation of radicals that can bind to lipids and proteins. Antibodies are formed against these altered proteins, and these antibodies can react against unaltered proteins (e.g., the E_2 moiety of the mitochondrial pyruvate dehydrogenase). Toxic mechanisms are therefore necessary for halothane-associated hepatotoxicity, and it remains unresolved whether the observed autoantobodies play a pathogenic role or only represent the result of liver injury.

Other Halogenated Hydrocarbons

Severe liver injury has been reported after exposure to methoxyflurane, enflurane, and rarely for isoflurane. The incidence is inversely proportional to the extent of microsomal metabolism of these agents, which is lowest for isoflurane. Significantly, cross-reactions between these substances may occur, making it advisable not to use halogenated hydrocarbons in patients recovered from severe halothane-induced hepatic injury.

Analgesics

Opiates

Liver injury has not been reported except for D-propoxyphene, which may rarely be hepatotoxic. Cholestatic liver injury has been described, developing 2 to 90 days after starting ingestion; idiosyncratic metabolic toxicity has been proposed as the likely mechanism.

Salicylates

Aspirin is a well documented cause of dose-dependent, hepatocellular liver injury. At doses higher than 3 g/day, up to 50% of the patients have elevated serum aminotransferases, whereas alkaline phosphatase and serum bilirubin are normal or only slightly elevated. Histologically, there is focal necrosis of hepatocytes. After the drug is discontinued, aspirin-associated liver injury is rapidly reversible.

A strong association has been established between the use of aspirin and the development of Reye's syndrome in children. This association may be caused by the fact that aspirin inhibits hepatic β-oxidation of long chain fatty acids.

Nonsteroidal Anti-Inflammatory Drugs (NSAIDs)

The incidence of acute or subacute liver injury (including acute and subacute liver necrosis, unspecified hepatitis, and jaundice according to ICD-9) has been estimated to be 3.7 per 100,000 NSAID users in England and Wales and 9 per 100,000 person years with a relative risk of 2.3 in Canada. The incidence was clearly highest for sulindac (148 per 100,000 users), lowest for ibuprofen (1.6 per 100,000 users), and intermediate for mefenamic acid (2.5 per 100,000 users), diclofenac (3.6 per 100,000 users), and naproxen (3.8 per 100,000 users). Symptoms were most often jaundice, malaise, abdominal pain, nausea, and vomiting and seldom systemic reactions compatible with an immunologic mechanism. The type of liver injury was most often hepatocellular and more seldom mixed or cholestatic. Risk factors for liver injury included concomitant hepatotoxic medication and rheumatoid arthritis but not age, sex, or duration of treatment.

Up to 15% of patients who ingest diclofenac develop a borderline elevation of serum aminotransferases (less than twice the upper limit of normal), whereas hepatocellular injury is rare. However, several cases of fulminant liver failure have been attributed to the ingestion of diclofenac. Its mechanism of toxicity is probably metabolic, but systemic features suggesting an allergic mechanism have also been described in some patients. Hepatic injury developed between 1 week and 14 months after patients began therapy with diclofenac. Monitoring of serum aminotransferases every 3 months is recommended in patients with prolonged ingestion of diclofenac.

Sulindac is a well-known hepatotoxin that leads most often to cholestatic liver injury. Systemic features such as fever as skin rash are often present, which suggests an immunologic mechanism. Because cholestasis is the prominent feature, recovery upon withdrawal may take several months.

Paracetamol (Acetaminophen)

When ingested at the recommended dose (up to 4 g/day for adults) hepatic toxicity is rare. Some individuals experience an idiosyncratic reaction that may be metabolic or immunologic with rash and eosinophilia. On the other hand, paracetamol is a well characterized, dose-dependent hepatotoxin that causes metabolic liver injury at doses exceeding 125 to 200 mg/kg or 10 to 15 g. Fulminant liver failure has also been described after the ingestion of doses below 10 g in chronic alcoholics; patients treated with enzyme inducers; impairment of the conjugation of paracetamol; geriatric patients; patients with renal, heart, or respiratory failure; and malnourished patients.

The typical clinical course after massive acute ingestion is the development of nonspecific symptoms such as nausea, vomiting, and diaphoresis. These symptoms subside, and the patient enters a symptom-free phase for approximately 24 hours. After this phase (normally 72 to 96 hours after ingestion), hepatocellular necrosis manifests first with nausea, vomiting, and abdominal pain. In severe cases, fulminant hepatic failure with jaundice, coagulopathy, and encephalopathy occurs. Patients with an arterial pH less than 7.30 regardless of the grade of encephalopathy or with a prothrombin time higher than 100 seconds and a serum creatinine higher than 300 mol/L in the case of grade III or IV encephalopathy have a bad prognosis and should be listed for transplantation.

Severe paracetamol toxicity can be prevented by the use of N-acetylcysteine (NAC), which prevents the hepatic glutathione stores from becoming depleted. In the studies by Prescott and associates, only 1 of 62 patients with paracetamol overdose developed severe liver failure (ALT levels >1000 U/L) when NAC was administered within 10 hours after ingestion of paracetamol; in contrast, 33 of 57 patients given only supportive care developed severe liver failure. There were no deaths in the group of patients treated within 10 hours, but three deaths occurred in the group with supportive care. Similar results were reported in a multicenter study conducted by the Rocky Mountain Poison Center in the United States. Recent reports suggest that the use of NAC may even be beneficial when started at later time points in paracetamol overdose; this beneficial effect of NAC is considered to be caused by improvement of the microcirculation with increased extraction of oxygen.

In addition to the administration of NAC, treatment with activated charcoal may help to reduce further absorption and to accelerate the elimination of paracetamol.

Anticonvulsants

Carbamazepine

Abnormalities in liver tests occur in approximately 10% of patients treated with carbamazepine. Granulomatous hepatitis is well known and may be accompanied by systemic features of hypersensitivity, suggesting an immunologic mechanism. Onset of granulomatous hepatitis is usually during the first 4 weeks of therapy. Bile duct injury with signs of acute cholangitis and destruction of bile ducts, finally leading to vanishing bile duct syndrome with secondary biliary cirrhosis, have also been described. Because carbamazepine is a strong inducer of CYP, it increases the toxicity of isoniazid and valproic acid.

Phenytoin

Phenytoin has been shown to be responsible for acute mixed hepatocellular/cholestatic or hepatocellular liver injuries that may have a fulminant course. Acute liver injury appears mainly during the first month of treatment and is frequently accompanied by systemic features of hypersensitivity such as fever, rash, lymphadenopathy, splenomegaly, eosinophilia, and a mononucleosis syndrome with atypical lymphocytes. In more severe cases, thrombocytopenia, arthritis, and exfoliative dermatitis may develop. Histologically, there is hepatocellular necrosis, usually with cellular infiltrates consisting of lymphocytes and eosinophils. Occasionally, granulomatous hepatitis may occur. In patients with a fulminant course, massive necrosis with centrizonal distribution is usually present, suggesting metabolic toxicity. Treatment is supportive; administration of steroids may improve systemic hypersensitivity but has no convincing effect on liver injury or survival.

Phenobarbital

Similar to carbamazepine and phenytoin, phenobarbital induces CYP and shares therefore the interactions with isoniazid and valproic acid described earlier. Rarely, cholestatic or hepatocellular liver injury may develop and are usually accompanied by systemic features of hypersensitivity.

Valproic Acid (Valproate)

Up to 40% of the patients develop mild hyperammonemia and transient increases in serum aminotransferases, usually during the first 3 months after the initiation of therapy. However, clinically overt liver injury is much less common. Between 1978 and 1984, the fatality rate from fulminant hepatic failure was approximately 1:500 in children up to 2 years of age and 1:12,000 in older children and adults receiving antiepileptic polytherapy. In patients treated with valproic acid as a monotherapy, the fatality rate was lower, reaching 1:7000 in children up to 2 years of age and 1:45,000 in older children and adults. Since 1984, the fatality rate has dropped, probably as a consequence of improved knowledge about the adverse effects of valproic acid. Risk factors for fulminant liver failure include concomitant treatment with enzyme inducers (e.g., carbamazepine, phenytoin, phenobarbital, and rifampicin), infancy, concomitant treatment with drugs that inhibit hepatic β-oxidation (e.g., aspirin), and pre-existing metabolic diseases associated with impaired hepatic fatty acid oxidation. The patients usually present with nonspecific symptoms including fever, anorexia, nausea, and development of seizures. Severely affected patients are jaundiced, and some develop fulminant liver failure. In these cases, liver histology shows microvesicular steatosis, suggesting decreased mitochondrial β-oxidation.

Valproic acid is principally metabolized by glucuronidation, mitochondrial oxidation, microsomal ω and ω-1 hydroxylation, and δ-dehydrogenation. Oxidative metabolism of valproate is associated with generation of several mitochondrial toxins and hepatocellular depletion of free coenzyme A, explaining the development of microvesicular steatosis of the liver. In addition, chronic administration of valproate has been shown to induce depletion of mitochondrial cytochrome a and a_3, leading to decreased activity of cytochrome oxidase and further impairing mitochondrial function.

There is no specific antidote for valproate-associated hepatotoxicity. Because most patients with valproate-induced fulminant liver failure have secondary carnitine deficiency, treatment with carnitine has been studied but its effectiveness remains unproved.

Antibiotics

Penicillins

Penicillin G

Penicillin G and phenoxymethyl penicillin have excellent safety records concerning hepatotoxicity and cause liver injury only rarely.

Amoxicillin/Clavulanic Acid

Amoxicillin rarely causes liver injury. In a recent retrospective cohort study, 14 of 329,213 patients treated with amoxicillin developed liver injury (incidence rate of 0.3 per 10,000 prescriptions), which was hepatocellular in half of the cases. Five patients were re-exposed, and liver injury only recurred in one of them.

In contrast, cholestatic liver injury during or after treatment with amoxicillin/clavulanic acid is an increasingly well recognized adverse reaction that occurs with a relative risk of 6.3. Bile duct lesions usually develop during therapy and resolve spontaneously in most patients but can also lead to vanishing bile duct syndrome with secondary biliary cirrhosis. Histologically, bile duct lesions are prominent, usually without cellular infiltrates. Interestingly, a patient was described with mixed hepatocellular/cholestatic liver injury during amoxicillin/clavulanic acid therapy and apparent cross-reactivity with erythromycin.

Other Penicillins

Cholestatic liver injury has also been described for cloxacillin, dicloxacillin, and flucloxacillin. The incidence is approximately 1:11,000 to 1:30,000 prescriptions. Female sex, advanced age, and high doses are risk factors. Liver injury was detected in most patients within 30 days after initiation of therapy and also 3 to 47 days after treatment was discontinued. Most patients were jaundiced and experienced pruritus. In liver biopsies, cholestasis was the predominant feature, sometimes with a moderate inflammatory infiltrate. After the drug was stopped, all patients treated with cloxacillin or dicloxacillin recovered in a few weeks, whereas 2 of 32 patients treated with flucloxacillin died. The clinical picture and the histologic findings were considered to be compatible with an idiosyncratic immunologic mechanism. Reversible cholestatic liver injury has also been reported in patients treated with nafcillin.

Fluoroquinolones

Asymptomatic elevation of aminotransferases have been reported frequently in studies from Europe, America, and Japan. Hepatocellular liver injury with spontaneous resolution has been reported for norfloxacin. Cholestatic liver injury was described for patients treated with ofloxacin, enoxacin, and ciprofloxacin. All patients recovered completely in 1 to 2 months after the drugs were stopped. Fulminant liver failure has been described in patients taking ciprofloxacin and enoxacin. In a recent report, five additional cases of fulminant liver failure in patients treated with ciprofloxacin and also in two patients treated with norfloxacin or ofloxacin are described. Significantly, patients with liver cirrhosis appear to have an increased risk for developing seizures during treatment with pefloxacin.

Erythromycin

Administration of erythromycin estolate is a well recognized cause of hepatocellular liver injury in up to 15% of patients. Some of these patients may develop jaundice, and reports about its incidence vary from approximately 3.6/100,000 up to 3%. Similar liver injuries have also been described for erythromycin propionate, ethylsuccinate, lactobionate, and troleandomycin. Liver injury appears typically 10 to 20 days after the initiation of therapy and may manifest earlier upon readministration of the drug. Symptoms are first nonspecific, but abdominal pain and jaundice may dominate later. Liver histology shows diffuse hepatocellular necrosis, a portal infiltrate containing eosinophils, and often centrilobular cholestasis. The prognosis is excellent with rapid normalization of liver injury after the drug is discontinued.

The frequency of the hepatocellular injuries suggests a toxic mechanism; indeed, erythromycin and its derivatives are metabolized by CYP to a nitrosoalkane derivative, which inhibits CYP by complexing Fe^{2+}. These nitrosoalkane derivatives are unstable intermediates that are normally detoxified by glutathione but may cause liver injury in susceptible individuals. A possible mechanism for erythromycin-associated liver injury is, therefore, initial toxicity by metabolites such as nitrosoalkanes that bind to SH-groups of proteins and lead to hepatocellular liver injury and to the development of an immune response. In a second phase, immunologic liver damage develops in susceptible patients and presents clinically as jaundice.

Tetracyclines

Oral administration of the recommended doses of tetracycline, chlortetracycline, doxycycline, and minocycline is only rarely associated with liver injury. However, 16 patients with hepatitis during minocycline therapy have been reported. Patients presented with symptomatic hepatocellular injury that clinically resembles autoimmune hepatitis. Most patients recovered completely after minocycline was discontinued, but two patients died. Some patients were re-exposed and developed liver injury again. Two patients were described with cholestatic liver injury during treatment with doxycycline or tetracycline. Both patients had only partially normalized liver tests 1 to 3 years after the cessation of treatment.

High intravenous doses of tetracycline have been shown to induce hepatocellular injury and frequently lead to fulminant liver injury and death. This type of liver injury has almost exclusively been observed in women, particularly during pregnancy. Nonspecific symptoms including nausea, vomiting, and abdominal pain usually develop 3 days after administration of 2 g of tetracycline and are followed by jaundice and encephalopathy. Histologically, hepatocytes show microvesicular steatosis, suggesting mitochondrial toxicity. Mitochondrial toxicity of tetracyclines may be caused by inhibition of mitochondrial fatty acid metabolism following the inhibition of mitochondrial protein synthesis.

Sulfonamides

Most sulfonamides have been described to cause cholestatic or mixed hepatocellular/cholestatic liver injury, which is frequently accompanied by systemic features of hypersensitivity including rash and fever. These types of liver disease can also appear in patients treated with sulfasalazine or sulfones. Fulminant liver failure can develop and has a bad prognosis. Patients infected with human immunodeficiency virus (HIV) carry a higher risk for immunologic toxic reactions, including liver injury. The risk for sulfonamide-induced liver injury appears to be increased in slow acetylators. The nonacetylated drug is converted to immunogenic hydroxylamines and nitrosometabolites by CYP isoenzymes.

Liver injury presents usually approximately within 2 weeks after the start of therapy or earlier after repeated exposure. Hepatocellular injuries are rapidly reversible after the drug is discontinued, whereas recovery from cholestatic injuries may last for 1 to 2 years. Corticosteroids have been used for treatment of sulfonamide-associated hepatitis but have shown no clear benefit.

Nitrofurantoins

Both acute and chronic liver injury is associated with the use of these antibiotics. Acute liver injury is usually mixed hepatocellular/cholestatic and accompanied by systemic features of hypersensitivity such as fever, rash and eosinophilia. After the drug is discontinued, most patients recover quickly. Upon rechallenge, liver injury reappears even after years.

The development of chronic liver disease that eventually leads to cirrhosis has clearly been documented in patients with long-term use of nitrofurantoin. Most patients affected have positive autoantibodies, which suggests an immunologic mechanism. Fatal outcome has been described, particularly in patients with continued treatment despite liver disease. In contrast to patients with autoimmune hepatitis, steroids are not effective in patients with nitrofurantoin-associated liver injury.

Antituberculous Agents

Isoniazid

Mild liver injury develops in up to 20% of patients during the first month of treatment and typically consists of an asymptomatic elevation of aminotransferases. In most patients, the aminotransferases normalize despite continued treatment, and there is no progression to more severe liver disease. All age groups are affected, but adults are affected slightly more often than are children.

Severe liver injury affects approximately 1% of patients, almost no children, but up to 2% of adults older than 50 years of age. Liver injury develops usually after 2 months of therapy or later; it is typically hepatocellular with submassive to massive necrosis resembling viral hepatitis. There are no features of hypersensitivity. Risk factors include age, alcohol, and enzyme-inducing agents, particularly rifampicin, malnutrition, and pre-existing liver disease.

Although earlier studies suggested that efficient acetylators are at increased risk for liver injury, more recent studies could not confirm a relationship between acetylator phenotype and isoniazid hepatotoxicity or even suggested that slow acetylators may be at increased risk. On the other hand, induction of CYP by rifampicin is a clearly established risk factor for isoniazid-induced hepatotoxicity. Isoniazid itself and its main metabolite N-acetyl-isoniazid can be metabolized by CYP to hydrazine and acetylhydrazine, respectively, which both are considered to be hepatotoxic.

Unfortunately, it is difficult to predict the subjects who are going to develop severe hepatocellular injury. Nevertheless, we and others believe that before antituberculous treatment is initiated, a detailed history should be obtained and that aminotransferases and alkaline phosphatase should be monitored at least for the first 3 months of therapy. Patients should also be informed exactly about signs and symptoms of liver disease. If the aminotransferases rise above three times the upper level of normal, isoniazid should be stopped and may be restarted slowly after normalization of the laboratory values. In patients with symptomatic liver disease, all antituberculous drugs should be stopped until laboratory values and symptoms are normal.

Rifampicin

As discussed earlier, rifampicin is a potent inducer of CYP and therefore increases the toxicity of isoniazid. Rifampicin interferes also with the hepatic uptake and excretion of bilirubin and bile acids and is, therefore, frequently associated with hyperbilirubinemia and increased serum bile acids. Rifampicin itself can induce hepatocellular liver injury, which may lead to fulminant liver failure. When isoniazid is combined with rifampicin, slow acetylators appear to be at higher risk for hepatotoxicity than efficient acetylators, possibly owing to the fact that the formation of hydrazine from isoniazid is increased in this situation.

Pyrazinamide

This drug is only rarely given alone but is also associated with the development of hepatocellular liver injury, which can progress to fulminant liver failure. One report suggests that the prognosis of liver failure is worse in patients treated with pyrazinamide in comparison with patients who do not receive this drug.

Antifungal Agents

Griseofulvin

Griseofulvin causes Mallory bodies in experimental animals, but this has not been observed in humans. Rarely, it is associated with hepatocellular and cholestatic liver injury in humans.

Imidazole Derivatives and Terbinafine

Ketoconazole is a well known hepatotoxin, causing predominantly hepatocellular and more seldom mixed or cholestatic liver injury in 5% to 10% of the patients. Normally, liver disease manifests during the second or third month of therapy and is only rarely accompanied by signs of hypersensitivity, suggesting metabolic toxicity. Liver histology shows centrilobular necrosis in most patients.

Fluconazole and itraconazole have both been associated with hepatocellular liver injury in certain patients; however, in comparison with ketoconazole, their hepatotoxic potential appears to be lower. One patient with fulminant liver failure associated with fluconazole has been described.

Terbinafine is an allylamine antifungal agent that is associated with predominantly cholestatic liver injury. Most patients recover after the drug is discontinued, but recovery may take months.

Antiviral Agents

A syndrome that consists of liver failure, lactic acidosis, and liver steatosis, mainly microvesicular but in some patients also macrovesicular, has been reported in HIV-positive patients treated with azidothymidine (AZT), didanosine (ddI), or zalcitabine (ddC). In patients treated with AZT, this syndrome did not develop before 6 months of treatment, whereas in patients treated with ddI it developed already after 13 to 15 weeks. A similar syndrome has been observed in patients with chronic hepatitis B treated with fialuridine for 8 to 12 weeks. The mechanism of toxicity is believed to originate from inhibition of the synthesis of mitochondrial DNA, leading to a disruption of oxidative phosphorylation with reduced mitochondrial synthesis of adenine triphosphate.

In addition, predominantly hepatocellular liver injury, which may be accompanied by jaundice, has been described in up to 10% of patients. This condition may not be related to mitochondrial dysfunction and may be fatal in some patients.

Antineoplastic and Immunosuppressants

Antimetabolites

Methotrexate

Chronic use of oral methotrexate in patients with psoriasis or rheumatoid arthritis is associated with fatty liver (liver injury grade 2 according to the classification of Roenigk), liver fibrosis (grade 3), and eventually liver cirrhosis (grade 4). The risk is greater in patients with psoriasis than rheumatoid arthritis, most likely owing to other liver toxins such as alcohol. Several studies show that the risk for development of fibrosis or cirrhosis is dose-dependent. For every gram of methotrexate ingested, the risk for progression of one histologic grade is approximately 6%.

Risk factors for the development of fibrosis include pre-existing liver disease, continued alcohol consumption, diabetes, obesity, advanced age, previous treatment with arsenic, and impaired renal function. Upon cessation of treatment, methotrexate-associated fibrosis or cirrhosis is usually stable but may progress in some patients, eventually necessitating liver transplantation.

Risk factors should be sought before treatment, and the risk is weighed against the possible benefit. Patients with chronic alcohol consumption or with pre-existing liver disease should be biopsied before treatment. During treatment, patients should be monitored clinically by measuring the aminotransferase, alkaline phosphatase, and albumin levels, and a further liver biopsy should be obtained when aminotransferases remain elevated despite the cessation of treatment, when serum albumin levels constantly decrease or when the patient experiences clinical symptoms of liver disease. Pre-existing chronic liver disease, development of fibrosis/cirrhosis, and alcohol consumption are considered to be contraindications for treatment with methotrexate.

Azathioprine, 6-Mercaptopurine, and 6-Thioguanine

Because azathioprine is a pro-drug of 6-mercaptopurine, these two drugs are discussed together. Azathioprine is associated with cholestatic liver injury, which develops in a dose-dependent fashion and is reversible upon dose reduction or cessation of the drug. After kidney transplantation, liver injury appeared 4 to 143 months after surgery at an average dose of 2.5 mg/kg/day in approximately 2% of the patients. Histology typically shows portal infiltrates and bile duct damage. Interestingly, chronic hepatitis B or C has been reported to be a risk factor for azathioprine-associated liver injury.

Azathioprine has been shown to be toxic for sinusoidal endothelial cells by interfering with glutathione metabolism. Endothelial damage is thought to lead to sinusoidal dilatation, peliosis hepatis, veno-occlusive disease, centrilobular necrosis, and nodular regenerative hyperplasia. Because these lesions can be detected in the same patient, it is believed that they all originate from endothelial damage. Endothelial damage may lead directly to peliosis hepatis and veno-occlusive disease with centrilobular necrosis and portal hypertension. Ischemic cell death may stimulate proliferation of well-perfused hepatocyte clusters, leading to nodular regenerative hyperplasia.

Thiopurine methyltransferase deficiency is a well-known cause for azathioprine-associated myelotoxicity. Because azathioprine-induced liver injury is dose-dependent, it can be expected that reduced thiopurine methyltransferase activity also represents a risk factor for liver injury.

Endothelial toxicity with veno-occlusive disease and portal hypertension has also been reported for 6-thioguanine, mainly in patients treated for acute leukemia or psoriasis.

5-Fluorouracil

Fluorouracil alone almost never induces liver injury. However, in combination with N-phosphono-acetyl-L-aspartate (PALA), an inhibitor of pyrimidine synthesis, many patients developed jaundice, coagulopathy, hypalbuminemia, and ascites, reflecting reduced hepatic protein synthesis.

Intra-arterial administration of floxuridine, a 5-fluorouracil derivative, for the treatment of hepatic metastases, induced cholestatic liver injury and jaundice in most patients. Most patients recovered upon cessation of therapy, but irreversible sclerosing cholangitis developed in some patients, probably owing to ischemia following toxic arteritis.

Alkylating Agents

Cyclophosphamide and Busulfan

Cyclophosphamide is a well-known cause for veno-occlusive disease in patients after bone marrow transplantation but can cause hepatocellular liver injury also when used as an immunosuppressant at lower doses.

Similarly, busulfan causes veno-occlusive disease when administered at high doses.

Nitrosoureas

The nitrosoureas (BCNU and CCNU) cause asymptomatic hepatocellular and cholestatic liver injury, which is rapidly reversible when the therapy is stopped.

Dacarbazine

Dacarbazine can cause rapidly progressive veno-occlusive disease, which occurs normally during the second cycle of therapy and is accompanied by signs of hypersensitivity such as eosinophilia and fever, suggesting an immunologic mechanism.

Other Immunosuppressants

Cyclosporine

In comparison with nephro- and neurotoxicity, hepatotoxicity is not an important problem and is not normally a cause for cessation of treatment. Nevertheless, both hepatocellular and cholestatic liver disease have been described in patients after transplantation of different organs or in patients with autoimmune disease.

Most patients have increased serum bile acids and some also have increased conjugated serum bilirubin concentrations, which may be caused by inhibition of canalicular excretion of anions. Cyclosporine-associated liver injury is dose-dependent and usually disappears upon reduction of the dose; only a few patients have developed chronic liver disease. Both cholestatic and hepatocellular liver injury was more pronounced in patients with parenteral nutrition, which may be a risk factor for cyclosporine-associated liver injury.

Tacrolimus (FK-506)

The spectrum of adverse drug reactions from tacrolimus is similar to those of cyclosporine, despite the different chemical structure. In a recent report, 6 of 50 patients with liver transplantation developed liver injury, necessitating dose reduction or cessation of therapy. Liver toxicity is predominantly cholestatic and considered to be dose-dependent. A decreased hepatic activity of CYP 3A has been identified as a risk factor for renal toxicity of tacrolimus. Because the development of liver injury is considered to be dose-dependent, decreased activity of CYP 3A could be a risk factor for liver injury.

Cardiovascular Drugs

Antihypertensive and Diuretic Drugs

ACE Inhibitors

Captopril, enalapril, and lisinopril have been associated with hepatocellular and cholestatic liver injury, which is frequently accompanied by systemic features of hypersensitivity, suggesting an immunologic mechanism. Liver failure can occur if treatment is not stopped, but liver injury improves in most patients upon cessation of treatment. Because cross-reactivity between different angiotensin-converting enzyme (ACE) inhibitors can occur, patients developing liver injury with an ACE inhibitor should not be treated with another member of this drug class.

α-Methyldopa

α-Methyldopa causes a wide spectrum of liver disease, ranging from asymptomatic elevation of aminotransferases to acute or chronic hepatitis with a considerable fatality rate. Asymptomatic elevation of aminotransferases occurs in up to 10% of patients and may disappear despite continued treatment.

Acute hepatitis is much rarer, occurs mainly during the first 3 months of treatment and is frequently accompanied by signs of hypersensitivity, suggesting an immunologic mechanism. Some patients are jaundiced, and liver histology shows necrosis of hepatocytes and cellular infiltrates indistinguishable from viral hepatitis. Liver injury is normally reversible after cessation of therapy but may lead to fulminant liver failure in up to 10% of patients.

Chronic hepatitis attributed to α-methyldopa is usually associated with autoimmune features including antinuclear and antismooth muscle antibodies. Histology is similar to chronic viral hepatitis and progression to cirrhosis has been described. After cessation of treatment, liver injury can regress, but recovery is slow. Although the pathogenesis of α-methyldopa–associated liver injury is not completely clear, clinical findings and in vitro investigations suggest an immunologic reaction induced by a metabolite that is generated by an oxidative metabolism.

Hydralazine and Dihydralazine

Liver injury is well known to occur in patients treated with hydralazines and typically presents with centrilobular necrosis, cellular infiltrates, and circulating autoantibodies; however, cholestatic injury has also been described. Women and slow acetylators are more susceptible. Typically, liver injury appears several months after the start of treatment and is reversible upon cessation. After re-exposure, liver injury recurs with a shortened interval. The postulated mechanism for liver injury includes the formation of a reactive metabolite by CYP 1A2, which binds covalently to this enzyme, forming a neoantigen and triggering an immunologic response.

Tienilic Acid

Tienilic acid was used as a uricosuric diuretic for treatment of arterial hypertension until it had to be withdrawn because of its hepatotoxic properties. Approximately 7% of the treated patients had elevated aminotransferases, whereas symptomatic hepatitis occurred in 0.1%. Hepatic injury occurred typically 1 to 5 months after the start of treatment and was fatal in up to 7%; rechallenge resulted in prompt recurrence of liver injury. Sera from patients with liver injury contained anti-LKM2 antibodies directed against CYP 2C9, the isoenzyme catalyzing sulfoxidation of tienilic acid, which suggests an immunologic mechanism. In support of this concept, deposition of tienilic acid-alkylated CYP 2C11 on the plasma membrane of hepatocytes has been shown in rats.

Antiarrhythmic Drugs

Amiodarone

Amiodarone is used frequently as an antiarrhythmic agent, because it has no negative inotropic effect. It causes two types of liver injury. One is asymptomatic elevation of aminotransferases, which appears in up to 50% of the patients and can normalize despite continued treatment.

It can also cause symptomatic hepatocellular liver injury in up to 3% of patients. Liver injury can develop after 1 month up to years after treatment is begun and shows no clear dose dependency. Because amiodarone has a long half-life, liver injury can develop even after cessation of the drug for several weeks. Liver histology reveals a picture resembling alcoholic hepatitis, including the presence of Mallory bodies being surrounded by a polymorphonuclear infiltrate. Occasionally, granulomas or cholangitis are present. Electron microscopy reveals myeloid figures in lysosomes, which reflect decreased degradation of phospholipids because of lysosomal accumulation of amiodarone. Myeloid figures can also be detected in patients without liver disease, indicating that they do not contribute to liver injury.

Quinidine

Quinidine can cause mild hepatocellular liver injury, which is reversible after cessation of treatment. Liver injury mani-fests usually 1 to 2 weeks after the start of treatment and is frequently combined with fever. Typical biopsy findings include diffuse necrosis and granuloma.

Hormones

Estrogens

Estrogens are associated with cholestatic liver injury, development of hepatic tumors, and thromboembolic complications.

In susceptible persons, cholestasis with pruritus, but without signs of hypersensitivity, develops usually within 2 months after the start of treatment. Conjugated bilirubin, serum bile acids, and alkaline phosphatase are increased, whereas serum aminotransferases remain normal. Liver histology shows an accumulation of bile in hepatocytes and canaliculi but no significant portal infiltrates or bile duct damage. Cholestasis is rapidly reversible after cessation of treatment. In patients with Dubin-Johnson syndrome or cholestasis of pregnancy, estrogens should be avoided, because the risk for the development of cholestasis is high.

The precise mechanism by which estrogens induce cholestasis remains unknown. A decrease in canalicular ATP-dependent transport of bile acids has been described in male rats treated with high estrogen doses.

Hepatic adenomas develop mainly in women who ingest oral contraceptives for more than 5 years. The relative risk for the development of an adenoma is approximately 30 for women ingesting oral contraceptives with a high (>50 mg ethinyl estradiol) and 3 with a low estrogen content. Important complications of adenomas include hemorrhage and progression to hepatocellular carcinoma. Therefore, estrogens should be avoided in these patients, and adenomas should be removed surgically if there is no contraindication.

Compared with adenomas, there is no clear evidence that the development of focal nodular hyperplasia is estrogen-dependent. However, growth of focal nodular hyperplasia depends on estrogens. Accordingly, the lesions can regress upon cessation and can become symptomatic or even rupture during treatment with estrogens. Therefore, patients with focal nodular hyperplasia should not be treated with estrogens.

Studies suggest that patients using estrogens for more than 5 years have an increased risk of hepatocellular carcinoma, which may be caused by conversion of adenomas into hepatocellular carcinomas. The incidence is low, however, and screening for hepatocellular carcinoma is not cost-effective in patients treated with estrogens.

Estrogens enhance the risk for venous thrombosis, and case reports suggest an association between estrogen consumption and Budd-Chiari syndrome.

Androgens and Anabolic Steroids

Similar to estrogens, androgens can cause cholestasis, hepatic adenomas, hepatocellular carcinomas, and vascular lesions.

Androgen-induced cholestasis is mainly associated with the use of 17-alkylated derivatives, such as methyltestosterone and norethandrolone. It is clinically and histologically indistinguishable from estrogen-induced cholestasis. Interestingly, compared with estrogen-induced cholestasis, pruritus appears to be rare, appearing in only about 10% of the patients with cholestasis. Androgen-induced cholestasis is also reversible after cessation of treatment, but it may last for several months.

Androgens have been associated with the development of hepatic adenomas, hepatocellular carcinomas, and hepatic angiosarcomas. The mechanism of the proliferative effect of androgens is unknown.

Several reports describe an association between the use of androgens and the development of peliosis hepatis; peliosis could be induced by proliferation of hepatocytes and endothelial cells, thus providing a possible link between peliosis and hepatic tumors.

Antiandrogens

Cyproterone

Cyproterone is an antiandrogenic with additional progestational effects. It can cause acute hepatocellular injury and can also induce growth of hepatocellular carcinoma.

Flutamide

Flutamide is a nonsteroidal antiandrogen. This drug is known to cause asymptomatic hepatocellular liver injury. Several patients have been described who developed fulminant liver failure. One patient died; three other patients have recovered over months.

Psychoactive Drugs

Neuroleptics

Chlorpromazine

Chlorpromazine induces symptomatic cholestatic liver injury in about 0.5% and asymptomatic liver injury in up to 20% of patients. Jaundice and pruritus develop typically 3 to 5 months after starting therapy and are often accompanied by eosinophilia and hypercholesterolemia. Aminotransferases may also be slightly elevated, but liver injury is cholestatic. Most patients recover within 3 months after cessation of treatment, but chronic cholestasis owing to the development of vanishing bile duct syndrome has been reported.

Liver histology shows centroacinar cholestasis and frequently a mononuclear portal infiltrate. Occasionally, there is diffuse necrosis of hepatocytes with a lobular, lymphocytic infiltrate and granulomas.

The mechanism of chlorpromazine-induced liver toxicity remains unclear. Eosinophilia suggests an allergic mechanism, but chlorpromazine and its hydroxymetabolites have been shown to induce cholestasis in perfused liver. These studies suggest that the metabolites 7,8-dihydroxychlorpromazine and 7-hydroxychlorpromazine are more toxic than chlorpromazine, which is more toxic than chlorpromazine sulfoxide. In line with this concept, patients with impaired sulfoxidation are at risk for chlorpromazine-induced cholestasis. Although immune responses to chlorpromazine have been described, their clinical significance is unclear.

Other Neuroleptics

Cholestatic liver injury has been described for many substances of this drug class, including fluphenazine, mepazine, perphenazine, promazine, thioridazine, trifluoperazine, triflupromazine, clopenthixol, chlorprothixene, and haloperidol. It is unclear, whether cross-reactions exist, but it is advisable to choose a neuroleptic agent from a different chemical class if therapy has to be continued in a patient with drug-induced hepatic injury.

Antidepressants

Monoamine Oxidase Inhibitors

Among the nonselective monoamine oxidase inhibitors, iproniazid is well known for its hepatotoxic effects. It can cause acute hepatocellular injury, histologically similar to acute viral hepatitis, which can progress to fulminant liver failure. In contrast, moclobemide, a selective monoamine oxidase inhibitor, is to date not known to cause symptomatic liver injury.

Tricyclic Antidepressants

Most tricyclic antidepressants are well known to cause hepatocellular or mixed hepatocellular/cholestatic liver injury, which is reversible when the drug is discontinued and which can progress to fulminant liver failure in rare cases. The mechanism is not clearly established with both immunologic and toxic mechanisms being proposed. Amineptine and tianeptine are activated to toxic metabolites by CYP-dependent reactions and cause microvesicular steatosis owing to inhibition of mitochondrial oxidation.

Other Antidepressants

Trazodone can cause acute hepatocellular and cholestatic liver injury, which can progress to fulminant liver failure. In most patients, the symptoms are rapidly reversible after cessation of the drug, but one patient with chronic hepatitis has been described.

In comparison, serotonin reuptake inhibitors appear not to induce severe hepatic adverse reactions.

Miscellaneous Drugs

Allopurinol

Allopurinol can induce hepatocellular liver injury, which manifests normally during the first month of treatment. Systemic features including fever, eosinophilia, and rash are common, and patients present occasionally with vasculitis or renal failure. Risk factors for allopurinol-induced hepatotoxicity and hypersensitivity include renal failure and concomitant use of diuretics. Histologically, centrilobular necrosis with eosinophilic infiltrates are predominant, and granulomas can be observed occasionally.

Table 23–4 Hepatotoxicity of Herbal Medicines

Species	Toxic Ingredients	Hepatotoxicity
Crotalaria, Senecio, Heliotropium, Symphytium officinale (comfrey)	Pyrrolizidine alkaloids	Veno-occlusive disease
Atractalis gummifera, Callilepsis laureola	Atractylate	Inhibition of oxidative phosphorylation → hepatic necrosis
Teucrium chamaedris (Germander)	Flavonoids, diterpenoids, saponins	Hepatocellular or cholestatic liver injury, fulminant liver failure
Larrea tridentata (Chaparral)	Nordihydroguaiaretic acid	Fulminant liver failure
Cassia angustifolia (Senna)	Anthrachinone derivatives	Hepatocellular liver injury
Chinese herbs, Jin Bu Huan	Not known	Hepatocellular liver injury, liver failure
Viscum album (mistletoe)	Not known	Possibly hepatocellular injury

Benzbromarone

Benzbromarone is a benzofurane derivative that is used as a uricosuric agent. Hepatocellular injury has been described in one patient who was rechallenged. Recently, one patient with subacute liver failure and two patients with chronic hepatitis and progression to cirrhosis have been reported. The mechanism of toxicity is unknown.

Disulfiram

Disulfiram has been reported to cause hepatocellular injury, which clinically resembles acute viral hepatitis and rarely progresses to fulminant liver failure. Most patients present within 2 months after the start of therapy. The mechanism of disulfiram-associated liver disease is unknown.

Retinoids

Both etretinate and its pro-drug acitretin can cause asymptomatic hepatocellular liver injury in up to 20% of patients at the beginning of therapy. In most patients, elevated aminotransferases normalize despite continued administration of the drug; liver histology is not available in such patients. However, some patients develop chronic hepatitis that can progress to cirrhosis and chronic liver failure, necessitating transplantation.

Tetrahydraminoacridine (Tacrine)

This drug is a centrally active noncompetitive inhibitor of acetyl cholinesterase, which is used for the treatment of patients with Alzheimer's disease. It is associated with hepatocellular liver injury in approximately 50% of patients but does not normally cause cholestatic liver injury. Liver injury manifests typically 6 to 8 weeks after exposure, and most patients stay free of symptoms. In patients with aminotransferases more than three times the upper limit of normal or jaundice, treatment should be withdrawn. The mechanism of toxicity is uncoupling of oxidative phosphorylation of hepatic mitochondria.

Herbal Medicines

Herbal medicines that cause liver injury have recently received more attention and should be carefully reviewed in patients presenting with liver disease of unknown origin.

The most important hepatotoxic herbs or herb mixtures are presented in Table 23–4.

SUGGESTED READINGS

Almdal TP, Sorensen TI: Incidence of parenchymal liver diseases in Denmark, 1981 to 1985: Analysis of hospitalization registry data. The Danish Association for the Study of the Liver. Hepatology 13:650–655, 1991.

Bass NM, Ockner RK: Drug-induced liver disease. In Zakim D, Boyer TD (eds): Hepatology: A Textbook for Liver Disease. Philadelphia: WB Saunders, 1996, pp 962–1017.

Benichou C: Criteria of drug-induced liver disorders: Report of an international consensus meeting. J Hepatol 11:272–276, 1990.

Bjorneboe M, Iversen O, Olsen S: Infective hepatitis and toxic jaundice in a municipal hospital during a five-year period: Incidence and prognosis. Acta Med Scand 182:491–501, 1967.

Bruppacher R: Epidemiological identification and evaluation of hepatic adverse drug reactions. Semin Liver Dis 15.301–308, 1995.

Danan G: Liver test abnormalities. In Benichou C (ed): Adverse drug reactions: A practical guide to diagnosis and management. Chichester, New York, Brisbane: John Wiley, 3–13, 1994.

Degott C, Feldmann G, Larrey D, et al: Drug-induced prolonged cholestasis in adults: A histological semiquantitative study demonstrating progressive ductopenia. Hepatology 15:244–251, 1992.

Dossing M, Sonne J: Drug-induced hepatic disorders. Incidence, management and avoidance. Drug Saf 1993; 9:441–449.

Edwards MJ, Keller BJ, Kauffman FC, Thurman RG: The involvement of Kupffer cells in carbon tetrachloride toxicity. Toxicol Appl Pharmacol 119:275–279, 1993.

Farrell GC: Drug-Induced Liver Disease. Edinburgh: Churchill Livingstone, 1994.

Fromenty B, Pessayre D: Inhibition of mitochondrial beta-oxidation as a mechanism of hepatotoxicity. Pharmacol Ther 67:101–154, 1995.

Garcia Rodriguez LA, Stricker BH, Zimmerman HJ: Risk of acute liver injury associated with the combination of amoxicillin and clavulanic acid. Arch Intern Med 156:1327–1332, 1996.

Glasgow JF, Moore R: Current concepts in Reye's syndrome. Br J Hosp Med 50:599–604, 1993.

Gut J, Christen U, Huwyler J: Mechanisms of halothane toxicity: Novel insights. Pharmacol Ther 58:133–155, 1993.

Halls H, Gram LF, Grodum E, et al: Drug-related admissions to medical wards: A population survey. Br J Clin Pharmacol 33:61–68, 1992.

Hoofnagle JH, Carithers RL Jr, Shapiro C, Ascher N: Fulminant hepatic failure: Summary of a workshop. Hepatology 21:240–252, 1995.

Kane JA, Kane SP, Jain S: Hepatitis induced by traditional Chinese herbs; possible toxic components. Gut 36:146–147, 1995.

King PD, Blitzer BL: Drug-induced cholestasis: Pathogenesis and clinical features. Semin Liver Dis 10:316–321, 1990.

Koff RS, Gardner RC, Harinasuta U, Pihl CO: Profile of hyperbilirubinemia in three hospital populations. Clin Res 79:524, 1971.

Larrey D, Pageaux GP: Hepatotoxicity of herbal remedies and mushrooms. Semin Liv Dis 15:183–188, 1995.

Lewis JH, Zimmerman HJ: Drug-induced liver disease. Med Clin North Am 73:775–792, 1989.

McMaster KR, Hennigar GR: Drug-induced granulomatous hepatitis. Lab Invest 44:61–73, 1981.

Mehendale HM, Roth RA, Gandolfi AJ, et al: Novel mechanisms in chemically induced hepatotoxicity. FASEB J 8:1285–1295, 1994.

Nelson SD: Molecular mechanisms of the hepatotoxicity caused by acetaminophen. Semin Liver Dis 10:267–278, 1990.

Perry MC: Chemotherapeutic agents and hepatotoxicity. Semin Oncol 9:551–565, 1992.

Pessayre D: Role or reactive metabolites in drug-induced hepatitis. J Hepatol 23 (Suppl 1):16–24, 1995.

Prescott LF: Paracetamol overdosage: Pharmacological considerations and clinical management. Drugs 25:290–314, 1983.

Roenigk HH Jr, Auerbach R, Maibach HI, Weinstein GD: Methotrexate in psoriasis: Revised guidelines. J Am Acad Dermatol 19:145–156, 1988.

Smilkstein MJ, Knapp GL, Kulig KW, Rumack BH: Efficacy of oral N-acetylcysteine in the treatment of acetaminophen overdose: Analysis of the national multicenter study (1976 to 1985). N Engl J Med 319:1557–1562, 1988.

Stricker BHC, Dukes MNG: Drug-Induced Hepatic Injury, 2nd ed. Amsterdam: Elsevier, 1992.

Van Pelt FNAM, Straub P, Manns MP: Molecular basis of drug-induced immunological liver injury. Semin Liver Dis 15:283–300, 1995.

Whiting O, QE, Fye KH, Sack KD: Methotrexate and histologic hepatic abnormalities: A meta-analysis. Am J Med 90:711–716, 1991.

24

Benign and Malignant Tumors of the Liver

Philip J. Johnson

In sub-Saharan Africa, the Mediterranean area, and the Far East, primary liver cancer (specifically hepatocellular carcinoma [HCC]) is one of the most common malignant tumors and represents a major public health problem. Throughout the world, the liver is the most frequent, and often the clinically predominant, site of metastatic disease. For these reasons, there are many situations in clinical hepatology in which malignant disease enters the differential diagnosis.

BENIGN LIVER TUMORS

Other than cavernous hemangiomas, benign liver tumors are uncommon tumors that seldom have clinical significance. Although hepatic adenomas have been associated with long-term use of oral contraceptive agents (and anabolic steroids), the association is, at best, weak and the absolute risk to an individual is very small. Hepatic adenomas may occasionally rupture or bleed into themselves, but they are usually asymptomatic and detected incidentally (Fig. 24–1 *A, B*). Focal nodular hyperplasia (FNH) is a tumor-like malformation that usually appears as an incidental solitary mass and is characterized by a central stellate scar with radiating septa that separate the mass into several smaller nodules (Fig. 24–2). It is probably unrelated to oral contraceptive usage. However, the latter may increase the vascularity of these lesions and lead occasionally to rupture or intratumoral bleeding. Hemangiomas occur in approximately 5% of the normal population and are the most common cause of a solid hepatic tumor. The distinction from malignant tumors is a frequent problem, and the best approach depends on the local facilities available. Magnetic resonance imaging (MRI) may prove ultimately to be the most useful technique, but tomographic tagged

red blood cell imaging and dynamic computed tomography (CT) scanning are also effective. Unless huge, hemangiomas do not cause symptoms.

Management

Only rarely when there is recurrent pain caused by intratumoral hemorrhage, or the patient's mobility is limited by the extreme size of the lesion, is any form of intervention indicated for hemangiomas or FNH. The management of incidentally found adenomas remains controversial. The discontinuation of the oral contraceptive may lead to tumor regression. When this does not occur, the best approach is to resect those cases in which the operative risk is considered minimal. This permits a confident diagnosis and removes any anxiety related to the very small risk of subsequent malignant transformation.

PRIMARY MALIGNANT LIVER TUMORS

Hemangiosarcomas are rare (representing ~1% of all primary liver tumors) and highly malignant tumors that have been associated with thorotrast (a radioactive contrast medium used for angiography between 1920 and 1950) and exposure to the vinyl chloride monomer during manufacture of polyvinyl chloride. Cholangiocarcinomas (which account for ~10% of primary liver tumors) are of two types. The first type, derived from small bile duct cells *(intrahepatic cholangiocarcinoma),* behaves clinically in a manner similar to hepatocellular carcinoma (HCC). The second type arises at, or around, the bifurcation of the common hepatic duct. This type is often known as a "hilar" cholangiocarcinoma or Klatskin tumor. The presentation is with pain, weight loss, and obstructive jaundice. In some areas of the

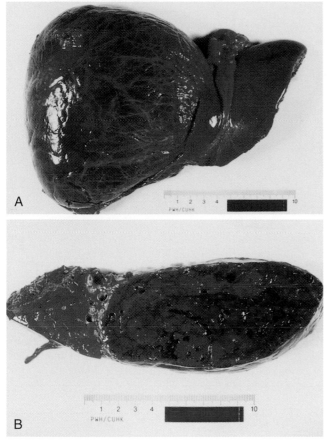

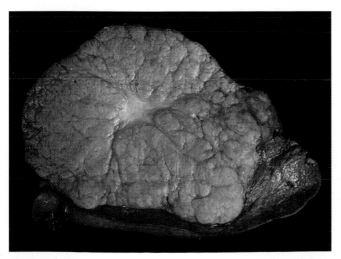

Figure 24–1
A and *B,* Macroscopic appearance of a huge hepatic adenoma. Note the normal appearances of the nontumorous liver and the areas of hemorrhage within the tumor. Note also the prominent capsular vascularity. (Courtesy of CT Liew, MD.)

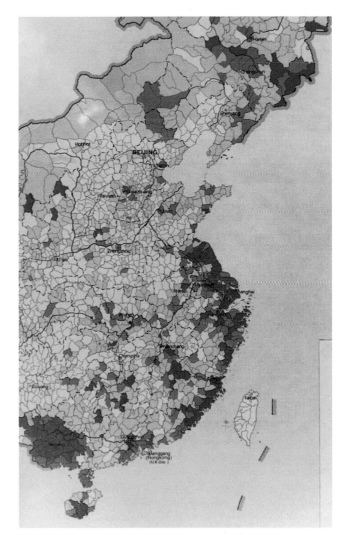

Figure 24–2
Section of a case of focal nodular hyperplasia. Note the pale nature of the tumor, its central scar, and radiating bands of fibrosis that form smaller nodules. (Courtesy of Bernard Portmann, MD.)

world cholangiocarcinomas are associated with liver fluke-infestation (such as *Clonorchis sinensis*) of the biliary system. Management is complex and patients should be referred to specialist centers. Options include drainage with internal stents, radiotherapy (both external and intra-luminal brachytherapy) surgical resection and liver transplantation.

Hepatocellular Carcinoma

HCC is one of the most common malignant tumors in the world today. The highest annual incidence rates, of more than 100 per 100,000 of the population, occur in parts of Southern Africa and the Far East (Figs. 24–3 and 24–4). Some estimates suggest that male Chinese carriers of the hepatitis B virus (HBV) (who may constitute up to 15% of men in certain populations) carry a lifetime risk of almost

Figure 24–3
Male liver cancer mortality in relation to the national rate in Eastern China. Red areas are in the highest decile; green areas are significantly lower than the national average. The carriage rate for hepatitis B virus is fairly consistent throughout China, and the variability may be best accounted for by aflatoxin exposure. (From Atlas of Cancer Mortality in the People's Republic of China.)

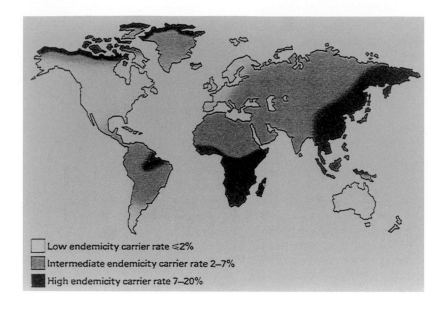

Figure 24–4
Worldwide carriage rate of the hepatitis B virus. Note that the areas with the highest carriage rates coincide with the areas that have the highest incidence of hepatocellular carcinoma (HCC).

☐ Low endemicity carrier rate ≤2%
▨ Intermediate endemicity carrier rate 2–7%
■ High endemicity carrier rate 7–20%

50% of developing the tumor. In contrast, HCC is much less common in Northern Europe, the United States, and Australia.

Etiology and Risk Factors

An understanding of the risk factors is important, because they are now well defined and form the basis for public health measures aimed at control. Chronic infection with HBV or hepatitis C virus (HCV) and exposure to mycotoxin and aflatoxin are definite risk factors. The relative risk for a man carrying HBV is approximately 100, and the figures for HCV carriage may be even higher. Most cases of HCC arise in a cirrhotic liver, although, particularly in high-incidence areas, cirrhosis is not always symptomatic and the development of HCC may be the first indication of the underlying cirrhosis (Figs. 24–5 *A, B*). Between 2% and 5% of patients with cirrhosis develop HCC each year. Men are affected much more commonly than women. The relative importance of these various risk factors varies greatly throughout the world. In Western countries, HCC arises most often as a complication of alcoholic cirrhosis, although cases involving both chronic HBV and HCV are of increasing importance. In sub-Saharan Africa and Southeast Asia, chronic hepatitis B is the major factor, whereas in Japan and much of Mediterranean Europe, hepatitis C is frequently implicated. Generally speaking, the median age of presentation is less in high incidence areas where tumor development in young adult life is common. In the West, the median age of presentation is between 55 and 65 years.

Aflatoxins are mycotoxins generated by the fungi *Aspergillus flavus* and *Aspergillus parasiticus*. Humans are exposed after they eat nuts and meal, which are stored in hot humid conditions and on which these molds grow. Studies that involve field estimates of exposure have consistently suggested a strong association and may account better for the variation in incidence of HCC than does any variation in the carriage of HBV. Recent studies in China, using biomarker techniques that can directly assess exposure to aflatoxin, suggest that exposure to

aflatoxin and carriage of HBV are synergistic risk factors. Routine vaccination at the time of birth against hepatitis B has been practiced for more than 10 years in many parts of Asia, and first indications are that the incidence of HCC is, as a result, starting to fall.

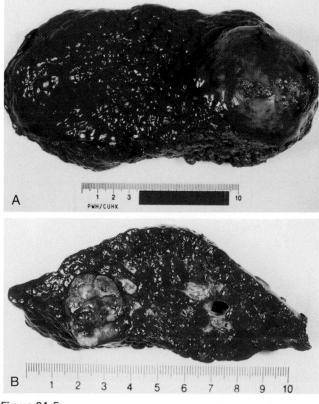

Figure 24–5
A and *B,* Typical appearances of a hepatocellular carcinoma arising as a well-circumscribed, solitary nodule in an extensively macrocirrhotic liver. (Courtesy of CT Liew, MD.)

Pathology

The tumors usually arise in a cirrhotic liver and may be solitary (see Fig. 24–5 *A, B*) or multiple. In the latter case, the multiple nodules usually represent "satellite" metastases from a primary tumor rather than from multiple primary tumors. Most show some degree of hepatocellular differentiation. The presence of bile in the tumor cells or dilated canaliculi is diagnostic of HCC. The histologic pattern is usually microtrabecular and may simulate normal liver, except that there are no portal tracts or bile ducts in evidence. Three histologically defined primary liver cancers that have specific clinical correlates deserve special consideration. The *fibrolamellar variant* of HCC has a better prognosis than the common form of HCC and consists of deeply eosinophilic cytoplasm and pyknotic nuclei interspersed with acellular collagen. The patients are young (mean age of 26 years); the male:female ratio is 1:1; the nontumorous liver is normal; and α-fetoprotein (AFP) is not produced in excess. The prognosis is much better than for the conventional HCC. Although resection rates are high, most patients will still die of their tumor. Median survival is approximately 5 years. Another variant with which fibrolamellar carcinoma may be confused has marked sclerosis histologically but does not have a better prognosis. It is often associated with hypercalcemia. *Epithelioid hemangioendothelioma* can be shown to be of endothelial origin by staining for factor VIII–associated antigen. Some patients with this tumor have survived for several years even without treatment, but resection or transplantation (as appropriate) is usually offered.

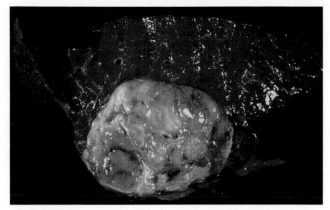

Figure 24–6
Hepatocellular carcinoma (HCC) resected from a patient presenting with spontaneous rupture 1 week previously. Note the large subcapsular hemorrhage on the surface of the liver. (Courtesy of CT Liew, MD.)

clot (hematobilia) in the biliary system. Spread to involve the portal or hepatic venous system may cause portal hypertension, and hepatic vein invasion is a cause of Budd-Chiari syndrome with massive tense ascites. HCC is increasingly being diagnosed presymptomatically in high-risk patients (those with cirrhosis or carriers of HBV) who are screened with serial estimates of AFP and ultrasound examination.

Natural History

HCC is one of the most rapidly growing of all tumors, and most untreated patients die within 12 months of the onset of symptoms. In Africa and the Far East, the tumor behaves particularly aggressively and in South African Bantu mine workers, has a mean duration of symptoms of 5 months. In China, the mean survival time from diagnosis is less than 3 months. In the West, those who do not have underlying cirrhosis survive longer. In general, survival is determined by the size of the tumor, the degree of vascular invasion, and the degree of underlying liver function impairment. The lung is the most common site of metastases from HCC (40% of cases coming to autopsy), but deposits can usually only be detected microscopically. However, as local treatment becomes more effective, symptomatic lung metastases are being detected more frequently.

Symptoms and Presentation

The most common mode of presentation is with the triad of abdominal pain in the right upper quadrant, weight loss, and the presence of an hepatic mass. Patients may also present with signs of decompensating cirrhosis with ascites, or variceal hemorrhage and cutaneous stigmata of chronic liver disease. A particularly dramatic presentation is spontaneous rupture of the tumor in which there is a sudden onset of severe abdominal pain with shock (Fig. 24–6). Paracentesis reveals blood-stained fluid. Rarer presentations include recurrent porphyria cutanea tarda, hypoglycemia, hypercalcemia, polycythemia, and jaundice caused by a tumor or blood

Diagnosis

Hepatomegaly, often massive, is an invariable feature of symptomatic malignant liver tumors, and vascular bruits can be detected in approximately 20% of cases. Currently, most reliance is placed on ultrasound examination or CT scanning. Ultrasound scanning shows the tumor as a hypoechoic lesion with ill-defined margins and can assess the patency of the portal and hepatic veins, particularly when Doppler flow studies are undertaken. It permits differentiation between solid and cystic space-occupying lesions and can allow accurate measurement of tumor size. It is particularly appropriate for regular screening of cirrhotic patients for the development of HCC, because lesions as small as 0.5 cm can be detected. Tumor and cirrhotic nodules can often be differentiated, but the whole examination is very operator dependent. CT scanning is equally sensitive but, in addition, a detailed search for primary or secondary lesions outside the abdomen is permitted, although examination time and expense may limit applicability. HCC is seen as a hypodense lesion that does not enhance with contrast. In most units, ultrasound examination is the first line of investigation. CT scanning is employed in cases that require more detailed assessment, particularly if surgical resection is contemplated. When doubt remains about the diagnosis, angiography is often useful, particularly when combined with lipiodol administration. As well as detecting small lesions, angiography is important before surgical resection is undertaken, because the vascular anatomy is displayed and the patency of the portal vein is confirmed. It is likely that MRI, which can detect extremely small lesions and gives excellent visualization of the vasculature, will become the investigation of choice within the next decade.

α-Fetoprotein

Serum AFP levels are elevated above the reference range (up to 10 ng/mL) in 50% to 80% of patients with HCC at the time of presentation. The median value is in the order of 3000 ng/mL in low incidence areas and 10,000 to 100,000 ng/mL in high incidence areas where levels may reach 10,000,000 ng/mL (10 g/L). The test is primarily of value in the diagnosis of HCC developing in patients with cirrhosis, in which a level above 500 ng/mL is, in the presence of a liver mass, virtually diagnostic. Levels between 10 and 500 ng/mL may occur in other, nonmalignant liver diseases, particularly severe untreated chronic hepatitis and fulminant liver failure. However, a steadily rising value over a 1- to 2-month period is very strongly suggestive of HCC. The test is less useful in distinguishing between primary and secondary tumors in the noncirrhotic normal liver—only 50% of such cases of HCC have elevated levels and up to 10% of patients with hepatic metastases will have elevated levels. Other tumor markers are valuable in the diagnosis of the fibrolamellar variant of HCC, and these include the vitamin B$_{12}$ binding protein and neurotensin.

Histologic Confirmation

Ideally histologic confirmation should always be obtained; however, at what stage of investigation biopsy should be undertaken remains contentious because of the small risk of tumor dissemination along the needle track. Provided the prothrombin time is not prolonged by more than 3 seconds, and the patient is not deeply jaundiced, the conventional percutaneous approaches using Menghini, Tru-Cut or fine-needle (depending on the availability of expert cytology) are usually safe. The frequency with which tumor tissue can be obtained can be increased by using ultrasound to guide the operator or by combining biopsy with laparoscopy. The former approach is now routine practice in most institutions. When there is reason to believe that the lesion may be resectable, many surgeons prefer to avoid preoperative biopsy, and the possible risks of tumor dissemination, and rely instead on frozen section histology at the time of operation.

Clinical Classification and Staging

The most practical staging procedure for HCC is that described by Okuda on the basis of observations on 229 untreated patients. Tumor size, the presence or absence of ascites and jaundice, and the serum albumin level are recorded and permit classification into stages one to three (Table 24–1 and Fig. 24–7), which have clear prognostic significance.

Treatment

Amid the numerous therapeutic options available, it is easy to lose track of the basic principles. Patients who have evidence of liver failure at presentation (encephalopathy, tense ascites, jaundice, recurrent variceal hemorrhage, or severe hypoalbuminemia) have an extremely poor prognosis and are seldom suitable for any active form of therapy. This group may constitute up to 50% of all patients in some re-

Table 24–1 Staging of Hepatocellular Carcinoma

Clinical Feature		Points
Tumor size (on anterior projection of a liver scan)	>50%	1
	<50%	0
Ascites	Present	1
	Absent	0
Serum albumin (mg/dL)	<3.0	1
	>3.0	0
Serum bilirubin (mg/dL)	>2	1
	<2	0

Total Score	Stage	Median Survival (Months)
0	1	28
1, 2	2	8
3, 4	3	1

Adapted from Okuda K, Ohtsuki T, Obata H, et al: Natural history of hepatocellular carcinoma and prognosis in relation to treatment. Cancer 56:918–928, 1985.

gions of the world. For the remainder, treatment can be divided into local and systemic. Local treatments, which include surgical resection, are effective in their aim of decreasing tumor mass and the choice of approach depends on local expertise. However, none has been conclusively and consistently shown to be better than no treatment, or superior in terms of overall survival, to any other. Their impact on the patient's quality of life has received little investigation.

Systemic therapy includes cytotoxic drugs, hormonal therapy, and biologic therapies. These approaches are usually ineffective in decreasing either tumor bulk or improving survival. It is generally agreed that only surgical resection (or liver transplantation) offers any chance of long-term survival or "cure." Although, for reasons enumerated later, this proves feasible in fewer than 15% of cases overall, the

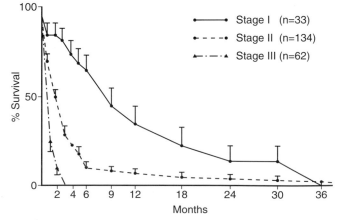

Figure 24–7
Survival of patients with hepatocellular carcinoma in relation to the stage. The staging procedure is shown in Table 24–1. (From Okuda K, Ohtsuki T, Obata H, et al: Natural history of hepatocellular carcinoma and prognosis in relation to treatment. Cancer 56:918–928, 1985.)

physician should consider the possibility in every patient in whom the diagnosis of this malignancy is established.

Surgical Approaches

Surgical resection of HCC is described in more detail in Chapter 30.

Preoperative Investigations

CT is useful in showing the site and extent of the disease but will miss up to one third of tumor nodules detected at laparotomy. Angiography helps to delineate the vascular anatomy, confirm patency of the portal vein, and detect a tumor that is not seen on CT. Intraoperative ultrasound may locate small tumors that may otherwise be undetected. It also helps to determine the resection margins and the plane of liver transection in relation to the hepatic vasculature, thus helping to preserve as much functioning liver tissue as possible. Liver tumors are considered unresectable if there is extrahepatic spread of the disease, extensive bilobar involvement, or tumor invasion of the major vessels including the inferior vena cava, main portal vein, and common hepatic artery. Approximately 10% of cases will come to operation, and the 5-year survival rate is between 35% (in patients with cirrhosis) and 50% (in those without cirrhosis). Failure is usually attributed to a local recurrence.

Liver Resection

Liver resection carries an operative mortality of approximately 5% in noncirrhotic and 10% to 15% in cirrhotic patients. A patient with a normal liver can tolerate resection of about three quarters of the liver, but in a cirrhotic liver a right lobectomy (55% resection) is probably the upper limit. Several attempts have been made to develop tests (or groups of tests) that will predict whether a patient will survive resection. However, to date none has been satisfactory, simply because many factors other than the preoperative liver function status also affect the patient's survival. These factors include the amount of intraoperative blood loss, the duration and degree of hypotension during surgery, and the extent of ischemia to the remaining liver remnant due to hilar clamping or injury to its blood supply.

Until recently, it was widely believed that patients with cirrhosis could not tolerate liver resection. However, it is now clear these strictures apply only to those with decompensated liver disease. Indeed, the presence of Child's grade C cirrhosis is still usually a contraindication to surgery. Furthermore and, again, contrary to earlier claims, the cirrhotic liver does regenerate to some degree (although not to the same extent as the normal liver). Many cirrhotic patients have coagulopathy with a prolonged prothrombin time or a low platelet count because of hypersplenism. Portal hypertension increases the risks of bleeding because of the high portal pressure and the opening up of portosystemic collaterals in the retroperitoneum behind the liver. A cirrhotic liver is firm, difficult to manipulate, and does not take stitches well. All these factors combine to increase the risk of surgery in the cirrhotic patient and emphasize the need for careful preoperative assessment by an experienced team.

Orthotopic Liver Transplantation

Orthotopic liver transplantation overcomes the problems of diffuse tumor spread throughout the liver and the development of hepatic insufficiency after major liver resection, especially for cirrhotic patients. In fact many of the first recipients to achieve long-term survival had malignant liver disease. In general, they tolerated the operation well and recovered rapidly. However, despite careful preoperative assessment that attempted to exclude those with extrahepatic spread, tumor recurrence, presumably arising from undetectable micrometastases, and perhaps favored by the requisite immunosuppression, was frequent. This led many groups virtually to abandon grafting for malignant disease other than when the tumor was found incidentally in a patient undergoing transplantation for advanced cirrhosis. Indeed, evidence is now emerging that tumor size or the degree of vascular invasion are the major factors influencing recurrence. Small tumors may have a very good prognosis after transplantation (~70% 5-year survival), whereas recurrence is the rule with tumors larger than 8 cm diameter or those that are multifocal, particularly if there is histologic or gross evidence of vascular invasion (Table 24–2). Adjuvant chemotherapy, administered either preoperatively or postoperatively, is practiced in many centers, but to date there is no conclusive evidence of its value.

Systemic Therapy

As noted earlier, systemic therapy has not had a major impact on survival, and it is therefore imperative that the physician does not add to the patient's problems with ineffective and toxic treatments. In this respect, careful objective

Table 24–2 Recurrence Rate and Survival in Relation to Tumor Size in Patients Undergoing Liver Transplantation

Tumor Dimensions (cm)	Recurrence No. (%)	Survival (%)		
		1 Year	3 Years	5 Years
<4	0 (0)	83.9	69.9	69.9
4–8	5 (33)	73.3	73	59
>8	7 (78)	66	0	0
Multifocal	14 (78)	33	14	14

Adapted from McPeake JR, O'Grady JG, Zaman S, et al: Liver transplantation for primary hepatocellular carcinoma: Tumor size and number determine outcome. J Hepatol 18:226–234, 1993.

assessment of response is particularly important. Results can be assessed clinically, radiologically, or biochemically. Clinical assessment of liver or tumor size is notoriously unreliable in terms of inter- and intraobserver variation so that only very large changes should be considered significant, and assessment by ultrasound examination or CT scanning is much more accurate. Serial estimation of AFP is widely used to assess a response.

Systemic Cytotoxic Chemotherapy for Inoperable Hepatocellular Carcinoma

Almost all the cytotoxic agents used in oncologic practice have been evaluated, and none has been shown (as a single agent or in combination with other agents) to improve survival or to achieve a consistent response rate of greater than 20%. The most widely used agent has been Adriamycin (doxorubicin). In a recent review of several published trials involving more than 600 patients, the objective response rate was 19% with a median survival of 4 months. This does not necessarily mean that systemic therapy should be completely abandoned, but rather it is important to identify that small percentage of patients who may gain some benefit. It is equally important to avoid undue toxicity among those who do not benefit. The standard regimen is 60 mg/m² given intravenously at three-weekly intervals. Because doxorubicin undergoes hepatic metabolism and biliary excretion, the dose is reduced to 50% if bilirubin is above normal and to 25% if more than twice normal. A reasonable approach is to administer three courses and to reassess at 2 months. If there is evidence of a response, in terms of a greater than 50% fall in serum AFP or a decrease in liver or tumor size as determined by ultrasound or CT scanning, then treatment should be continued to a maximum dose of 550 mg/m². Above this cumulative dose, cardiotoxicity becomes increasingly frequent. In the absence of response, active treatment should be abandoned or changed. Recently a regimen known as PIAF (platinum, interferon, adriamycin, and 5-fluorouracil) has been shown to convert about 20% of unresectable tumors to resectable ones, but this regimen should remain experimental until controlled trials are completed.

It is noteworthy that the most common primary liver tumor in childhood, hepatoblastoma, is significantly more chemosensitive, and it is now common practice to administer chemotherapy before surgical resection. The most usual regimen is PLADO (cisplatin 80 mg/m² over 24 hours by continuous infusion) and doxorubicin (60 mg/m² as an intravenous infusion over 48 hours). Using this regimen, more than 80% of cases of hepatoblastoma will achieve remission, and initially unresectable tumors can often be resected after four courses.

Hormonotherapy and Biotherapy

Estrogen receptors (ER) have been detected in normal, hyperplastic, and neoplastic liver tissues. To date, most studies using tamoxifen have shown no evidence of tumor regression. Recent large prospective randomized trials have shown no evidence of improved survival. Side effects appeared tolerable in most cases, and interferons may, in the future, become more widely used in combination with cytotoxic drugs.

Intra-arterial (Regional) Therapy—The Theoretical Basis

With the disappointing results seen with systemic therapy, several approaches that aim to target the tumor specifically have been developed. There are three ways in which targeting may be achieved. The first approach is based on the observation that primary and secondary liver tumors derive the bulk of their blood supply from the hepatic artery. Direct infusion of agents into the hepatic artery may allow an increase of the exposure of the tumor to the drug. Depending on the agent used, the time/concentration interval may increase by up to 400-fold. Dose-limiting toxicity may then become "regional" (i.e., hepatic and not systemic). A second approach is the use of lipiodol as a vehicle for cytotoxic chemotherapy. This oily based contrast medium, when injected into the hepatic artery at the time of arteriography, is cleared from normal hepatic tissues but accumulates in malignant tumors. This is probably because of the leaky character of neovascular tissue, combined with the lack of lymphatic clearance from tumor tissue. Thirdly, the agent may be injected directly (percutaneously) into the tumor.

Regional Therapy—Results in Practice

There seems no doubt that, compared with systemic administration, drugs given intra-arterially are more effective, although it must not be forgotten that patients treated in this manner are invariably in considerably better condition than are those treated with systemic therapy. For this reason, better results would be expected regardless of any inherent increased efficacy of the treatment. Embolization of the hepatic artery does lead to tumor necrosis and any of several direct attacks on the tumor are also effective in causing tumor necrosis. Some of these regional approaches, which have often been used in combination, are described later.

Transcatheter Oily Chemoembolization (TOCE)

TOCE has been the most widely used approach. A drug (usually doxorubicin or cisplatin) is mixed with lipiodol and injected into the tumor-feeding arteries, followed by embolization with 0.5 to 1 mm of gelatin cubes or similar material. Effective embolization is often associated with fever, pain, and vomiting for 3 to 5 days after which it subsides spontaneously. It should be noted that different operators induce widely different degrees of embolization and, therefore, different severities of side effects. The best approach is not yet defined, and these observations should be taken into account when assessing clinical trials. Antibiotic prophylaxis is required for 1 week, starting on the day before the procedure, together with adequate analgesia. Other side effects are uncommon but include accidental embolization of other organs including the gallbladder and spleen. Portal vein thrombosis is usually a contraindication, because the cirrhotic liver is crucially dependent on the hepatic artery in this situation, and any further interruption thereof may lead to liver failure. The presence of Child's grade C cirrhosis is also a relative contraindication. Although regarded as standard treatment, the only controlled trials to date do not show an increase in survival. The initial optimism for TOCE is perhaps starting to wane, and in a prospective study of various approaches based on embolization with gelatin sponge, a consensus is emerging that although the "primary effect" (i.e., causing tumor volume reduction) is good, there is little effect on long-term survival for which other factors such as the tumor type, degree of spread, and serum AFP level are more significant than the treatment. Although these data probably counsel against the routine use of such therapy, they do, nonetheless, form a basis for future studies. Furthermore, in the search for prolongation of survival, it should not be forgotten that patients are often more interested in the relief of symptoms, and in this capacity, embolization can be very effective.

Percutaneous Alcohol Injection

Ultrasound-guided percutaneous injection of absolute alcohol into liver tumors has been practiced for more than 10 years. The most suitable patients are those with small solitary tumors with good underlying liver function (Child's grade A or B). The procedure causes extensive tumor necrosis, and one report suggests that over a 3-year follow-up period, survival is similar to that obtained by surgical resection. Other ablative approaches include cryotherapy, radiofrequency thermal ablation, laser photocoagulation, and focused ultrasound.

Radiotherapy

The application of external beam irradiation for the treatment of liver tumors has been severely limited by the radiosensitivity of normal hepatocytes. Maximum tolerance of normal liver to radiation is generally accepted to be between 2500 and 3000 cGy; above this level, the risk of radiation hepatitis (veno-occlusive disease with perivenular congestion and fibrosis) increases rapidly.

Internal Irradiation with Intra-arterial Radioisotopes

Therapeutic doses of radioisotopes can be administered into the hepatic artery using ^{90}Y tagged to resin-based or glass microspheres or ^{131}I in conjunction with lipiodol. Lipiodol-^{131}I emits mainly γ-radiation. The volume of radioactive lipiodol administered is limited by the size and vascularity of the tumor; thus in practice, radioactive lipiodol is used only in patients with tumors less than 5 cm in diameter. About 40% of patients will gain objective remissions with minimal toxicities while keeping the radiation dose to a normal liver below 2000 cGy. ^{90}Y, a pure β-emitter, is more powerful than ^{131}I with a mean tissue penetration of about 2.5 mm. Optimal tumor regression and reduction of serum AFP level are seen when the average radiation dose to the tumor is above 12,000 cGy. The partial response rate is more than 50%. Despite the presence of cirrhosis, there is little evidence of radiation hepatitis, even when the nontumorous liver receives up to 7000 cGy. Leakage of the microspheres into the right gastric artery or gastroduodenal artery may occasionally cause radiation gastritis or duodenitis. Systemic leakage of the microspheres to involve the lungs, which are also sensitive to irradiation, may occur if there is extensive arteriovenous shunting within the tumor. For this reason, the degree of lung shunting must be determined before administration of the radioisotope by using a ^{99m}Tc macroaggregated albumin (^{99m}Tc-MAA) scan with

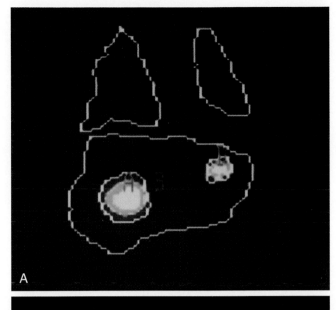

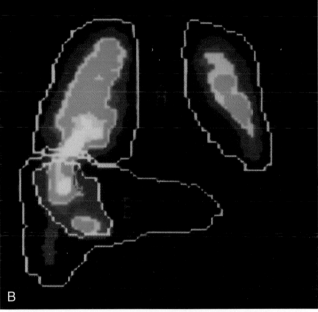

Figure 24–8
A and *B*, ^{99m}Tc macroaggregated albumin scan in two patients with hepatocellular carcinoma. *A*, The technetium macroaggregated albumin (Tc-MAA) scan is confined to the liver tumor, predicting a high tumor to normal ratio and a good therapeutic effect for ^{99}Y therapy. *B*, There is extensive shunting to the lungs, predicting that any administration of radiotherapy to the tumor would pass to the lungs with a very high chance of radiation pneumonitis.

γ-camera scanning as a simulation to predict the percentage of lung shunting (Fig. 24–8 *A, B*).

SECONDARY LIVER TUMORS

At autopsy, liver metastases are found in approximately 1% of all cases, and approximately 40% of adult patients with primary extrahepatic malignancy. Up to 75% of primary tumors drained by the portovenous system (pancreas, large bowel, and stomach), will have spread to involve the liver before death occurs. The tumors are less vascular than HCCs, are often umbilicated, and tend to be more infiltrative (Fig. 24–9 *A, B*). Approximately 50% of patients survive 3 months from the onset of symptoms from secondary liver tumors, and fewer than 10% of patients survive for more than 1 year. Metastases from primary carcinoid tumors are the only secondary tumors to exhibit a significantly better prognosis, and survival periods of up to 10 years are common. With the widespread use of more sophisticated radiologic techniques, the diagnosis is being established earlier (often while the patient is asymptomatic), and this makes for an apparent increase in survival. The percentage of liver involved is probably the major influence on survival time.

Surgical Resection for Secondary Liver Tumors

The only large series of resection for secondary liver cancer relates to patients with metastases from colorectal cancer. Among those patients who appear to have disease confined to a single lobe of the liver (~5% of all patients with colorectal metastases), and in whom curative resection is attempted, about 30% will be alive and 25% disease free at

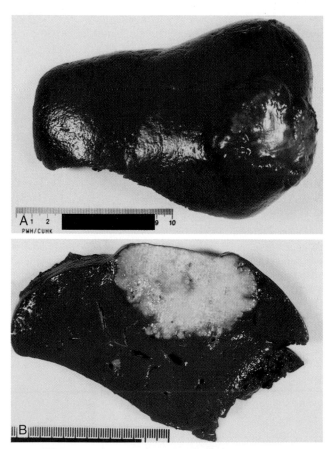

Figure 24–9
A and *B,* Secondary liver tumor. Note the umbilicated appearance and the poorly defined borders of the tumor compared with hepatocellular carcinoma. (Courtesy of CT Liew, MD.)

2 years. These statistics are better than those achieved with any other form of therapy.

Systemic Chemotherapy for Secondary Liver Tumors

Metastases from colorectal carcinoma account for most cases in which chemotherapy is considered. Most experience has been gained with 5-fluorouracil (5-FU), the standard drug against which new agents are compared. A typical regimen is a bolus of 500 mg/m^2/day (to a maximum of 1 g) for 5 days with courses repeated every 5 weeks. The objective response rate is on the order of 15%, and there is probably a modest overall improvement in survival. In the absence of new, more effective drugs, and waning enthusiasm for the combination of other drugs such as the nitrosoureas with 5-FU, attention has focused on methods of enhancing or modulating the effects of 5-FU.

The combination of 5-FU and folinic acid (leucovorin) is consistently superior to 5-FU alone in terms of response rates that increase from 15% to almost 25%. This combination is becoming the most widely used treatment regimen. Some of the remissions are prolonged and complete, and there is a trend toward an increased rate of survival when compared with therapy using 5-FU alone. Complications include stomatitis, bone marrow depression, and diarrhea, depending on the dose of leucovorin used. The most appropriate regimen to date is probably the so-called "low-dose" regimen. Leucovorin is given at a dose of 20 mg/m^2 and is immediately followed by 5-FU at a dose of 425 mg/m^2. Both drugs are given by rapid intravenous injection for 5 consecutive days with courses repeated every 4 weeks.

The optimal management of patients with inoperable colorectal cancer metastatic to the liver remains contentious, but there is a move away from an entirely nihilistic approach. Certainly patients in poor clinical condition, with a large tumor load or with extensive extrahepatic disease, will gain little from systemic therapy. However, a consensus is starting to emerge that, in patients who have a good performance score (although there may be little to choose between the various regimens), treatment does increase survival by approximately 6 months. Treatment should be started before symptoms occur, and it is cost effective when compared with supportive care alone.

Intra-arterial Infusion Chemotherapy for Metastatic Liver Cancer

When FUDR (floxuridine) is infused chronically into the hepatic artery (0.15 to 0.3 mg/kg/day), response rates of more than 50% are consistently obtained in controlled trials, compared with only approximately 15% in control arms in which the drug was given intravenously. The drug is administered over 14-day periods using an implantable pump designed and pioneered by Blackshear in the 1970s. Many responses are dramatic, and there is a strong impression that quality of life is improved significantly. Survival is improved compared with no active treatment (Fig. 24–10). Although time to tumor progression is significantly prolonged, convincing proof of improvement in overall survival, compared with standard intravenous treatment, remains elusive. In patients with isolated hepatic metastases, who are in good

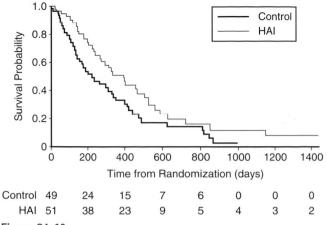

Figure 24–10

Survival in patients with colorectal metastases treated with hepatic artery infusion, administered via an implanted pump, compared with a control group receiving supportive therapy alone. The difference is statistically significant ($P < .03$), and the median survival was 405 versus 226 days in the two groups. The control group illustrates the natural history of untreated inoperable colorectal metastases; those with very extensive disease were excluded (>60% of liver replaced by a tumor). (From Allen-Mersh TG, Earlam S, Fordy C, et al: Quality of life and survival with continuous hepatic-artery floxuridine infusion for colorectal liver metastases. Lancet 344:1255–1260, 1994.)

clinical condition and who are symptomatic, intra-arterial chemotherapy is now a practical and reasonable treatment, although still limited in its application by expense. The toxicity is distinct from that seen with systemic administration of 5-FU with nausea, vomiting, diarrhea and myelosuppression all being uncommon. The most common toxicity is a chemical hepatitis and, in the longer term, sclerosing cholangitis, probably caused by damage of the blood vessels feeding the bile ducts, which also derive their blood supply from the hepatic artery.

Use of Chemotherapy in an Adjuvant Setting

Because of the high recurrence rate (particularly to the liver) in patients with stage B_2 or C colorectal cancer, the role of adjuvant chemotherapy among these groups has been extensively investigated, with a view to decreasing the incidence of subsequent metastatic disease, which is most frequently to the liver. The evidence that postoperative 5-FU and levamisole or 5-FU and leucovorin decrease mortality by approximately 30% in stage C patients is convincing. The latter combination is now considered standard therapy. Equally good results have been reported for the combination of 5-FU and irradiation in patients with rectal cancer.

Hepatic Metastases from Other Primary Sites

Early trials employing the FAM regimen (5-FU, Adriamycin, and mitomycin C) in metastatic disease originating from stomach, pancreas, or bile duct were encouraging, but more recent reports fail to confirm any increased activity

over the single agents alone. Metastases from breast cancer are considerably more sensitive to chemotherapy; response rates are in the order of 50%, particularly with doxorubicin, and, more recently, taxol-based regimens. Other tumors that are sensitive to cytotoxic chemotherapy, such as small cell carcinoma of the lung, germ cell tumors, and lymphomas, may all involve the liver, although isolated hepatic metastases are most unusual and the liver involvement is usually part of widespread metastatic disease.

Hepatic Metastases from an Unknown Primary Site

All too frequently, patients present with malignant liver disease (usually adenocarcinoma on the biopsy), but no obvious primary extrahepatic site can be detected after full physical examination. Extensive radiologic investigations such as barium meal, barium enema, and intravenous pyelography are not indicated, because the occult tumor is seldom in the gut or kidney and both false-positive and false-negative results are common. CT scanning of the abdomen may be more rewarding. It is increasingly recognized that by using various histologic methods involving special stains, immunocytochemistry, and electron microscopy, the origin of certain highly anaplastic tumors can be ascertained. For example, identification of a lymphoma on the basis of positive B or T cell surface markers is particularly gratifying as specific therapy is available.

Carcinoid Syndrome

The development of the carcinoid syndrome (facial flushing and diarrhea, less commonly wheezing, cardiac complications, osteoarthropathy, and pellagra) invariably implies metastatic spread from the small bowel to involve the liver. Abdominal pain may be caused by obstruction by the primary small bowel tumor. The diagnosis is based on an elevated level of urinary 5-hydroxyindole acetic acid (5-HIAA) and the characteristic histologic pattern of a neuroendocrine tumor involving the liver. It is highly characteristic of this tumor that the patient's clinical state appears remarkably good in relation to the extent of liver involvement. In the absence of symptoms, there is little indication for active treatment of hepatic carcinoid metastases unless complete surgical resection is feasible. When the characteristic carcinoid syndrome does develop, the symptoms may be mitigated by reduction of tumor mass (through surgery, arterial embolization, or cytotoxic chemotherapy), pharmacologic interference with production or action of the tumor products, or by nonspecific symptomatic control. It should be emphasized that most of these approaches have unpleasant side effects and should be used only when symptoms are severe.

By the time that the carcinoid syndrome has developed, the tumor is usually too widespread for curative resection to be attempted. It may be successful occasionally, and liver transplantation has been used in carefully selected cases. Surgery (shelling out individual deposits) has now been mostly superseded by hepatic artery embolization (HAE). With this approach, approximately 80% of patients achieve complete resolution of symptoms, and these remissions last from 1 month to 3 years. A major advantage of HAE over ligation of the hepatic artery is that the procedure can be repeated over several years. Cytotoxic therapy with streptozotocin is the last resort. When rapid symptomatic improvement does not occur, treatment should not be continued. The addition of other agents (e.g., Adriamycin and 5-FU) may give rather higher response rates but at the cost of much greater toxicity. All these approaches to decreasing tumor bulk may be associated with the massive release of vasoactive peptides from the tumor tissue. To prevent the resultant complications, patients are treated with blocking agents for 2 days before and 3 days after the procedure.

Early approaches including drugs such as methyldopa and parachlorophenylalanine have now been mainly superseded by the long-acting somatostatin analogue, octreotide, which is often dramatically effective against the diarrhea. The disadvantage is that it needs to be administered subcutaneously three times per day, but most patients learn to administer the drug themselves, and long-acting somatostatin analogues such as lanreotide are becoming available. Octreotide is also very effective in managing carcinoid crises during surgery. The aim of therapy is symptom control, and early reports that there was tumor shrinkage have not been substantiated.

SUGGESTED READINGS

Allen-Mersh TG, Earlam S, Fordy C, et al: Quality of life and survival with continuous hepatic-artery floxuridine infusion for colorectal liver metastases. Lancet 344:1255–1260, 1994.

Altaee MY, Johnson PJ, Farrant JM, Williams R: Etiological and clinical characteristics of peripheral and hilar cholangiocarcinomas. Cancer 68:2501–2505, 1991.

Beasley RP: Hepatitis B virus. The major etiology of hepatocellular carcinoma. Cancer 61:1942–1956, 1988.

Bismuth H, Houssin D, Ornowski J, Meriggi F: Liver resection in cirrhotic patients—a Western experience. World J Surg 10:311–317, 1986.

Carr BI, Iwatsuki S, Starzl TE, et al: Regional cancer chemotherapy for advanced stage hepatocellular carcinoma. J Surg Oncol (Suppl) 3:100–103, 1993.

Castells A, Bruix J, Bru C, et al: Treatment of small hepatocellular carcinoma in cirrhotic patients: A cohort study comparing surgical resection and percutaneous ethanol injections. Hepatology 18:1121–1126, 1993.

Chen HSG, Gross JF: Intra-arterial infusion of anticancer drugs: Theoretic aspects of drug delivery and review of responses. Cancer Treat Rep 64:31–40, 1980.

Craig JR, Peters RL, Omata M: Fibrolamellar carcinoma of the liver: A tumor of adolescents and young adults with distinctive clinicopathologic features. Cancer 46:372–379, 1980.

Farinati F, De Maria N, Chiaramonte M: Hormonal treatment of hepatocellular carcinoma. J Hepatol 12:402–406, 1991.

Ishak K, Sesterhenn IA, Goodman MZD, et al: Epithelioid haemangioendothelioma of the liver: A clinical pathologic and follow-up study of 32 cases. Hum Pathol 15:839–852, 1984.

Jaffe BM: Factors influencing survival in patients with untreated hepatic metastases. Surg Gynaecol Obstet 127:1–11, 1968.

Johnson PJ, Williams R: Serum alphafetoprotein estimations in hepatocellular carcinoma: Influence of therapy and possible value in early detection. J Natl Cancer Inst 64:1329–1332, 1980.

Kasugai H, Kojima J, Tatsuta M, et al: Treatment of hepatocellular carcinoma by transcatheter arterial embolization combined with intra-arterial infusion of a mixture of cisplatin and ethiodized oil. Gastroenterology 97:965–971, 1989.

Klatskin GK: Adenocarcinoma of the hepatic duct at its bifurcation within the porta hepatis. Am J Med 38:241–256, 1965.

Lai CL, Lau JYN, Wu PC, et al: Recombinant interferon-alpha in inoperable hepatocellular carcinoma: A randomised controlled trial. Hepatology 17:389–394, 1993.

Lau WY, Leung WT, Ho SKW, et al: Adjuvant intra-arterial iodine–131-labelled lipiodol for resectable hepatocellular carcinoma: A prospective randomized trial. Lancet 353:797–801, 1999.

McPeake JR, O'Grady JG, Zaman S, et al: Liver transplantation for primary hepatocellular carcinoma: Tumor size and number determine outcome. J Hepatol 18:226–234, 1993.

Moertel CG, Fleming TR, MacDonald JS: Levamisole and fluorouracil for adjuvant therapy of resected colon carcinoma. N Engl J Med 322:352–358, 1990.

Nerenstone SR, Ihde DC, Friedman MA: Clinical trials in primary hepatocellular carcinoma: Current status and future directions. Cancer Treat Rep 15:1–31, 1998.

Oberg K, Norheim I, Theodosson E: Treatment of malignant carcinoid tumors with a long-acting somatostatin analogue octreotide. Acta Oncol 30:503, 1991.

O'Connell MJ, Laurie JA, Kahn M, et al: Prospectively randomised trial of postoperative adjuvant chemotherapy in patients with high-risk colon cancer. J Clin Oncol 16:295–300, 1998.

Okuda K, Ohtsuki T, Obata H, et al: Natural history of hepatocellular carcinoma and prognosis in relation to treatment. Cancer 56:918–928, 1985.

Ortega JA, Krailo MD, Haans JE: Effective treatment of unresectable or metastatic hepatoblastoma with cisplatin and continuous infusion of doxorubicin chemotherapy: A report from the Children's Cancer Study Group. J Clin Oncol 9:2167–2176, 1991.

Rougier P, Pelletier G, Ducreux M, et al: Unresectable hepatocellular carcinoma: Lack of efficacy of lipiodol chemoembolization. Final results of a multicenter randomized trial. Proc Annu Meet Am Soc Clin Oncol 16:A989, 1997.

Simonetti RG, Liberati A, Angiolini C, Pagliaro L: Treatment of hepatocellular carcinoma: A systematic review of randomized controlled trials. Ann Oncol 8:117–136, 1997.

Sobrero AF, Herrmann R, Rischin D, Zalcberg J: Current controversies in cancer. Does biomodulation of 5-fluorouracil improve results? Eur J Cancer 335:186–194, 1999.

Stewart JF, Tattersall MHN, Woods RL, Fox RM: Unknown primary adenocarcinoma: Incidence of over investigation and natural history. BMJ 1:1530–1533, 1979.

Waterhouse JAH, Muir C, Shanmugaratnam K, Powell J: Cancer incidence in five continents. In International Agency for Research on Cancer (IARC Scientific Publications no. 42), Lyon, 1982, Vol 5.

Willis RA: Secondary tumors of the liver. In The Spread of Tumors in the Human Body. London: Butterworths, 1973.

Yamashita Y, Takahashi M, Koga Y, et al: Prognostic factors in the treatment of hepatocellular carcinoma with transcatheter arterial embolization and arterial infusion. Cancer 67:85–91, 1991.

25

Cystic Disorders of the Liver and Biliary Tree

Gregory T. Everson
Roshan Shrestha

This chapter introduces the reader to the clinical and pathologic features of a group of hepatic conditions known collectively as the fibrocystic diseases of the liver. The fibrocystic diseases are characterized by ectasia of intrahepatic bile ducts, cysts of biliary epithelial cell origin, portal fibrosis, and persistence or lack of remodeling of the embryonic ductal plate (ductal plate malformation). The disorders included in this category of hepatic diseases are autosomal dominant polycystic disease (AD-PKD), solitary hepatic cysts, congenital hepatic fibrosis, Caroli's disease, and choledochal cysts. Historical perspective, demography, genetics, clinical associations, and radiologic imaging are provided, and controversies in management and treatment are emphasized. The discussion of polycystic liver disease is highlighted because there have been many recent advances in the natural history, genetics, and molecular biology of this relatively common, inherited disorder.

POLYCYSTIC LIVER DISEASE

Background

Polycystic liver disease may occur in association with ADPKD1 and ADPKD2 or in isolation. ADPKD is one of the most common inherited disorders (10 times more common than sickle cell disease and 15 times more common than cystic fibrosis) and second only to hemochromatosis in inherited disorders involving the liver. As polycystic patients survive for longer periods of time, owing to improvements in management of renal cystic disease, dialysis, and transplantation, complications arising from hepatic cysts are recognized with increased fre-

quency. Many patients may be completely asymptomatic, with normal renal function, and unaware of their underlying disease. The largest and most recent study employed ultrasonography to screen families of index cases of patients with polycystic disease. In this study, several key observations regarding the expression of hepatic cystic disease were made: the frequencies of hepatic and renal cystic disease were similar in men and women, renal cysts could be detected in the early neonatal period, or in utero, but liver cysts were rarely detected before the onset of puberty. After puberty, the number and size of hepatic cysts were significantly greater in women, and the relative overexpression of hepatic cystic disease in women correlated strongly with the number of pregnancies. Hepatic cystic disease also correlated with age, severity of renal cystic disease, and worsening of renal function. Exogenous use of female steroid hormones, as either contraceptive steroids or postmenopausal hormonal replacement, may accelerate the growth or expand the size of hepatic cysts.

The treatment of polycystic liver disease has gone through evolutionary changes. Early attempts at therapy included open laparotomy with surgical fenestration of hepatic cysts. Some have advocated more aggressive surgery, such as hepatic resection or even liver transplantation. Radiologic intervention with aspiration of cyst fluid is only temporarily effective because fluid reaccumulates rapidly in all cases. If cyst aspiration is followed by sclerotherapy, obliteration of the cyst cavity may be achieved, but the technique has limited benefit because only a few cysts can be treated in a single session. Recent progress in laparoscopic surgery has led to the emergence of laparoscopic cyst fenestration and decompression as an alternative and, in some cases, preferred initial therapeutic approach.

Natural History

Little is known of the natural history, associated anomalies, and risk factors of isolated polycystic liver disease. For this reason, the natural history of hepatic cysts occurring in the setting of polycystic kidney disease is described. Hepatic cysts occur uncommonly before puberty, but prevalence of hepatic cysts increases dramatically from the onset of puberty through the early, child-bearing years of adult life. Most patients are asymptomatic without clinical consequences; they possess only a few hepatic cysts or have hepatic cysts whose diameters range from a few millimeters to 1 or 2 cm. Some patients develop massive hepatic cystic disease (almost exclusively restricted to women) during early adult life, and many of these patients become symptomatic, usually with abdominal pain or discomfort, early postprandial fullness, or shortness of breath. As patients live into late adult life, there is the risk of renal failure owing to renal cystic disease and the need for either hemodialysis or renal transplantation. Complications arising in hepatic cysts may occur more frequently in this population. In series of hemodialysis patients, 10% to 15% experienced complications in hepatic cysts, usually hemorrhage or infection, and, rarely, cyst carcinoma.

Risk Factors

The four major risk factors for development of hepatic cysts in ADPKD are increasing age, female gender, severity of renal cystic disease, and severity of renal dysfunction. Hepatic cysts are the most common extrarenal manifestation of ADPKD but are rarely detected before puberty. The prevalence of hepatic cysts increases dramatically during the early, child-bearing years of adult life, and by age 60 almost 80% of patients with ADPKD have hepatic cysts (Fig. 25–1). Although the age-related prevalence of hepatic cysts is similar in men and women, women have greater numbers and larger

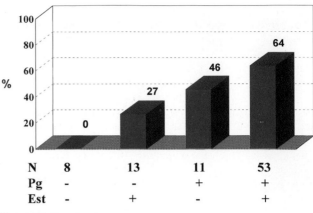

Figure 25–2
The prevalence of hepatic cystic disease as detected by screening ultrasonography is shown for women stratified by history of prior pregnancy (Pg) or prior use of female steroid hormones (Est). The number above each bar is the percent prevalence, and N = the number of subjects in each group. (Adapted from Shrestha R, McKinley C, Russ P, et al: Postmenopausal estrogen therapy selectively stimulates hepatic enlargement in women with autosomal dominant polycystic kidney disease. Hepatology 26:1282–1286, 1997.)

sizes of hepatic cysts. This female tendency to develop massive hepatic cystic disease correlates with both pregnancy (Fig. 25–2) and the use of exogenous female steroid hormones. In one analysis, women who had never been pregnant had numbers and sizes of hepatic cysts that were similar to those found in men.

Genetics

ADPKD1: The autosomal dominant inheritance of polycystic disease was established by Dalgaard in 1957 in a study of 284 patients and their family members. Subsequent reports confirmed this pattern of inheritance and indicated that spontaneous mutations accounted for only a few cases, less than 10%. However, it was not until almost 30 years later, in 1985, that Reeders and colleagues localized the first gene for ADPKD, ADPKD1, to the short arm of chromosome 16 by linkage techniques. Eight years later, the same group of investigators identified, cloned, and sequenced the ADPKD1 gene. The protein encoded by this gene is designated as polycystin-1. The amino acid sequence for polycystin-1 has been determined from knowledge of the nucleotide sequence of the ADPKD1 gene and protein structure has been inferred from the amino acid sequence. This analysis has suggested that polycystin-1 is a ubiquitous protein, found in almost all tissues in the body, and is likely to be an integral membrane protein involved with calcium flux and cell signaling.

ADPKD2: In 1988, 3 years after the discovery of the chromosomal localization of ADPKD1, two publications described polycystic families that did not exhibit linkage to markers on the short arm of chromosome 16. Five years later, in 1993, the location of the ADPKD2 gene was assigned to chromosome 4q. Three years later, in 1996, the

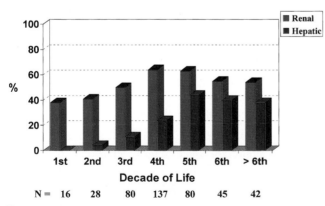

Figure 25–1
The frequency of renal and hepatic cysts is displayed by age in a population at risk for autosomal dominant polycystic kidney disease (ADPKD). Cysts were detected by real-time ultrasonography. The population at risk included 239 patients with ADPKD and 189 unaffected family members. The number of subjects in each decade is indicated at the bottom (From Gabow PA, Johnson AM, Kaehny WD, et al: Risk factors for the development of hepatic cysts in autosomal dominant polycystic kidney disease. Hepatology 11:1033–1037, 1990.)

ADPKD2 gene was identified, sequenced, and cloned. The protein encoded by the ADPKD2 gene is called polycystin-2. Polycystin-2 shares little sequence homology with polycystin-1 but is ubiquitous and also thought to be a membrane-embedded protein that works in concert with polycystin-1 to regulate calcium flux and cell signaling.

Isolated Polycystic Liver: It was long suspected that some families had a form of polycystic disease that was uniquely restricted to the liver. Typically, affected family members had extensive hepatic cystic disease with either no or only a few renal cysts. Proof of a liver-restricted form of polycystic disease was provided in a 1996 study by Pirson and colleagues. They described a Dutch family with isolated polycystic liver disease that was transmitted through three generations. None of the affected family members exhibited linkage to the genetic markers for either ADPKD1 or ADPKD2. As of this writing, the chromosomal location, gene, and encoded protein have not been identified.

Clinical Features

Symptoms: Most patients with polycystic liver are asymptomatic or may note only a protuberant abdomen. In our studies we arbitrarily divided patients with polycystic liver disease into two groups, massive or minimal, based on a definition for massive of a total liver cyst:parenchyma volume ratio greater than 1. Using this definition, we found that most symptomatic cases were restricted to the patients with massive hepatic cystic disease. In one study, we reported that abdominal pain and discomfort and shortness of breath correlated with severity of hepatic cystic disease. Pain related to hepatic cystic disease is dull and aching and may be positional. Patients commonly describe abdominal fullness and often resort to ingestion of frequent small meals, because they experience early postprandial fullness when they eat larger meals. Although γ-glutamyl-transferase (GGT) may be slightly increased in those with massive disease, liver enzymes are typically normal and patients rarely exhibit any features of hepatic decompensation. Likewise, biliary complications are rare.

The major consequence of growth of hepatic cysts is the development of abdominal symptoms without any major clinical manifestations of hepatic failure. Rarely, a patient with polycystic liver disease experiences hepatic decompensation and variceal hemorrhage, ascites, or encephalopathy. Quantitative tests of hepatic function indicated that almost all polycystic patients, including those with massive hepatic cystic disease, have preserved hepatic metabolic capacity as judged from the clearance of caffeine and antipyrine. In contrast, there is a slight but significant increase in portosystemic shunting in those with massive hepatic cystic disease (Fig. 25–3). However, the increase in portosystemic shunt is modest and not usually associated with either variceal bleeding or other features of portal hypertension.

The most common, clinically relevant complications arising in hepatic cysts are intracystic hemorrhage, infection, or post-traumatic rupture. Rare reports of cyst adenocarcinoma, biliary obstruction, Budd-Chiari syndrome, or hepatic failure exist. Table 25–1 lists the complications, the preferred method of diagnosis, and options for medical or surgical management.

In addition to these complications, patients with polycystic disease may have a variety of other associated conditions, including mitral valve prolapse, diverticulosis, inguinal hernias, and berry aneurysms of the cerebral circulation.

Laboratory Studies: Blood count and standard biochemical tests of liver disease are usually normal. Some patients with hepatic cystic disease exhibit elevations in GGT; there is a weak, but significant, correlation of GGT with severity of hepatic cystic disease. Plain radiographs of chest and abdomen are usually normal, except for elevation of the right hemidiaphragm in those with massive disease. Barium studies are unremarkable except for the observance of mass effects caused by the compression of the column of barium by the enlarged liver and kidneys. Polycystic patients may have extensive diverticular disease expressed at a relatively early age.

Modern imaging methods (ultrasonography, computed tomography [CT], nuclear scans, and magnetic resonance imaging [MRI]) easily demonstrate hepatic cysts. Ultrasonography is preferred as the initial screening test, and other scans are reserved for specific indications or research applications. Hepatic cysts appear as thin-walled cavities without intraluminal echogenicity on ultrasonography. CT

Figure 25–3
Portosystemic shunt is slightly increased in patients with the most severe hepatic cystic disease (mean ± SD). (Adapted from Everson GT: Hepatic cysts in autosomal dominant polycystic kidney disease. Am J Kidney Dis 22[4]:520–525, 1993.)

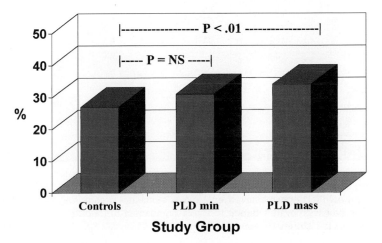

Table 25–1 Clinical Complications Arising in Hepatic Cysts in Patients with Polycystic Disease

Complication	Diagnosis	Treatment
Cyst infection	CT, MRI, In-WBC scan	Antibiotics (fluoroquinolones); drainage, if not responding
Cyst hemorrhage	CT, MRI	Medical management, pain control
Cyst adenocarcinoma	CT, MRI, aspiration cytology	Surgical resection
Portal hypertension		
Hepatic failure	Endoscopy, hepatic angiography	EST/EVL, P-S shunt, OLTx
Budd-Chiari	Hepatic venography	Cyst decompression, if unsuccessful then OLTx
Rupture of cyst	Clinical suspicion	Medical management, pain control
Biliary obstruction	ERCP	Stent placement, cyst decompression

CT, computed tomography; MRI, magnetic resonance imaging; In-WBC scan, indium-labeled white blood cell scan; EST, endoscopic sclerotherapy; EVL, endoscopic variceal ligation; P-S shunt, portosystemic shunt; OLTx, orthotopic liver transplantation; ERCP, endoscopic retrograde cholangiopancreatography.

scans reveal similar findings with minor differences in Hounsfield's units between cysts (Fig. 25–4). In contrast, MRI scans may exhibit significant heterogeneity between cysts. Standard liver-spleen scans have little diagnostic value; biliary scintigraphy (HIDA) is normal; and indium-labeled white blood cell scans may be useful in diagnosing hepatic cyst infection.

Cyst Fluid: There have been several analyses of hepatic cyst fluid and all demonstrate that the composition is consistent with a biliary origin for hepatic cysts. Electrolytes reflect plasma levels; glucose is low to nondetectable; secretory IgA is present; and fluid is relatively enriched in GGT. In vivo, cyst secretion studies suggest that hepatic cysts may secrete fluid in response to intravenously administered secretin. In vitro studies have further confirmed the biliary origin and nature of hepatic cystic epithelium.

Therapy

Medical Treatments: There are no effective medical therapies for polycystic liver disease. The finding of secretin-induced secretion by hepatic cysts prompted clinicians to attempt to reduce cyst volume using long-acting somatostatin analogue. However, this anecdotal experience has failed to demonstrate any major significant effect on hepatic cyst growth or size.

As indicated earlier, hepatic cystic disease may be influenced by the female gender, pregnancy, and use of exogenous female steroid hormones. One prospective study quantitated liver (cyst and parenchymal) and kidney volumes at baseline and after 1 year of follow-up in women with ADPKD on and off estrogen replacement therapy. There was no difference in renal cyst growth, but the growth of hepatic cysts was significantly greater on estrogen therapy (Fig. 25–5).

Should women with polycystic liver disease take estrogen replacement therapy despite the risk of accelerating their hepatic cystic disease? The clinician must individualize treatment by weighing this potential deleterious effect

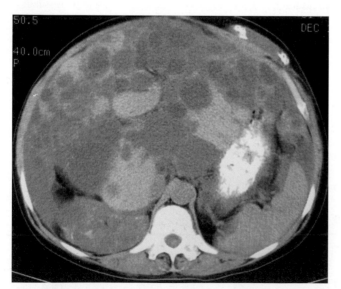

Figure 25–4
An abdominal computed tomography image from a patient with ADPKD1 and massive hepatic cystic disease is shown. The liver with cysts extends to the lateral aspect of the left side of the abdomen.

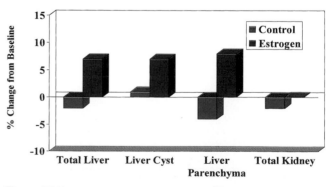

Figure 25–5
Percentage of volume change in the liver and kidney at the end of 1 year of follow-up is shown. Estrogen-treated patients are depicted by a *blue bar* and the nontreated group are indicated by the *red bar*. (Adapted from Shrestha R, McKinley C, Russ P, et al: Postmenopausal estrogen therapy selectively stimulates hepatic enlargement in women with autosomal dominant kidney disease. Hepatology 26:1282–1286, 1997.)

against the potential for other benefits (e.g., bone metabolism, amelioration of estrogen withdrawal symptoms, lipid metabolism) or risks (thromboembolism, uterine or breast cancer).

Radiologic Cyst Aspiration and Sclerosis: Most patients with polycystic disease have too many cysts of insufficient size to warrant percutaneous aspiration and sclerotherapy (alcohol, doxycycline). Those who have one or a few dominant cysts may be considered for this treatment. Success in obliterating individual cysts in polycystic patients is higher than 90%.

Cyst Fenestration: Cyst fenestration is the most commonly applied surgical treatment in the management of symptomatic massive hepatic cystic disease. Two approaches have been used: open laparotomy and, recently, laparoscopy. Several series of open laparotomy, encompassing large numbers of patients, indicate that this approach results in satisfactory resolution of symptoms. However, open laparotomy is associated with prolonged hospitalization and the morbidity of major abdominal surgery. Operative mortality is low (<1%), and reported rates of postoperative complications (bleeding, infection, bile leak, ascites) range up to 50%. Because of its less invasive nature, laparoscopic cyst fenestration is gaining increased acceptance as an alternative surgical technique. Advantages of laparoscopic surgery include less morbidity, reduced hospital stay, and the potential for outpatient surgical management. Individual center experience with laparoscopic cyst decompression is rather limited, but the sum of the results in the reported literature suggests that this approach is effective and associated with low mortality (<1%) and morbidity (up to 25%). At the University of Colorado we have performed nine laparoscopic cyst fenestrations in five patients. Two patients experienced significant complications during the procedure, including gallbladder trauma, which resulted in biliary leak and cholecystectomy, and cyst hemorrhage, which required conversion from laparoscopy to open laparotomy. The other three have had successful amelioration of symptoms and reduction in liver volume (Fig. 25–6).

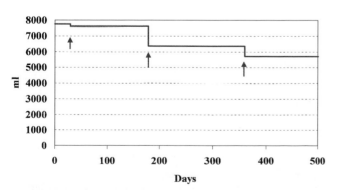

Figure 25–6
The reduction in liver volume achieved by sequential laparoscopic cyst fenestration in a single patient is shown. The initial liver volume was 7710 mL and the final liver volume, after three procedures (green ↑ indicates the days of laparoscopic cyst decompression), was 5677 mL.

Liver Resection: One center reported its experience with partial liver resection in the management of 31 patients with highly symptomatic, massive hepatic cystic disease. The age of the patients ranged from 34 to 69 years of age; the gender ratio (male:female) was 3:28; and renal function varied from normal to dependence on dialysis. Almost all patients experienced significant relief from symptoms, and long-term sustained reduction in symptoms was common (>95%). However, more than 50% experienced significant perioperative morbidity, and there was one perioperative death (caused by rupture of an intracranial aneurysm). We currently reserve hepatic resection for patients who fail to respond or are refractory to cyst decompression.

Liver Transplantation: Polycystic patients with hepatic failure may be considered for hepatic transplantation using standard criteria that are applied to all patients with end-stage liver disease. However, as noted earlier, most patients with polycystic liver disease have preserved hepatic function, and hepatic failure sufficient to warrant transplantation is rarely encountered. It is more likely that the patient with massive hepatic cystic disease would be considered for hepatic transplantation for abdominal symptoms, when other options are unavailable or have failed. Combined liver and kidney transplantation should be considered in patients with end-stage renal disease, on or near dialysis, with symptomatic massive hepatic cystic disease that is not amenable to radiologic, laparoscopic, or alternative surgical interventions. Isolated liver transplantation is considered for patients with preserved renal function but who have massive hepatic cystic disease with symptoms or complications not amenable to other interventions. Cyst infection, hemorrhage, and adenocarcinoma are not indications for hepatic transplantation. Cyst reduction procedures (fenestration, resection, sclerosis) are preferred in the initial management of Budd-Chiari syndrome or biliary obstruction caused by hepatic cysts.

SOLITARY HEPATIC CYST

Background

Solitary hepatic cysts are relatively common and usually asymptomatic. They are most often discovered during the evaluation of a wide variety of abdominal symptoms or disorders and are almost always incidental. Exact prevalence of solitary hepatic cysts for the United States population is unknown, but the female:male ratio is approximately 4:1. A Taiwanese study used ultrasonography in a large-scale community-based screening for simple hepatic cysts to explore the age- and sex-specific prevalence and also in a hospital-based study to record the size of simple hepatic cysts. A total of 3600 subjects in eight communities underwent screening ultrasonography, and 156 simple hepatic cysts were detected in 132 study subjects. The overall prevalence was, therefore, 3.6%. Prevalence increased with age, ranging from 0.8% in patients younger than 40 years of age to 7.8% in subjects older than 60 years of age. The sizes of 219 hepatic cysts in 167 hospitalized patients were measured; 53% had diameters between 1 and 3 cm, and only 7% were larger than 5 cm. Cysts occurred more commonly in the right lobe and were twice as prevalent in women.

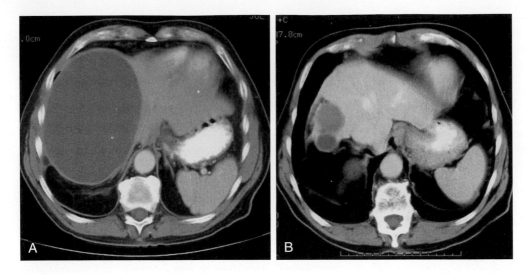

Figure 25–7
A, A large solitary hepatic cyst.
B, The residual after successful alcohol sclerotherapy.

Clinical Features

Most solitary hepatic cysts are found incidentally, are less than 5 cm in diameter and asymptomatic, and do not require any therapeutic intervention. The most common symptom attributed to large hepatic cysts (diameter >5 cm) is localized pain in the right upper quadrant of the abdomen. Rarely, solitary hepatic cysts may develop intracystic hemorrhage, infection, or neoplasia. The latter complications may be diagnosed by radiologic imaging studies or cyst aspiration, cytologic and chemical analysis of cyst fluid, and culture.

Treatment

Asymptomatic solitary hepatic cysts are best managed conservatively using a "watch and wait" approach. The preferred treatment of symptomatic cysts is ultrasound- or CT-guided percutaneous cyst aspiration followed by alcohol (or doxycycline) sclerotherapy (Fig. 25–7 *A, B*). This approach is more than 90% effective in controlling symptoms and ablating the cyst cavity. The recurrence rate after successful ablation is only 5% to 15%. If the radiologically guided, percutaneous approach is ineffective or unavailable, treatment may include either laparoscopic or open surgical cyst fenestration. The laparoscopic approach is used increasingly for anatomically accessible cysts, and greater than 90% efficacy is reported.

CONGENITAL HEPATIC FIBROSIS

Background

Congenital hepatic fibrosis is a rare, inherited, autosomal recessive disorder that is most often associated with autosomal recessive polycystic kidney disease. Congenital hepatic fibrosis may also be observed in adult ADPKD, renal dysplasia, nephronophthisis, Meckel-Gruber syndrome, Ivemark's syndrome, Jeune's syndrome, vaginal atresia, and tuberous sclerosis. Patients with congenital hepatic fibrosis may have other liver malformations, including Caroli's disease and choledochal cyst. Although the histopathologic

features vary, in almost all cases there is fibrous enlargement of the portal tracts, which contain abnormally shaped bile ducts. Congenital hepatic fibrosis typically involves all lobes of the liver equally, but occasionally only one lobe of the liver will be affected. Von Meyenburg complexes (VMCs), also referred to as bile duct microhamartomas, are dilated, ectatic, intra- and interlobular bile ducts embedded in a fibrous stroma and occur in almost all patients with congenital hepatic fibrosis. (VMCs are commonly found in both polycystic disease and Caroli's disease.)

Clinical Features

Congenital hepatic fibrosis presents in three clinical forms: (1) complications related to portal hypertension, (2) recurrent cholangitis, and (3) asymptomatic or latent disease. The first two forms usually present in early childhood with variceal hemorrhage and unexplained biliary sepsis, respectively. In contrast, many patients are detected later, even into early adult years, for other reasons, such as unexplained hepatomegaly or portal hypertension encountered during exploratory laparotomy. Some patients may present with evidence of both portal hypertension and cholestasis, the latter caused by either associated biliary anomalies (Caroli's disease) or intrinsic destructive cholangiopathy. In general, hepatic function is well preserved, despite portal hypertension or bouts of cholangitis, although some patients experience progressive hepatic failure in long-term follow-up.

Treatment

Variceal Hemorrhage: The first line of treatment for this complication is the institution of β-adrenergic blockade or endoscopic variceal eradication (either sclerotherapy or ligation treatment). In most cases, varices may be successfully obliterated by the endoscopic approach, thus controlling this potentially life-threatening complication. Surgical or transjugular intrahepatic portosystemic shunt (TIPS) are reserved for patients who fail endoscopic therapy or bleed from gastric varices or portal hypertensive gastropathy. Occasionally, patients experience progressive hepatic fibrosis and hepatic dysfunction that necessitates their consideration for liver transplantation.

Cholangitis: Radiologic imaging (ultrasonography, biliary radioscintigraphy, CT, or MRI) is required to determine whether the patient with congenital hepatic fibrosis has concomitant biliary cystic disease. If the latter is present, the treatment of cholangitis is centered around provision of adequate biliary drainage, relief of obstruction (papillotomy with stone extraction or stricture dilation), and control of infection with antibiotics. In the absence of biliary cystic disease or cholangiocarcinoma (which may occur in as many as 6% of cases of congenital hepatic fibrosis), cholestasis may be related to idiopathic inflammatory destructive cholangiopathy and respond to ursodeoxycholate therapy.

Liver Transplantation: In general, patients with congenital hepatic fibrosis lack evidence of significant hepatic dysfunction or hepatic failure and they respond to the management of complications as noted earlier. Indications for hepatic transplantation include:

1. Variceal hemorrhage or hemorrhage from portal hypertensive gastropathy not responsive to endoscopic treatment or amenable to portal-systemic shunt surgery or TIPS
2. Recurrent cholangitis not amenable to medical, endoscopic, radiologic or surgical therapy
3. Hepatic failure (development of coagulopathy, biochemical deterioration, ascites, or portosystemic encephalopathy)

Because patients with congenital hepatic fibrosis often have autosomal recessive polycystic kidney disease, one may need to consider combined liver-kidney transplantation in suitable candidates.

CHOLEDOCHAL CYST

Background

Choledochal cysts are cystic dilatations that may occur throughout the macroscopic intra- and extrahepatic biliary tree. Although the term choledochal cyst has been used for any cystic dilatation of the biliary tree, isolated choledochal cysts are usually restricted to only the common hepatic or bile duct. Despite the uncommon occurrence of choledochal cysts, there are hundreds of reports in the literature encompassing more than 3000 cases. The first report was in 1723 by Vatano, with the first large series published in 1909 by Lavenson (28 cases). Several small series have subsequently been reported by different authors during the past several decades. Choledochal cyst is a rare condition in the Western hemisphere; however, it is relatively more common among Asian populations. Several classifications of choledochal cysts have been proposed, but the most commonly cited in the medical literature is by Todani (Fig. 25–8). The pattern of inheritance is unclear, and there have been no definitive studies of either the genetic markers or molecular biology of choledochal cysts.

Although the pathogenesis is unknown, several theories regarding the formation of choledochal cysts have been proposed. The most favored theory is that congenital weakness of the common bile duct and relative distal obstruction, caused by congenital pancreatobiliary malformation, facilitate ascending infection of the bile duct (cholangitis) or chronic reflux of pancreatic enzymes. Support for this theory is found in experimental models where choledochal cysts have been produced by removing epithelium, ligating the distal portion of the bile duct, and anastomosing the pancreatic duct directly to the biliary system. Histologically, the cyst walls are made up of fibrous tissue representing a chronic inflammatory process, and the epithelial lining is either partially or completely absent.

Clinical Features

The most common clinical presentation of a choledochal cyst is a relatively young patient (child or adolescent) with pain, a mass in the right upper quadrant or epigastrium, and jaundice. In one series of 740 cases, jaundice was the most common and consistent presenting feature. In infants, jaundice is often the only sign, and the disorder may be difficult to distinguish from biliary atresia. Most patients have been diagnosed before 30 years of age, and the male:female ratio in most series is approximately 1:4.

Patients with choledochal cysts have abnormal liver enzymes, mainly elevations in bilirubin, alkaline phosphatase, and γ-glutamyl transferase and elevation in pancreatic enzymes, amylase, and lipase. Patients with more extensive disease, who experience marked stasis of bile within cysts and cholangitis, may also have elevated aminotransferases.

Reported complications include spontaneous and traumatic rupture, rupture during pregnancy, liver abscess, cirrhosis, and complications related to portal hypertension including esophageal varices and cholangiocarcinoma. The incidence of cholangiocarcinoma ranges from 2.5% to 17.5%, which is 5 to 35 times higher than the general population. The incidence of carcinoma is 0.7% in affected children younger than 10 years of age. It increases throughout life and approaches 50% by 50 years of age. Internal drainage procedures without cyst excision appear to accelerate the development of cholangiocarcinoma. Bacterial overgrowth and increased levels of secondary bile acids may contribute to cyst metaplasia and carcinoma.

Diagnosis

The diagnosis of a choledochal cyst should always be suspected in a child presenting with recurrent abdominal pain, jaundice, and raised serum amylase. Initial imaging of the biliary tree by ultrasonography or radioscintigraphy (HIDA scans) is usually diagnostic. Confirmation and anatomic definition may require CT, endoscopic retrograde cholangiopancreatogram (ERCP), or percutaneous transhepatic cholangiogram (PTC).

Patients with extrahepatic choledochal cysts have an increased incidence of anomalous pancreaticobiliary junction, which requires ERCP when planning for excision of the cyst. In recent years, endoscopic ultrasonography (EUS) has been a useful imaging method for patients with a suspected anomalous pancreaticobiliary junction. When intrahepatic cysts are detected by ultrasonography, one should determine whether they communicate with the biliary tree by ra-

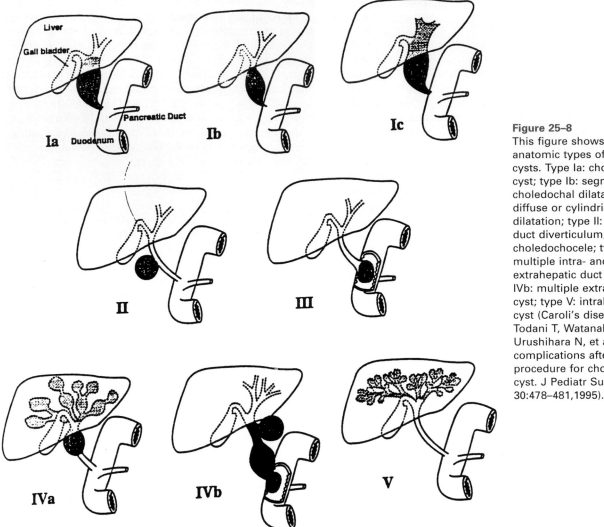

Figure 25–8
This figure shows the various anatomic types of choledochal cysts. Type Ia: choledochal cyst; type Ib: segmental choledochal dilatation; type Ic: diffuse or cylindrical duct dilatation; type II: extrahepatic duct diverticulum; type III: choledochocele; type IVa: multiple intra- and extrahepatic duct cyst; type IVb: multiple extrahepatic duct cyst; type V: intrahepatic duct cyst (Caroli's disease.) (From Todani T, Watanabe Y, Urushihara N, et al: Biliary complications after excisional procedure for choledochal cyst. J Pediatr Surg 30:478–481,1995).

dioscintigraphy (HIDA), CT scan after intravenous administration of biliary contrast agent (Cholegraffin), or ERCP. Prenatal ultrasonography can detect choledochal cysts in utero, which may help antenatal counseling because early neonatal cyst excision and duct revision may be required.

Treatment

The preferred surgical treatment of choledochal cysts is complete cyst excision with Roux-en-Y hepaticojejunostomy. This eliminates any opportunity for stasis, infection, stone formation, and possible development of cholangiocarcinoma, and the procedure provides excellent long-term results with low morbidity and mortality. Nonetheless, lifelong follow-up is necessary to avoid potential problems such as biliary cirrhosis. Internal cyst drainage procedures (cystoduodenostomy, cystojejunostomy) have often been unsatisfactory with a complication rate as high as 50%, and this procedure may actually accelerate the development of cholangiocarcinoma. Unilobar intrahepatic cystic disease is usually treated by resection of the affected lobe of the liver. Radiologic and endoscopic drainage procedures are used to

stabilize patients with acute or recurrent cholangitis. However, recurrent symptoms are common, and the risk of development of cholangiocarcinoma is not eliminated. When features of end-stage liver disease develop, or when endoscopic, radiologic, or surgical therapy has failed to resolve the biliary infectious complications, orthotopic liver transplantation should be considered.

CAROLI'S DISEASE

Background

In 1958, Jacques Caroli described this disease as a congenital malformation of intrahepatic bile ducts characterized by segmental cystic dilatation of the intrahepatic ducts, increased incidence of biliary lithiasis, cholangitis and liver abscesses, absence of cirrhosis and portal hypertension, and association of renal cystic disease. Subsequent to Caroli's report, two distinct disease entities associated with Caroli's disease have been recognized: (1) simple type associated with medullary sponge kidney in 60% to 80% of cases;

(2) periportal fibrosis type associated with congenital hepatic fibrosis, cirrhosis, portal hypertension, and esophageal varices (see discussion earlier regarding congenital hepatic fibrosis).

Clinical Features

The most common presenting symptoms of Caroli's disease are recurrent episodes of fever, chills, and abdominal pain caused by cholangitis; with peak incidence in early adult life. Men and women are equally affected, compared with the female predominance of both polycystic disease and choledochal cysts. More than 80% present with symptoms before 30 years of age. Rarely, the disease presents later in life with evidence of portal hypertension and its complications, most commonly bleeding esophageal varices. The risk of development of cholangiocarcinoma in Caroli's disease is approximately 7%. Biliary lithiasis is found in one third and predisposes patients to recurrent episodes of cholangitis due to obstruction and ascending infections. Patients also occasionally experience multiple liver abscesses. The genetics are unclear, with both autosomal dominant and autosomal recessive patterns of inheritance proposed.

Diagnosis

Caroli's syndrome is typically discovered by ultrasonography performed during evaluation of biliary obstruction or cholangitis. Communication of the intrahepatic cysts with the biliary tree is confirmed by scintigraphy, CT scan after biliary contrast, ERCP, or PTC. Some studies have suggested that CT is superior to ultrasonography in the initial evaluation of adult patients. Ultrasonography is preferred in children. PTC and ERCP provide a detailed examination of the biliary tree and may aid in therapy (Fig. 25–9).

Treatment Options

Biliary Drainage: In most cases, the primary approach to management is restoration of normal or adequate biliary drainage. Endoscopic therapy with ERCP is effective in removing sludge or stones from the common bile duct but has limited use in providing adequate drainage of intrahepatic cysts. In contrast, PTC is more effective in draining these cysts and avoids recurrent episodes of cholangitis especially if patients comply with periodic flushing and changing of drainage catheters. However, the multiple instrumentations and frequency of visits to the interventional radiology suite makes this option less desirable for many patients.

Rarely, the cystic disease is confined to one hepatic lobe, and, in this case, hepatic lobectomy is often curative. Although some have advocated hepaticojejunostomy after partial hepatectomy as primary therapy, the long-term efficacy of this procedure is uncertain, and the extensive surgery could compromise the outcome from hepatic transplantation.

Liver Transplantation: There are two main indications for hepatic transplantation in Caroli's disease: hepatic decompensation and recurrent cholangitis unresponsive to endoscopic or radiologic interventions. Most patients with

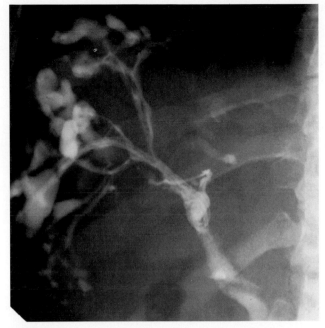

Figure 25–9
This percutaneous transhepatic cholangiogram demonstrates the typical intrahepatic biliary cysts of Caroli's disease and the position of a percutaneously placed pigtail drainage catheter.

Caroli's disease have preserved hepatic function, but some have associated congenital hepatic fibrosis and portal hypertension. Bleeding from esophageal varices is usually controlled by endoscopic therapy (sclerotherapy or ligation) or TIPS. If, however, variceal bleeding recurs despite these measures or if the patient develops cirrhosis (biliary type) and experiences ascites or encephalopathy then transplantation is preferred. The most common indication for transplantation is recurrent cholangitis despite prior interventions. Transplantation should be considered if patients have two or more bouts of cholangitis despite maximum radiologic or endoscopic therapy.

SUGGESTED READINGS

Bean WJ: Hepatic cysts: Treatment with alcohol. Am J Radiol 144:237–241, 1985.

Belloli G, Battaglino F, Guglielmini C, Cappellari F. Long-term (over 22 years) follow-up of four familial cases of Caroli's disease. Ital J Gastroenterol Hepatol 27:185–188, 1995.

Chapman AB, Rubinstein D, Hughes R, et al: Intracranial aneurysms in autosomal dominant polycystic kidney disease. N Engl J Med 327:916–920, 1992.

Chen HM, Jan YY, Chen MF, et al: Surgical treatment of choledochal cyst in adults: results and long-term follow-up. Hepatogastroenterology 43:1492–1499, 1996.

D'Agata ID, Jonas MM, Perez-Atayde AR, et al: Combined cystic disease of the liver and kidney. Semin Liver Dis 14:215–228, 1994.

Desmet VJ. Congenital diseases of intrahepatic bile ducts: Variations on the theme "ductal plate malformation." Hepatology 16:1069–1083, 1992.

Everson GT: Hepatic cysts in autosomal dominant polycystic kidney disease. Mayo Clin Proc 65:1020–1025, 1990.

Everson GT: Hepatic cysts in autosomal dominant polycystic kidney disease. Am J Kidney Dis 22:520–525, 1993.

Everson GT, Emmett M, Brown WR, et al: Functional similarities of hepatic cystic and biliary epithelium: Studies of fluid constituents and in vivo secretion in response to secretin. Hepatology 11:557–565, 1990.

Everson GT, Scherzinger A, Berger-Leff N, et al: Polycystic liver disease: Quantitation of parenchymal and cyst volumes from computed tomography images and clinical correlates of hepatic cysts. Hepatology 8:1627–1634, 1988.

Fabiani P, Mazza D, Toouli J, et al: Laparoscopic fenestration of symptomatic non-parasitic cysts of the liver. Br J Surg 84:321–322, 1997.

Fick GM, Gabow PA: Natural history of autosomal dominant polycystic kidney disease. Annu Rev Med 45:23–29, 1994.

Gabow PA: Autosomal dominant polycystic kidney disease. N Engl J Med 329:332–342, 1993.

Gabow PA, Johnson AM, Kaehny WD, et al: Risk factors for the development of hepatic cysts in autosomal dominant polycystic kidney disease. Hepatology 11:1033–1037, 1990.

Gigot JF, Legrand M, Hubens G, et al: Laparoscopic treatment of nonparasitic liver cysts: Adequate selection of patients and surgical technique. World J Surg 20:556–561, 1996.

Harris RA, Gray DW, Britton BJ, et al: Hepatic cystic disease in an adult polycystic kidney disease transplant population. Aust N Z J Surg 66:166–168, 1996.

Kabbej M, Sauvanet A, Chauveau D, et al: Laparoscopic fenestration in polycystic liver disease. Br J Surg 83:1697–1701, 1996.

Kerr DNS, Harrison CV, Sherlock S, Walker RM: Congenital hepatic fibrosis. Q J Med 1961; 30:91–117

Kerr DNS, Okonkwo S, Choa RG: Congenital hepatic fibrosis: The long-term prognosis. Gut 9:514–520, 1978.

Klingler PJ, Gadenstatter M, Schmid T, et al: Treatment of hepatic cysts in the era of laparoscopic surgery. Br J Surg 84:438–444, 1997.

Lipsett PA, Pitt HA, Colombani PM, et al: Choledochal cyst disease: A changing pattern of presentation. Ann Surg 220:644–652, 1994.

Mall JC, Charhemani GG, Boyer JL: Caroli's disease associated with congenital hepatic fibrosis and renal tubular ectasia. Gastroenterology 66:1029–1053, 1974.

Miyano T, Yamataka A, Kato Y, et al: Hepaticoenterostomy after excision of choledochal cyst in children: A 30-year experience with 180 cases. J Pediatr Surg 1996; 31:1417–1421

Parfrey PS, Bear JC, Morgan J, et al: The diagnosis and prognosis of autosomal dominant polycystic kidney disease. N Engl J Med 323:1085–1090, 1990.

Pirson Y, Lannoy N, Peters D, et al: Isolated polycystic liver disease as a distinct genetic disease, unlinked to polycystic kidney disease 1 and polycystic kidney disease 2. Hepatology 23:249–252, 1996.

Rha SY, Stovroff MC, Glick PL, et al: Choledochal cysts: A ten year experience. Am Surg 62:30–34, 1996.

Sans M, Rimola A, Navasa M, et al: Liver transplantation in patients with Caroli's disease and recurrent cholangitis. Transpl Int 10:241–244, 1997.

Shrestha R, Mckinley C, Russ P, et al: Postmenopausal estrogen therapy selectively stimulates hepatic enlargement in women with autosomal dominant polycystic kidney disease. Hepatology 26:1282–1286, 1997.

Telenti A, Torres VE, Gross JB, et al: Hepatic cyst infection in autosomal dominant polycystic kidney disease. Mayo Clin Proc 65:933–942, 1990.

Tikkakoski T, Makela JT, Leinonen S, et al: Treatment of symptomatic congenital hepatic cysts with single-session percutaneous drainage and ethanol sclerosis: Technique and outcome. J Vasc Intervent Radiol 7:235–239, 1996.

Todani T, Watanabe Y, Urushihara N, et al: Biliary complications after excisional procedure for choledochal cyst. J Pediatr Surg 30:478–481, 1995.

Torres VE, Rastogi S, King BF, et al: Hepatic venous outflow obstruction in autosomal dominant polycystic kidney disease. J Am Soc Nephrol 5:1186–1192, 1994.

Uddin W, Ramage JK, Portmann B, et al: Hepatic venous outflow obstruction in patients with polycystic liver disease: Pathogenesis and treatment. Gut 36:142–145, 1995.

vanSonnenberg E, Wroblicka JT, D'Agostino HB, et al: Symptomatic hepatic cysts: percutaneous drainage and sclerosis. Radiology 190:387–392, 1994.

Ward CJ, Turley H, Ong ACM, et al: Polycystin, the polycystic kidney disease 1 protein, is expressed by epithelial cells in fetal, adult, and polycystic kidney. Proc Natl Acad Sci U S A 93:1524–1528, 1996.

Chapter

26

Disorders of the Hepatic Venous System, Peliosis, and Sinusoidal Dilatation

Dominique Valla
Jean-Pierre Benhamou

Vascular disorders of the liver include diseases of the hepatic veins, hepatic venules, and sinusoids, which will be considered in this chapter, and diseases of the portal vein or venules and hepatic artery or arterioles for which the reader is referred to Chapters 16 and 28, respectively.

Obstruction of the hepatic veins is commonly but inappropriately equated to Budd-Chiari syndrome or hepatic venous outflow block. In fact, there are two types of hepatic venous outflow block. The predominant type is characterized by the obstruction of the main hepatic veins or suprahepatic inferior vena cava. The other type of hepatic venous outflow block is diffuse obstruction of the hepatic venules without involvement of the main hepatic veins.

OBSTRUCTION OF THE HEPATIC VEINS OR INFERIOR VENA CAVA

Epidemiology

Obstruction of the hepatic veins or inferior vena cava is a rare disease, because surveys in Japan and France could identify only a few hundred cases over 1 to 2 decades. However, in some places, such as Nepal, a very high prevalence has been recorded.

Pathophysiology

In patients with nontumorous obstruction, the usual lesion is a concentric thickening of the vein wall by noninflammatory, subintimal fibrosis. As a result, the lumen of the hepatic vein is greatly reduced or obliterated. This lesion can involve the whole length of a main hepatic vein, which ap-

pears as a fibrous cord remnant. In other cases, fibrous thickening is limited to the terminal, juxtaostial portion of the main hepatic vein, forming short stenoses or hepatic vein webs (Fig. 26–1). Recent and old (i.e., organized and recanalized) thrombi are superimposed on fibrous lesions. Pure thrombosis is uncommon. There has been debate as to whether the primary event is thrombosis or fibrosis of the venous wall. The discussion has been obscured by the cause of hepatic vein occlusion not being identified in most of the necropsied cases. In our experience, obstruction of the hepatic veins is commonly associated with thrombogenic disorders. It is tempting to hypothesize that the adherence of abnormal platelets to areas of damaged endothelium in the terminal portion of the hepatic veins might be responsible for the fibrous lesions; a conjectural cause of damaged endothelium might be the mechanical distortion of the terminal portion of the hepatic veins by the diaphragm during the respiratory movements. There are various associated lesions of the small hepatic veins. There is either no lesion or dilatation, thrombosis, fibrosis, endophlebitis, or disappearance of the small hepatic veins.

The obstruction of a single main hepatic vein is clinically silent and only recognized at necropsy. The obstruction of the venous drainage of a region corresponding to two or to the three main hepatic veins has two main effects (Fig. 26–2). Blood pressure increases in the corresponding sinusoids, and blood flow through these sinusoids drops. Raised sinusoidal pressure induces sinusoidal dilatation and congestion, which predominates in the central area of the hepatic lobules (Fig. 26–3). Increased sinusoidal pressure enhances the filtration of interstitial fluid. When the drainage capacity of hepatic lymphatics is exceeded, filtration of fluid through the liver capsule occurs. The filtered fluid has a high protein content because of the high perme-

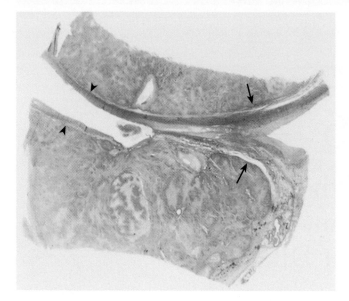

Figure 26–1
Membranous stenosis of the left hepatic vein ostium. Low magnification view of the termination of the left hepatic vein *(small arrows)* into the inferior vena cava *(arrowheads)* in a patient with a myeloproliferative disorder. There is a "web" occluding the ostium.

ability to proteins of the sinusoidal wall, but this fluid is diluted by an admixture of a protein-poor fluid that originates in the mesentery. Rapid massive production of ascitic fluid can induce hypovolemia and subsequent functional renal failure. Raised sinusoidal pressure is transmitted to the portal vein and results in portal hypertension. The elevated sinusoidal pressure induces the development of gross and microscopic collateral venous channels between the obstructed areas and the contiguous patent areas of the liver or the contiguous parietal or diaphragmatic veins. The "spider-web network," a pattern visible at angiography, corresponds with these intrahepatic and extrahepatic collaterals. These collateral channels can ultimately diminish the

sinusoidal pressure and thus prevent the development of clinical manifestations.

Ischemia caused by the reduced sinusoidal perfusion is not always present. The more sudden the obstruction, the more marked will be the ischemia. Ischemic liver cell necrosis is visible as a loss of centrilobular hepatocytes (see Fig. 26–3). Liver failure resulting from ischemic liver cell necrosis is rarely fulminant. The consequences of ischemia are usually transient. Reversibility may be explained by the development of collaterals between the obstructed areas and the neighboring patent areas.

Within a few weeks after an obstruction of the hepatic veins, centrilobular fibrosis develops as a result of sinusoi-

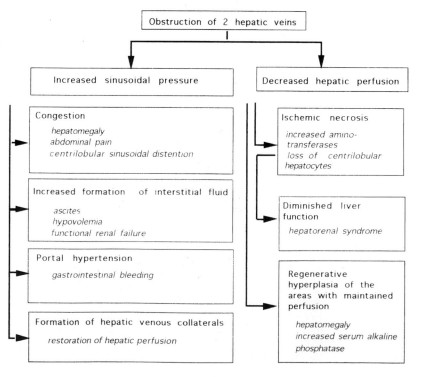

Figure 26–2
Diagrammatic representation of the pathophysiologic consequences of hepatic venous outflow block. On the left, the consequences of increased sinusoidal pressure are constant and permanent. On the right, consequences of impaired liver perfusion are inconstant and usually transient.

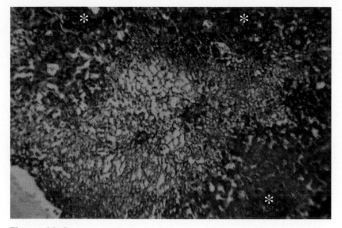

Figure 26–3
Histologic features of hepatic venous outflow block. Centrilobular necrosis visible as a loss of hepatocytes in the center of the photograph while hepatocytes are preserved in the periportal areas (indicated by asterisks). There is also a marked dilatation of the centrilobular sinusoidal remnants (Masson trichrome).

dal hypertension and ischemia. Within a few months, nodular regeneration may take place, predominantly in the periportal area. Moderate portal fibrosis can be present. Cirrhosis can eventually develop.

In approximately one half of the cases of obstruction of the main hepatic veins, the caudate lobe is hypertrophic. Hypertrophy can be quite marked, resulting in compression of the inferior vena cava. Hypertrophy of the caudate lobe is explained by the preservation of its independent outflow tract, which allows compensatory hypertrophy. Usually, the obstruction of the hepatic veins is not synchronous. As a re-

sult, atrophy of the formerly obstructed liver segments coexists with hypertrophy of the later obstructed ones.

Etiology

Compression by Space Occupying Lesions

Obstruction is more likely to complicate compression by infectious space-occupying lesions than by benign or malignant neoplastic tumors. Amebic and pyogenic liver abscesses, hydatid disease caused by *Echinococcus granulosus,* alveolar hydatid disease caused by *E. multilocularis,* secondary liver cancer, and polycystic dominant kidney disease have been reported to cause compression of the hepatic veins.

Endoluminal Invasion by a Tumor

Some malignant tumors tend to progress inside the lumen of their venous outflow tract, toward the inferior vena cava, up to the point where they obstruct the hepatic vein ostia, producing an acute or fulminant variant of Budd-Chiari syndrome. These malignant tumors include Wilms' tumor and renal cell carcinoma, hepatocellular carcinoma, adrenocortical carcinoma, leiomyosarcoma of the inferior vena cava, and myosarcoma of the right atrium.

Thrombosis

This is the most common lesion that affects the hepatic veins. Table 26–1 lists the thrombogenic conditions reported in association with obstruction of the main hepatic veins or suprahepatic inferior vena cava. Their relative prevalence is derived from our experience but does not differ greatly from that of several Western series published in the last few

Table 26–1   Causes of Obstruction of the Hepatic Veins

Condition	Relative Prevalence*	Specific Diagnostic Test
Primary myeloproliferative disorders		
Full-blown form	36%	Set of conventional criteria
Occult form	36%	Culture of bone marrow cells
Paroxysmal nocturnal hemoglobinuria (flow cytometry)	10%	Counts of CD55 and CD59 positive blood cells
Lupus anticoagulant and anticardiolipin antibodies	15%	Activated partial thromboplastin time
		Specific radio- or enzyme-linked immunoassay
Disorders of coagulation or fibrinolysis	Rare	Specific measurements
Drugs		
Dacarbazine	Rare	Clinical history
Oral contraceptives	30%†	Clinical history
Pregnancy	4%†	Clinical history
Miscellaneous conditions		
Behçet's disease	6%	Set of conventional criteria
Sarcoidosis	Rare	Tissue biopsy
Ulcerative colitis	Rare	Endoscopy
Connective tissue diseases	Rare	Serologic tests
Immunoallergic vasculitis	Rare	Biopsy of skin lesions

*In 80 patients admitted to Hôpital Beaujon in whom systematic appropriate investigations for detecting a thrombogenic condition were performed (including bone-marrow culture for demonstrating a latent primary myeloproliferative disorder).
†In most of the patients, oral contraceptives and pregnancy act in exacerbating a pre-existing thrombogenic condition.

years. The etiology of occlusion of the main hepatic veins may be different in other parts of the world.

Primary Myeloproliferative Disorders

Hepatic venous outflow block can complicate (and can be the presenting manifestation of) primary myeloproliferative disorders with a frequency of approximately 1% to 3%. Primary myeloproliferative disorders of any type are the cause of about two thirds of the cases of hepatic vein thrombosis in recent prospective studies. This high prevalence has been recognized only since the identification of occult myeloproliferative disorders, which are characterized by the lack of characteristic peripheral blood changes together with a specific abnormality of bone marrow progenitor cells. A spontaneous formation of erythroid colonies occurs when progenitor cells are cultured in an erythropoietin-poor medium. Several factors may explain the absence of peripheral blood changes in occult myeloproliferative disorders when hepatic vein thrombosis is present: (1) an increase in red blood cell volume can be masked by a parallel increase in plasma volume; and (2) iron deficiency of unclear origin can interfere with erythropoiesis. However, in most patients with occult myeloproliferative disorders demonstrated by spontaneous formation of erythroid colonies, there are various suggestive abnormalities, such as a bone marrow biopsy showing dystrophic megakaryocytes or hyperplasia of bone marrow cells or a liver biopsy or histologic examination of a splenectomy specimen showing myeloid metaplasia.

Paroxysmal Nocturnal Hemoglobinuria

Paroxysmal nocturnal hemoglobinuria is an acquired clonal disorder of the blood cells that is characterized by a deficiency in the glycosyl-phosphatidyl-inositol residue through which various surface proteins are anchored in the plasma membrane. For unknown reasons, hepatic vein thrombosis is a very common complication of this rare disease. Manifestations and prognosis are related to the extent of hepatic vein obstruction: manifestations are absent or transient when thrombosis is limited to a few small hepatic veins; chronic ascites results from partial occlusion of the main hepatic veins; a fatal course is a consequence of a complete obstruction of the main hepatic veins.

Antiphospholipid Syndrome

We recently reported that the antiphospholipid syndrome ranked as the second cause of hepatic vein thrombosis, accounting for almost 20% of the cases. In most of the reported cases, the American Rheumatism Association criteria for the diagnosis of systemic lupus erythematosus were not fulfilled. Frequently, interruption of anticoagulant therapy is followed by the development or the exacerbation of manifestations of hepatic venous outflow obstruction.

Disorders of Coagulation and Fibrinolysis

A congenital deficiency of antithrombin III, protein C, or protein S is difficult to document in patients with liver disease, because liver failure per se induces a nonspecific decrease in the serum level of these factors. The newly identified resistance to activated protein C (factor V Leiden)

may well prove to be a common cause of hepatic vein thrombosis.

Drugs

Dacarbazine may cause fulminant hepatic vein occlusion. The mechanism of the vascular lesion may be an initial immunoallergic injury that affects the small- and medium-sized hepatic veins. Extension of thrombosis to the main hepatic vein has been reported.

Use of oral contraceptives increases the risk of hepatic vein occlusion approximately by two. Circumstantial evidence suggests that oral contraceptives act by exacerbating the thrombogenic potential of an underlying thrombogenic disorder, the investigation of which should always be carried out.

Pregnancy and Postpartum Period

Several cases of hepatic vein occlusion have been reported during pregnancy or in the postpartum period. In several cases, an associated thrombogenic condition was also present, such as paroxysmal nocturnal hemoglobinuria or primary myeloproliferative disorder. Thus, in pregnant women, an underlying thrombogenic condition must be suspected.

Miscellaneous Systemic Thrombogenic Conditions

Behçet's disease, ulcerative colitis, celiac disease, sarcoidosis, connective tissue disease in the absence of lupus anticoagulant or antiphospholipid autoantibodies, and idiopathic hypereosinophilic syndrome have each been reported in a few cases of hepatic venous outflow block. All of these disorders are known to affect vessels or to precipitate thrombosis.

Association of Thrombogenic Conditions

It is increasingly recognized that the association of two thrombogenic conditions and a triggering factor might be necessary in order for thrombosis to develop. This possibility has not yet been appropriately evaluated in patients with hepatic vein obstruction. However, there are isolated cases of such an association. Therefore, a systematic investigation of all the recognizable thrombogenic conditions should be performed in any patients with hepatic or inferior vena cava obstruction.

Hepatic and Inferior Vena Cava Obstruction of Unknown Cause

In most retrospective studies, this category accounts for 25% to 50% of cases of hepatic venous outflow block. However, when all the tests listed in Table 26–1 are performed, the proportion of idiopathic cases falls to less than 20%. This is mainly due to the identification of occult myeloproliferative disorders.

Membranous Obstruction of Inferior Vena Cava

Membranous obstruction of the inferior vena cava is the major cause of hepatic venous outflow block in South Africa

Table 26–2 Clinical Manifestations of Hepatic Venous Outflow Block Due to Hepatic Vein or Inferior Vena Cava Thrombosis in 1970–1987 and 1987–1991*

Signs and Symptoms	1970–1987 (No. = 47) (%)	1987–1991 (No. = 34) (%)
Ascites	95	65
Liver enlargement	95	76
Abdominal pain	80	53
Leg edema	47	15
Jaundice	43	21
Fever	40	18
Hepatic encephalopathy	20	3
Gastrointestinal bleeding	16	6
None of the above symptoms	0	24

*Adapted from Hadengue A, Poliquin M, Vilgrain V, et al: The changing scene of hepatic vein thrombosis: Recognition of asymptomatic cases. Gastroenterology 106:1042–1047, 1994.

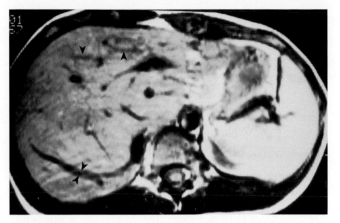

Figure 26–4
Magnetic resonance imaging of the liver in an asymptomatic patient with obstruction of the hapatic veins. The numerous vascular channels that are indicated by *arrowheads* are abnormal collateral veins, which should not be mistaken as normal hepatic veins.

and Japan and, to a lesser extent, in India. The inferior vena cava is obstructed at or above the level of the hepatic vein ostia. One of the main hepatic veins usually remains patent and drains into the caudal portion of the inferior vena cava. Blood from the inferior vena cava is returned to the right atrium through large lumbar and azygous collateral veins. The other main hepatic veins are usually obstructed.

This lesion has long been considered of congenital origin, but there are several lines of circumstantial evidence suggesting the acquired nature of membranous obstruction of the inferior vena cava. The prominent caval-caval collateral circulation usually develops in adulthood, which is not consistent with a congenital malformation. When systematically investigated, an associated thrombogenic disorder is usually found. In most of the other reported cases of membranous obstruction, investigation for demonstrating an underlying thrombogenic condition had not been systematically carried out. In a patient with lupus anticoagulant, inferior vena cava thrombosis was shown to transform into membranous obstruction. Histopathology of membranous obstruction strongly suggests a thrombotic origin. An associated obstruction of the hepatic vein consists of various types: the termination of one, two, or three hepatic veins may be obliterated; the hepatic vein opening can be located below or above the membranous obstruction. Such a variety is less compatible with a congenital malformation than with one that has an acquired origin.

Clinical Features

The prevalence of the main manifestations of hepatic venous outflow block in a series of 87 patients admitted to Hôpital Beaujon is described in Table 26–2. Manifestations differ according to the date at which patients were seen, because a noninvasive imaging procedure now allows easy recognition of previously overlooked cases. Patients can be assigned to one of three main categories of clinical variants (Table 26–3).

Asymptomatic Variant

This entity has now been individualized. These patients have no ascites, hepatomegaly, or abdominal pain. Hepatic outflow obstruction is either fortuitously discovered by imaging investigation of other complaints or documented by the investigation for abnormal liver tests. Persistent patency of one large hepatic vein or the development of a large venous collateral probably explains the absence of clinical manifestations in these patients (Fig. 26–4). Approximately 20% of patients with hepatic venous outflow block seen since 1990 can be placed in this category.

Acute/Subacute Variants

This entity is characterized by the rapid development of ascites with hepatomegaly, functional renal failure, and jaun-

Table 26–3 Obstruction of Hepatic Veins: Clinical Variants

	Asymptomatic	Acute	Chronic
Ascites	Absent	Present	Present
Prothrombin	Normal	<50%	>50%
Alanine aminotransferase	Normal	>5 times the upper limit of normal	<2 times the upper limit of normal
Functional renal failure	Absent	Usually Present	Usually Absent
Relative prevalence	20%	25%	55%

dice. Serum aminotransferase is higher than five times the upper limit of the normal range. The prothrombin level is less than 40% of normal. This syndrome develops within 1 month. Approximately 25% of patients with hepatic outflow block fall into this group. The prognosis is good in the short term, but it could be worse than in the chronic variant in the long term. In exceptional cases, fulminant liver failure may occur.

Chronic Variants

This entity is characterized by progressive formation of ascites over 2 months or more. Serum aminotransferase is slightly increased or normal. Jaundice is absent. The prothrombin level is higher than 40% of normal. A functional renal failure is present only in half of the cases. Approximately 55% of the patients with hepatic outflow block can be ascribed to this group.

The spontaneous outcome is not well known, because many patients undergo surgery. There have been reports of spontaneous regression of severe acute manifestations. Three major complications may occur: (1) Rapidly developing liver failure is uncommon; (2) Gastrointestinal bleeding occurs in approximately 15% of patients and was responsible for most deaths observed before the introduction of the portosystemic shunt in the therapy of hepatic venous outflow block; and (3) Ascites is the main complication; in our experience, ascites is resistant to medical therapy at the time of presentation in one third of the patients or is associated with functional renal failure; in one third of the patients, ascites can be controlled initially by medical therapy; however, within 6 months, ascites becomes resistant; in one third of the patients, ascites is and remains easily controlled by medical therapy.

Several features of membranous obstruction of the inferior vena cava are distinct from those of hepatic vein obstruction: (1) The clinical manifestations develop much more insidiously; ascites is usually absent; prominent subcutaneous thoracic, lumbar, and abdominal collaterals are common; all these manifestations have been present for several years before patients seek medical attention; (2) Centrilobular congestion is not as marked as in cases of primary lesions of the hepatic veins; portal fibrosis and cirrhosis are more common; and (3) Hepatocellular carcinoma may develop although this complication has been exceptionally encountered in patients with a pure large hepatic vein obstruction.

Diagnosis

The diagnosis of hepatic venous outflow block should be suspected in the following circumstances: (1) whenever ascites and liver enlargement and upper abdominal pain are simultaneously present; (2) in patients with signs of chronic liver disease, whenever intractable ascites contrasts with mildly altered liver function tests; (3) whenever liver disease is documented in a patient with a known thrombogenic disorder; (4) whenever fulminant hepatic failure is associated with liver enlargement and ascites; and (5) whenever chronic liver disease remains unexplained after alcoholism, chronic viral hepatitis, autoimmunity, iron overload, Wilson's disease, and α_1-antitrypsin

deficiency have been excluded. In most cases, noninvasive imaging procedures give evidence of an obstruction of the hepatic outflow. In patients in whom the noninvasive imaging procedures fail to establish the diagnosis, a liver biopsy should be performed. Rarely, opacification of the hepatic veins is needed.

Ultrasonography

In 75% of the patients with an obstruction of the main hepatic veins, the diagnosis can be based simply on ultrasonography. The specific features are: echogenic material in the lumen of the main hepatic veins or inferior vena cava, stenosis on inferior vena cava or main hepatic veins with upstream dilatation, hyperechogenic cord replacing one of the main hepatic veins, and intrahepatic venous collaterals (Fig. 26–5). Occlusion limited to a hepatic vein ostium may give a false-normal aspect of that vein. Nonvisualization, tortuosity, and reduced diameter of the main hepatic veins are frequently noted; however, these abnormalities are also present in cirrhosis in the absence of obstruction of the main hepatic veins.

The patency of the portal vein and superior mesenteric vein can be well evaluated by ultrasonography. This information is essential for the choice of therapeutic options.

Pulsed Doppler and color Doppler imaging improve the diagnostic accuracy of ultrasound (see Fig. 26–5).

Computed Tomography

Contrast infusion produces characteristic images: in the early phase, there is a mottled enhancement of the liver, predominating in the peripheral and perihilar regions. In the late phase, opacification of the liver becomes homogeneous. Tumors that invade or compress the hepatic veins are well delineated by computed tomography.

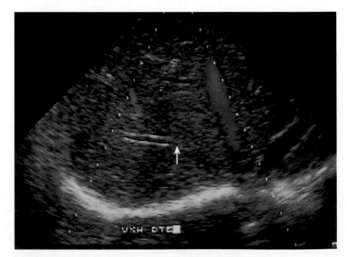

Figure 26–5
Demonstration by color Doppler ultrasound of an abnormal collateral (colored in red, i.e., flowing toward the probe at the top) connecting an obstructed right hepatic vein (*arrow*) to a patent middle hepatic vein (colored in blue, i.e., flowing off the probe).

Magnetic Resonance Imaging

The main hepatic veins are well recognized by magnetic resonance imaging. Small series have suggested that magnetic resonance imaging is as efficacious as ultrasonography for recognizing hepatic vein obstruction and intrahepatic collateral circulation (see Fig. 26–4); it might be better than ultrasonography for studying the inferior vena cava.

Liver Biopsy

According to our experience, in about half of the cases of hepatic vein occlusion, coagulation disorders preclude percutaneous needle biopsy of the liver; however, in 90% of our patients, noninvasive imaging procedures render liver biopsy unnecessary. The characteristic histologic lesions (i.e., centrilobular congestion) (see Fig. 26–3) may not be obvious in needle biopsy specimens, especially in patients with long-standing hepatic venous outflow block and cirrhosis.

Angiography

Opacification of the hepatic veins can be obtained by using transhepatic thin needle puncture of a hepatic vein radicle or by retrograde cannulation of the hepatic veins via the superior or inferior vena cava. The former procedure is preferred to the latter procedure, because it gives better delineation of hepatic vein lesions. When severe coagulation disorders or massive ascites are present, the only feasible procedure is retrograde cannulation. Angiographic abnormalities indicating hepatic vein occlusion are: (1) segmental obliteration or stenosis of a main hepatic vein (Fig. 26–6); (2) luminal filling defects; and (3) opacification of a collateral network.

Failure to cannulate the hepatic vein ostia is only presumptive evidence for hepatic vein occlusion. A drawback of retrograde cannulation is the risk of aggravating thrombosis or dislodging a recent thrombus.

Patency of the inferior vena cava is a major determinant of the treatment. Inferior vena cavography must be performed whenever patency cannot be clearly demonstrated by noninvasive imaging procedures (Fig. 26–7). Inferior vena cavography must be combined with a measurement of inferior vena cava pressure to assess the hemodynamic consequences of compression by an hypertrophied caudal lobe.

Prevention of renal failure induced by contrast agent is essential in patients with hepatic venous outflow block. Whenever pharmacologic thrombolysis is envisaged, the invasive angiographic procedures should not be done.

Treatment and Prognosis

Treatment aims at four goals: (1) eradication or control of the cause, (2) prevention of venous thromboses, (3) control of manifestations with nonspecific measures, and (4) restoration of the hepatic venous outflow in the hope that this is associated with improved survival.

Treatment of the Cause

This essential part of the therapeutic strategy is beyond the scope of this chapter.

Prevention of Other Venous Thromboses

Prevention of the development of thrombosis in still patent hepatic veins, the inferior vena cava, the portal vein, and

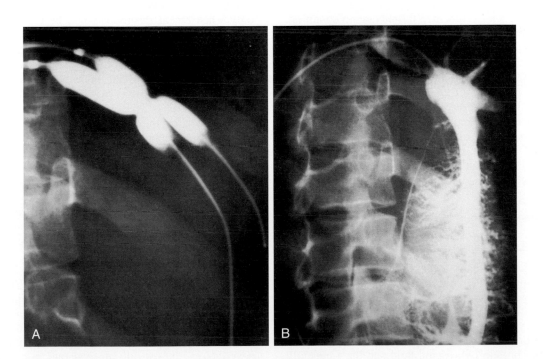

Figure 26–6
A, Retrograde hepatic venography in a patient with myeloproliferative disease and a short length of stenosis on the trunk of the middle and left hepatic veins. *B,* The stenosis is better outlined during an unsuccessful attempt at percutaneous angioplasty.

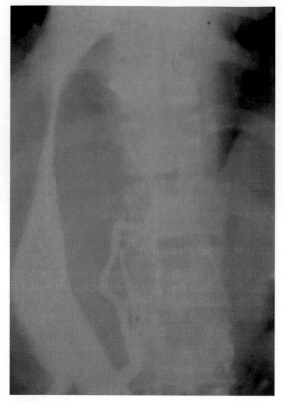

Figure 26–7
Characteristic compression of the inferior vena cava by the enlarged caudate lobe in a patient with hepatic venous obstruction. This compression may lessen the efficacy of a portacaval shunt in decreasing the intrahepatic pressure.

also other venous territories is very important. It is justified in the patients with a documented thrombogenic condition. It is also justified when no cause has been identified, on the assumption that a thrombogenic condition is probably present but has been overlooked. In our experience, heparin in the early phase and a vitamin K antagonist in the long term can be used safely. Overt primary myeloproliferative disorders must be treated urgently.

An additional justification for anticoagulation is the observation that treatment with heparin alone has allowed recanalization of thrombosed hepatic veins and of a thrombosed portal vein associated with thrombosed hepatic veins to take place without the need for an operation.

Control of Manifestations with Nonspecific Measures

Treatment of Ascites

Control of ascites is usually achieved with diuretics. When diuretics are inefficient, paracentesis with an infusion of albumin is indicated. Peritoneovenous shunting should be done only when ascites is resistant to medical therapy and portosystemic shunting is not feasible; obstruction of the valve and thrombosis of the recipient vein are common, because of the protein-rich ascitic fluid and the frequently associated thrombogenic condition. When control of ascites requires permanent diuretic therapy, an operation

aimed at restoration of hepatic blood outflow must be considered.

Treatment of Gastrointestinal Bleeding Due to Portal Hypertension

The procedures that have proved to be efficient in cirrhosis can be used in patients with hepatic vein thrombosis with the following particularities. During active bleeding, balloon tamponade or endoscopic therapy should be preferred to vasoconstrictor agents, because the reduction in splanchnic blood flow might precipitate mesenteric or portal vein thrombosis and intestinal infarction in patients with a thrombogenic disorder. Prevention of first or recurrent bleeding should rely first on β-adrenergic blocking agents, because the associated anticoagulant therapy may make endoscopic therapy difficult. When bleeding recurs or is difficult to control, an operation aimed at restoration of hepatic blood outflow must be considered.

Restoration of Hepatic Blood Outflow

This aspect of the treatment aims to correct sinusoidal and portal venous hypertension, thus controlling ascites and preventing gastrointestinal bleeding. Another theoretical goal is to reduce hepatic ischemia and therefore the severity of liver failure. There are three ways to restore hepatic blood outflow: (1) repermeation of obstructed hepatic venous outflow, (2) portosystemic shunting, and (3) transplantation.

Restoration of Obstructed Hepatic Venous Outflow

Thrombolytic therapy has achieved good results in selected cases of hepatic vein or inferior vena cava thrombosis. However, failure has also been reported. Series of consecutive cases are awaited. This therapy should be used early, only when recent thrombosis can be clearly documented. The criteria for recent thrombosis could be an increase in serum aminotransferase activity to values higher than fivefold the upper limit of normal values. When thrombolytic therapy is considered, no invasive diagnostic procedure should be done.

Angioplasty has been attempted in patients with a short length stenosis of the hepatic veins, usually using the percutaneous endoluminal route. Although an immediate relief of obstruction was obtained in most reported cases, recurrence was common. Insertion of metallic stents may prevent restenosis. Several procedures have been used for direct treatment of membranous obstruction of the inferior vena cava—transcardiac membranotomy and percutaneous transluminal angioplasty using dilatation balloons or laser. A recurrence of stenosis can occur but may be prevented by the insertion of an expandable metallic stent. Various reconstructive or caval-atrial bypass operations have also been used and associated with extracorporeal circulation, but preference is now given to percutaneous angioplasty. These procedures are justified only when at least one main hepatic vein remains patent and drains into the caudal segment of the inferior vena cava. Mortality can be high, up to 20%; nevertheless, the overall survival rate in operated patients seems to be better than the spontaneous outcome.

Dorsocranial liver resection with direct hepatoatrial anas-

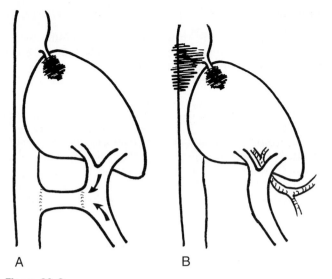

Figure 26–8
Schematic representation of the effect of laterolateral portosystemic shunting in hepatic venous outflow obstruction. *A,* Laterolateral portacaval shunting turns the portal vein into an outflow tract. *B,* Marked compression or occlusion of the inferior vena cava precludes construction of a portacaval shunt. Portosystemic shunting is still possible using a radicle of the superior vena cava or the right atrium as a termination for the shunt.

tomosis was proposed on the basis of the observation that hepatic veins are usually occluded in their terminal portion. Late results do suggest that it is as good an operation as portosystemic shunting in patients with a patent portal vein and a compressed or occluded inferior vena cava. The results in patients with a thrombosed portal vein are less impressive.

Portosystemic Shunting

Transformation of the portal vein into an outflow tract is the rationale for portosystemic shunting (Fig. 26–8).

A side-to-side portacaval shunt and a mesocaval shunt have given the best results. Interposition of a venous graft is usually necessary. In-hospital mortality ranges from 0 to 30%. Most of the patients have no ascites at 1 year of follow-up. Shunt thrombosis occurs in approximately 25% of patients and is usually an early complication. Although the level of pressure in the inferior vena cava has little value in predicting the outcome of surgery; it is usually accepted

that a pressure in the inferior vena cava exceeding 20 mm Hg precludes portacaval or mesocaval shunting.

Portoatrial and mesoatrial shunts using a long prosthetic graft are a logical solution to cope with simultaneous occlusion of the hepatic veins and occlusion of the inferior vena cava, when the portal vein is patent. The initial results have been disappointing: The mortality was close to 60% at 1 year of follow-up; the risk of thrombosis of the long prosthetic graft ranges from 30% to 40%, but recent series have achieved results similar to those of portacaval or mesocaval shunts. Anastomosis of the portal vein to the innominate vein has been proposed to avoid the opening of the pericardium and the ensuing risk of tamponade.

Transjugular intrahepatic portosystemic shunting (TIPS) has been proposed. If long-term patency is achieved, it may represent a valuable alternative to surgical shunting.

Liver Transplantation

Liver transplantation has been used as an alternative to portacaval and mesocaval shunts. Overall results are similar to those of portosystemic shunting. There are three critical issues in the debate regarding whether or not to perform a transplantation in patients with hepatic venous outflow block. The first issue pertains to the risk of thromboses of the vascular anastomoses and of recurrent thrombosis of the hepatic veins. This risk has been controlled with systematic early postoperative anticoagulation. The second issue relates to the risk that immunosuppression exacerbates the myeloproliferative disorder that is commonly associated with a transplant. At present, no data can substantiate this fear. The third issue, which is still unresolved, is to determine whether hepatic transplantation is an alternative to portosystemic shunting, a rescue operation after a failing portosystemic shunt, or a primary operation in patients with predictably bad results after portosystemic shunting. Because portacaval and mesocaval shunting have achieved good results in patients without severe liver lesions, hepatic transplantation should be reserved for patients with severe cirrhosis or with fulminant liver failure.

Indications

The indications for the currently available procedures mainly depend on three conditions: the presence or the absence of manifestations, the patency of the portal vein and of the inferior vena cava, and the presence or absence of severe liver failure (Table 26–4).

Table 26–4 Obstruction of the Hepatic Veins or Suprahepatic Inferior Vena Cava: Proposed Treatment

Manifestations Absent or Easily Controlled	Anticoagulation Symptomatic Treatment		
Manifestations not easily controlled	Portal vein patent	No severe liver failure	Angioplasty (preferably percutaneous) If impossible: portosystemic shunting
		Severe liver failure	Transplantation
	Portal vein obstructed	No severe liver failure	Angioplasty (preferably percutaneous) If impossible: hepatoatrial anastomosis
		Severe liver failure	Transplantation if possible

In asymptomatic patients and in patients in whom manifestations have been easily controlled, no operation is justified. When permanent treatment is necessary for ascites or when gastrointestinal bleeding recurs, an operation can be considered. When the portal vein is patent, several therapeutic options can be discussed.

When severe liver failure is present, liver transplantation should be envisaged first. When signs of liver failure are not prominent, percutaneous or surgical angioplasty should be preferred whenever the venous lesions can be corrected. In other cases, a portosystemic shunt can be constructed, the type of which will depend on the patency of the inferior vena cava. When the portal vein is obstructed, liver transplantation can still be done if the mesenteric vein is patent. Otherwise, repermeation of the hepatic veins is critical, because portosystemic shunting cannot be considered. Hepatoatrial anastomosis would theoretically be indicated in this last situation.

Prognosis

The natural history of hepatic venous outflow block is unknown. In most recent series of unselected patients, the survival rate was approximately 60% after a 5-year follow-up. Most of the deaths occur in the first year of follow-up. These series include unselected patients treated with various modalities. The prognosis is dismal in patients with endoluminal tumorous invasion. In patients with nontumorous obstruction the influence of the underlying thrombogenic disease on the prognosis has been well evaluated.

OBSTRUCTION OF THE HEPATIC VENULES: VENO-OCCLUSIVE DISEASE

Epidemiology and Pathophysiology

Obstruction of hepatic venules without involvement of large hepatic veins may be observed in some of the conditions already mentioned (e.g., paroxysmal nocturnal hemoglobinuria, and treatment with dacarbazine). In addition, various lesions of the hepatic venules have been described in alcoholic liver disease: lymphocytic phlebitis, perivenular fibrosis, and veno-occlusive changes. In hepatic sarcoidosis, granulomas can be found within the wall of hepatic venules.

Veno-occlusive disease of the liver must be distinguished from the lesions mentioned earlier and is characterized by a nonthrombotic, concentric, luminal narrowing of the central or intercalated (sublobular) veins by loose connective tissue, without an obstruction of the large hepatic veins. This definition can be extended to include the earlier stage of the lesion (subendothelial edema with entrapped blood cells) as well as the later stage (perivenular fibrosis and dense fibrous scar replacing the central vein). The venular lesions are always associated with severe hemorrhagic congestion and hepatic cell necrosis affecting the central area of the lobules. In contrast with the rarity of true thrombosis, features suggesting the activation of the coagulation seem to be common. The disease can progress to an extensive central fibrosis with central-to-central or central-to-portal bridging, nodular regeneration, and, ultimately, cirrhosis.

The physiopathologic consequences of hepatic venule obstruction are akin to those of a large vein obstruction.

Etiology

Pyrrolizidine alkaloids, irradiation, antineoplastic drugs, and conditioning for bone marrow transplantation are the main causes of veno-occlusive disease.

Veno-Occlusive Disease Caused by Pyrrolizidine Alkaloids

These alkaloids are found in many plant species. When poisoning is caused by ingestion of flour contaminated with alkaloid-containing plants, the disease may be epidemic. Ingestion of alkaloid-containing plant infusion or decoction (as a herbal tea or an enema) is responsible for most endemic and sporadic cases. Experimental hepatotoxicity is dose dependent. This is relevant to the natural history of the human disease. The acute form results from recent ingestion of large amounts of pyrrolizidine alkaloids, whereas chronic disease results from prolonged ingestion of small amounts of these toxins. The term "veno-occlusive" might be inappropriate to describe the early lesions caused by pyrrolizidine alkaloids. Injury to the perivenular hepatic cells and sinusoids may actually be the initial lesion in the absence of central vein occlusion.

Veno-Occlusive Disease Caused by Irradiation

The clinical onset occurs 2 to 5 weeks after liver irradiation. The level of severity ranges from an asymptomatic to a fatal course. Although sensitivity to liver irradiation varies from one patient to another, a direct relationship is suggested by the limitation of the lesion to the irradiated part of the liver and by the dose-dependent prevalence of the lesion. Veno-occlusive disease rarely occurs below 30 Gy, if irradiation is not associated with administration of antineoplastic drugs.

Veno-Occlusive Disease Caused by Antineoplastic Drugs

Several antineoplastic drugs have been reported to cause veno-occlusive disease. At a cumulative dose ranging from 150 to 2500 g, urethane (ethyl carbamate) induced either an acute or a subacute type of veno-occlusive disease. Most cases were fatal. The drug is no longer used, but a case resulting from surreptitious administration has recently been reported.

Azathioprine and the closely related compounds 6-mercaptopurine and 6-thioguanine have been implicated in several cases of centrilobular hemorrhagic necrosis, which was attributed to veno-occlusive disease. Several features distinguish veno-occlusive disease caused by azathioprine from veno-occlusive disease attributed to other causes. The clinical onset takes place after 6 to 108 months of continuous administration. Most patients are renal transplant recipients who also receive corticosteroids. The initial manifestations are jaundice or liver enlargement rather than ascites. Serum alkaline phosphatase is often increased. Perivenular and perisinusoidal fibrosis are prominent. Veno-occlusive lesions are often associated with peliosis and nodular regenerative hyperplasia.

Several other antineoplastic drugs have been implicated, such as mitomycin C, BCNU (carmustine), indicine-*N*-

oxide, mustine hydrochloride, vincristine, and doxoru-bicin; however, their role has not always been clearly established.

Veno-Occlusive Disease Caused by Conditioning for Bone Marrow Transplantation

Conditioning for bone marrow transplantation has become the major cause of veno-occlusive disease. Conditioning usually includes the administration of cyclophosphamide with or without other alkylating agents, together with total body irradiation. The features of the disease have been reviewed. The clinical onset takes place within 4 weeks after transplantation, with rapidly rising serum bilirubin, upper abdominal pain, liver enlargement, ascites, and weight gain. Liver failure causes or contributes to death in almost half of the patients. The prevalence of veno-occlusive disease is related to elevated aminotransferase values before transplantation, cytoreductive therapy with a high-dose regimen, and previous therapy to the abdomen.

Clinical Manifestations

Similar to an obstruction of the large hepatic veins, acute, subacute, and chronic clinical types of veno-occlusive disease have been recognized. In the acute type, there is sudden abdominal distention caused by enlargement of the liver and ascites. Complete recovery can occur, or the clinical course can be fulminant with early death from liver failure. The subacute type results from incomplete recovery of the acute type. The chronic type is clinically indistinguishable from cirrhosis of any cause.

Diagnosis

The diagnosis of an obstruction of the hepatic venules should be suspected in the same circumstances as those envisaged for the diagnosis of an obstruction of the large hepatic vein and whenever liver disease is documented in a patient with known exposure to pyrrolizidine alkaloids, with recent irradiation, chemotherapy, or bone marrow transplantation. The diagnosis requires that both patency of the large hepatic veins and congestion in the centrilobular area are demonstrated. In the bone marrow transplantation setting, a liver biopsy may be difficult to obtain. When the diagnosis is based on clinical criteria including hepatomegaly, weight gain, and jaundice, the prevalence of veno-occlusive disease after bone marrow transplantation is approximately 54% in recent series. The prevalence of veno-occlusive disease after bone marrow transplantation ranges from 13% to 20% in older series. Clinical criteria tend to overestimate the prevalence of histologically documented criteria. There is a good clinicopathologic correlation when the definition of veno-occlusive disease is extended to include fibrosis and necrosis in acinar zone III.

Treatment

Established veno-occlusive disease might benefit from the prompt administration of thrombolytic agents, although a controlled study to document this is awaited. Prevention of the disorder has been attempted with various pharmacologic agents. A controlled, but unrandomized, study suggested a reduced mortality after the administration of prostaglandin E_2. Benefit from the intravenous infusion of heparin has also been reported.

PELIOSIS HEPATIS

Peliosis hepatis is characterized by blood-filled cavities of various sizes, bordered by hepatocystic plates, and randomly distributed throughout the hepatic lobule. The hepatocytes that border the peliotic cavities are often atrophic or compressed. Peliosis hepatis, sinusoidal dilatation, perisinusoidal fibrosis, and nodular regenerative hyperplasia may coexist. The peliotic cavities consist of dilated sinusoids and the space of Disse (Fig. 26–9).

Epidemiology and Pathophysiology

The pathogenesis is unknown. Indirect evidence suggests two mechanisms: (1) obstruction at the junctions of sinusoids and central veins; and (2) a primary lesion of the sinusoidal (mainly endothelial) cells.

Peliosis hepatis is frequently associated with extrahepatic diseases (listed in Table 26–5). Most of these associated diseases share the following features: (1) a chronic debilitating condition, (2) frequently associated with severe infections, and (3) leading commonly to the administration of androgenic-anabolic steroids. Several drugs and chemicals have been incriminated; however, rather than a direct toxic effect, these substances may only potentiate the action of yet unidentified endogenous factors. In patients with acquired immunodeficiency syndrome (AIDS), an infectious form of peliosis hepatis has been characterized under the name of bacillary peliosis hepatis. It is related to infection by a newly identified pathogen: *Bartonella henselae*.

Peliosis hepatis is associated with portal hypertension attributed to an intrahepatic block as demonstrated by an increased hepatic venous pressure gradient. The mechanism for increased intrahepatic resistance is unknown. Perisinusoidal fibrosis is a late sequela after resolution of the peliotic cavities but can be demonstrated at electron microscopy in the early stages. Perisinusoidal fibrosis could thus explain the intrahepatic block observed in peliosis hepatis.

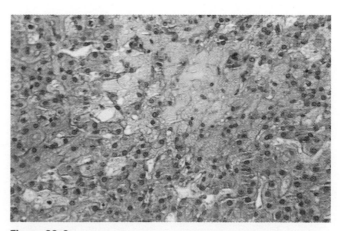

Figure 26–9
Histologic features of peliosis hepatis (Masson trichrome). (Courtesy of Professor Claude Degott.)

Table 26–5 Reported Conditions Associated with Peliosis Hepatis and Sinusoidal Dilatation

Peliosis Hepatis	Sinusoidal Dilatation
Drugs and Chemicals	**Drugs and Chemicals**
Androgenic-anabolic steroids	Contraceptive steroids
Contraceptive steroids	Azathioprine
Antineoplastic drugs	Thorium dioxide
Azathioprine-6 thiocyanine	
Corticosteroids	
Arsenic	
Thorium dioxide	
Vinyl chloride	
Copper sulfate	
Toxic oil syndrome	
Bacterial Infections	**Bacterial Infections**
Endocarditis	Brucellosis
Pneumonia, bronchopneumonia	Tuberculosis
Cellulitis	
Tuberculosis	
Monoclonal Gammopathies	
Multiple myeloma	
Waldenström's macroglobulin- emia	
Systemic light chain deposition	
Myeloproliferative Disorders	
Myelofibrosis	
Polycythemia vera	
Malignancies	**Malignancies**
Solid tumors	Solid tumors
Hodgkin's disease	Hodgkin's disease
	Lymphoma
Anemias	
Fanconi's anemia	
Sideroblastic anemia	
Other Conditions	**Other Conditions**
Renal transplantation	Renal transplantation
Chronic hemodialysis	Pregnancy
Diabetes	Cirrhosis
Acquired immunodeficiency syn- drome	Amyloidosis
	Infectious mononucleosis
	Histiocytosis X

Clinical Manifestations

Manifestations of peliosis hepatis are related to the severity of the lesions: mild lesions induce no sign or symptom, whereas in severe lesions, hepatomegaly, ascites, esophageal varices, or liver failure are present. Liver tests are usually mildly impaired. A marked increase in serum alkaline phosphatase and γ-glutamyl transpeptidase activities can occur. Death results from intraperitoneal bleeding, liver failure, or a complication of the associated conditions but not from portal hypertension.

Diagnosis

Clinical diagnosis is extremely difficult. Liver biopsy is required to demonstrate the blood lakes. In rare cases, macro- scopic blood-filled cavities can be demonstrated at imaging by magnetic resonance imaging, computed tomography scan, or ultrasound.

Treatment and Prognosis

There is no specific treatment. Symptomatic peliosis hepatis should be regarded as a feature of an extremely bad prognosis, even though it is rarely the direct cause of death.

SINUSOIDAL DILATATION

The lesion of sinusoidal dilatation differs from peliosis hepatis in the following characteristics: (1) the ectatic sinusoids do not take the cystic appearance that is typical of peliosis hepatis; (2) the dilatation is not randomly distributed but affects a distinct part (pericentral and midzonal or periportal) of the lobule (Fig. 26–10). However, the separation between the two entities may be difficult to make morphologically and etiologically.

Epidemiology and Pathophysiology

As in peliosis hepatis, sinusoidal dilatation has been reported alone or in association with nodular regenerative hyperplasia and perisinusoidal fibrosis. Table 26–5 lists the conditions that have been reported to be associated with sinusoidal dilatation; these conditions are almost similar to those associated with peliosis hepatis and nodular regenerative hyperplasia.

A distinction should be made between sinusoidal dilatation induced by oral contraceptives and pregnancy, which predominates in the periportal region (zones I and II) and sinusoidal dilatation associated with the other conditions, which predominates in the centrilobular region (zones II and III). The pathogenesis is unknown.

Hemodynamic findings may further distinguish periportal from centrilobular sinusoidal dilatation. In the former, the hepatic venous pressure gradient was normal, whereas in the latter, it was increased.

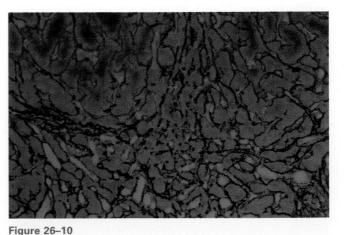

Figure 26–10
Histologic features of sinusoidal dilatation (Reticuline stain). (Courtesy of Professor Claude Degott.)

Clinical Manifestations

Manifestations of sinusoidal dilatation may be absent or include right upper quadrant pain, fever, and hepatomegaly. Ascites and esophageal varices have been reported. The erythrocyte sedimentation rate and serum γ-globulin are almost constantly raised. Liver function test results are moderately abnormal. Perisinusoidal fibrosis may persist as a late sequela. In a few cases, the disease progresses to fibrosis and cirrhosis with esophageal varices, splenomegaly, and hypersplenism.

Diagnosis

The diagnosis of sinusoidal dilatation raises the same difficulties as that of peliosis hepatis. A liver biopsy cannot be avoided. The differential diagnosis of right upper quadrant pain with fever and mild or absent abnormalities of liver tests includes acute cholecystitis, perihepatitis, acute hepatic venous outflow block, and right heart failure. Ultrasound plays a major role in this differential diagnosis.

Treatment and Prognosis

There is no specific treatment for this benign condition. The manifestations disappear with the resolution of the associated acute or chronic disease.

SUGGESTED READINGS

Bellin MF, Challier E, Valla D, et al: Budd-Chiari syndrome: Value of duplex sonography and color Doppler imaging for diagnosis and follow-up. Eur Radiol 5:379–386, 1995.

Blum U, Rössle M, Haag K, et al: Budd-Chiari syndrome: Technical, hemodynamic and clinical results of treatment with transjugular intrahepatic portosystemic shunt. Radiology 197:805–811, 1995.

Dilawari JB, Bambery P, Chawla Y, et al: Hepatic outflow obstruction (Budd Chiari syndrome): Experience with 177 patients and review of the literature. Medicine 73:21–36, 1994.

Gupta S, Barter S, Phillips GWL, et al: Comparison of ultrasonography, computed tomography, and ^{99m}Tc: Liver scan in diagnosis of Budd-Chiari syndrome. Gut 28:242–247, 1987.

Hadengue A, Poliquin M, Vilgrain V, et al: The changing scene of hepatic vein thrombosis: recognition of asymptomatic cases. Gastroenterology 106:1042–1047, 1994.

Kage M, Arakawa M, Kojiro M, Okuda K: Histopathology of membranous obstruction of the inferior vena cava in the Budd-Chiari syndrome. Gastroenterology 102:2081–2090, 1992.

Kohli V, Pande GK, Dev V, et al: Management of hepatic outflow obstruction. Lancet 342:718–722, 1993.

Ludwig J, Hashimoto E, McGill DB, van Heerden JA: Classification of hepatic venous outflow obstruction: Ambiguous terminology of the Budd-Chiari Syndrome. Mayo Clin Proc 65:51–55, 1990.

McDonald GB, Hinds MS, Fisher LD, et al: Veno-occlusive disease of the liver and multiorgan failure after bone marrow transplantation: A cohort study of 355 patients. Ann Intern Med 118:255–267, 1993.

Menu Y, Sebag G, Vigrain V, Nahum H: Budd-Chiari syndrome: MR evaluation. Diagn Interv Radiol 2:23–28, 1990.

Menu Y, Alison D, Lorphelin JM, et al: Budd-Chiari syndrome: US evaluation. Radiology 157:761–764, 1985.

Mitchell MC, Boitnott JK, Kaufman S, et al: Budd-Chiari syndrome: Etiology, diagnosis, management. Medicine 61:199–218, 1982.

Nishikawa N, Miyoshi S, Imai Y, et al: Treatment of Budd-Chiari syndrome in polycythemia vera by repeated percutaneous transluminal angioplasty of the hepatic vein stenosis. Postgrad Med J 58:511–514, 1982.

Orloff MJ, Orloff MS, Daily PO: Long-term results of treatment of Budd-Chiari syndrome with portal decompression. Arch Surg 127:1182–1188, 1992.

Panis Y, Belghiti J, Valla D, et al: Portosystemic shunt in Budd-Chiari syndrome: Long-term survival and factors affecting shunt patency in 25 patients in Western countries. Surgery 115:276–281, 1994.

Parker RGF: Occlusion of the hepatic veins in man. Medicine (Baltimore) 38:369–402, 1959.

Rector WG, Xu Y, Goldstein L, et al: Membranous obstruction of inferior vena cava in the United States. Medicine 64:134–143, 1985.

Ringe B, Lang H, Oldhafer KJ, et al: Which is the best surgery for Budd-Chiari syndrome: Venous decompression or liver transplantation? A single-center experience with 50 patients. Hepatology 21:1337–1344, 1995.

Shafer AI: Hypercoagulable states: Molecular genetics to clinical practice. Lancet 344:1739–1742, 1994.

Valla D, Dhumeaux D, Babany G, et al: Hepatic vein thrombosis in paroxysmal nocturnal hemoglobinuria: A spectrum from asymptomatic occlusion of hepatic venules to fatal Budd-Chiari syndrome. Gastroenterology 93:569–575, 1987.

Valla D, Le MG, Poynard T, et al: Risk of hepatic vein thrombosis in relation to recent use of oral contraceptives: A case-control study. Gastroenterology 90:807–811, 1986.

Valla D, Benhamou JP: Drug-induced vascular and sinusoidal lesions of the liver. Baillières Clin Gastroenterol 2:481–500, 1988.

Valla D, Benhamou JP: Obstruction of the hepatic veins or suprahepatic inferior vena cava. Dig Dis 14:99–118, 1996.

Valla D, Casadevall N, Lacombe C, et al: Primary myeloprolifcrative disorders and hepatic vein thrombosis: A prospective study of erythroid colony formation in vitro in 20 patients with Budd-Chiari syndrome. Ann Intern Med 103:325–334, 1985.

Voinchet O, Degott C, Scoazec JY, et al: Peliosis hepatis, nodular regenerative hyperplasia of the liver, and light chain deposition in a patient with Waldenström's macroglobulinemia. Gastroenterology 95:482–486, 1988.

Wang Z, Zhu Y, Wang S, et al: Recognition and management of Budd-Chiari syndrome: Report of one hundred cases. J Vasc Surg 10:149–156, 1989.

Wanless IR, Peterson P, Das A, et al: Hepatic vascular disease and portal hypertension in polycythemia vera and agnogenic myeloid metaplasia: A clinicopathological study of 145 patients examined at autopsy. Hepatology 12:1166–1174, 1990.

Winkler K, Poulsen H: Liver disease with periportal sinusoidal dilatation: A possible complication to contraceptive steroids. Scand J Gastroenterol 10:699–704, 1975.

27

Liver Disease and Pregnancy

Grace L. Su
Rebecca Van Dyke

L iver disease that occurs during pregnancy can be divided into three categories: liver diseases that are unique to pregnancy; liver diseases that occur more commonly with or because of pregnancy; and acute or chronic liver diseases that exist coincidentally with pregnancy (Table 27–1). The first category contains diseases such as intrahepatic cholestasis of pregnancy (IHCP), pre-eclampsia/eclampsia/HELLP syndrome, and acute fatty liver of pregnancy. The latter two categories include many types of liver diseases; however, in this chapter we will focus on liver diseases that are affected by the pregnant state or liver diseases that have special therapeutic implications in the setting of pregnancy. For example, the pregnant state is a risk factor for common problems such as the development of gallstones and biliary colic as well as rare diseases, such as herpes hepatitis and Budd-Chiari syndrome. Other liver diseases can be more devastating for the pregnant woman (e.g., hepatitis E) or may have, like hepatitis B, implications for the newborn infant. Finally, in any patient with chronic liver disease, the consequences of pregnancy must be considered carefully, both for the mother and the child.

EPIDEMIOLOGY

Liver disease is uncommon during pregnancy; however, jaundice, which is often a sign of significant liver disease, is reported in approximately 1 in 1500 to 1 in 5000 pregnancies. The most common reason for jaundice during pregnancy in the United States is viral hepatitis, a reflection of the prevalence of viral hepatitis in the general population. Other than hepatitis E, which is rarely encountered in the United States, the incidence and course of hepatitis A, B, and C are not different in the pregnant patient as opposed to

the nonpregnant patient. The next most common cause of jaundice is a disease unique to pregnancy, IHCP, which varies in prevalence worldwide. IHCP is seen more often in Chile where, at least in the past, up to as many as 10% of pregnancies are affected; it also occurs in patients of Scandinavian or Polish descent. This disease is rare in African-Americans and Asian-Americans.

NORMAL CHANGES IN LIVER TESTS DURING PREGNANCY

Various laboratory and physical findings that occur during normal pregnancy can be mistaken for evidence of liver disease. On physical examination, normal pregnant women may have peripheral edema as a result of a decrease in lymphatic and venous drainage from the lower extremities caused by pressure exerted by a gravid uterus or as a result of lower limb venous incompetence. Spider nevi and palmar erythema are common findings in normal pregnancy (particularly in the second and third trimester) and are related to increases in serum estrogen level. During pregnancy biochemical liver tests may also be affected (Table 27–2). Plasma albumin levels are decreased as a result of increasing plasma volume. Alkaline phosphatase normally increases throughout pregnancy to as much as 2 times the upper limits of normal as a result of both placental production and increased bone mobilization. These findings thus are not reliable indicators of liver disease. On the other hand, the liver and spleen are not easily palpable in mid- to late pregnancy owing to displacement by the gravid uterus; therefore, palpation of these organs likely reflects abnormal hepatosplenomegaly. There have been a few reports that blood levels of serum alanine aminotransferase (ALT) and serum aspartate aminotransferase (AST) may be slightly increased

Table 27–1 Liver Diseases in Pregnancy

Liver Diseases Unique to Pregnancy	Liver Diseases Occurring More Commonly in Pregnancy	Pre-existing Liver Diseases Coincident with Pregnancy
Hyperemesis gravidarum	Gallstones (symptomatic)	Hepatitis B and C
Intrahepatic cholestasis of pregnancy	Fulminant hepatitis E	Autoimmune hepatitis
Preeclampsia/HELLP	Budd-Chiari syndrome	Wilson's disease
Acute fatty liver of pregnancy	Herpes hepatitis	Cirrhosis
		Alcoholic liver disease

in later pregnancy compared with normal nonpregnant women, but these values do not exceed the upper limits of normal and therefore clear, consistent increases in AST and ALT are reliable clues to liver disease. Other liver function tests such as 5′ nucleotidase, γ-glutamyl transpeptidase, and bilirubin remain either unchanged or may actually decrease with normal pregnancy.

PATHOPHYSIOLOGY AND CLINICAL FEATURES

Liver Diseases Unique to Pregnancy

Hyperemesis gravidarum is an idiopathic syndrome of severe nausea and vomiting that generally occurs in the first trimester of pregnancy, typically before 10 weeks of gestation. Risk factors for hyperemesis gravidarum include young age, obesity, nulliparity, tobacco use, and twin gestation. The severity of the nausea and vomiting can lead to dehydration, malnutrition, and metabolic acidosis. In up to 50% of patients, abnormal biochemical liver tests may be noted, usually elevation of both serum bilirubin and aminotransferases. The elevations tend to be mild with bilirubin levels usually less than 4 mg/dL and aminotransferases up to 200 U/L. Liver biopsy shows only mild fatty change or no abnormality. Because liver injury appears only in severe disease (i.e., cases in which there is dehydration and malnutrition requiring hospitalization), the liver abnormalities found in these patients may be caused by malnutrition and dehydration.

There is no specific treatment for liver abnormalities found in hyperemesis gravidarum other than general supportive care with rehydration and correction of electrolyte imbalance and metabolic acidosis. Cessation of oral feedings may be necessary to reduce nausea and vomiting, but malnutrition will need to be carefully assessed. Total parenteral nutrition may be necessary in severe cases.

IHCP is also known by several other names, including

benign cholestasis of pregnancy, cholestasis of pregnancy, and obstetric cholestasis. The disease usually presents in the third trimester at a mean gestation time of 30 weeks. Patients typically present with generalized pruritus that affects the trunk, extremities, palms, and soles. As with other pruritic syndromes, the itching is usually worse at night and can become very intense. Patients often have a general sense of malaise and fatigue. Patients may have a family or personal history of pruritus during pregnancy or prior oral contraceptive use. Frank jaundice occurs in about one third to one half of patients, usually after the onset of pruritus. The jaundice is generally not severe, and bilirubin levels rarely rise above 6 mg/dL. Alkaline phosphatase usually rises above what is expected from normal pregnancy to 3 to 4 times the upper limits of normal. Serum aminotransferases can also increase variably from 2- to 10-fold. Serum bile acids are increased to 10- to 100-fold. In severe cases, with clinically obvious jaundice, steatorrhea and vitamin K deficiency may occur owing to intestinal bile salt deficiency. Liver biopsy shows a "bland" cholestasis with minimal or no inflammation (Fig. 27–1).

The pathophysiology of IHCP is unknown, but a role for inherited hypersensitivity to the cholestatic effects of estrogen has been postulated. The observations of unequal ethnic distribution support a role for genetic predisposition. A role for hypersensitivity to the cholestatic effects of estrogen is supported by observations that in both humans and animals, exogenous estrogen impairs hepatic uptake as well as biliary secretion of both bilirubin and bile salts and by the occurrence of this disease in the third trimester when serum estrogen levels peak. Interestingly, even in high prevalence areas, IHCP is now much less common now than a decade ago, suggesting that other factors may also play a role.

The treatment of choice for IHCP is delivery of the infant, which is followed by resolution of pruritus, although this may not always be feasible because of fetal immaturity. If the pruritus is severe, therapy with ursodeoxycholic acid (10 to 15 mg/kg/day) in divided doses (2 to 3 times daily) or cholestyramine (8 to 16 g/day) in divided doses (3 to 4 times

Table 27–2 Expected Changes in Liver Function Tests in Pregnant Women

Test	First Trimester	Second Trimester	Third Trimester
Albumin	Decreased	Decreased	Decreased
Alkaline phosphatase	Unchanged	Unchanged	Increased
Serum alanine aminotransferase-ALT	Unchanged	Unchanged or increased (but within normal limits)	Unchanged or increased (but within normal limits)

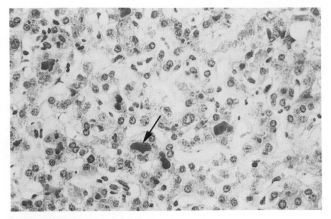

Figure 27-1
Liver biopsy from a patient with intrahepatic cholestasis showing cholestatic changes including bile accumulation in canalicular spaces *(arrow)*.

daily) has been helpful. No maternal or fetal toxicities related to these agents have been observed. Cholestyramine is most effective if given early, at the time of symptom onset, and may take more than 2 weeks to become fully effective. Other treatments that have been tried with initial success but that did not show efficacy in randomized prospective studies include s-adenosyl-L-methionine and dexamethasone. In addition to the debilitating symptom of pruritus, infants of mothers with IHCP appear to be at some increased risk of fetal distress, low birthweight, perinatal mortality, and stillbirth. Thus, pregnancies should be monitored closely, and delivery should be initiated when feasible. The use of vitamin K has been advocated in jaundiced patients, especially those receiving cholestyramine, to decrease postpartum bleeding.

Preeclampsia, a common disease in pregnancy, has been associated with a spectrum of liver injury. Preeclampsia, which is characterized by the triad of hypertension, proteinuria, and edema, occurs in the late second trimester or third trimester. Eclampsia is a more severe stage of the disease with extreme hypertension ($\geq$160/100), proteinuria ($\geq$5 g/24 hr), and evidence of symptomatic organ damage (e.g., seizures, headaches, visual disturbances, epigastric or right upper quadrant pain, congestive heart failure, pulmonary edema, azotemia, or oliguria). Often the distinction between preeclampsia and eclampsia is difficult to discern, because they represent parts of a spectrum of disease. Preeclampsia/eclampsia occurs in approximately 5% to 10% of pregnancies. Risk factors for the development of preeclampsia/eclampsia include pre-existing hypertension, extremes of childbearing age, first pregnancy, and the presence of multiple gestations.

Although its pathogenesis is unknown, preeclampsia/eclampsia is a systemic disease of abnormal endothelial reactivity that can affect multiple organs. The initial event may be abnormal trophoblastic implantation leading to reduced tissue perfusion and endothelial dysfunction. Mothers exhibit decreased, or normal, cardiac output in the face of decreased plasma volume, accompanied by an increased systemic vascular resistance; decreased perfusion of the placenta, kidney, liver, and brain; abnormal endothelial reactiv-

ity with vasospasm; deposition of fibrin in vascular spaces; and activation of the coagulation cascade. These lead to ischemic damage of multiple organs, including the liver. On liver biopsy, one can see fibrin thrombi in the periportal sinusoids, hepatocyte necrosis, and periportal hemorrhage (Fig. 27-2).

Liver disorders associated with preeclampsia include a range of abnormalities from mildly abnormal liver tests to hepatic infarction, subcapsular hematoma, and hepatic rupture. The frequency and severity of liver function test abnormalities, such as aminotransferase elevations, is correlated with the severity of preeclampsia/eclampsia. This likely reflects the degree of hepatocellular necrosis that occurs with the increasing severity of disease. HELLP syndrome (*h*emolysis, *e*levated *l*iver enzymes, and *l*ow *p*latelet count), the most common clinical manifestation of preeclampsia-related liver disease, denotes a subset of women who exhibit evidence of microangiopathic hemolytic anemia, thrombocytopenia, and elevated liver tests. In patients with HELLP syndrome, serum transaminases are elevated from 2 to 50 times normal. Because of associated hemolysis, serum lactic dehydrogenase (LDH) and bilirubin are also elevated to a variable degree. Characteristically, the prothrombin time is usually normal despite these elevated liver enzymes. HELLP syndrome occurs in 4% to 12% of patients with severe preeclampsia with an overall incidence of 0.1% to 0.6% of pregnancies.

Hepatic infarction, subcapsular hematoma, and hepatic rupture, which are estimated to occur in 1:45,000 pregnancies, are rarer complications of preeclampsia/eclampsia with significant morbidity and mortality. Patients usually present in the third trimester or the immediate postpartum period with abdominal pain, hypotension, fever, leukocytosis, nausea, vomiting, and abnormal liver tests. It is likely that these disorders represent a progression from hepatic infarction to subcapsular hematoma, and subsequently, to uncontrolled hepatic rupture. Because it may be difficult to differentiate on clinical grounds a contained subcapsular hematoma from free hepatic rupture, abdominal imaging, particularly with computed tomography, can be very helpful in the evaluation of these patients (Fig. 27-3). The treatment

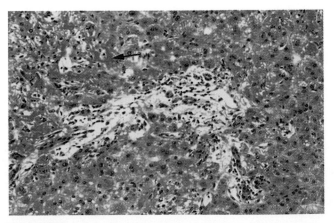

Figure 27-2
Liver biopsy from a patient with preeclampsia/eclampsia. Characteristic fibrin thrombi *(arrow)* are seen in the periportal sinusoidal space.

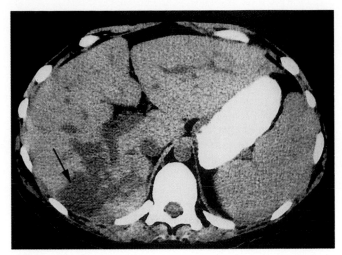

Figure 27–3
Computed tomography scan of a patient with preeclampsia/eclampsia who developed hepatic infarction *(arrow)*.

of choice for preeclampsia–related liver diseases is early delivery of the infant. For acute hepatic rupture, a cesarean section should be performed emergently with surgical drainage and packing of the liver. Some selected cases can be treated with hepatic artery embolization. Contained subcapsular hematomas do not need specific treatment and resolve slowly after delivery.

Acute fatty liver of pregnancy is a potentially devastating microvesicular fatty liver disease that occurs primarily in the third trimester or the first few days postpartum. A rare disorder, it is estimated to occur in approximately 1 in 13,000 pregnancies. Patients usually note the onset of nausea and vomiting accompanied by abdominal pain, particularly in the right upper quadrant or epigastrium. Viral-like symptoms such as malaise, headache, and anorexia may predominate. Rarely, patients present with symptoms of polydipsia and evidence of diabetes insipidus. Acute renal failure is common, possibly owing to fat deposits in renal tubular cells. Patients typically develop progressive jaundice, but pruritus is rare. The liver is a normal size or small. Acute liver failure may ensue with the onset of severe coagulopathy and hypoglycemia. The serum transaminases are elevated but are relatively unimpressive, especially in view of other laboratory evidence of fulminant hepatic failure and do not usually rise above 10-fold the upper limit of normal. Levels higher than this should prompt consideration of other diagnoses, such as hepatic ischemia. The development of hepatic encephalopathy with somnolence progressing to coma portends a poor outcome. On liver biopsy, the pathognomonic finding is that of centrilobular microvesicular fatty infiltration with little or no inflammation (Fig. 27–4*A*). The preportal hepatocytes are relatively spared. A frozen section of the liver biopsy stained for fat with an oil red O stain can be very helpful, especially if fatty infiltration is not obvious on a hematoxylin and eosin stain (see Fig. 27–4*B*).

The pathogenesis of acute fatty liver of pregnancy is unknown, although in as many as half of the cases, there are associated symptoms characteristic of preeclampsia. Furthermore, some cases occur in mothers of fetuses homozygous for genetic defects in hepatic mitochondrial

β-oxidation of long chain fatty acids. At this time, the only treatment for acute fatty liver of pregnancy is early delivery (because the disease appears to subside spontaneously after delivery) and supportive care.

Liver Diseases Occurring More Commonly with Pregnancy

Pregnancy is a risk factor for the development of biliary sludge and *cholesterol gallstones*. This may be related to pregnancy-induced decreases in motility of gallbladder smooth muscle due to elevated progesterone levels and an increase in biliary cholesterol secretion caused by higher estrogen levels. Indeed, transient formation of sludge and stones occurs commonly during normal pregnancy, when monitored by ultrasound examination. In addition, during pregnancy, gallstones are more likely to cause symptoms. Clinically, patients with gallstone disease present in a manner similar to that of the nonpregnant patient, and the management is the same, although elective cholecystectomy is usually deferred until after delivery.

Budd-Chiari syndrome, or hepatic vein thrombosis, is a rare disease that may occur in some women during pregnancy. Pregnancy, like the use of oral contraceptives, is thought to contribute to a hypercoagulable state that increases the risk of thrombotic diseases. In addition to

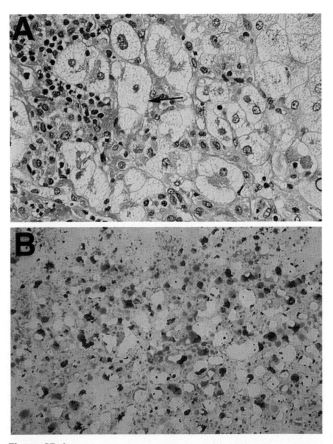

Figure 27–4
Liver biopsy from a patient with acute fatty liver of pregnancy. *A,* Microvesicular fatty change in hepatocytes *(arrow)*. *B,* Oil red O stain.

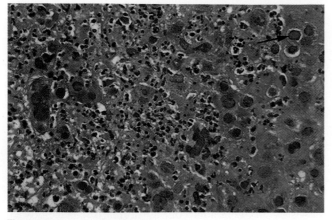

Figure 27-5
Liver biopsy from a patient with *Herpes simplex* hepatitis. There is widespread hepatocyte necrosis with many characteristic eosinophilic intranuclear viral inclusions *(arrow)*.

pregnancy, however, patients with Budd-Chiari syndrome may also have other underlying hypercoagulable states (e.g., myeloproliferative disorders) that are uncovered during pregnancy. The syndrome typically occurs shortly postpartum with the sudden onset of abdominal pain and ascites. As in patients with Budd-Chiari syndrome without pregnancy, the diagnosis is confirmed by venography. Liver biopsy shows centrilobular congestion. Treatment options are unsatisfactory.

Herpes simplex virus (HSV) hepatitis is a rare form of hepatitis that has been reported to occur predominantly in pregnant women and immunocompromised patients. It represents a form of disseminated primary herpes infection, and most cases are caused by herpes simplex type 2. All of the reported cases have occurred in the second or third trimester. Systemic symptoms are very common, including fever, chills, malaise, and nausea. Mucocutaneous lesions characteristic of HSV, if present, are helpful in making the diagnosis. Anicteric liver failure is the hallmark of this disease. The serum aminotransferases are usually extremely elevated, rising to levels of 25- to 40-fold normal. In contrast, serum bilirubin is only mildly elevated to a level about 2- to 3-fold that of normal. Marked hepatocellular dysfunction is evident as indicated by an increased prothrombin time. Although a computed tomography scan may show multiple nonenhancing low-density lesions, these are not specific enough to confirm the diagnosis. A liver biopsy is usually diagnostic, and both immunoperoxidase staining for HSV and viral culture should be performed in addition to routine histologic staining. Histologically, the liver shows patchy and confluent hepatic necrosis with hemorrhage but little inflammation. At the periphery of the necrosis, there may be intranuclear eosinophilic Cowdry type A inclusions (Fig. 27-5). Although this disease occurs rarely, early recognition is essential and treatment with acyclovir is effective. Maternal and fetal mortality are approximately 50%.

Other Liver Diseases That Occur Coincidentally with Pregnancy

Any liver disease can exist concurrently with pregnancy, and the pathogenesis of these diseases is discussed else-

where in this book. Patients with pre-existing liver disease, such as Wilson's disease, autoimmune hepatitis, hepatitis C, chronic hepatitis B, and alcoholic liver disease, have lower rates of fertility; however, cases of pregnancy do occur. In general, the pregnancy does not change the course of the underlying liver disease. The outcome of the pregnancy can depend on the clinical condition of the patient. Bearing this in mind, in Wilson's disease and autoimmune hepatitis, it is important not to stop prior medications. Drugs like penicillamine may have rare teratogenic effects on the fetus, but the risk of this possibility is far outweighed by the benefit of continued therapy. In general, a higher incidence of fetal wastage and premature births occurs in these pregnancies, probably related to the poorer clinical condition of the mothers.

Pregnancy in a cirrhotic patient has additional implications. Pregnant women with cirrhosis have approximately a 20% to 25% chance of experiencing variceal bleeding during the pregnancy, especially in the latter half of gestation, and this risk is higher in patients with demonstrable varices. This increased risk probably reflects the increased circulatory volume in late pregnancy. In addition, as the gravid uterus enlarges, there may be an obstruction of the inferior vena cava with peripheral venous return forced through collateral systems. Despite the risk of variceal bleeding and associated maternal and fetal mortality, no clear guidelines are available regarding therapy. Patients should be aware of the risk, and the option of a therapeutic abortion should be considered. In patients with documented varices, multiple different therapies have been performed with variable results. β-Blocker therapy, shunt surgery, and elective sclerotherapy during pregnancy have all been used successfully to treat variceal bleeding, but no prospective trials are available to assess the true efficacy of these treatments. There have been no reports, as yet, of using transjugular intrahepatic portosystemic shunts (TIPS) or esophageal banding in pregnancy, but these therapeutic modalities may also be considered. In patients who are actively bleeding from esophageal varices, standard therapy with resuscitation, intravenous octreotide, sclerotherapy, a Sengstaken-Blakemore tube, and placement of TIPS should be used. The use of Pitressin has been avoided, given the risk of inducing labor with this medication.

In the case of infectious diseases such as viral hepatitis, although the outcome of the liver disease is not affected by pregnancy, vertical transmission from mother to child needs to be considered. Transplacental transfer of hepatitis A has not been reported. The infant is at risk of infection during delivery if the acute infection occurs within 2 weeks of delivery. If that is the case, a single intramuscular injection of immune serum globulin shortly after birth is recommended. Transplacental transmission of hepatitis B has not been reported, but vertical transmission at the time of delivery is common with the risk estimated to be approximately 25% if the mother is HBsAg+ and approximately 80% to 90% if she is also HBeAg+. Many infants infected at birth develop chronic infections and perpetuate infection to the next generation. Hepatitis B is a common infection worldwide, and because of lifelong risks of infections, universal vaccination has been recommended for all infants. Infants born to HBsAg+ mothers, regardless of HBeAg status, should be given both active and passive immunization with hepatitis B vaccine and immune globulin (HBIG), respectively at the

Table 27–3   Hepatitis B Immunoprophylaxis for the Neonate

HBsAg Status of Mother	Passive Immunoprophylaxis	Active Immunoprophylaxis
Positive	Intramuscular injection of hepatitis B immune globulin (HBIG) at birth; 0.5 mL (250 IU)	• Hepatitis B vaccine at birth, at 1 to 2 months, and at 6 to 18 months of age • 0.5 mL of recombinant vaccine or 1 mL of plasma-derived vaccine • First dose can be given concurrently with HBIG but should be given at a different site • HBsAg and anti-HBs can be checked at 12 to 15 months of age to document the success of vaccination
Negative	None	• Hepatitis B vaccine at birth, at 1 to 2 months, and at 6 to 18 months of age • Hepatitis B vaccine at 1 to 2 months, at 4 months, and at 6 to 18 months of age • 0.5 mL of recombinant vaccine or 1 mL of plasma-derived vaccine

time of birth (Table 27–3). With hepatitis C, there is, at this time, no available vaccination or immune globulin. Fortunately, the rate of vertical transmission appears to be very low unless there is concomitant maternal infection with the human immunodeficiency virus (HIV).

DIFFERENTIAL DIAGNOSIS

The differential diagnosis of liver disease in pregnancy includes all types of liver diseases, but in this section we focus on diseases that are either unique to pregnancy or more common in pregnancy. Diagnosis can be divided based on the stage of pregnancy (Table 27–4). In the first trimester of pregnancy, the only disease unique to pregnancy is hyperemesis gravidarum, which should be easily differentiated from acute viral hepatitis by more severe nausea and vomiting in the former and much more elevated AST/ALT values in the latter. If there is a significant elevation in serum transaminases, serologic testing may be needed to exclude viral hepatitis. Gallstone disease, like hyperemesis gravidarum, may present with nausea and vomiting and mild liver test abnormalities, but significant abdominal pain should only be present in the former. In the second trimester of pregnancy, the possibility of herpes hepatitis should be considered in patients with marked elevations in serum aminotransferases and mild elevations of bilirubin. This disease may present similar to other causes of viral hepatitis (e.g., hepatitis A and B) but can be differentiated by serology, liver biopsy and, if present, skin lesions.

In the third trimester of pregnancy, various diseases can occur, which may be differentiated based on clinical presentation (Table 27–5). A cholestatic pattern of liver tests in the setting of pruritus will differentiate IHCP from other liver diseases (e.g., HELLP, acute fatty liver of pregnancy, and viral hepatitis). Fulminant hepatic failure can result from acute fatty liver of pregnancy, viral hepatitis, or severe HELLP syndrome, but these can be differentiated with either serology or liver biopsy. Differentiations of acute viral hepatitis from IHCP, HELLP syndrome, and acute fatty liver of pregnancy are particularly important, because the treatment for the latter three is early delivery. A summary of the treatments for liver disease unique to pregnancy is shown in Table 27–6.

PROGNOSIS

For patients with chronic liver disease who become pregnant, the maternal outcome and prognosis depend greatly on the underlying liver disease. Pregnancy does not alter the outcome of most liver diseases, but the presence of cirrhosis and portal hypertension greatly increases the risk of gastrointestinal bleeding, which then portends a poor prognosis. For the fetus, the perinatal mortality is increased, with a higher incidence of prematurity, stillbirth, and intrauterine growth retardation, but there is no increased risk of birth defects.

For patients with hyperemesis gravidarum, maternal survival is excellent if dehydration, metabolic disorders, and

Table 27–4   Differential Diagnosis of Liver Disease According to the Stage of Pregnancy

First Trimester	Second Trimester	Third Trimester
Acute viral hepatitis	Acute viral hepatitis	Acute viral hepatitis
Hyperemesis gravidarum	Gallstone disease	Intrahepatic cholestasis of pregnancy*
Gallstone disease	Herpes hepatitis	Acute fatty liver of pregnancy*
		Preeclampsia-related liver disease (HELLP, hepatic infarction, hepatic hematoma, hepatic rupture)*
		Gallstone disease
		Herpes hepatitis

*This can rarely occur in the second trimester or shortly postpartum.

Table 27–5 Diagnostic Features Distinguishing Causes of Jaundice in the Third Trimester

Diagnostic Tools	Intrahepatic Cholestasis of Pregnancy	Preeclampsia/Eclampsia–Related Liver Disease	Acute Fatty Liver of Pregnancy	Viral Hepatitis
Recurrent disease with subsequent pregnancy	• Likely	• Possible	• Rare	• No
Family history	• Yes	• No	• No	• No
Symptoms	• Pruritus	• Malaise, nausea, vomiting, abdominal discomfort, fever	• Malaise, anorexia, nausea, vomiting, abdominal discomfort • Somnolence	• Malaise, nausea, vomiting
Signs	• Skin excoriations	• Preeclampsia (hypertension, proteinuria, edema) • Evidence of shock should lead to suspicion for hepatic rupture	• Can be associated with preeclampsia in as many as 50% • Hepatic encephalopathy • Bleeding (GI, GU) due to coagulopathy	• Signs of liver failure
Serum tests: liver function tests	• Bilirubin rarely >6 mg/dL • Alkaline phosphatase up to 4 times normal • Serum aminotransferase level variable 2- to 10-fold × normal	• Variable elevations of AST/ALT • Extreme elevations of aminotransferases should point to the possibility of hepatic infarction	• Variable increases in bilirubin of up to 10× normal, serum aminotransferase levels rarely exceed greater than 10× normal • Increased PT • Renal failure	• Significant elevations of aminotransferases from 5 to 25 × normal • Variable degree of liver dysfunction
Serum tests: other	• Serum bile acid 10 to 100× normal	• Hemolysis and thrombocytopenia • Increased uric acid • DIC	• Hypoglycemia • Increased uric acid • DIC • Leukocytosis	• Hepatitis serology: anti-HAV IgM, anti-HBc IgM, HBsAg, HBeAg, anti-HCV, and HCV RNA
Hepatic imaging	• Normal	• Useful for diagnosing hepatic infarcts, hematomas, and rupture	• Can show fatty liver but not very sensitive	• Not useful
Liver biopsy	• Cholestasis with little or no inflammation	• Periportal hemorrhage with fibrin deposit in the periportal sinusoids	• Microvascular fatty infiltration of centrilobular hepatocytes	• Intense portal and periportal inflammation with lobular necrosis

DIC, disseminated intravascular coagulation; PT, prothrombin time; GI, gastrointestinal; GU, genitourinary; HCV, hepatitis C virus.

Table 27–6 Treatment of Liver Diseases Unique to Pregnancy

Disease	Treatment
Hyperemesis gravidarum	• Supportive care with rehydration; correction of underlying metabolic and electrolyte imbalance • Nutritional support with total parenteral nutrition in severe cases
Intrahepatic cholestasis of pregnancy	• Ursodeoxycholic acid (10–15 mg/kg/day) • Cholestyramine, phenobarbital • Parenteral vitamin K, especially near the time of delivery • Early delivery
Preeclampsia-related liver disease/HELLP	• Treatment of preeclampsia • Early delivery
Hepatic hematoma/rupture	• Cesarean section for patients with suspected rupture • Laparotomy with drainage and packing in cases of rupture • Hepatic artery embolization in selected cases • Early delivery when feasible
Acute fatty liver of pregnancy	• Early delivery • Supportive care of liver failure

HELLP, hemolysis, elevated liver enzymes, and low platelet count.

Table 27–7   Prognosis of Liver Diseases Unique to Pregnancy

Disease	Maternal Outcome	Fetal Outcome
Hyperemesis gravidarum	• Excellent maternal outcome with good supportive care	• Decreased mean birthweight in severe cases
Intrahepatic cholestasis of pregnancy	• Pruritus and abnormal liver function tests resolve with delivery • Increased risk of postpartum hemorrhage • Recurrence is common with subsequent pregnancies and use of oral contraceptives	• Increased risk of meconium staining, spontaneous preterm labor, and intrapartum fetal distress resulting in increased perinatal mortality
Preeclampsia-related liver disease/HELLP	• Adverse effect on maternal outcome with mortality of 3–25%. • No long-term sequelae	• Increased perinatal mortality related to severity of maternal disease
Acute fatty liver of pregnancy	• Poor maternal outcome with 10–33% mortality • No long-term sequelae • Recurrence is rare	• >30% fetal mortality related to the severity of maternal disease

HELLP, hemolysis, elevated liver enzymes, and low platelet count.

malnutrition are treated (Table 27–7). Mean infant birthweight is decreased if the hyperemesis is severe, for example, with a greater than 3% decrease in maternal body weight. In intrahepatic cholestasis of pregnancy, maternal survival is not affected, but there is a 70% chance of a recurrence with subsequent pregnancies. Furthermore, there is some perinatal morbidity and mortality, owing to prematurity, stillbirth, and fetal death. The prognosis for HELLP and acute fatty liver of pregnancy is much less optimistic, with maternal mortality rates up to 25%. This is an improvement on historical reports, likely caused by advances in intensive care, early diagnosis, early delivery, and recognition of milder cases. Recurrence has been variable with rates of 3% to 27% for HELLP and is rare, but not absent, for acute fatty liver of pregnancy.

SUGGESTED READINGS

Abell TL, Riely CA: Hyperemesis gravidarum. Gastroenterol Clin North Am 21:835–849, 1992.

Bacq Y, Zarka O, Brechot J, et al: Liver function tests in normal pregnancy: A prospective study of 103 pregnant women and 103 matched controls. Hepatology 23:1030–1034, 1996.

Cheng Y: Pregnancy in liver cirrhosis and/or portal hypertension. Am J Obstet Gynecol 128:812–822, 1977.

Davis A, Katz VL, Cox R: Gallbladder disease in pregnancy. J Reprod Med 40:759–762, 1995.

Diaferia A, Nicastri PL, Tartagni M, et al: Ursodeoxycholic acid therapy in pregnant women with cholestasis. Int J Gynecol Obstet 52:133–140, 1996.

Fagan EA: Intrahepatic cholestasis of pregnancy. BMJ 309:1243–1244, 1994.

Floreani A, Paternoster D, Melis A, Grella PV: S-adenosylmethionine versus ursodeoxycholic acid in the treatment of intrahepatic cholestasis of pregnancy: Preliminary results of a controlled trial. Eur J Obstet Gynecol 67:109–113, 1996.

Freund G, Arvan DA: Clinical biochemistry of preeclampsia and related liver diseases of pregnancy: A review. Clin Chim Acta 191:123–152, 1990.

Klein NA, Mabie WC, Shaver DC, et al: Herpes simplex virus hepatitis in pregnancy: Two patients successfully treated with acyclovir. Gastroenterology 100:239–244, 1991.

Lee WM: Pregnancy in patients with chronic liver disease. Gastroenterol Clin North Am 21:889–903, 1992.

Mudido P, Marshall GS, Howell RS, et al: Disseminated *Herpes simplex* virus infection during pregnancy. J Reprod Med 38:964–968, 1993.

Reyes H, Sandoval L, Wainstein A, et al: Acute fatty liver of pregnancy: A clinical study of 12 episodes in 11 patients. Gut 35:101–106, 1994.

Reyes H, Simon FR: Intrahepatic cholestasis of pregnancy: An estrogen-related disease. Semin Liver Dis 13:289–301, 1993.

Smith LG, Moise KJ, Dildy GA, Carpenter RJ: Spontaneous rupture of liver during pregnancy: Current therapy. Obstet Gynecol 77:171–175, 1991.

Treem WR, Shoup ME, Hale DE, et al: Acute fatty liver of pregnancy, hemolysis, elevated liver enzymes, and low platelets syndrome, and long chain 3-hydroyacyl-coenzyme A deficiency. Am J Gastroenterol 91:2293–2300, 1996.

Watson WJ, Seeds JW: Acute fatty liver of pregnancy. Obstet Gynecol Surv 45:585–591, 1990.

28

The Liver and Systemic Diseases

Vinod K. Rustgi

The liver has played a central role in the popular imagination and mythology since ancient times. The Greeks and the Egyptians believed that it was the seat of the soul and even relied on it for divination.

The liver is the most biochemically complex organ within the body. Complex interactions exist between the liver and other organ systems. In turn, the liver may be involved in diffuse processes. This chapter reviews liver involvement in some of these systemic diseases. It is limited in its review to those processes not covered in more detail in other chapters.

ENDOCRINE DISORDERS

Diabetes Mellitus

Patients with metabolic disorders such as obesity and diabetes mellitus may present with abnormal liver tests or even with massive hepatomegaly (Table 28–1). The most common histologic abnormality observed in these individuals is fatty change or "steatosis," reflected by an obvious demonstrable deposition of large, macronodular fat droplets in liver parenchymal cells. These histologic findings may be found in asymptomatic, obese, or diabetic patients without liver enzyme abnormalities. The accumulation of fatty acids may add significantly to the toxic effects of fat deposition. In poorly controlled type 1 diabetic patients, hepatomegaly may also be caused by a cytoplasmic accumulation of glycogen.

Under normal conditions, there is a constant cycling of fatty acids between the liver and the adipose tissue. This balance is subtle and distorts easily in favor of net transfer of triglycerides from adipose tissue to the liver. Diabetes

mellitus may lead to an enhanced rate of lipolysis in the adipose tissue, a reaction that is normally suppressed by insulin. In adult-onset diabetes mellitus, insulin insensitivity and obesity are the major factors responsible for the fatty infiltration.

Fatty infiltration of the liver is generally diffuse, although focal changes may also be seen. Computed tomography may show areas of low attenuation, which cause no mass effect and may present as nonspherical, subsegmental, or poorly marginated lesions. In addition, there may be multiple, rounded lesions suggestive of liver metastases. Other conditions associated with hepatic steatosis are listed in Table 28–2.

Nuclear glycogenation, producing a vacuolated appearance of the nucleus at the light microscopic level, may be found in the liver in up to 75% of diabetics (Fig. 28–1). This feature is not pathognomonic of diabetes and may also occur normally, in septic inflammation, tuberculosis, cirrhosis, hepatitis, and Wilson's disease.

A peculiar type of subcapsular focal fatty change is found in diabetic patients on continuous ambulatory peritoneal dialysis (CAPD). It is thought that glucose and insulin from the dialysis solutions diffuse through the hepatic capsule and reach their highest concentrations in the thin rim of subcapsular hepatocytes. By inhibiting the oxidation of free fatty acids and by stimulating the synthesis of triglycerides, the high insulin concentration in the subcapsular hepatocytes results in localized steatosis (Table 28–2).

Thyroid Disease

The liver has an important role in thyroid hormone metabolism because it manufactures proteins such as thyroxine-binding globulins (TBGs), prealbumin, and albumin. It is

Table 28–1   Diabetes and Associated Liver Diseases

Hepatic disease caused by diabetes
  Glycogen deposition (Mauriac syndrome)
  Fatty liver
  Cirrhosis
  Biliary tract disease
Liver diseases associated with therapy of diabetes
  Viral hepatitis (needle stick)
  Injury due to oral hypoglycemic drugs
Liver disease associated with diabetes
  Hemochromatosis
  Chronic active autoimmune hepatitis
  Hepatogenic diabetes

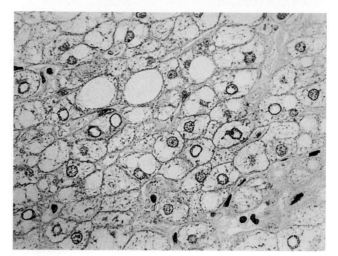

Figure 28–1
Glycogenated nuclei. Microvesicular and macrovesicular fat are present.

also the major site of thyroid hormone peripheral metabolism and is involved in its conjugation, biliary excretion, oxidative deamination as well as the extrathyroidal deiodination of thyroxine (T_4), triiodothyronine (T_3), and conversion to reverse T_3. The level of thyroid hormones is also important in normal hepatic function and bilirubin metabolism.

Liver damage may be seen secondary to the systemic effects of hormone excess or direct toxic effects. Some patients with chronic liver diseases may have thyroiditis, which results in hyperthyroidism or hypothyroidism through autoimmune mechanisms. Alterations of thyroid hormone metabolism or tests may be seen secondary to liver disease. Liver or thyroid disorders may be related to therapy for thyroid or liver disease.

Hyperthyroidism

During thyroid storm, hepatic injury is frequent. This is usually due to excess oxygen requirements by mitochondrial-based metabolic activity within hepatocytes. Liver biopsies in patients with thyrotoxicosis show vacuolization of hepatocytes, balloon degeneration, nuclear glycogen, mild infiltration of mononuclear cells, centrilobular cholestasis, and Kupffer cell hyperplasia. It is unclear whether these are the

Table 28–2   Causes of Liver Steatosis

Increased fatty acid mobilization
  Obesity
  Insulin deficiency
  Corticosteroid excess
  Starvation
  Alcohol
  Inflammatory bowel disease
Increased fatty acid synthesis
  Alcohol
  Hyperalimentation
Decreased synthesis of apoproteins
  Tetracycline
  Yellow phosphorus
Decreased transport and release of lipoproteins
  Colchicine
  Ethanol
  Orotic acid

results directly of the thyroid abnormality or because of associated conditions such as congestive heart failure, infection, or malnutrition. Abnormal laboratory values that can be seen include decreased albumin, increased bromosulfophthalein (BSP) retention, elevated aspartate aminotransferase (AST), and serum alanine aminotransferase (ALT) as well as γ-glutamyl transpeptidase (GGTP) and alkaline phosphatase. These may be related to thyroid dysfunction, because they tend to return to normal soon after restoration of a euthyroid state.

Hypothyroidism

ALT may be slightly elevated compounded by hypercholesterolemia, resulting in a fatty liver. Myopathy may cause confusion with AST elevation. Ascites may be seen with myxedema. A specific central congestive fibrosis of the liver has been described, particularly in cases of ascites due to myxedema.

Thyroid abnormalities may be present with autoimmune hepatitis or primary biliary cirrhosis on an autoimmune basis. This may also be seen with hepatitis C and again may be on an autoimmune basis. Interferon therapy for viral hepatitis has been associated with both hyper- and hypothyroidism, possibly caused by unmasking of autoimmune thyroiditis.

Liver Injuries Associated with Antithyroid Therapy

Methimazole or carbimazole can induce cholestatic liver injuries that usually recover upon their withdrawal. Women older than 50 years of age are most commonly affected. Propylthiouracil (PTU) can induce hepatocellular injury, which may occasionally be severe and is sometimes associated with hepatic failure or death. It usually occurs in women younger than 30 years of age during the first few months of therapy, but these women usually recover completely after therapy is discontinued. It has been suggested that PTU may form active metabolites, which interact with the macromolecules of the endoplasmic reticulum and lead to centrilobular hepatic necrosis. Analogous to the situation with isoniazid, PTU therapy may be continued with caution in case of minor hepatic injury, unless overt hepatitis occurs; in this case, PTU should be stopped immediately.

Thyroid Laboratory Test Abnormalities

The most consistent findings in liver disease are an elevated T_4 and TBG with normal levels of free T_4 and TSH. T_4 elevation may be secondary to TBG elevation, and hepatitis may be caused by increased TBG synthesis in regenerating hepatocytes, release of TBG by damaged hepatocytes, or decreased TBG degradation. At least in hepatocellular carcinoma, it seems that TBG elevation may occur to increased synthesis and secretion by hepatocellular carcinoma cells. Low serum T_3 levels may be due to diminished conversion of T_4 to T_3.

Acromegaly

Acromegaly represents the clinical expression of long-standing unrestrained growth hormone excess (hypersomatotropism) usually secondary to a pituitary adenoma. There are an estimated 17,000 people with acromegaly currently in the United States.

Despite the fact that visceromegaly is a common finding on autopsy examination in acromegaly, clinical hepatomegaly or splenomegaly should be viewed with greater suspicion. Hepatic function tests are uniformly normal even in those patients with enlarged livers except for an increased maximal excretory rate of BSP.

Liver Involvement in HIV Infection

The liver plays an important role in the pathogenesis of human immunodeficiency virus (HIV) (Table 28–3). It serves

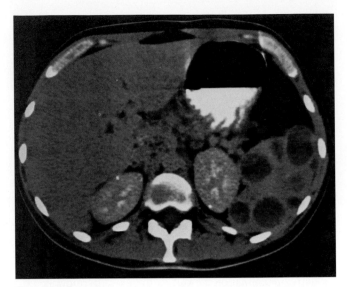

Figure 28–2
A computed tomography scan of splenic involvement in non-Hodgkin's lymphoma.

as a reservoir of hepatotropic viruses and opportunistic infections. Because it is so rich in blood flow, it is often the target of disseminated, blood-borne opportunistic infections. The most common symptoms for which gastroenterologists are asked to see patients with acquired immunodeficiency syndrome (AIDS) are hepatomegaly, abnormal liver enzymes, or fever with consideration of a liver biopsy. Granulomas are the most frequent findings on liver biopsy in patients with AIDS. These are usually caused by *Mycobacterium avium*–complex (MAC) (Fig. 28–3) but rarely can also be from other mycobacterial species including *M. tuberculosis* and *M. kansasii*. Granulomas tend to be small, histiocyte-predominant, and poorly formed. Standard stains may also reveal fungal organisms. In a retrospective series of 501 HIV-seropositive patients who underwent liver biopsy, Poles and associates found granulomas in 17.4% of biopsies and *M. tuberculosis* in 2.6% of biopsies.

If no infectious etiology such as *Candida*, histoplasmosis, or cryptococcosis (Fig. 28–4) is found, granulomas may be attributed to drug-related liver disease. Sulfamethoxazole-trimethoprim and zidovudine may cause

Table 28–3   Diseases Affecting the Hepatobiliary System and Histologic Changes in AIDS

Viral hepatitis	AIDs cholangiopathy
Hepatitis A	Acalculous cholecystitis
Hepatitis B	Sclerosing cholangitis
Hepatitis C	Papillary stenosis
Hepatitis D	Lymphoma of the biliary
CMV	tree
EBV	Neoplasms
HSV	Kaposi's sarcoma
HIV	Non-Hodgkins' B cell lym-
Opportunistic infections	phoma (see Fig. 28–2)
MAC	Drug-induced hepatitis
Cryptosporidium	Histologic findings
Pneumocystis carinii	Steatosis (fatty liver)
MTB	Granulomatous hepatitis
Coccidioides immitis	Portal inflammation
Candida albicans	Sinusoidal dilatation
Histoplasma capsulatum	Peliosis hepatis
Cryptococcus neoformans	
Rochalimaea henselae	

AIDS, acquired immunodeficiency syndrome; EBV, Epstein-Barr virus; CMV, cytomegalovirus; HSV, herpes simplex virus; MAC, *Mycobacterium avium* complex; MTB, *Mycobacterium tuberculosis*.

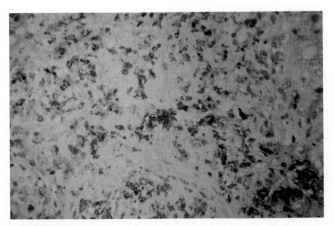

Figure 28–3
Mycobacterium avium-complex in the liver.

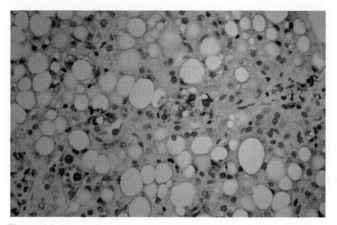

Figure 28–4
Cryptococcus infection in a patient with AIDS.

Table 28–4   Liver Findings in Systemic Lupus Erythematosus (SLE)

Number of patients	551
Number with evidence of liver disease	146 (26.5%)
Etiology	
Drug-related	50 (9%)
Liver disease not related to SLE	17 (3%)
Venous congestion	8 (1.5%)
Unknown	72 (13%)
Clinically significant liver disease	22 (4%)
Death due to liver disease	3 (<1%)

hepatic steatosis and rarely hepatitis. Dapsone may cause hepatic failure, and hepatic toxicity can also be seen associated with the use of 2′,3′-dideoxyinosine (ddI). Kaposi's sarcoma may appear as solid red-purple nodules seen in the liver at laparoscopy but almost always occurs in the presence of cutaneous Kaposi's sarcoma.

Significant steatosis of the liver is not an uncommon finding in AIDS. Histologically, the fat is macroscopic, panlobular, and without any zonal predilection. Steatosis may occur due to increased levels of tumor necrosis factor, interleukin-1, and interferons.

HIV may affect the natural history of chronic viral hepatitis. Cirrhosis is seen infrequently. Epstein-Barr virus (EBV) infection may be ameliorated due to the increased T-suppressor cell activity seen in AIDS. The interactions with hepatitis B and hepatitis C are controversial. There are good reasons to believe, based on immunologic grounds, that there is a higher degree of hepatitis B viral replication associated with lower aminotransferase levels and milder histologic activity in HIV-infected individuals compared with patients who are anti-HIV negative. Hepatitis C virus (HCV) load increases over time and is enhanced by HIV. HCV-RNA may increase as immune deficiency progresses.

Finally, sinusoidal abnormalities, including a nonspecific dilatation, may also be seen. Pathogenic mechanisms are unknown, but an increased presence of hyperplastic sinusoidal macrophages has been noted. Injury to endothelial cells has been postulated. Peliosis hepatitis, which represents a blood-filled space that may or may not have an endothelial lining, has been reported.

Collagen Vascular Disorders

The incidence and significance of hepatic abnormalities in collagen-vascular disorders are poorly defined, because, although clinical and laboratory assessment of hepatic dysfunction is easy, definite diagnosis of liver abnormalities is difficult without biopsy.

Systemic Lupus Erythematosus

Systemic lupus erythematosus (SLE) is a multisystem inflammatory disease associated with the development of au-

toantibodies to various self-antigens, particularly nuclear antigens. It is likely there are several different factors that induce the disease by impairing normal immune regulatory processes and by breaking self-tolerance. In some individuals, genetic predisposition may be the determining factor. In other cases, environmental triggers such as viral infections may play the most important role.

Mild liver dysfunction and hepatomegaly are not uncommon in typical cases of SLE. Rare cases develop severe immunologically mediated liver disease and overlap with autoimmune hepatitis. In addition, patients with active SLE seem particularly susceptible to drug-induced hepatic damage. Liver disease can also develop secondary to vascular occlusion, which is related to the hypercoagulable states that occur in SLE. Common liver involvement in SLE can include fatty infiltration and necrosis of central hepatocytes. On a composite basis, two retrospective studies and a prospective study are summarized in Table 28–4.

Patients with SLE may develop antibodies directed against phospholipids. These antibodies include the lupus anticoagulant, antibodies to cardiolipin, and those causing a biologic false-positive test for syphilis. The lupus anticoagulant is an immunoglobulin that inhibits the conversion of prothrombin to thrombin and thus prolongs the activated partial thromboplastin (APTT). It paradoxically is associated in vivo with an increased tendency to venous or arterial thrombosis. This may lead to Budd-Chiari syndrome. Hepatic arterial occlusion has been associated with hepatic infarction. Rarely, hepatic veno-occlusive disease has also been reported.

Many patients with SLE are treated with drugs that may have hepatic side effects. Corticosteroids may cause steatosis, whereas azathioprine may cause cholestatic hepatitis. Aspirin is a particular offender, and liver biopsies of patients with aspirin hepatotoxicity may show hepatocyte injury and necrosis. The injury appears to be dose-related; patients taking 3 to 5 g of aspirin daily are at particular risk.

Nodular regenerative hyperplasia (NRH) of the liver, characterized by a diffuse nodular area of liver produced by many regenerative nodules without associated fibrosis, has been frequently described in rheumatoid arthritis but has also been described in patients with SLE.

Rheumatoid Arthritis

NRH has been described in association with a variety of diseases, most of them rheumatic or hematologic disorders. This may be a prominent feature in liver involvement with rheumatoid arthritis. NRH was also described in the toxic oil syndrome, a scleroderma-like disorder caused by toxic oil intoxication in Spain.

Vascular injuries probably play a primary pathogenic role. Direct vessel injury of the hepatic vascular bed has been observed in patients with NRH and rheumatoid vasculitis. NRH may be the morphologic response to atrophy of the liver parenchyma caused by vascular obstruction of small hepatic arteries or portal veins. Hyperplastic nodules may arise in those acini with maintained blood supply. The prevalence may be up to 2.5% as reported in a series of 2500 autopsies.

Sjögren's Syndrome

Skopouli and associates investigated 300 patients with primary Sjögren's syndrome for liver involvement using clinical, biochemical, immunologic, and histologic data. Seven percent of patients showed evidence of liver disease with elevated liver enzymes. Of patients with antimitochondrial antibody, 92% showed liver involvement with features of chronic cholangitis similar to stage 1 primary biliary cirrhosis. The presence of an antimitochondrial antibody is the most sensitive indicator of underlying liver pathology in patients with Sjögren's syndrome.

Lipid Storage Diseases

Gaucher's Disease, Niemann-Pick Disease

This is the most common lysosomal storage defect with an autosomal recessive inheritance. It is characterized by a deficiency of the specific β-glucosidase, glucocerebrosidase, leading to an excess accumulation of glucosylceramide in the lysosomes of reticuloendothelial cells. Hepatosplenomegaly, osteopenic degeneration of the skeleton, and central nervous system dysfunction are the major chronic manifestations of this disease. Gaucher's disease is now treated by intravenous administration of a modified glucocerebrosidase (alglucerase), which has exposed mannose residues to promote uptake by target macrophages.

Since treatment is available for patients with Gaucher's disease, methods of follow-up have become important in making treatment decisions. Bone abnormalities (infarct and avascular necrosis) tend to be irreversible, whereas visceral volumes are not, suggesting that it may be useful to follow patients with visceral volume determinations. Magnetic resonance imaging has shown a statistical relationship between marrow changes, liver size and avascular necrosis.

Niemann-Pick disease is caused by sphingomyelinase deficiency, leading to excess deposition of sphingomyelin, bis (monoacylglycerol) phosphate, cholesterol, glycosphingolipids, and lysosphingolipids in visceral and brain tissues. The enzyme deficiency is inherited as an autosomal recessive trait with considerable heterogeneity in the phenotype of affected patients. Prolonged survival into adulthood is associated with cirrhosis, hypersplenism, and respiratory infections. Liver transplantation has been attempted without long-term success.

Amyloidosis

"Amyloid" as a term was first coined by Matthias Schleiden, a German botanist in 1838, to describe a normal amylaceous constituent of plants. In 1854, Rudolph Virchow used the term amyloid because the iodine-sulfuric acid test indicated that the substance was similar to cellulose.

Primary amyloidosis (AL) is characterized by the deposition of an abnormal extracellular protein in the form of fibrils, which are derived from monoclonal immunoglobulin-like chains. One of the most important properties of these fibrils is their continuous accumulation, which is responsible for the functional damage to organs and tissues. AL diagnosis requires a demonstration of amyloid deposits in tissues. The most commonly used stain is Congo red, which produces an apple-green birefringence under polarizing light. Although the tissue diagnosis can be made from other locations, the results of a liver biopsy are almost always positive. The procedure may cause bleeding, and in rare cases the liver has ruptured. Physical findings are presented in Figure 28–5.

In a series of 474 patients reviewed by Kyle and Gertz, the serum alkaline phosphatase was increased in almost 25%. The AST value was increased in one third, whereas hyperbilirubinemia was an infrequent finding but indicated a short survival when present. Hypalbuminemia was common with albumin levels less than 2 g/dL in 12%.

In another series, Kyle and Gertz found low globulin levels and occasionally a high platelet count, both of which are unusual in chronic liver disease with splenomegaly. It was thought that hypogammaglobulinemia probably signified increased urinary losses or suppression of normal immunoglobulin synthesis, whereas the raised platelet count probably represented a degree of functional hyposplenism. Jaundice can be difficult to explain, although it has been hypothesized that modified light chains might be able to induce functional alterations of the liver (Table 28–5).

Orthotopic liver transplantation has been used for familial amyloidotic polyneuropathy (FAP). This rare autosomal-dominant disease has a metabolic origin that lies in an abnormal protein synthesized primarily in the liver. This hereditary form of amyloidosis is the rarest form affecting kindreds of specific ethnic backgrounds. The true incidence in the United States is unknown. The mutant protein, transthyretin or prealbumin, forms amyloid fibrils that accumulate in vital tissues. Liver transplantation leads to the

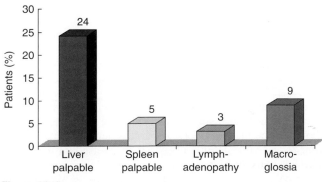

Figure 28–5
Physical findings in 474 patients with primary amyloidosis. (From Kyle RA, Gertz MA: Primary systemic amyloidosis: Clinical and laboratory features in 474 cases. Semin Hematol 32(1):45–59, 1995.)

Table 28–5   Liver Function Tests in Amyloidosis

	No. of Patients	Value Median	Range	Other
Alkaline phosphatase (U/L) (normal, <250)	468	169	79–3660	>250 = 26%
AST U/L (normal, <31)	470	27	9–351	>31 = 34%
Bilirubin (mg/dL)				>0.3 = 8%
Direct	466	0.1	0–11.3	>1.1 = 11%
Total	466	0.6	0.1–15.7	>2 = 3%
				<3 = 51%
Serum albumin (g/dL)	463	2.9	0.8–4.6	<2 = 12%
Prothrombin time (seconds)	332	12	9–33	>13 = 16%

AST, aspartate aminotransferase.

production of normal transthyretin protein, and this theoretically should arrest the disease process. Gene therapy for familial amyloidotic polyneuropathy, using recombinant retrovirus factors that carry the full length human cDNA for transthyretin, is a future possibility.

Systemic Mastocytosis

Mastocytosis is often associated with hepatic mast cell hyperplasia, fibrosis, and in some cases nodular regenerative hyperplasia, portal venopathy, or veno-occlusive disease. Abnormal liver function tests are usually minimal; however, further evaluation may indicate a cause other than mastocytosis in patients with minimal disease with skin involvement only. Those patients with more systemic involvement may have comparatively more infiltrates, fibrosis, hepatomegaly, and splenomegaly and they may develop ascites. Severe liver disease in association with ascites carries a serious prognosis in these patients.

Cardiac Cirrhosis

Hepatic fibrosis is found in most patients with prolonged congestive heart failure (CHF). Congestive hepatic fibrosis varies from mild deposition of sinusoidal collagen to broad fibrous septa with distortion of the architecture (cirrhosis). The pathogenesis of congestive fibrosis and cirrhosis is generally thought to be a reaction of the hepatic stroma to hypoxia, pressure, or hepatocellular necrosis. However, this does not explain why congestive fibrosis can be variable despite similar degrees of cardiac decompensation or why the degree of fibrosis varies from one region of the liver to another. Sinusoidal thrombosis exacerbates stasis and augments fibroblast activation and collagen deposition. The critical event causing necrosis and subsequent parenchymal extinction may be propagation of thrombosis into medium hepatic veins. When cardiac ascites is seen, constrictive pericarditis should be considered as well.

Henri and associates studied the acute effects of cardiac events on the liver by studying high-risk patients for 1 year in a coronary care unit. The incidence of hypoxic or ischemic hepatitis was noted to be about 2.6% of the 766 patients admitted during this period and was associated with a decrease in hepatic blood flow and passive hepatic venous congestion. Hypoxic hepatitis was defined as a serum aminotransferase activity of at least 20 times the upper limit of normal without any other cause for hepatic necrosis. The pathologic correlate is a centrilobular necrosis.

SUGGESTED READINGS

Ezzat S: Hepatobiliary and gastrointestinal manifestations of acromegaly. Dig Dis 10:173–180, 1992.
Ghany MG, Leissinger C, Lagier R, et al: Effect of human immunodeficiency virus infection on hepatitis C virus infection in hemophiliacs. Dig Dis Sci 41(6):1265–1272, 1996.
Gibson T, Myers AR: Subclinical liver disease in SLE. J Rheumatol 8:752–759, 1981.
Grunfeld C, Kotler DP: Wasting and the acquired immunodeficiency syndrome. Semin Liver Dis 12:175–187, 1992.
Harrison RF, Hawkins PN, Roche WR, et al: Fragile liver and massive hepatic hemorrhage due to hereditary amyloidosis. Gut 38:151–152, 1996.
Henri NJ, Descamps O, Luwaert R, et al: Hypoxic hepatitis in patients with cardiac failure: Incidence in a coronary care unit and measurement of hepatic blood flow. J Hepatol 21(5):696–703, 1994.
Huang MJ, Liaw YF. Thyroxine-binding globulin in patients with chronic hepatitis B virus infection: Different implications in hepatitis and hepatocellular carcinoma. Am J Gastroenterol 85:281–284, 1990.
Huang M-J, Liaw Y-F: Clinical associations between thyroid and liver diseases. J Gastroenterol Hepatol 10:344–350, 1995.
Jeffers LJ, Alzate I, Aguliar H, et al: Laparoscopic and histologic findings in patients with human immunodeficiency virus. Gastrointest Endosc 40(2):160–164, 1994.
Kyle RA, Gertz MA: Primary systemic amyloidosis: Clinical and laboratory features in 474 cases. Semin Hematol 32(1):45–59, 1995.
Lefkowitch JH: Pathology of AIDS-related liver disease. Dig Dis 12:321–330, 1994.
Lewis WD, Skinner M, Simms RW, et al: Orthotopic liver transplantation for familial amyloidotic polyneuropathy. Clin Transpl 8 (2 Part 1):107–110, 1994.
Matsumoto T, Yoshimine T, Shimouchi K, et al: The liver and systemic lupus erythematosus: Pathologic analysis of fifty-two cases and review of Japanese autopsy registry data. Human Pathol 23(10):1151–1158, 1992.
Mican JM, DiBisceglie AM, Fong T-L, et al: Hepatic involvement of mastocytosis: Clinical pathologic correlations in 41 cases. Hepatology 22:1163–1170, 1995.
Miller MH, Urowitz MB, Gladman DD, Blendis LM: The liver and systemic lupus erythematosus. Q J Med 211:401–409, 1984.
Olano JP, Borucki MJ, Wen JW, et al: Massive hepatic steatosis and lactic acidosis in a patient with AIDS who was receiving zidovudine. Clin Infect Dis 21(4):973–976, 1995.
Peters RA, Koukoulis G, Gimson A: Primary amyloidosis and severe intrahepatic cholestatic jaundice. Gut 35:1322–1325, 1994.
Poles MA, Dieterich DT, Schwarz ED, et al: Liver biopsy findings in 501 patients infected with human immunodeficiency virus (HIV). J Acquir Immune Defic Synd Hum Retrovirol 11:170–177, 1996.

Runyon BA, Labrecque DR, Anuras S: The spectrum of liver disease in systemic lupus erythematosus. Am J Med 69:187–194, 1980.

Rustgi VK, Hoofnagle JH, Gerin JL, et al: Hepatitis B virus infection in the acquired immunodeficiency syndrome. Ann Intern Med 101:795–797, 1984.

Skopouli FN, Barbatis C, Moutsopouls HM: Liver involvement in primary Sjogren's syndrome. Br J Rheumatol 33 (8):745–748, 1994.

Terk MR, Esplin J, Lee K, et al: MR imaging of patients with type I Gaucher's disease: Relationship between bone and visceral changes. Am J Roentgenol 165 (3):599–604, 1995.

Tran A, Quaranta JF, Benzaken S, et al: High prevalence of thyroid autoantibodies in a prospective series of patients with chronic hepatitis C before interferon therapy. Hepatology 18:253–257, 1993.

Van Steenberg NW, Lanckmans S: Liver disturbances in obesity and diabetes mellitus. Int J Obesity Relat Metab Disord 19 (Suppl 3):S27–S36, 1995.

Wanless IR, Liu JJ, Butany J: Role of thrombosis in the pathogenesis of congestive hepatic fibrosis (cardiac cirrhosis). Hepatology 21:1232–1237, 1995.

Wanless IA: Micronodular transformation (nodular regenerative hyperplasia) of the liver: A report of 64 cases among 2500 autopsies and a new classification of benign hepatocellular nodules. Hepatology 11:787–797, 1990.

Part

Specialized Evaluation and Treatment of Liver and Biliary Disease

29

Evaluation of Surgical Risk in Patients with Liver Disease

Lisa A. Mueller
Lawrence S. Friedman

The liver is an organ with numerous functions: synthesis of plasma proteins and coagulation factors, metabolism of nutrients and drugs, excretion and detoxification of endogenous toxins and exogenous agents, and a functional filtering system for portal venous blood. Any or all of these functions may be impaired in patients with liver disease. It is easy to understand why there is increased morbidity and mortality in patients with liver disease who undergo surgery. The pharmacokinetic parameters of anesthetics and perioperative medications are affected by the changes in plasma protein binding, detoxification, and excretion that result from liver disease. Increased perioperative bleeding may accompany coagulopathy. Impaired filtering of antigens by hepatic reticuloendothelial cells and other changes in the immune system contribute to an increased propensity toward postoperative infections. Finally, a diseased liver is particularly susceptible to subtle hemodynamic changes that accompany any surgical procedure.

The importance of recognizing and assessing the inherent risks of surgery in patients with liver disease cannot be overemphasized. In this chapter we consider the impact of surgery on the liver and present an approach to assessing operative risk in patients with various liver diseases. In addition, guidelines for managing patients with liver disease in the perioperative period are provided.

ANESTHETIC AND SURGICAL CONSIDERATIONS

The medications used in the perioperative period, anesthetic agents, and the surgical procedure itself all have the potential to affect liver function adversely. Indeed, mild postoperative liver function test abnormalities are common even in surgical patients without pre-existing liver disease. Patients

with liver disease are particularly sensitive to such insults; therefore, an understanding of various stressors in the perioperative period is essential when evaluating surgical risk in these patients.

Perioperative Medications

Inhaled Anesthetics

Inhalational agents of the halothane family (haloalkanes) are lipid soluble and are metabolized by the liver to more hydrophilic substances that can be excreted in bile. The degrees of hepatic metabolism of methoxyflurane (no longer used), halothane, enflurane, and isoflurane are 50%, 20%, 2%, and 0.2%, respectively. In addition, these volatile anesthetics may decrease hepatic blood flow. This effect results from decreases in portal vein and hepatic artery blood flow as well as a negative inotropic effect of these agents. It appears from animal studies that hepatic blood flow is least affected by isoflurane. Because it undergoes negligible hepatic metabolism and interferes least with hepatic blood flow, isoflurane is now considered the anesthetic agent of choice in patients with liver disease.

Halothane hepatitis is a dreaded but rare complication of halothane administration. Retrospective studies have found that it occurs in about 1 in 35,000 exposures. The mechanism of halothane-induced hepatic necrosis is unclear but may relate to the formation of trifluoroacetylated proteins formed by oxidative metabolism of halothane. These proteins then become the target of immune-mediated injury. Large retrospective studies have identified obesity, female gender, multiple exposures to halothane, and a family history of similar occurrences as risk factors for halothane hepatitis compared with other haloalkanes. Enflurane and isoflurane have also been reported to cause hepatitis, but less frequently. Sevoflurane and desflurane are under investigation as anesthetic agents and appear to have even less hepatotoxic potential than do other haloalkanes. Nitrous oxide, which is commonly used as an adjunct to the haloalkanes, is not hepatotoxic.

Neuromuscular Blocking Agents

Commonly used neuromuscular blocking agents generally have an increased volume of distribution in patients with liver disease, as a result of fluid retention. Because liver dysfunction is associated with reduced plasma cholinesterase activity, agents such as succinylcholine and mivacurium, which are inactivated by plasma cholinesterase, have a prolonged duration of action. This is also true for agents such as pancuronium and vecuronium, which are excreted in the bile. Atracurium has been recommended as the agent of choice in patients with liver disease, because its metabolism does not depend on the liver or kidneys, and its pharmacokinetics and pharmacodynamics are similar to those in healthy persons. Doxacurium is recommended for prolonged surgical procedures, such as liver transplantation. It is a long-acting, nondepolarizing skeletal muscle relaxant that is excreted unchanged in urine and bile, and its pharmacokinetics are not significantly altered during liver transplantation.

Narcotics

Narcotics such as morphine and meperidine undergo extensive first-pass metabolism by the liver. As a result, patients with liver disease and altered hepatic blood flow are exquisitely sensitive to these agents, and they generally require doses that are lower than usual. Fentanyl and sufentanil are preferred because their metabolism is not affected significantly by liver disease.

Hypnotics and Sedatives

Sedatives carry the risk of precipitating hepatic encephalopathy in patients with chronic liver disease. Benzodiazepines that undergo glucuronidation, such as oxazepam and lorazepam, are preferred in patients with liver disease because their elimination is not prolonged, in contrast to diazepam and chlordiazepoxide. Barbiturates do not seem to affect hepatic blood flow significantly but must be used with caution in patients with liver disease, because they bind to γ-aminobutyric acid (GABA) receptors and can precipitate encephalopathy.

Benzodiazepines can occasionally cause cholestatic (and rarely hepatocellular) liver injury. Barbiturates, like phenytoin and carbamazepine, are rarely associated with a syndrome of fever, hepatitis, lymphadenopathy, eosinophilia, and dermatitis. The risk of such reactions is no greater in patients with liver disease than in others.

Hemodynamic Effects

One of the most critical ways in which surgery can adversely affect the liver is by diminishing hepatic blood flow, thus decreasing the supply of oxygenated blood. Three

quarters of the hepatic blood flow comes from the portal vein; the remainder comes from the hepatic arterial system. Both blood supplies can be influenced by surgery itself as well as by the pharmacologic agents used in the perioperative period.

Independent of the nature of the surgical procedure, the induction of anesthesia may reduce hepatic blood flow by 30% to 50%. This is true for inhalational anesthetics as well as for spinal and epidural anesthesia. However, not all inhalational anesthetic agents affect hepatic blood flow to the same degree. Halothane and enflurane decrease both portal and hepatic arterial blood flow. In contrast, isoflurane reduces portal blood flow but increases hepatic arterial blood flow. Nitrous oxide does not seem to affect hepatic blood flow as long as ventilation is adequate.

Another pharmacologic agent that may affect hepatic blood flow is morphine, which reduces splanchnic blood flow at low doses but can actually increase splanchnic blood flow at higher doses. Barbiturates do not affect hepatic blood flow.

Ventilatory support during anesthesia must be monitored closely in patients with liver disease, because hypoperfusion of the liver may occur if hypercarbia is allowed to develop. This results in splanchnic vasodilatation and diminished hepatic blood flow. Regardless of the mechanism, when the delivery of oxygenated blood to the liver is reduced, there is a risk of ischemic injury to the hepatocyte. This effect is usually subtle in patients with a normal liver who undergo surgery but can lead to acute hepatic decompensation in patients with pre-existing liver disease.

Type of Surgery

The type of surgical procedure and other surgical factors are important variables in assessing operative risk in a patient with liver disease (Table 29–1). Laparotomy results in greater reduction in hepatic blood flow than does extra-abdominal surgery. Visceral traction may result in reflex systemic hypotension from dilatation of capacitance vessels and can thus diminish hepatic blood flow. When surgery is complicated by hemorrhage, decreased blood volume may precipitate a fall in hepatic blood flow and ischemic injury to the liver. In patients with cirrhosis, previous abdominal

Table 29–1   Potential Effects of Anesthesia and Surgery* on the Liver

Hemodynamic alterations caused by
Blood loss
Anesthetics
Medications
Mechanical ventilation
Abdominal surgery

Medication-related complications
Precipitation of encephalopathy
Haloalkane hepatitis
Increased sensitivity to sedatives

*High-risk surgery includes emergent surgery, upper abdominal surgery, cholecystectomy, colectomy, cardiac surgery, and hepatic resection.

surgery can result in adhesions that are highly vascular, making repeat abdominal surgery particularly difficult technically, with an increased risk of intraoperative bleeding. Emergent surgery is associated with markedly higher morbidity and mortality than elective surgery. Cholecystectomy and gastric surgery are particularly hazardous in patients with cirrhosis and extensive upper abdominal collaterals. Colectomy in patients with cirrhosis is also associated with high rates of morbidity (up to 48%) and mortality (up to 24%). Moreover, stomal varices, which can bleed, may ultimately develop in patients with an ileostomy.

OVERALL APPROACH TO ASSESSING OPERATIVE RISK IN PATIENTS WITH LIVER DISEASE

History

The evaluation of perioperative risk in any patient should include a complete and detailed medical history. This is particularly true when considering hepatic diseases, because liver function tests are not routinely ordered preoperatively. Risk factors for hepatitis should be identified, including previous blood transfusions, tattoos, intravenous drug abuse, and homosexual intercourse. Careful attention should be paid to a personal or family history of postoperative jaundice after an inhalational agent such as halothane, in which case use of another anesthetic agent may be advisable. Excessive alcohol intake or a history of hepatitis may raise the question of chronic occult liver disease. A family history of early onset cirrhosis raises considerations of diseases such as hemochromatosis and α_1-antitrypsin deficiency. A complete medication history should be obtained, including use of over-the-counter medications and herbal remedies. Finally, a thorough review of systems may identify symptoms of chronic liver disease such as fatigue, pruritus, or increased abdominal girth.

Physical Examination

A careful physical examination may provide clues to the diagnosis of chronic liver disease or cirrhosis, even in asymptomatic persons with normal liver function tests. Palmar erythema, spider telangiectases, splenomegaly, and gynecomastia and testicular atrophy in men are just a few characteristic physical findings associated with chronic liver disease. The presence of jaundice, ascites, or encephalopathy is of particular prognostic importance. Mild encephalopathy may be suggested by insomnia with daytime somnolence, asterixis, or constructional apraxia. A careful assessment of nutritional status is essential, because malnutrition may increase surgical risk.

Laboratory Data

Whether liver function tests should be ordered routinely on preoperative evaluation is controversial. The frequency of unsuspected liver function test abnormalities has been estimated to be about 1 in 700 preoperative patients. However, if clues are found in the history or physical examination, a full panel of liver function tests should be ordered. Eleva-

tions in serum aspartate aminotransferase (AST) and alanine aminotransferase (ALT) are indicators of hepatic inflammation and may influence the decision to postpone surgery. Hypoalbuminemia and prolongation of the prothrombin time are markers of the severity of chronic liver disease, although neither parameter is specific for liver disease. When associated with liver disease, both reflect impaired hepatocellular function. Hyperbilirubinemia, in the presence of other evidence of hepatocyte dysfunction, also has prognostic importance. However, Gilbert's syndrome, which is characterized by isolated unconjugated hyperbilirubinemia, is not associated with increased surgical risk. Similarly, isolated elevations in alkaline phosphatase and 5′ nucleotidase levels are of little importance when assessing perioperative risk, and further diagnostic testing to determine the cause of these abnormalities may be deferred until the postoperative period. The decision to include additional testing, such as radiologic imaging studies of the liver and liver biopsy, as part of the preoperative evaluation must be made on an individual basis.

ASSESSMENT OF OPERATIVE RISK IN SPECIFIC TYPES OF LIVER DISEASE

Acute Hepatitis

The presence of acute hepatitis is considered to be a contraindication to elective surgery. This recommendation is based on older studies that found an operative mortality of 9.5% to 13% in icteric patients who underwent laparotomy as part of their diagnostic work-up and who were subsequently found to have acute viral hepatitis.

Alcoholic hepatitis, particularly when alcoholic hyaline is present in liver biopsy specimens, has also been associated with a high operative mortality. In one study comparing percutaneous and open liver biopsy in patients with alcoholic hepatitis, a 5-fold increase in mortality was found in those undergoing open liver biopsy, in whom the mortality rate was 58%. In general, elective surgery should be deferred until liver function test results have returned to normal.

Chronic Hepatitis

The impact chronic hepatitis has on operative outcome seems to be related to the clinical, biochemical, and histologic severity of the hepatitis. Patients with what was previously referred to as chronic active hepatitis have been reported to have greater morbidity than those with chronic persistent hepatitis. A new classification of chronic hepatitis proposed by the International Working Party on the Terminology of Chronic Hepatitis is based on etiology, grade (degree of portal, periportal, and lobular inflammation), and stage (degree of hepatic fibrosis) and may prove useful in assessing prognosis in patients with chronic hepatitis who undergo surgery (see Chapter 5). In general, elective surgery can be performed in patients with asymptomatic, mild chronic hepatitis. Patients with symptomatic chronic hepatitis have an increased surgical risk, particularly if hepatic synthetic or excretory function is impaired, portal hypertension is present, or hepatic inflammation is severe (bridging or multilobular necrosis). In these patients, surgery should be postponed, if possible, until liver function improves.

Alcoholic Liver Disease

The spectrum of alcoholic liver disease includes fatty liver, a benign, reversible condition that is not a contraindication to elective surgery, and acute alcoholic hepatitis, which can be associated with unacceptable surgical mortality. Hepatic inflammation in alcoholic hepatitis may be protracted, despite abstinence, and if there is any question of ongoing inflammation, a liver biopsy may be helpful before proceeding with elective surgery. Surgery in patients with alcoholic cirrhosis is discussed later.

Autoimmune Hepatitis

The mainstay of therapy for autoimmune hepatitis is corticosteroids with or without azathioprine. As for patients on chronic corticosteroid therapy for any reason, surgery is a significant stressor, and perioperative hydrocortisone boluses are recommended in a dose of 100 mg intravenously every 8 hours starting the night before surgery until the patient can take medications orally, followed thereafter by a rapid taper to the maintenance dose. Azathioprine may be discontinued during the time when the patient takes nothing by mouth. Because of the additional suppression of the immune system by chronic corticosteroids, prophylactic broad-spectrum antibiotics may be considered in the perioperative period.

Cirrhosis

Most available data on the risk of surgery in patients with liver disease pertain to patients with cirrhosis. There is clearly increased operative morbidity and mortality in patients with cirrhosis, but assessment of the degree of risk in an individual patient presents a challenge. First, the severity of cirrhosis is difficult to quantitate because of the multiplicity of functions that may be involved. Second, there are multiple causes of cirrhosis, and the prognostic implications of each cause with regard to surgical risk are not well defined. Third, available data for defining risk factors in cirrhotic patients undergoing surgery are derived from small studies that have methodologic weaknesses, especially retrospective designs and selection biases. Nonetheless, several parameters have been found in more than one study to be associated with increased surgical morbidity and mortality (Table 29–2).

As discussed earlier, emergent surgery carries a higher risk in cirrhotic patients than elective surgery. Abdominal procedures, particularly biliary tract surgery, are associated with increased morbidity and mortality when compared with nonabdominal surgery. For obvious reasons, hepatic resection is associated with a substantial risk in persons with cirrhosis, and the outcome depends on the degree of hepatic reserve and the ability of the remaining liver to regenerate.

The most widely used measures of hepatic function are adapted from the Child-Turcotte classification, which was published initially in 1964. This classification predicted the outcome in patients who had cirrhosis and who were under-

Table 29–2 Risk Factors for Morbidity and Mortality in Patients with Cirrhosis Undergoing Surgery

Type of Surgery

Emergent
Abdominal
Hepatic resection
Cardiac surgery

Patient Profile

Child's classification (see Table 29–3)
Ascites
Encephalopathy
Infection
Anemia
Malnutrition
Jaundice
Hypoalbuminemia
Portal hypertension
Prolongation of prothrombin time that does not correct with vitamin K
Abnormal quantitative liver function tests
 Galactose elimination capacity
 Aminopyrine breath test
 Monoethylglycinexylidide test

going portosystemic shunt surgery. Often, the Child-Pugh classification is used, in which prolongation of the prothrombin time replaces nutritional status, and the other four parameters—serum albumin, serum bilirubin, the degree of ascites, and the severity of encephalopathy—are identical to the original classification proposed by Child and Turcotte.

There are several inherent problems with the Child-Pugh classification in general and its use in assessing operative risk in particular. First, the degree of encephalopathy is a subjective assessment. Second, the absence of ascites on clinical assessment may not correspond with findings on ultrasonography. Third, no significance is placed on whether a prolonged prothrombin time corrects with administration of vitamin K. Finally, the Child-Pugh classification does not take into account other important variables such as the type or urgency of surgery, which have been shown to affect operative risk.

Despite these inadequacies, the Child-Pugh classification is the most widely used predictor of surgical risk in patients with cirrhosis. Use of this classification to assess surgical risk is supported by several small studies, most notably that of Garrison and associates in 1984. They found that among 100 patients with predominantly alcoholic cirrhosis undergoing abdominal surgery, the operative mortality was 10%, 31% and 76% for patients classified as Child's class A, B, and C, respectively, and that the Child classification was the best predictor of surgical mortality and morbidity among 52 parameters assessed.

Attempts have been made to assess liver function quantitatively by using dynamic tests such as the galactose elimination capacity, aminopyrine breath test, indocyanine green clearance, and rate of metabolism of lidocaine to monoethylglycinexylidide (MEGX) (see Chapter 3). These tests, although of some value in assessing hepatic reserve, have not

Table 29–3   Assessment of Surgical Risk in Relation to Child-Turcotte-Pugh Classification (see also Table 31–3)

Child-Turcotte-Pugh Class	A	B	C
Child-Turcotte-Pugh Score	5–6	7–9	≥10
Perioperative mortality rates	0–10%	4–31%	19–76%
Operability	Good	Possible	Poor
Hepatic reserve	Adequate	Moderate	Minimal

yet gained widespread clinical acceptance, and it has not been shown that they provide any additional prognostic information over that already derived from the Child-Pugh classification (Table 29–3).

In general, surgery is well tolerated in patients with Child's A cirrhosis. In patients with Child's B cirrhosis, surgery is not contraindicated, but attempts should be made to improve hepatic function before surgery (although the benefit of this approach has never been evaluated prospectively), and certain types of surgery, such as extensive hepatic resections or cardiac surgery, should be avoided. Child's C cirrhosis should generally be regarded as an absolute contraindication to elective surgery.

MANAGEMENT OF COMPLICATIONS OF LIVER DISEASE IN THE SURGICAL PATIENT

Impaired Hemostasis

Coagulopathy with impaired hemostasis has the potential to affect outcome adversely in patients with liver disease who undergo surgery. Impaired hepatic synthetic function results in diminished production of most coagulation factors with prolongation of the prothrombin time and, with severe coagulopathy, the partial thromboplastin time. Cholestasis can result in vitamin K deficiency, as can malnutrition and use of certain antibiotics. Parenteral vitamin K should be administered to any patient with liver disease and prolongation of the prothrombin time. If the coagulopathy cannot be corrected, it may be necessary to postpone surgery, because this implies significant impairment of hepatocellular function. Certain types of surgery, such as vascular surgery involving major arteries, may be particularly hazardous in patients with coagulopathy.

Thrombocytopenia frequently accompanies liver disease and results from portal hypertension with hypersplenism, impaired hepatic synthesis of thrombopoietin, and bone marrow suppression by alcohol. In addition to quantitative abnormalities, there may be qualitative defects in platelet function. Platelet transfusions are indicated preoperatively when the platelet count is less than 50,000/mm^3. Although the accuracy and usefulness of the bleeding time are debated, prolongation of the bleeding time may also be an indication for platelet transfusions and the administration of desmopressin acetate (DDAVP), a synthetic analogue of vasopressin that causes the release of endogenously produced von Willebrand factor, which is essential for platelet function in primary hemostasis.

Ascites

Ascites in patients with cirrhosis reflects advanced liver disease and of itself has the potential to complicate surgical procedures. Ascites may lead to delayed healing of abdominal wall incisions, wound dehiscence, and incisional hernias. Because ascites restricts diaphragmatic mobility, mechanical ventilation is more difficult in patients with ascites. Perioperative fluid management is more complex in patients with ascites because of the potential for large fluid shifts that can result from the intraoperative loss of ascitic fluid. Moreover, loss of ascitic fluid can lead to depletion of ascitic proteins and opsonins, which may contribute to infectious complications in the perioperative period. It is well recognized that patients with liver disease are more susceptible than patients without liver disease to septic sequelae of surgery, particularly peritonitis and intra-abdominal abscesses as a result of direct contamination of ascites at laparotomy or seeding of ascites due to bacteremia associated with surgery at remote sites. In general, before elective surgery it is prudent to minimize the amount of ascites by large-volume paracentesis with or without medical therapy. In any patient with ascites undergoing surgery, a diagnostic paracentesis to exclude occult peritonitis is worthwhile.

Encephalopathy

Encephalopathy should be evaluated and treated before elective surgery. Close attention to fluid and electrolyte management, correction of metabolic abnormalities such as alkalosis, avoidance of sedatives, and control of gastrointestinal bleeding and other factors that can precipitate encephalopathy in the perioperative period are essential (Table 29–4). Modest dietary protein restriction, correction of constipation, and treatment of any infections will also help minimize the chance of recurrent encephalopathy postoperatively (Table 29–5). Refractory encephalopathy that persists, despite correction of precipitating factors and the administration of lactulose, is a contraindication to elective surgery.

Portal Hypertension

The presence of portal hypertension and intra-abdominal varices has important technical implications for abdominal surgery, in addition to reflecting significant underlying liver disease. As mentioned earlier, vascular adhesions can pose a challenge to surgical dissection and lead to catastrophic intra-abdominal bleeding. Postoperative anastomotic and

Table 29–4 Common Perioperative Precipitants of Hepatic Encephalopathy

Infection
Constipation
Gastrointestinal hemorrhage
Alkalosis
High protein diet
Hypoxia
Central nervous system depressants
Progressive hepatic dysfunction
Azotemia
Dehydration
Portosystemic shunt surgery
Hepatic resection

stomal varices can also result in bleeding. If liver transplantation is contemplated in the future, the decision to undertake intra-abdominal surgery must take into account the possibility that the technical difficulty of liver transplantation may be increased by prior abdominal surgery, particularly in the right upper quadrant. When possible, elective surgery should be deferred.

Hepatocellular Carcinoma

Hepatocellular carcinoma is a well-established complication of long-standing cirrhosis, with an estimated annual incidence of 3% to 5% in patients with cirrhosis. In the past, cirrhosis was considered a contraindication to hepatic resection. Reported perioperative mortality rates were in the order of 50%. With better patient selection, meticulous preoperative preparation of the patient, intensive intra- and postoperative monitoring, and improved surgical techniques, recent studies have reported a perioperative mortality rate for hepatic resection (usually for hepatocellular carcinoma) of 3% to 16%. Postoperative morbidity is still high, with rates in cirrhotic patients up to 60%. Hepatic failure (jaundice, ascites, or encephalopathy), gastrointestinal hemorrhage, and sepsis are the most common postoperative complications. The Child classification is still the most widely used measure of operability, but studies have failed

Table 29–5 Preoperative Preparation of Patients with Advanced Cirrhosis

Maximize nutritional status
Salt restriction and diuretic therapy of ascites
Diagnostic paracentesis to exclude peritonitis
Large-volume paracentesis when ascites is substantial
Correct coagulopathy with vitamin K, fresh frozen plasma
Modest protein restriction and lactulose for hepatic encephalopathy
Correct potential precipitants of encephalopathy such as electrolyte abnormalities, constipation, and alkalosis
Perioperative antibiotics
Consider intraoperative hemodynamic monitoring

to confirm its value in predicting morbidity and mortality because of selection bias and the small number of patients with Child's class B and C cirrhosis studied. A general rule has been that patients with Child's A cirrhosis tolerate hepatic resection quite well; patients with Child's B cirrhosis need to be assessed individually after aggressive therapy to optimize their medical condition; and patients with Child's C cirrhosis should not undergo hepatic resection. However, one study suggests that as many as 60% of patients with Child's A cirrhosis, when associated with portal hypertension as measured by a hepatic venous pressure gradient higher than 10 mm Hg, experience unresolved hepatic decompensation after hepatic resection for hepatocellular carcinoma. If this finding is confirmed in larger studies, routine preoperative identification of portal hypertension by measurement of the hepatic venous pressure gradient may be warranted to assess the feasibility of hepatic resection.

As indicated previously, quantitative liver function tests such as the galactose elimination capacity are used in some centers to assess hepatic reserve, but they are not widely available and their advantage over the Child classification as a prognosticator is not established. In the assessment of surgical risk, particularly in patients undergoing hepatic resection, advanced age and comorbid conditions must also be considered.

MANAGEMENT OF EXTRAHEPATIC COMPLICATIONS OF LIVER DISEASE

Several forms of liver disease are associated with extrahepatic manifestations that warrant special consideration in the perioperative period. For example, patients with hemochromatosis may have diabetes that needs close monitoring in the perioperative period. They may have a cardiomyopathy that may affect surgical risk. In fact, recent experience suggests that the outcome of liver transplantation in patients with hemochromatosis may be less favorable than that for other types of liver disease because of an increased rate of cardiac and infectious complications post-transplantation.

Patients with Wilson's disease may have a number of extrahepatic manifestations. Neuropsychiatric involvement may interfere with the ability to provide informed consent; cardiomyopathy and hemolytic anemia may warrant additional perioperative evaluation; and renal dysfunction necessitates close attention to fluid and electrolyte status. Moreover, some patients with Wilson's disease do not tolerate major surgery, which may precipitate or aggravate neurologic symptoms. Therefore, elective surgery should be performed only if absolutely necessary. Cholecystectomy, which is required with increased frequency in patients with Wilson's disease because of pigment stone formation as a result of hemolysis, should be undertaken only after careful consideration of the fact that subsequent liver transplantation may be made technically more difficult.

When patients with Wilson's disease undergo surgery, the dose of D-penicillamine should be decreased in the first 1 to 2 postoperative weeks, because this agent interferes with cross-linking of collagen and may impair wound healing. Nephrotic syndrome may complicate therapy with

Table 29–6   Relative Contraindications to Elective Surgery in Patients with Liver Disease

Acute viral hepatitis
Acute alcoholic hepatitis
Fulminant hepatic failure
Child's class C cirrhosis
Severe or symptomatic chronic hepatitis
Potential liver transplantation candidate
Prolongation of the prothrombin time of $>$ 3 seconds despite administration of vitamin K
Severe extrahepatic abnormalities including:
  Hypoxemia
  Cardiomyopathy
  Acute renal failure

Table 29–7   Factors Reported to be Associated with Increased Operative Mortality in Patients with Obstructive Jaundice

Hematocrit value $<30\%$
Serum bilirubin $>$ 11 mg/dL
Malignant cause of obstruction
Azotemia
Hypoalbuminemia
Cholangitis

D-penicillamine, and the possibility of an associated hypercoagulable state should be kept in mind. Aggressive perioperative measures to prevent thromboembolism are recommended in this group of patients.

The hepatopulmonary syndrome can occasionally complicate cirrhosis. This entity is defined as the triad of liver disease, an increased alveolar-arterial gradient on room air with hypoxemia, and intrapulmonary vascular dilatations. When severe, elective surgery may be precluded (Table 29–6). Pulmonary hypertension and pleural effusions may also complicate cirrhosis and may interfere with oxygenation and the ability to tolerate anesthesia.

SPECIAL PROBLEM OF SURGERY IN PATIENTS WITH OBSTRUCTIVE JAUNDICE

Obstructive jaundice of any cause, from choledocholithiasis to malignancy, is associated with increased surgical morbidity and mortality. The perioperative mortality rate in patients with obstructive jaundice has been estimated to be in the range of 8% to 20%. Several factors have been reported to contribute to this poor outcome, including a malignant cause of biliary obstruction, the degree of hyperbilirubinemia, and endotoxemia resulting from bacterial translocation across the intestinal wall.

Risk Factors

Attempts have been made to stratify patients preoperatively according to operative risk. One of the largest studies was a retrospective review by Dixon and associates of 373 patients undergoing surgery for obstructive jaundice. They found a perioperative mortality rate of 9.1%, and on multivariate analysis they identified three predictors of postoperative mortality: (1) an initial hematocrit value less than 30%, (2) an initial serum bilirubin level higher than 200 mol/L (11 mg/dL), and (3) a malignant cause of obstruction. When all three factors were present, the mortality rate was approximately 60%, whereas when none were present, the mortality rate was only 5%. Other preoperative predictors of poor surgical outcome identified in other studies include azotemia, hypoalbuminemia, and cholangitis (Table 29–7).

Complications

Infection is an important cause of perioperative morbidity and mortality in patients with obstructive jaundice. Bacterial colonization of the biliary tree is often the source, and cholangitis has been reported in up to 25% of patients who have undergone endoscopic retrograde cholangiopancreatography (ERCP) in the presence of biliary obstruction. In addition, the immune system is depressed in icteric individuals. Impairment in both Kupffer cell function and delayed hypersensitivity have been demonstrated. More recently, defective neutrophil function has been observed in patients with obstructive jaundice. Endotoxemia has been found in as many as 60% of patients with obstructive jaundice. It is not surprising that postoperative wound infections and other septic complications are common (Table 29–8).

Renal failure is a frequent complication in the perioperative period in patients with obstructive jaundice. The etiology is probably multifactorial and may relate to perioperative volume depletion and redistribution of intrarenal blood flow mediated through prostaglandins and other vasoactive substances. To what extent bilirubin is directly toxic to the kidney is not clear; however, the risk of renal failure is directly related to the serum bilirubin level. Endotoxemia as a result of depressed immune function and bacterial translocation across the gut has been proposed as a pathogenic factor. Fibrin has been shown to deposit in glomeruli, and the creatinine clearance decreases. Acute tubular necrosis is common. When renal failure complicates surgery for obstructive jaundice, the mortality rate may exceed 50%.

Other postoperative complications seen in patients with obstructive jaundice that may be related to endotoxemia include disseminated intravascular coagulation and gastroin-

Table 29–8   Postoperative Complications in Patients with Obstructive Jaundice

Cholangitis/infection
Renal failure
Disseminated intravascular coagulation
Gastrointestinal hemorrhage
Delayed wound healing
Wound dehiscence
Incisional hernia
Prolonged ileus

testinal bleeding from stress ulcers. In animal models and in humans, obstructive jaundice has also been shown to lead to delayed wound healing. Additionally, there appears to be an increased risk of wound dehiscence, wound infection, and incisional hernias. It is not clear whether this is related to hyperbilirubinemia per se or to associated malnutrition.

Perioperative Management

Oral administration of bile salts, such as ursodeoxycholic acid, to patients with obstructive jaundice has been reported to prevent endotoxemia and reduce the likelihood of postoperative azotemia. Lactulose 30 mL every 6 hours starting 2 to 3 days before surgery may also be beneficial.

Given the relatively high frequency of postoperative infections, intravenous antibiotics are generally recommended in the perioperative period. Gram-negative and anaerobic coverage is essential.

Maintenance of intravascular volume is important to prevent postoperative renal failure. Intravenous administration of mannitol has been advocated to maintain urine output in excess of 1 mL/min. Potentially nephrotoxic drugs, such as nonsteroidal anti-inflammatory agents and aminoglycosides, should be avoided.

Biliary Decompression

Because many of the postoperative complications seen in patients undergoing surgery for obstructive jaundice are thought to be related either directly or indirectly to hyperbilirubinemia, preoperative biliary decompression is often considered. However, several prospective randomized controlled studies have shown that preoperative external biliary drainage (i.e., via a transhepatic approach) does not improve surgical morbidity or mortality. Although preoperative endoscopic biliary drainage has the advantages of restoring enterohepatic circulation of bile salts and avoiding percutaneous puncture, evidence is lacking to support its routine use before abdominal surgery in patients with a malignant cause of obstruction.

Therapeutic Options

Malignant causes of biliary obstruction are often incurable, and regardless of the approach taken to decompress the biliary tree, the aim of therapy is often palliative. There continues to be debate as to the optimal palliative approach. One study comparing endoscopic placement of a plastic biliary endoprosthesis and surgical decompression for malignant distal bile duct obstruction found similar efficacy rates and similar overall survival rates, though lower early morbidity and mortality rates in the group treated endoscopically. Whether endoscopic placement of metallic stents offers an advantage over surgical palliation remains uncertain. For lesions higher in the bile duct, percutaneous decompression may be used alone or in combination with an endoscopic approach.

Choledocholithiasis is successfully managed endoscopically in up to 90% of cases, depending on a number of variables including stone size and technical expertise. Management of large calculi occasionally requires additional endoscopic interventions such as mechanical or laser litho-

tripsy. Extracorporeal lithotripsy is another nonsurgical option. In patients who are not good surgical candidates, biliary endoprostheses may be placed as palliative treatment of large bile duct stones that cannot be removed. In patients who have not undergone cholecystectomy, the risk of cholecystitis after endoscopic papillotomy for choledocholithiasis is approximately 10% over the next 5 to 10 years.

For patients with acute cholecystitis who are not good surgical candidates, cholecystostomy is an alternative to open cholecystectomy. Choledocholithiasis complicated by cholangitis is treated with intravenous antibiotics and endoscopic decompression; surgical decompression is associated with higher morbidity and mortality rates.

POSTOPERATIVE JAUNDICE (see Chapter 4)

As described earlier, there are many factors that contribute to postoperative liver function test abnormalities, including hemodynamic changes, drugs, infections, and occasionally extrahepatic obstruction. Benign postoperative jaundice is a well-described entity that may follow major abdominal surgery. It is characterized by hyperbilirubinemia that usually develops during the first three postoperative days and typically peaks between days 3 and 10. There may be a 2- to 3-fold increase in the serum alkaline phosphatase level, but the serum aminotransferases, albumin, and prothrombin time usually remain normal. The diagnosis is usually made after exclusion of extrahepatic obstruction by ultrasonography and, if necessary, ERCP, and after the time course and pattern of liver function test abnormalities become apparent. Patients with liver disease are more likely to develop this entity, and unlike centrilobular necrosis that results from acute hypoperfusion of the liver, benign postoperative jaundice is, as the name implies, benign and self-limiting. Its pathophysiology is probably multifactorial, including increased pigment load from blood transfusions and resorption of hematomas and impaired hepatocyte function in the immediate postoperative setting. A list of potential causes of postoperative jaundice is outlined in Table 29–9.

Table 29–9 Causes of Postoperative Jaundice

Increased bilirubin load
  Transfusions of red blood cells (hemolysis)
  Resorption of hematomas
  Gilbert's syndrome
  Underlying hemolytic anemia

Hepatocellular dysfunction
  Anesthetic hepatotoxicity
  Hypoperfusion injury with centrilobular necrosis
  Hepatotoxins (e.g., phenothiazines, antibiotics)
  Total parenteral nutrition
  Sepsis
  Benign postoperative intrahepatic cholestasis

Extrahepatic obstruction
  Choledocholithiasis
  Cholecystitis
  Pancreatitis
  Biliary stricture, leak, tumor, or clot

SUGGESTED READINGS

Bruix J, Castells A, Bosch J, et al: Surgical resection of hepatocellular carcinoma in cirrhotic patients: Prognostic value of preoperative portal pressure. Gastroenterology 111:1018–1022, 1996.

Chijiiwa K, Kozaki N, Naito T, et al: Treatment of choice for choledocholithiasis in patients with acute obstructive suppurative cholangitis and liver cirrhosis. Am J Surg 170:356–360, 1995.

Child CG, Turcotte JG: Surgery and portal hypertension. In Child GC (ed): The Liver and Portal Hypertension. Philadelphia: WB Saunders, 1964, pp 1–85.

Diamond T, Parks RW: Perioperative management of obstructive jaundice. Br J Surg 84:147–149, 1997.

Dixon JM, Armstrong CP, Duffy SW, Davies GC: Factors affecting morbidity and mortality after surgery for obstructive jaundice: A review of 373 patients. Gut 24:845–852, 1983.

Friedman LS, Maddrey WC: Surgery in the patient with liver disease. Med Clin North Am 71:453–476, 1987.

Garrison RN, Cryer HM, Howard DA, et al: Clarification of risk factors for abdominal operations in patients with hepatic cirrhosis. Ann Surg 199:648–655, 1984.

Gholson CF, Provenza JM, Bacon BR: Hepatologic considerations in patients with parenchymal liver disease undergoing surgery. Am J Gastroenterol 85:487–496, 1990.

Grande L, Garcia-Valdecasa JC, Fuster J, et al: Obstructive jaundice and wound healing. Br J Surg 77:440–442, 1990.

Greig JD, Krukowski ZH, Matheson NA: Surgical morbidity and mortality in one hundred and twenty-nine patients with obstructive jaundice. Br J Surg 75:216–219, 1988.

Greve JW, Gouma DJ, Soeters PB, Buurman WA: Suppression of cellular immunity in obstructive jaundice is caused by endotoxins: A study with germ-free rats. Gastroenterology 98:478–485, 1990.

Harville DD, Summerskill WHJ: Surgery in acute hepatitis. JAMA 184:257–261, 1963.

Holt C, Csete M, Martin P: Hepatotoxicity of anesthetics and other central nervous system drugs. Gastroenterol Clin North Am 24:853–874, 1995.

Hunter JM: New neuromuscular blocking drugs. N Engl J Med 332:1691–1699, 1995.

Lai ECS, Chu KM, Lo CY, et al: Surgery for malignant obstructive jaundice: Analysis of mortality. Surgery 112:891–896, 1992.

Lai ECS, Mok FPT, Fan ST, et al: Preoperative endoscopic drainage for malignant obstructive jaundice. Br J Surg 81:1195–1198, 1994.

LaMont JT, Isselbacher KJ: Postoperative jaundice. N Engl J Med 288:305–307, 1973.

Lehnert T, Herfarth C: Peptic ulcer surgery in patients with liver cirrhosis. Ann Surg 217:338–346, 1993.

MacIntosh EL, Minuk GY: Hepatic resection in patients with cirrhosis and hepatocellular carcinoma. Surg Gynecol Obstet 174:245–254, 1992.

Mansour A, Watson W, Shayani V, Pickleman J: Abdominal operations in patients with cirrhosis: Still a major surgical challenge. Surgery 122:730–736, 1997.

Metcalf AMT, Dozois RR, Wolff BG, Beart RW: The surgical risk of colectomy in patients with cirrhosis. Dis Colon Rectum 30:529–531, 1987.

Pain JA, Cahill CJ, Bailey ME: Perioperative complications in obstructive jaundice: Therapeutic considerations. Br J Surg 72:942–945, 1985.

Plusa S, Webster N, Primrose J: Obstructive jaundice causes reduced expression of polymorphonuclear leukocyte adhesion molecules and a depressed response to bacterial wall products in vitro. Gut 38:784–787, 1996.

Pugh RNH, Murray-Lyon IM, Dawson JL, et al: Transection of the oesophagus for bleeding oesophageal varices. Br J Surg 60:646–649, 1973.

Runyon BA: Surgical procedures are well tolerated by patients with asymptomatic chronic hepatitis. J Clin Gastroenterol 8:542–544, 1986.

Smith AC, Dowsett JF, Russell RCG, et al: Randomised trial of endoscopic stenting versus surgical bypass in malignant low bile duct obstruction. Lancet 344:1655–1660, 1994.

Stone HH: Preoperative and postoperative care. Surg Clin North Am 57:409–419, 1977.

Wait RB, Kahng KU: Renal failure complicating obstructive jaundice. Am J Surg 157:256–263, 1989.

Ziser A, Plevak DJ, Wiesner RH, et al: Morbidity and mortality in cirrhotic patients undergoing anesthesia and surgery. Anesthesiology 90:42–53, 1999.

30

Hepatobiliary Surgery

Henri Bismuth
Annie Fecteau

A good understanding of liver anatomy, especially vascular planes, is crucial to hepatobiliary surgery. Even though Caprio performed the first lobectomy in 1932, it is only since the publication of the landmark anatomic study by Couinaud in 1957 that modern liver surgery has evolved. The application of segmental anatomy of the liver to surgery, which was made possible through the popularization of intraoperative ultrasound, led to a new way of conceptualizing and performing liver resections. During the past decade, the principles of segmental anatomy have been widely applied. This, combined with the remarkable advances in techniques and tools, has allowed surgeons to perform resections with increasing safety and efficacy and to diminish the incidence of local complications, such as postoperative bleeding, necrosis, and biliary fistula. Improved techniques of vascular control, in some cases derived directly from liver transplantation, have allowed access to the most awkwardly placed lesions.

Laparoscopic surgery has revolutionized gallbladder surgery in the last 10 years but has also been associated with a resurgence of bile duct injuries. Laparoscopic techniques are beyond the scope of this chapter.

HEPATIC SURGERY

Classification of Liver Resections

Hepatic resections can be divided into three large categories:

1. Anatomic resections are performed following the segmental anatomy of Couinaud which identifies, according to the distribution of the branches of the portal vein and of the hepatic veins, eight segments, four sectors, and two hemilivers. Anatomic resections can be named depending on the number of neighboring segments that are removed. A right hepatectomy is a resection of segments 5, 6, 7, and 8, whereas a left hepatectomy removes segments 2, 3, and 4 (Fig. 30–1). In both cases, the line of transection is the plane of the middle hepatic vein. Both of these hepatectomies are considered major hepatectomies and thus are trisegmentectomies (removal of three segments in Couinaud's nomenclature). Common trisegmentectomies are the combined resection of segments 4, 5, and 6 or centrally of segments 4, 5, and 8 or 4, 5, and 1. The extended right hepatectomy includes the removal of segment 1 or 4; the extended left hepatectomy includes segments 1 or 5 and 8 (Fig. 30–2). A superextended hepatectomy would involve the removal of six segments. Limited or minor hepatectomies involve less than one, one, or two segments (Fig. 30–3). Each of the eight segments described by Couinaud can be resected separately as a unisegmentectomy, although the elective resection of segments 2 or 3 has no practical value and a left lobectomy, involving both segments in which the line of transection is the umbilical fissure, is preferably performed. A subsegmentectomy designates the removal of an important volume of a segment guided by the distribution described by subsegmental vascular structures. The most common subsegmentectomies are the anterior resection of segment 4 and the anterior, middle, or posterior resection of segment 8. Limited hepatectomies are particularly useful in patients with cirrhosis, because they combine the advantages of being more economical in the functional parenchyma removed and of reducing the operative blood loss by being performed under vascular control.

2. Atypical resections are not guided by vascular intrahepatic anatomy, and thus the plane of resection is not in an anatomic plane.

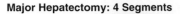

Major Hepatectomy: 4 Segments

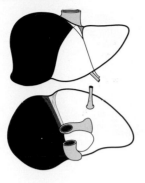

Right Hepatectomy

Major Hepatectomy: 3 Segments

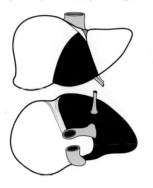

Left Hepatectomy   Trisegmentectomy 4–5–6

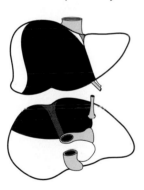

Trisegmentectomy 8–5–4   Trisegmentectomy 5–4–1

Figure 30–1
Major hepatectomies.

Extended Hepatectomies: 5 segments on the right

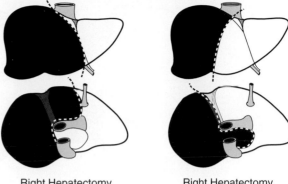

Right Hepatectomy   Right Hepatectomy
Segment 4   Segment 1

Extended Hepatectomies: 4 segments on the left

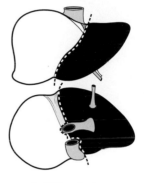

Left Hepatectomy
Segment 1

Figure 30–2
Extended hepatectomies.

3. Tumorectomies remove only the tumor without any functional parenchyma per se.

Operative Aspects of Hepatic Surgery

It is the meticulous attention to details in the preoperative assessment of the patient, surgical technique, and postoperative care that have allowed the decrease in mortality and morbidity of liver surgery. The operative blood loss has been recognized as the main factor associated with morbidity and mortality in liver resections. Techniques of parenchymal dissection and of vascular control have evolved so as to permit minimal blood loss associated with maximal

security when dealing with the main blood vessels. There are three basic techniques for anatomic hepatectomies.

Hepatectomy with Preliminary Vascular Ligation

This technique was described by Lortat-Jacob at the time of the first typical right hepatectomy in 1952. With this technique, the hepatectomy is begun with the ligation and division of the left or right side of the portal pedicle at the hilum and then continues with the ligation and division of the appropriate hepatic veins and lastly the sectioning of the liver parenchyma. The dissection of the hepatic veins can be hazardous. There is a risk of entering the veins themselves or the inferior vena cava, resulting in hemorrhage, which is difficult to control, or an air embolism. For this reason, in the initial technique of Lortat-Jacob, it was suggested that the dissection of the right hepatic vein should be preceded by control of the suprahepatic and infrahepatic inferior vena cava.

This technique has two advantages: (1) it reduces intraoperative blood loss, and (2) it shows clearly the line of division between the ischemic and the normally vascularized liver. The disadvantage of this technique, besides the risk of injury to major veins, is the danger of erroneous ligation of an element in the porta hepatis, which supplies a portion of

Minor Hepatectomy: 2 Segments

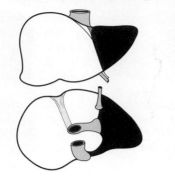
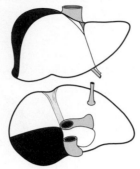
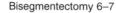
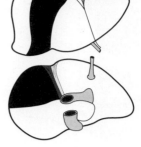

Left Lobectomy   Bisegmentectomy 6–7   Bisegmentectomy 5–8

Minor Hepatectomy: 1 Segment

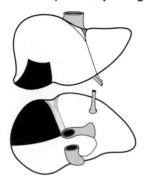

Segmentectomy 5   Segmentectomy 6   Segmentectomy 4

Minor Hepatectomy: Subsegmentectomy

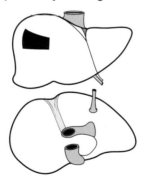
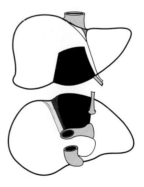

Subsegmentectomy 8 Anterior   Subsegmentectomy 4 Anterior

Figure 30–3
Minor hepatectomies.

the remaining liver, and poses an increased risk by the frequency of anatomic variations in this area.

Hepatectomy by Primary Parenchymal Transection

In this technique, described by Ton That and Tung Nguyen-Duong-Quang, the hepatic tissue is divided along the line of the middle hepatic vein, and glissonian elements are then approached and ligated within the liver, without prior control. Section of the hepatic vein is performed in the same fashion within the liver toward the end of the procedure. The technique has two advantages: (1) the liver tissue is excised as required according to the nature and location of the lesion, and (2) the risk from anatomic variants is minimized as the portal elements are approached above the hilum and within the liver to be resected. The disadvantage of this technique is that bleeding can be considerable if the resection is not performed quickly, and continuous or intermittent clamping of the hepatic pedicle may be necessary.

Hepatectomy with Extrahepatic Vascular Control and Intrahepatic Ligation

These two basic techniques of hepatectomy have been incorporated in this technique, which is used at the authors' institution and aims to benefit from the advantages while seeking to avoid their disadvantages. The principle is to start with the hilar dissection to gain control of the arterial and portal elements of the side to be resected and to clamp without ligating them. The appropriate side of the vena cava is freed without dissecting the hepatic vein. The liver is then divided along the main scissural line and, as in the technique of Ton That, the portal elements are located as the parenchyma is transected. Ligation of the vessels is, therefore, performed distal to the clamps. At the end of the liver transection, the hepatic vein is ligated within the liver and the clamps are removed. This technique has the advantages of minimizing blood loss by prior vascular control and of safe, accurate division and ligation of the vessels and biliary branches within the liver.

Techniques of Vascular Control

Liver resections are performed on richly irrigated tissue, and blood loss can be reduced by temporary interruption of the vascular supply to the liver. This can be performed at various levels, from the hepatic pedicle in the hepatoduodenal ligament to the segmental portal branches (Fig. 30–4). The definition of the indications for each particular type of vascular control and the tolerance of the liver to each have been some of the most important developments in hepatic surgery in the last decade (Table 30–1).

Clamping of the Vascular Pedicle

Occlusion of the hepatic inflow by clamping of the hepatic pedicle is the oldest method to reduce bleeding from a cut or torn liver tissue. Pringle used it first in patients with liver trauma and reported it with the results of his experimental observations in a remarkable publication in 1908. Although not affecting bleeding from the hepatic veins, clamping of the hepatic pedicle alone is simple and quick and is usually not accompanied by hemodynamic instability, despite some degree of congestion in the territory drained by the portal vein. It may be complicated by pancreatitis. The normal liver can tolerate continuous

pedicular clamping for up to 60 minutes and periods exceeding 1 hour have been reported in patients with cirrhosis. Although the experimental evidence in favor of intermittent clamping is not unequivocal, in most cases intermittent clamping is preferred, with a period of 15 minutes of occlusion alternating with a 5- to 10-minute period during which the pedicle is unclamped. In cirrhotic patients or patients with abnormal liver function from previous chemotherapy, continuous clamping should be avoided, periods of intermittent clamping should be reduced to 10 minutes, and total ischemia time should be kept under 30 minutes as much as possible.

Selective Portal Clamping and Suprahilar Vascular Control

This method of hemihepatic vascular control can be extended to segmental liver resection. It has the double advantage of allowing a virtually bloodless operative field and of diminishing the splanchnic congestion associated with the Pringle maneuver. The perfusion of different sectors or segments can be interrupted at the suprahilar level by ligation or temporary occlusion of the portal pedicles after having lowered the hilar plate and dissected superficially into the liver parenchyma following closely the portal vein branches. Clamping is usually followed by an ischemic demarcation on the liver surface that limits the resection.

Balloon Exclusion of Segmental Portal Branches

Balloon occlusion of segmental portal branches is the most refined application of the concept of intraparenchymal vascular control (Fig. 30–5). Using intraoperative ultrasound, the portal branch supplying the segment to be resected is punctured and, through an introducer, a balloon catheter is inserted in the portal vein and the balloon is inflated, stopping the portal inflow. By clamping the appropriate arterial branch at the hilum, total vascular exclusion of the segment is achieved. The boundaries of the excluded segment can be

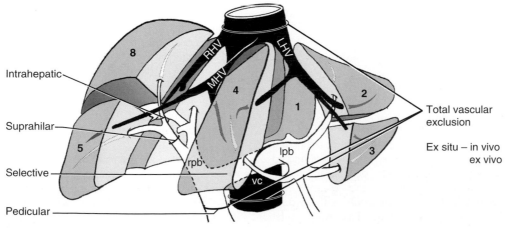

Figure 30–4
Different methods of clamping.

Table 30–1 Hepatic Vascular Clamping: Methods, Tolerances, and Indications

Clamping Method	Maximum Reported Period of Clamping	Particular Points
Pedicular	Normal liver: • Continuous clamping: 60 min* • Intermittent clamping: (20 min and 5 min unclamping) 90–140 min† (15 min and 5 min unclamping)‡ 120 min Cirrhotic liver: • Continuous clamping: to be avoided • Intermittent clamping: (10 min and 5 min unclamping) >30 min§	An anomalous left artery should be clamped as well
Selective	Duration not delimited but not unlimited	Different levels of clamping: • Hemihepatic: hilar • Sectorial: hilar or suprahilar • Segmental: intraparenchymal
Total vascular exclusion	Normal liver: 60‖; 90 min¶ Cirrhotic liver: 30 min§	Indications are related to the characteristics of the tumor If not well tolerated hemodynamically, extracorporeal circulation can be used Not used by the authors in cirrhotic patients
Total vascular exclusion and cold perfusion	In situ: 90 to 120 min** Ex situ in vivo: 3 to 5 hours†† Ex vivo: 9 hours of the anhepatic phase‡‡	Indications are related to the characteristics of the tumor Extracorporeal circulation mandatory for ex situ in vivo and ex vivo surgery Contraindicated in cirrhotic livers Indications to be evaluated for steatotic livers, chronic hepatitis, and postchemotherapy livers

*From Hannoun L, Borie D, Delva E, et al: Liver resection with normothermic ischemia exceeding an hour: A ten-year experience. Br J Surg 80:1161–1165, 1993.

†From Elias D, Desruennes E, Lasser P: Prolonged intermittent clamping of the portal triad during hepatectomy. Br J Surg 78:42–44, 1991.

‡From Isozaki H, Adam R, Gigou M, et al: Experimental study of the protective effect of intermittent hepatic pedicle clamping in the rat. Br J Surg 79:310–313, 1992.

§From Nagasue N, Yukaya H, Suehiro S, Ogawa Y: Tolerance of the cirrhotic liver to normothermic ischemia: A clinical study of 15 patients. Am J Surg 147:772–775, 1984.

‖From Bismuth H, Castaing D, Garden OJ: Major hepatic resection under total vascular exclusion. Ann Surg 210:13–19, 1989.

¶From Huguet C, Nordlinger B, Galopin JJ, et al: Normothermic hepatic vascular exclusion for extensive hepatectomy. Surg Gynecol Obstet 147:160–163, 1978.

**From Fortner JG, Shiu MH, Kinne DW, et al: Major hepatic resection using vascular isolation and hypothermic perfusion. Ann Surg 180:644–652, 1974.

††From Hannoun L, Panis Y, Balladur P, et al: Ex situ-in vivo liver surgery. Lancet 1:1616, 1991.

‡‡From Pichmayr R, Grosse H, Hauss J, et al: Technique and preliminary results of extracorporeal liver surgery (bench procedure) and of liver surgery on the in situ perfused liver. Br J Surg 77:21–26, 1990.

defined by injecting methylene blue through the introducer, staining the portion of tissue supplied by the occluded branch. This technique is especially useful in cirrhotic patients in whom the maximum amount of functioning liver tissue must be preserved.

Total Vascular Exclusion

In the case of very large tumors when an extended hepatectomy is indicated and in the case of tumors in close relation to the retrohepatic vena cava or the confluence of the hepatic veins, hemorrhage can be reduced by complete vascular exclusion of the liver. This procedure was first described by Heaney and Jacobson in 1966. It is achieved by simultaneous clamping of the hepatic pedicle and of the suprahepatic and infrahepatic vena cava. Huguet and coworkers showed that the human liver would withstand up to 65 minutes of ischemia. This technique has proved to be both efficient and safe during major hepatic resection in a

series of 51 patients in whom the mean duration of the vascular exclusion was 46.5 ± 5.0 minutes, with a mean transfusion requirement of 1.4 ± 0.4 unit of blood and a mortality of 2.6%. The main limitation of its use is the danger of hemodynamic instability associated with diminished venous return from clamping both the portal vein and the inferior vena cava. External venovenous bypass is indicated for patients with altered cardiac and renal function, which in our experience has been necessary in 10% of cases of total vascular exclusion. Modification of this technique by clamping the hepatic veins and the portal pedicle only, without interrupting the caval flow, has been described by Elias.

When extended periods of ischemia are anticipated or when vascular reconstruction is necessary, some authors have suggested combining total vascular exclusion with cold perfusion of the liver with preservation solution through both the gastroduodenal artery and a branch of the portal vein to be resected.

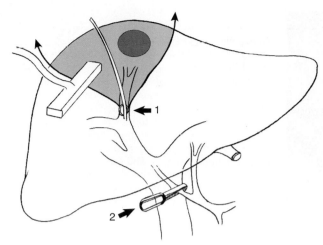

Figure 30–5
Principles of hepatic surgery with portal clamping by segmental balloon exclusion. (1) Occlusion of the segmental portal branch guided by ultrasound and (2) selective arterial clamping allow the demarcation of the segment to be resected.

Ex Situ Surgery

Surgery on a totally removed liver and cooled with preservation solution (ex situ, ex vivo), with the external venovenous bypass, is the logical application of the techniques learned in liver transplantation. A simpler approach is the disconnection of the suprahepatic inferior vena cava only with the insertion of perfusion cannulas in the nonsevered hepatic vessels (ex situ, in vivo). Although very useful in selected cases, the indications for these techniques are very limited.

Techniques of Dissection and Hemostasis

The liver tissue may be divided by several methods, including the finger fracture technique, the Kelly clamp, and the Cavitron ultrasonic dissector (Cavitron Surgical Systems, Stamford, CT). The aim of all these methods is to divide only the parenchymal tissue, exposing the vessels and the biliary structures. The ultrasonic dissector consists of a vibrating device that oscillates at a frequency of 23 kHz. It fragments preferentially the water-filled parenchymal cells that are removed by a coaxial irrigation apparatus. The collagen and elastic tissue of the vessels are preserved so that they can be dissected clean before accurate coagulation or ligation.

In most cases nothing more is needed than meticulous suture or ligation of the larger vessels and coagulation of smaller vessels as the resection proceeds. Bile channels run with the portal pedicles and are simultaneously dealt with by suture ligation during the resection. Small bile leaks on the raw surface should be actively looked for and oversewn with fine sutures. Diluted methylene blue can be injected under slight pressure in the biliary system, through the gallbladder or the cystic duct, to reveal leaks, which may otherwise escape detection.

Mortality Rate for Hepatectomy

The analysis of the mortality rate of 1193 hepatectomies of the 30-year experience at Paul Brousse Hospital has shown that hepatectomies done under elective conditions in noncirrhotic patients are extremely safe. There was a 0.9% operative and 2-month postoperative mortality rate in 1014 patients who underwent hepatectomies for primary and metastatic tumors, benign lesions, and various other indications (unpublished data) (Fig. 30–6). Resection of hepatocellular carcinoma in cirrhotic patients carried a much higher mortality rate of 7.6%. Hepatectomies for trauma were also associated with a higher mortality rate of 8.8%.

Intraoperative Ultrasound

With 5-MHz T-shaped probes intraoperative ultrasound can be performed easily by the surgeon after mobilization of the liver and does not add much to the operative time. The benefit of the intraoperative ultrasound is two-fold—diagnostic and therapeutic.

The ultrasound allows the surgeon to establish the position of all the important vessels within the liver parenchyma and mark the surface of the liver as appropriate. It permits the recognition of accessory suprahepatic veins, especially the accessory right suprahepatic vein which, if present, may allow for an easier isolated resection of the anterior of posterior segments of the right liver. The glissonnian pedicles can be followed from the hilum, and their sectorial and segmentary division and branching can be defined accurately. Anatomic variation of these pedicles is common and must be looked for and recognized.

Localizing tumors by palpation can be difficult if cirrhosis hardens the liver or if the tumor has the same consistency as the liver parenchyma. A thorough examination of the liver parenchyma by ultrasound can precisely localize a known tumor but can also define unrecognized tumors. A prospective study has shown that 32% of tumors less than 1 cm were discovered only by intraoperative ultrasound. Intraoperative ultrasound may sufficiently enhance the available information so as to modify the surgical plan by allowing a more limited resection, increasing the extent of the resection to ensure a total excision of the tumors, or demonstrating unresectable disease. Intraoperative ultrasound also ensures good positioning of the line of resection as the surgeon is progressing in the parenchymal division.

Portal Vein Embolization and Two-Step Hepatectomies

With the resection of large amounts of hepatic parenchyma, which may occur in cases of right hepatectomy, the risk of postoperative liver failure is increased significantly. When resection is feasible but not practical because of the amount of functional reserve in the remaining liver, preoperative left hepatic hypertrophy induced by right portal vein embolization has been reported to have promising results. The subsequent compensatory hypertrophy of the left liver enables a more confident resection of a tumor with clear margins and reduces the potential for postoperative hepatic failure. Portal vein embolization is performed under general anesthesia.

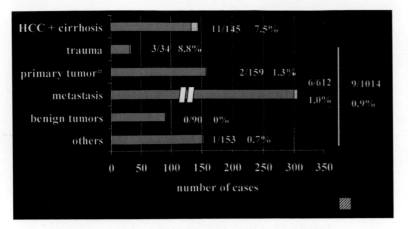

Figure 30–6
Mortality rate of hepatectomies at Paul Brousse Hospital: operative and 2 months' postoperative mortality. Resection of hepatocellular carcinoma in cirrhotic patients and hepatectomies for trauma are considered high risk, with a respective mortality of 7.6% and 8.8%. Hepatectomies in patients with noncirrhotic livers have a much lower mortality rate of 0.9%. Asterisk indicates primary tumors resected in noncirrhotic patients. The *hatched area* on each bar represents the number of deaths. The metastasis *bar* has been interrupted to represent the 612 patients.

Under ultrasound guidance, a superficial tributary of the left portal vein is identified and percutaneously entered with a 22 gauge Chiba needle through a transhepatic route. Under fluoroscopic control, the portal trunk is catheterized using the Seldinger technique. After a venous portography, the right portal branch is selectively catheterized. Embolization is done under fluoroscopic control with a mixture of N-butyl-2-cyanoacrylate (Histoacryl, Braun Lab, Hamburg, Germany) and lipiodol (Lipiodol ultra fluide, Guerbet Lab, Paris, France) in proportions of 1:4 to delay polymerization and cast formation. The portal vein trunk is then catheterized, and the absence of reflux into the left portal branch and the preferential flow to the left portal branch are demonstrated. The catheter is removed while injecting 2 mL of fibrin glue (Tissucol, Immuno AG, Vienna, Austria) into the needle tract within the liver parenchyma. Hepatic volumes are followed using tomographic image volume measurements before and every 2 weeks after embolization. The hepatic resection is performed when optimal liver hypertrophy of the left liver has occurred.

In a series reported from Paul Brousse Hospital, right portal vein embolization was performed for malignant hepatic disease in 16 patients with an 88% technical success rate and no complications. The failure in two cases was caused by an excessive angle of the right portal branch, which prohibited access of the catheter from the right side. No morbidity or mortality was associated with the procedure. Of the 16 patients, 13 underwent laparotomy, of whom 9 were resected successfully. The other four patients had been found to have extrahepatic disease. The remaining patients were still being evaluated and awaiting surgery.

In patients with a significant bilobar metastatic disease burden, a planned *two-step hepatectomy* also counts on the postresection remaining liver hypertrophy to achieve complete tumor resection with the minimization of the risk of postresection liver insufficiency. The metastases in the more involved lobe are resected; liver parenchyma is preserved as much as possible; and the remaining metastases in the other lobe are subsequently resected at a second operation after the postresection hypertrophy has been achieved. This strategy has the potential risk of favoring tumor growth in the hypertrophying lobe, but many of these patients would otherwise be considered unresectable.

Cryosurgery

In some patients with diminished hepatic reserve from cirrhosis or previous liver resection (especially in cases of lesions deeply seated inside the liver), conventional surgical resection may represent too big a sacrifice of functional hepatic tissue or an excessive operative risk. In some cases, alcohol injection or surgical cryotherapy can be used. Cryosurgery is a recent technique that provides a new therapeutic approach for unresectable liver tumors or acts as a complementary treatment in an attempt to achieve tumor eradication when combined with surgical resection. With the new refinements of cryosurgery and the widespread use of intraoperative ultrasound, reports have shown the potential benefit of cryosurgery in patients who were not amenable to resection. The efficacy of cryosurgery in unresectable liver tumors is still under scrutiny, because most reports include different tumors, different criteria for selection of patients, and different treatment protocols.

Surgical cryotherapy is done under ultrasound guidance, after complete immobilization of the liver, by introducing into the tumor a probe that is cooled with liquid nitrogen to −196°C. Two freezing-thawing cycles are usually performed on the tumor. The extent of the destruction can be monitored accurately by the progression of the area of frozen tissue, which appears intensely hypoechogenic on the ultrasound. One published series from Paul Brousse Hospital explored the possible benefits of cryosurgery in the treatment of unresectable hepatocellular carcinomas. During a 3-year period, 13 of 251 patients with hepatocellular carcinoma were treated with cryosurgery. Four patients who had undergone partial liver resection had cryosurgery applied to their resection margin because of small tumor margins (<1 cm). Local recurrence was not observed in any of these patients after a mean follow-up of 17 months. Of the 191 patients who were considered unresectable, 9 (5%) were treated either with cryosurgery alone or in association with liver resection. Cryosurgery was considered for these patients only if it was thought to achieve complete macroscopic treatment of the liver tumor. None of these patients had extrahepatic metastases, and the unresectability was related to technical considerations (large, inaccessibly located, multiple bilateral lesions). Chemoembolization with lipiodol (Lipiodol ultra fluide, Guerbet Lab, Paris, France) was a mandatory pretreatment evaluation to ensure that no lipiodol-retaining nodule had been missed by ultrasound or abdominal computed tomography (CT) scan. For these nine patients, 9 of 15 nodules were treated by cryotherapy and the others were resected. There was no notable technical difficulty and no intraoperative mortality. A temporary elevation in serum aminotransferases and a diminution in platelets and prothrombin time were commonly observed and were related to the duration of the cryotherapy and the number of treated lesions. Normalization of the values was observed within 5 days. A partial response (50% reduction in the size of the tumor) was observed in five of the nine patients (55%). In the other four patients, the tumor was reduced by less than 50% and was thus considered stable. The local recurrence rate was 0%, and the overall recurrence rate was 33% at 16 months. The overall survival was 77% at 12 months and 63% at 24 months. Six patients (63%) were considered to be free of tumors.

Even though cryosurgery could not be applied to a large number of patients with unresectable tumors, the authors concluded that cryosurgery was safe and showed encouraging results because there were no local recurrences. The best survival was achieved in patients treated with a multimodality associating cryosurgery, resection, and either systemic chemotherapy or chemoembolization. The benefit was related to complete treatment of the tumor, which is a goal that is rarely obtained in patients with widespread multinodular disease.

BILIARY SURGERY

Cholangiocarcinoma

Hilar cholangiocarcinoma, despite its slow growth and its low propensity for metastasis, is usually not diagnosed until the bile duct is occluded, and the patient is jaundiced. Even though the lesion may be small, its location and close proximity to important structures in the liver hilum make curative excision technically difficult and often impossible. Most reports have shown disappointing overall improvements in long-term survival with excision; however, some studies have suggested that in a small but significant percentage of patients, improved survival can be obtained after excision. Most of the controversy concerning the excision to achieve a cure surrounds the ability of a local resection to completely remove all tumor tissue. Cholangiocarcinoma has a tendency to grow into perineural tissue and thus spread for a considerable distance along the bile duct wall.

Classification of Cholangiocarcinoma

Cholangiocarcinoma can be divided into four anatomic types using a modification of the original Bismuth-Corlette classification (Fig. 30–7).

- Type I: The tumor does not obstruct the confluence.
- Type II: The tumor reaches the primary confluence, which is obstructed.
- Type III: The tumor extends beyond the primary confluence to either the right (type IIIa) or left (type IIIb) secondary confluence.
- Type IV: The tumor extends to the secondary confluence of both the right and left bile ducts.

Principles of Resection

A recent series from Paul Brousse Hospital has suggested that, with complete excision of the tumor, it is possible to alter the natural history of this disease in terms of progression of the tumor and long-term survival. To achieve a curative resection, all tumor tissue must be removed, with free resection margins. This emphasizes the importance of extensive preoperative and perioperative assessment so that resection is only performed when it can be potentially curative, and inappropriate extensive resection is avoided.

In type I lesions, local excision without hepatic resection is an appropriate treatment. In type II cases, there is no communication between the right and the left duct systems on the cholangiogram, and the superior aspect of the confluence is involved. In this situation, the bile ducts that drain the caudate lobe (segment 1) are almost inevitably involved by the tumor. For these lesions, local excision of the tumor should probably always be accompanied by the resection of the caudate lobe. For some large type II lesions, tumor extension may involve the parenchyma of segment 4, and resection of segment 4 may also be necessary.

When the lesion involves the superior aspect of the biliary confluence and extends into one of the main hepatic ducts (type III), a radical tumor clearance cannot be achieved by local excision, because there will invariably be ductal involvement of the caudate lobe and of the secondary bile ducts of the involved side. Treatment should thus consist of local resection, which should be complemented by resection of the caudate lobe and a hemihepatectomy of the involved side. For some large type IIIa lesions, with tumor extension involving the parenchyma of segment 4, a resection of segment 4 may also be necessary.

In these patients, the feasibility of extensive liver resection depends on the remaining volume of functioning hepatic parenchyma. In particular, an extended right hepatec-

Figure 30–7
Classification of hilar tumors: I: The tumor does not obstruct the confluence; II: The tumor reaches the primary confluence, which is obstructed; IIIa: The tumor extends beyond the primary confluence to the right; IIIb: The tumor extends beyond the primary confluence to the left; IV: The tumor extends to the secondary confluence of both the right and the left bile ducts.

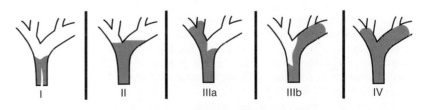

tomy for type IIIa lesion may not leave sufficient functioning parenchyma. In some cases, however, tumor extension with involvement of the major branch of the portal vein may result in unilateral liver atrophy, with corresponding hypertrophy of the other hemiliver, thus making major resection possible. As discussed earlier, preoperative portal vein embolization may also be used to favor liver hypertrophy in the remaining liver. In some cases, with deteriorating preoperative liver function or sepsis, preoperative percutaneous transhepatic biliary drainage may be indicated to improve the hepatocellular function and reduce the risk of liver failure in the immediate postoperative period.

When the tumor has extended to involve the secondary bile ducts or hepatic parenchyma bilaterally, or the main trunk of the hepatic artery or the portal vein (type IV), resection techniques almost always fail to achieve a radical excision of all tumor tissue. For type IV lesions, hepatectomy and liver transplantation may be indicated. This offers the only chance of complete tumor removal and potential cure in these cases, although results have been generally poor, with a high incidence of tumor recurrence.

Repair of Biliary Injuries

Injuries to the bile ducts are seen most often after a cholecystectomy but can also complicate many other surgeries such as gastectomy; hepatic, pancreatic, and duodenal surgery; or surgery for portal hypertension. Injuries to the common bile duct (CBD) are best avoided by careful dissection when performing an open or laparoscopic cholecystectomy. Many authors have advocated first the dissection of Calot's triangle and the identification of the cystic duct and artery and the hepatic duct. The surgeon must then perform the dissection of the neck of the gallbladder before any sectioning.

The most common mechanisms of injuries to the CBD are the confusion of the CBD and the cystic duct when performing cholangiography or dissection of the cystic duct (Fig. 30–8 [1.A,B,C]). This injury is seen mainly when the cystic duct is short or the common bile duct is small. The CBD can also be at risk when too much traction is placed on the neck of the gallbladder and pulls the CBD in line with the gallbladder (see Fig. 30–8 [1.C,D]). When the neck of the gallbladder is adherent to the CBD and the pedicle is severely inflamed, the CBD can be difficult to recognize. It is then injured laterally in its high portion, causing a complete transection or a partial loss of tissue (see Fig. 30–8 [2.A]). This is also seen when a biliobiliary fistula is forming with a large stone impacted in the neck of the gallbladder (see Fig. 30–8 [2.B]). The CBD, and especially the right hepatic duct, can also be confused for the cystic artery, which is usually seen again when too much traction is applied to the neck of the gallbladder (see Fig. 30–8[3.]). Many CBD injuries are the result of difficulties in hemostasis when blind clipping or clamping is done (see Fig. 30–8[4.]). The CBD can be torn when large stones are extracted through a choledochotomy (see Fig. 30–8[5.]), or the CBD can be perforated by the cholangiography cannula (see Fig. 30–8[6.]). Anatomic anomalies, such as the implantation of a right hepatic duct in the cystic duct, certainly increase the risk of injuries (see Fig. 30–8 [7.A,B]).

The first attempt at repair has the best chance of being successful. Even when recognized, biliary tract injuries are

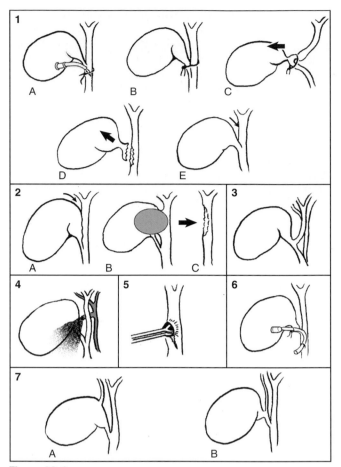

Figure 30–8
The different mechanisms of iatrogenic common bile duct (CBD) trauma.
1. During the dissection of the cystic duct: (A): wrong placement of the cholangiography cannula; (B): ligation of both ducts; (C): excessive traction on the gallbladder pulling the CBD in line with the cystic duct; (D): avulsion of the lateral wall by excessive traction; (E) confusion of the CBD for the short cystic duct.
2. During the dissection of the gallbladder neck: (A) in an inflamed pedicle with adherence of the gallbladder to the CBD; (B): erosion of a large stone; (C): resulting in CBD trauma.
3. Due to the compression of the CBD by a vascular structure.
4. During the attempt at hemostasis.
5. During difficult extraction of common bile duct stones.
6. Injury due to instruments.
7. Due to anatomic anomalies: (A) segmental canal inserting in the gallbladder neck; (B) segmental canal inserting in the cystic duct.

best repaired immediately; they still have a 30% risk of complication or failure. These failures are usually operated on again within 2 years, but 20% are still recognized later, even up to 10 years. Immediate repair (as opposed to secondary repair) is almost always done on fine ducts with healthy mucosa. Partial injuries can be repaired by simple sutures over a drain. Right hepatic duct injuries can also be repaired using the same technique. When an accessory canal is injured, it can be ligated after confirmatory cholangiography. When there is a complete transection of the CBD without loss of tissue, most surgeons would agree that an end-to-end repair is the best option. This should be done by freshening the edges without extensive dissection, so as not to devascularize the two ends. The repair should be done without tension and with close, small bites, thus ensuring good apposition of the mucosa. When tissue is lost and a tensionless repair cannot be achieved, a terminolateral hepaticojejunal anastomosis is the only option available to the surgeon.

Secondary Repair

There are three possible courses of events when the bile duct injury is unrecognized at the time of the first operation: (1) the appearance of jaundice early in the postoperative period, (2) the development of an external bile fistula, or (3) the development of biliary ascites. Jaundice usually starts within 2 to 4 days postoperatively and progresses rapidly. Pruritus begins between postoperative days 7 and 12. There is a rapid rise in the alkaline phosphatase to three to four times its normal value accompanied by an elevation of the serum aminotransferases to five to eight times their normal levels by postoperative day 10. This is usually easily distinguished from benign postoperative intrahepatic cholestasis, which is seen in patients who required large intraoperative transfusions or who had halothane-induced hepatitis. The external biliary fistula usually becomes apparent early in the postoperative course when the wound dressing becomes soaked with bile. The bile is usually not completely drained, and bile drainage must be completed by the percutaneous insertion of a drain to prevent sepsis. Biliary ascites is usually present with abdominal pain, fever, and an ileus, suggesting peritonitis, which often requires a re-exploration and a simple external drainage without any attempt at repair.

Experience suggests that the optimal delay for a secondary repair is about 2 months, except for the uncomplicated ligation of the common bile duct associated by jaundice, in which case an earlier intervention can be done. Early repairs of bile duct injuries are rendered more difficult by the inflammation in the hepatoduodenal ligament and by the absence of bile duct dilatation. Optimally, the repair should be undertaken when the pedicular region has healed and scarred from all the inflammation related to the injury and when the bile ducts above the injury have had time to dilate. As well as an important thickening of the peritoneum in the hepatoduodenal ligament, bile duct injuries are usually characterized by a progressive retraction of the bile duct stump, as if the dilatation of the bile ducts was compensated by a loss of length. The key element in the secondary repair of bile duct injuries is to ensure that the repair is done at the level of healthy bile mucosa and that there is true apposition of the mucosa.

Classification of Bile Duct Strictures

Bile duct strictures have been classified by Bismuth according to the level of the stricture in relation to the hepatic duct confluence (Fig. 30–9). Five types have been described:

- Type I: The stricture is more than 2 cm away from the confluence. This is a low or pedicular stricture.
- Type II: The common bile duct stump is shorter than 2 cm. This is a mid- or subhilar stricture.
- Type III: There is no common bile duct stump. The stricture is at the level of the hepatic duct confluence but the two ducts still communicate. This is a high or hilar stricture. This is the most common type.
- Type IV: The stricture reaches the origin of the two hepatic ducts, and their communication is destroyed, with a varying distance between the two ducts. This is a lesion of the confluence.

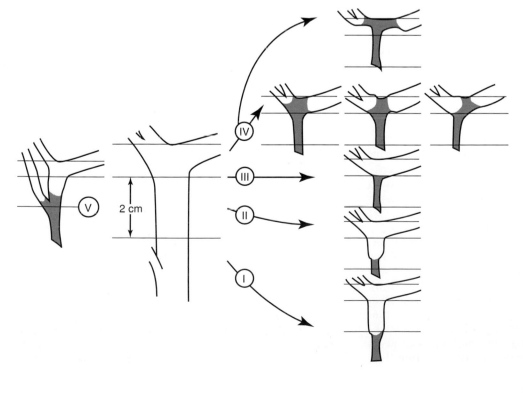

Figure 30–9
Classification of biliary strictures using three landmarks: 2 cm under the confluence; the inferior level of the confluence; the roof of the confluence. Type I: low or pedicular stricture; type II: mid or subhilar stricture; type III: high or hilar stricture; type IV: confluence lesion: ducts in contact, ducts apart; type V: isolated right sectorial duct from the CBD by a stricture.

• Type V: This type is seen in a patient with a low confluence of a right sectorial duct, which is involved in the stricture, isolating one hepatic sector from the bile duct.

Preoperative Work-up

Obtaining and reading the old operative reports is the first step in the understanding of the patient's bile duct injury. Four investigations seem most useful in the better comprehension of the total picture. Hepatic ultrasound helps to appreciate the degree of bile duct dilatation and the liver volume in its defined sectors. It also recognizes the presence of aerobilia from either a previous anastomosis or a spontaneous biliointestinal fistula and intrahepatic stones. A CT scan adds little to a good ultrasound. Upper gastrointestinal endoscopy is done to look for esophageal varices and to check the duodenum for any signs of a biliary fistula. Mesenteric angiography is indicated when there is the possibility of bleeding at the time of the cholecystectomy. The angiography detects any associated injury to the hepatic artery. Revascularization of the hilum through collateral vessels renders the dissection and the repair more difficult and hemorrhagic. The venous phase of the test is used to assess the degree of portal hypertension. The percutaneous transhepatic cholangiogram (PTC) must be done under antibiotic prophylaxis and with a small needle, because cholangitis and a bile leak present complications. It is important not to overfill the bile ducts during the examination. The cholangiogram must be interpreted with caution because the incomplete filling of the bile ducts or the presence of stones may cause the erroneous impression of a very high stricture.

Principles and Techniques of Repair

There are three types of repair:

1. The end-to-end bile duct repair is used in only optimal conditions where there is no loss of tissue and a tensionless mucosa-to-mucosa anastomosis can be done. This technique is impeded by the discrepancy in the size of the two ends of the bile duct but mainly by the distance that separates the two stumps after both ends have been freshened back to healthy mucosa. A Kocher maneuver is always necessary to allow the inferior stump to reach the superior one. Dissection of each stump may lead to a partial devascularization of the bile duct wall. This, added to traction exerted by the anastomosis, may be the main reason for a recurrent stricture at the site of repair.

2. The most common type of repair used today is the Roux-en-Y hepaticojejunal anastomosis. The objective is to create a mucosa-to-mucosa anastomosis between a wide biliary opening and the 70- to 80-cm loop of jejunum that has been brought up in a retrocolic fashion.

   In type I and II lesions, this is a straightforward endeavor after the pedicular adhesions have been lysed. For the higher stricture, the simple dissection of the pedicle is not sufficient for the creation of a wide anastomosis on healthy mucosa. It is only possible after the hilar plate has been dissected.

   The hilar plate, as described by Couinaud, is a thickening of the Glisson capsule at the hilar level to create an adherent plate, which forms the roof of the hilum (Fig.

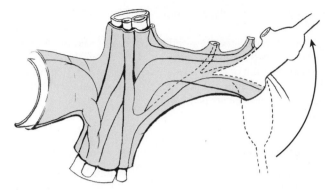

Figure 30–10
Hilar anatomy: The hilar plate is shown by *hatched bars.* It covers the hilar elements and is continuous with the gallbladder plate on the right and the umbilical plate on the left. On the entire hilar width, the biliary structures are just beneath the hilar plate without any interposition of vessels.

30–10). This plate extends to the right and separates the gallbladder from the liver and to the left above the round ligament. All the vascular and biliary pedicles that enter the liver parenchyma will drag with them an invagination of this plate as a fibrous sheath. The important point is that the separation of the hilar plate from the liver parenchyma allows the superior side of the hilum to be lowered, making it anterior (Fig. 30–11). One must also remember the discrepancy in length between the right duct, which is almost vertical and short and is 1 cm on average, and the left duct, which travels more horizontally and measures 3 cm on average.

The first step in the repair is the localization of the superior biliary stump. This is confirmed by an intraopera-

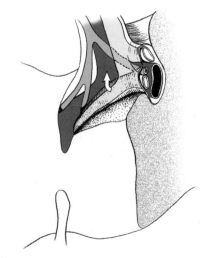

Figure 30–11
Lowering of the hilar plate. This allows the superior surface of the left duct, the right duct and the confluence to be moved to a more accessible anterior position.

tive cholangiogram, which best defines the level of the stricture. It is very important to ensure that the cholangiogram is complete, that all the branches are opacified, and that no sector is excluded. The first few films with low pressure filling of the bile ducts are the best to recognize intrahepatic stones, common sequela of bile duct stricture. The stump is then opened toward the left duct for 2 to 3 cm and, if necessary, toward to right branch for ½ to 1 cm, creating a V-shaped opening and exposing the entire confluence. If there is any suspicion of a missing duct, its opening must be looked for by exploring the inside of the opening with a fine dissector or stylet. If no orifice is found, the missing canal must be looked for outside the hilar sclerosis. An undrained segment exposes the patient to repeated episodes of cholangitis.

The Roux-en-Y loop is then created. It should be long, approximately 70 to 80 cm, to avoid reflux into the intrahepatic duct and diminish the risk of cholangitis. The loop is brought up in a retrocolic fashion just right of the duodenum. An end-to-side anastomosis is then fashioned, ensuring complete apposition of both mucosas. No drain is left in the anastomosis.

In types IV and V, the opening of the confluence is not sufficient to ensure the presence of healthy mucosa at the level of the anastomosis. The lowering of the hilar plate is essential here and must be extended along the two hepatic ducts. If the two ducts are still within proximity of each other, they may be reunited medially if this can be done without tension, thus creating a single opening. If this is not possible, two separate anastomoses should be created on the Roux-en-Y limb. If, after complete lowering of the hilar plate and enlargement of the opening, healthy biliary mucosa is still not found (most often right-sided occurrence), a transanastomotic stenting drain should be left in place. The favored drain is a silicone U transanastomotic and transhepatic drain as described by Praderi, which can easily be changed, washed, and unobstructed.

3. The Rodney-Smith biliary anastomosis was proposed for cases where no healthy bile duct mucosa can be recognized (Fig. 30–12). This anastomosis consists of a jejunal mucosal graft done by the invagination of the exposed mucosa of a Roux-en-Y loop into the bile duct. A transhepatic drain is placed in the left or right bile duct exiting in the common bile duct. A ring of seromuscular tissue is excised from the jejunal loop that is brought up. The drain is placed through its center and fixed to the loop. The drain is then pulled back, driving the mucosa into the bile duct.

Smith has pointed out contraindications to his technique: biliary cirrhosis, severe infections of the bile ducts, and intrahepatic bile duct stones. A few criticisms can be made of this method. The principle of this technique relies on the fact that the stricture is so high within the liver that healthy mucosa cannot be reached. This intrahepatic confluence is often the result of postoperative changes, and dissection of the hilar plate usually allows sufficient lowering of the biliary stump. The pulling of the mucosa into the bile duct is done in a blind fashion, and it is impossible to know where the biliary mucosa stops. The jejunal mucosa can then be positioned under the biliary mucosa without obtaining mucosal apposition or can go beyond the healthy biliary mucosa and obstruct a secondary duct.

Thus, the Rodney-Smith technique should be considered as a salvage technique, when even after a thorough dissection along the bile ducts, healthy biliary mucosa is not reached. It is the case of type IV stricture involving mainly the short right branch, where a very high stricture results in the loss of mucosa high up into the liver parenchyma.

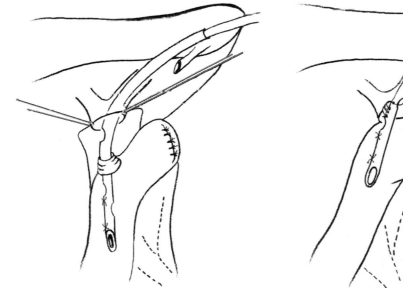
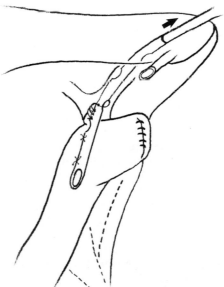

Figure 30–12
The technique of the jejunal graft as described by Rodney Smith.

Bile duct stones above the stricture are a common additional complication of bile duct stricture. These stones are pigmented, caused by stasis, and vary in size from mere concretions of 1 to 2 mm to real stones of ½ to 1 cm in diameter. They can be isolated to the stump but are found most often to be intrahepatic. It is important to extract as many stones as possible with repeated washings, Fogarty catheters, stone forceps, and so forth. One can never ensure complete clearance of the intrahepatic ducts, and thus the anastomosis must be as large as possible to prevent future obstruction by remaining stones.

At the time of the initial cholecystectomy, a concomitant arterial injury may be reported. Bile duct injury often occurs during a blind attempt at hemostasis. It is, therefore, not surprising that arterial injuries at the level of the pedicle are associated with biliary injuries. Most of the arterial injuries are of the right branch and are much less often of the hepatic artery proper. Arterial lesions are associated particularly with high biliary lesions, types III or IV. The arterial interruption of the right branch is always followed by revascularization of the concerned hepatic territory by hilar collateral vessels developed from the left branch. The revascularization after the severance of the hepatic artery comes from an anomalous right hepatic artery or the formation of collateral vessels from the inferior diaphragmatic artery, the superior mesenteric artery, or even from jejunal arteries after a bilioenteric anastomosis has been created. The knowledge of this arterial injury prepares the surgeon for a more difficult operation in view of the hypervascular hilum. Caution must be taken while enlarging the left duct opening after a right arterial branch injury, because the new arterioles that supply the caudate and right lobe may cross that left bile duct.

Injuries to the bile duct may result in global hypertrophy of the liver or of one lobe in response to the atrophy of the obstructed side. The hypertrophied liver is often hard and may cause real operative difficulty. The hilum seems then to ascend and is literally engulfed by the liver. The surgeon is then confronted with an exposure problem, which may be resolved only by a thoracoabdominal incision. This incision allows the subluxation of the liver out of the right upper quadrant and the opening of the operative field. When one lobe atrophies in response to the biliary obstruction, the hilum's position changes. It ascends and rotates toward the atrophied side. This should be suggested by the preoperative ultrasound and may push the surgeon to modify the operative approach.

Secondary biliary cirrhosis is the last stage in the evolution of a benign biliary stricture. The biliary retention results in a few months in fibrosis of the portal space. This evolves slowly, over 3 to 7 years on average, toward cirrhosis. The treatment of the stricture is then complicated by three factors: (1) the repair is made more difficult by the usually repeated previous attempt at repair, increasing the adhesions in the hilum; (2) portal hypertension renders the dissection more hemorrhagic and may be complicated by variceal bleeds; (3) cirrhosis with its associated hepatocellular insufficiency, ascites, and coagulation problems worsen the surgical risk. In the face of well-established cirrhosis, liver transplantation then becomes the only real option to offer these patients (who are often young) a decent quality of life.

Results of Biliary Repair

The results of repairs of biliary stricture are influenced by many factors. The most important factors bearing on the chance of a satisfactory repair are the number of previous attempts at repair, the level of the stricture, and the method of repair. Operative mortality is also influenced by these factors but also by a history of major infections, the preoperative liver function, and particularly the presence of liver fibrosis and portal hypertension.

A 10% morbidity is reported in biliary tract repair, which is most often related to bile leaks and wound infections. A mortality rate of less than 2% is reported in large series. Results should be judged over a 10-year period, because many recurrent strictures are only diagnosed after a 3- to 5-year period. A good result would be defined as a 10-year period free of any biliary symptoms. In a series of 121 patients who had undergone a hepaticojejunal anastomosis and who were followed for more than 10 years, 88% had good results, 6% had satisfactory results after a transient period of problems or discrete late troubles, and 6% failed. Of the failures, two were recurrent strictures, five had secondary biliary cirrhosis, and one had a distant small bowel obstruction.

CONCLUSION

Over the years, hepatobiliary surgery (including liver transplantation) has become a surgical subspecialty of its own. The ever-evolving surgical techniques and the better understanding of the anatomy and physiologic consequences related to liver surgery have pushed back the limits of liver tumor resectability. An aggressive approach to liver resection can now be undertaken more safely.

SUGGESTED READINGS

Adam R, Akpinar E, Johann M, et al: Place of cryosurgery in the treatment of malignant liver tumors. Ann Surg 225:39–50, 1997.

Azoulay D, Raccula JS, Castaing D, Bismuth H: Right portal vein embolization in preparation for major hepatic resection. J Am Coll Surg 181:267–269, 1995.

Bismuth H: Surgical anatomy and anatomical surgery of the liver. World J Surg 6:3–9, 1982.

Bismuth H, Corlette MB: Intrahepatic cholangioenteric anastomosis in carcinoma of the hilus of the liver. Surg Gynecol Obstet 140:170–178, 1975.

Bismuth H, Nakache R, Diamond T: Management strategies in resection of hilar cholangiocarcinoma. Ann Surg 215:31–38, 1992.

Castaing D, Bismuth H: Apport de l'echographie per-opératoire dans la chirurgie des tumeurs du foie. Chirurgie 116:738–741, 1990.

Castaing D, Garden J, Bismuth H: Segmental liver resection using ultrasound-guided selective portal venous occlusion. Ann Surg 210:20–23, 1989.

Couinaud C: Le Foie: Études Anatomiques et Chirurgicales. Paris: Masson, 1957.

Elias D, Lasser P, Debaene B, et al: Intermittent vascular exclusion of the liver (without vena cava clamping) during major hepatectomy. Br J Surg 82:1535–1539, 1995.

Huguet C, Nordlinger B, Galopin JJ, et al: Normothermic hepatic vascular exclusion for extensive hepatectomy. Surg Gynecol Obstet 147:160–163, 1978.

Lortat-Jacob JL, Robert HG, Henry C: Un cas d'hepatectomie reglée. Mem Acad Chir 78:244–251, 1952.

Ton That, Tung Nguyen-Duong-Quang: L'hepatectomie reglée par ligature vasculaire intra-parenchymateuse. Presse Med 73:3015–3017, 1965.

Chapter

31

Liver Transplantation: Indications, Pretransplant Evaluation, and Short-Term Post-Transplant Management

Frederick A. Nunes
Kim M. Olthoff
Michael R. Lucey

Liver transplantation has become the treatment of choice in the developed world for many patients with life-threatening liver failure. Table 31–1 lists conditions for which liver transplantation is an appropriate therapy. The improved survival statistics after liver transplantation are due to improvements in surgical technique and greater understanding of the immunosuppression requirements that are unique to liver transplantation. The prospect of success is governed in part by the underlying disease. As shown in Table 31–2, the 5-year patient survival rate is 80.7% among patients transplanted for chronic cholestatic disorders such as primary biliary cirrhosis and primary sclerosing cholangitis, but the survival rate is only 35.4% among patients undergoing liver transplantation for malignant neoplasms.

DONOR ORGAN SHORTAGE

Liver transplantation, like all solid organ transplantation, requires a source of donor organs. In the Western World, the source for donor livers is almost exclusively from heart-beating brain-dead donors. Wherever liver transplantation has become established, donation of livers is dependent on altruism. Sophisticated schemes are required to identify potential donors, harvest their organs, and transport the organs to the location of the potential recipient. At the same time, the number of potential recipients awaiting liver transplantation continues to grow rapidly, outstripping the modest increases in donor numbers. This has meant that there are many more recipients for every donor liver in the United States. The disparity between the availability of donors and the number of recipients has led to growing numbers of patients on the waiting list for liver transplant. These patients then experience longer waiting times. As shown in Figure

31–1, it follows that increasing numbers of patients are dying while on the liver transplant waiting list. Great hopes rest with xenotransplantation and cellular transplantation to correct the liver donor shortage in the future.

The increasing imbalance between the available donors and the number of candidates with life-threatening liver disease has led to strategies to expand the pool of donor organs. Such strategies have included requiring by law that families of brain-dead persons are asked to consent for organ donation ("mandatory request"), or even presuming that the brain-dead person has consented to organ donation, rather than requiring consent by the donor family ("presumed consent"). An alternative approach is to supplement altruism with payments to donor families, usually characterized as small sums to assist in funeral expenses.

Innovative responses to the donor shortage have included the division of a cadaveric organ between two recipients (often referred to as a split liver transplant), or the harvesting of liver segments from living donors. Unfortunately, not all donor livers are suitable for splitting, and living related segmental liver transplantation poses real risks for the donor.

Finally, the donor organ shortage has led to the more frequent use of donor organs that hitherto would have been discarded: so-called marginal donor organs. Marginal organs include those from older donors or from patients infected with present or past hepatitis B virus (HBV) or hepatitis C virus (HCV). The latter are matched to a recipient already infected by the same virus, albeit only after the recipient is appraised and has given consent. An example would be putting an anti-HCV–positive liver into an HCV–positive recipient or an anti-HBV–core-positive liver into an HBsAg-positive recipient. Other marginal grafts include steatotic livers, in which frozen biopsy demonstrates greater

Table 31–1 Conditions Suitable for Liver Transplantation

Acute Parenchymal Disorders

Fulminant hepatic failure	Idiopathic
	Drug toxicity
	Acute viral hepatitis
	Amanita poisoning
	Wilson's disease

Chronic Parenchymal Disorders

Cryptogenic cirrhosis	
Chronic viral hepatitis	Chronic hepatitis B
	Chronic hepatitis C
Toxic/metabolic liver disease	Alcohol
	Hemochromatosis
	Wilson's disease
	α_1-Antitrypsin deficiency

Cholestatic Disorders

	Primary biliary cirrhosis
	Primary sclerosing cholangitis
	Biliary atresia
	Cystic fibrosis

Rare Indications

	Budd-Chiari syndrome
	Hyperoxalosis
	Niemann-Pick disease
	Crigler-Najjar syndrome
	Tyrosinemia
	Alagille's syndrome
	Polycystic liver disease

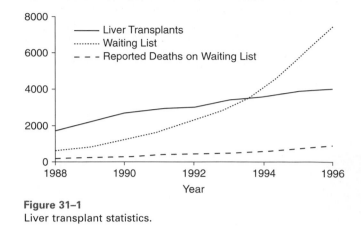

Figure 31–1
Liver transplant statistics.

than 25% microvesicular or macrovesicular fat. These grafts are associated with a higher incidence of primary nonfunction of the allograft (see later for a definition).

IMMUNOLOGY OF LIVER TRANSPLANTATION

Rejection is the term used to describe the immune-mediated response of the host (the recipient) to the donor antigens in the transplanted organ. The rejection response has been subdivided into separate forms. These forms include hyperacute rejection, which is caused by preformed antibodies and occurs immediately after transplantation. This is rarely a problem in orthotopic liver allographs, although it is a major ob-

stacle to the clinical utility of porcine xenografts. Acute cellular rejection is the term that encompasses: cellular-mediated immune responses involving the presentation of donor antigens to host (recipient) lymphocytes; clonal expansion of host lymphocytes with accompanying cytokine elaboration and further recruitment to the donor liver of host lymphocytes and other cells of the circulating cellular immune system; and consequent injury of target donor liver constituent cells. The clinical features of acute cellular rejection will be described later in the section on post-transplant clinical course. When the term *chronic rejection* is used in relation to liver transplantation, it refers to cholestatic injury with bile duct loss and vasculopathy and is sometimes called vanishing bile duct syndrome (VBDS), or chronic ductopenic rejection. This clinicopathologic phenomenon is the corollary of endarteritis obliterans in heart or lung transplants. The immune mechanisms, which are presumed to underlie chronic rejection, are poorly understood, but many cases are preceded by an overt episode of acute cellular rejection.

The immune response to the transplanted liver is a dynamic process. The period of greatest immunogenicity occurs in the first few weeks after transplantation. All liver allograft recipients require initial immunosuppression to forestall graft injury and loss due to acute cellular rejection. Even with use of prophylactic immunosuppression, approximately 50% of liver transplant recipients will experi-

Table 31–2 Outcome of Liver Transplantation in the United States

Primary Diagnosis	No. (94–95)	1-Year Survival (%)	Standard Error	No.	5-Year Survival (%)	Standard Error
Noncholestatic cirrhosis	3520	86.2	0.6	10734	70.1	0.6
Cholestatic liver disease	939	89.4	1.1	3477	80.7	0.8
Biliary atresia	337	91.9	1.6	1549	82.1	1.2
Acute hepatic necrosis	392	77.5	2.2	1367	67.1	1.5
Metabolic disease	274	88.7	2.0	978	79.9	1.5
Malignant neoplasms	151	76.3	3.9	796	35.4	2.2
Overall	6271	87	0.5	20063	72.3	0.4

Based on the 1997 Annual Report of U.S. Scientific Registry for Transplant Recipients and the Organ Procurement and Transplantation Network—Transplant Data: 1988–1996. UNOS, Richmond, VA, and the Division of Transplantation, Office of Special Programs, Health Resources and Human Services Administration, U.S. Department of Health and Human Services, Rockville, MD.

ence at least one episode of clinical acute cellular rejection. This is treated by a temporary increase in immunosuppression. The protocols for treatment of acute episodes of cellular rejection vary from center to center. Eighty per cent of clinical episodes of acute cellular rejection occur in the first 10 weeks after transplantation. Thereafter the requirement for immunosuppression declines toward a baseline in which the donor appears to be partially tolerant. However, most liver transplant recipients require lifelong immunosuppression.

The ideal management of a liver allograft would be to induce a state of tolerance to the donor organ with preservation of the immune response to other non–self-antigens. The immunosuppressive agents in use currently ameliorate the immune response nonspecifically and have a damping effect on the immune response to disparate antigenic stimuli. This translates into an increased susceptibility to viral, bacterial and fungal infection, and to an increased propensity to cancer development. Oncogenesis is often linked to viral infection, especially infection by Epstein-Barr virus (EBV), resulting in post transplant lymphoproliferative disorder and human papillomavirus (HPV) with consequent cervical, vulvar or anorectal carcinoma. In addition, many immunosuppressive agents produce side effects that limit their use and result in significant morbidity.

There is no consensus on what constitutes the best immunosuppressive protocol, and every center devises its own protocols, which are modified when new immunosuppressive agents become available. Most liver transplant centers use a calcineurin inhibitor (cyclosporin A or tacrolimus) as the principal agent plus either one or two other agents. Corticosteroids constitute the main additional agent, and many programs also use azathioprine. There has been a trend to withdraw corticosteroids in order to ameliorate their harmful side effects. Mycophenolate mofetil, an inhibitor of inosine monophosphate dehydrogenase, an essential enzyme for purine synthesis and thus T lymphocyte activation, has replaced azathioprine in some circumstances. The place, if any, of newer agents including rapamycin, or monoclonal antibodies directed at interleukin-2 receptors, remains to be established.

SELECTION FOR TRANSPLANTATION

General Considerations

Evaluation of patients for liver transplantation can be reduced to three main questions:

- What is the severity and prognosis of the patient's liver disease?
- Are there confounding medical, surgical, or psychological factors that would reduce the expectation of a successful liver transplant?
- What are the wishes of the patient with regard to liver transplantation?

These questions are best addressed in a multidisciplinary process. The evaluation is usually carried out in an outpatient setting in which the prospective candidate is examined by transplant surgeons and physicians, social workers, and selected subspecialists including psychiatrists, cardiologists, pulmonologists, and nephrologists. Previous investigations

Table 31–3 Child-Turcotte-Pugh Scoring System

Clinical and Biochemical Measurements	Points Scored for Increasing Abnormality		
	1	*2*	*3*
Encephalopathy (grade)	None	1 and 2	3 and 4
Ascites	Absent	Slight	Moderate
Bilirubin (mg/dL)	1–1.9	2–2.9	≥3
Albumin (g/dL)	>3.5	2.8–3.5	<2.8
Prothrombin Time (sec. Prolonged)	1–4	4–6	>6
For PBC bilirubin (mg/dL)	1–4	4–10	>10

Child Grade	Total Score
A	5–6
B	7–9
C	≥10

*PBC, Primary biliary cirrhosis.

including radiographs and biopsies are retrieved, and new investigations are ordered when necessary. When the information-gathering segment of the evaluation is complete, the patient is presented to the transplantation evaluation committee and a decision is made regarding placement of the patient's name on the transplant waiting list.

Assessment of Severity and Prognosis

Assessment of acute liver injury/fulminant hepatic failure is described in Chapter 22 and is not considered further here. Liver transplantation is a suitable therapy for many forms of chronic liver disease. Assessment of the severity and prognosis of patients with chronic liver failure differs according to the nature of the liver injury. Liver failure due to cirrhosis is assessed by the Child-Turcotte-Pugh classification (Table 31–3). This scoring scheme is an empiric compilation of five features of end-stage liver failure (ascites, encephalopathy, prothrombin time, serum bilirubin, and serum albumin). Survival of cirrhotic patients declines with worsening Child's class. Although the Child's class is useful for segregation of patients according to risk of dying, it does not indicate the prognosis for an individual patient with cirrhosis. A complementary approach is to consider compensated (or stable) and decompensated cirrhosis. Stable cirrhosis is defined by biopsy-proven cirrhosis in a patient who has never experienced variceal hemorrhage, accumulation of ascites, jaundice associated with cirrhosis, or encephalopathy. Conversely, cirrhosis and the onset of at least one of these clinical phenomena define decompensated cirrhosis. It has been shown both in heterogeneous groups of cirrhotics and also in cirrhosis secondary to chronic hepatitis C infection that the onset of decompensation is associated with significantly impaired survival. The onset of decompensation in a previously stable cirrhotic patient indicates the need to evaluate for liver transplantation. Similarly, spontaneous bacterial peritonitis and hepatorenal failure are indicators of significantly worsened prognosis and should prompt transplantation evaluation.

The liver allocation scheme in use in the United States at present gives priority to those patients with the most accumulated time on the waiting list. Therefore, justice requires some parity between liver transplant centers with regard to policy as to when it is appropriate in the course of chronic liver disease for a patient to be placed on the transplant waiting list. It has been agreed that any patient with fulminant hepatic failure, or any cirrhotic patient who has experienced an episode of decompensation or is in Child's class B who meets minimal criteria (Child's score >7), will be placed on the transplant waiting list. There is less consensus on minimal criteria for chronic cholestatic disorders, or special cases such as primary hepatocellular carcinoma, Budd-Chiari syndrome, or polycystic disease. Primary biliary cirrhosis and primary sclerosing cholangitis are the disorders with the best characterized prognostic scoring schemes. These are described in greater detail in Chapters 14 and 15.

Assessment of Medical, Surgical, and Psychological Suitability

Cardiopulmonary Evaluation

A history of systemic hypertension, angina pectoris, myocardial infarction, or age greater than 45 years necessitates a cardiology evaluation. This includes stress cardiography, echocardiography, and in selected cases coronary angiography. Evidence of pulmonary hypertension on echocardiography requires right-sided heart catheterization. Patients whose systolic pulmonary artery pressure exceeds 45 mm Hg should not undergo liver transplantation. A chest radiograph is standard in all patients, and selected patients require pulmonary function studies.

Assessment for Malignancy

As shown in Table 31–2, the 1996 UNOS data show a 5-year survival for all patients undergoing liver transplantation for malignant neoplasms to be 35.4% (No. = 796), compared with 72.3% for all liver transplants (No. = 20,063). In contrast, small unifocal hepatocellular carcinomas, defined as less than 5 cm in greatest diameter, or small multifocal hepatocellular carcinomas (defined as up to three tumors, whose greatest diameter is no more than 3 cm) without evidence of vascular invasion or extrahepatic spread, may be cured by timely liver transplantation. Their survival statistics are similar to those for transplantation for benign disease. Biopsy confirmation of a small tumor is rarely necessary and is likely to spread the tumor along the biopsy track. Hepatoblastomas and neuroendocrine tumors are also occasionally considered appropriate for transplantation. There is general agreement that patients with cholangiocarcinoma should not receive liver transplantation, except within a defined research protocol.

All candidates for liver transplantation should undergo a careful evaluation for cancer, including measurement of serum α-fetoprotein and imaging of the liver parenchyma. The choice of cross-sectional image of the abdomen includes ultrasonography plus Doppler studies, spiral computed tomography (CT) or magnetic resonance (MR) imaging. A past history of malignancy provides a difficult challenge for the transplant assessment team to determine how many disease-free years are required to reduce the chance of recurrence to an acceptable minimum. All adult women need a gynecologic assessment including a Papanicolaou cervical cytology smear. Women older than 40 years should undergo mammography. All patients older than 40 years should be assessed for occult colon cancer with hemoccult testing followed by colonoscopy whenever the result of the screening is positive. All men older than 45 years should undergo testing for prostate-specific antigen (PSA).

Assessment for Infection

Screening for tuberculosis includes chest radiograph and placement of purified protein derivative (PPD). Candidates who are PPD positive may be treated with antituberculosis monotherapy (e.g., isoniazid for 6 months) before transplantation, or treatment may be postponed until after the transplant. All patients should be screened for antibodies to human immunodeficiency virus (HIV). The role of liver transplantation in HIV-infected patients with end-stage liver failure is controversial. Antibodies to cytomegalovirus (CMV), EBV, and herpes simplex virus (HSV) are measured as baseline studies. In the case of CMV, the viral status of the donor and recipient predict the risk of CMV disease after transplant. Chronic hepatitis C infection has become the most common indication for liver transplantation in the United States. Persistence of HCV after transplant is invariable. The outcome after transplantation is significantly worse in patients with greater than 1 million copies of hepatitis C RNA in serum before transplantation. The viral genotype, quasi-species, and mode of acquisition appear less important as predictive factors. Serologic markers for hepatitis B infection are estimated in all patients. Markers for active viral replication such as HBeAg and HBV DNA used to be considered relative contraindications to liver transplantation. The advent of antiviral agents, including lamividudine, and postoperative management protocols using HBIg have allowed successful transplantation in high-risk patients. Antibodies to hepatitis D should be measured in HBsAg-positive patients. Coinfection by hepatitis D ameliorates the severity of post-transplant hepatitis B infection. Candidates without circulating antibodies to hepatitis A or hepatitis B should receive appropriate vaccination.

Nutritional Assessment

Many patients with end-stage liver failure are malnourished. Unfortunately, it is difficult to restore nutritional well-being in outpatients with liver failure. Many liver patients are already on restricted diets: sodium restriction to diminish poorly controlled ascites, protein restriction to control recurrent hepatic encephalopathy, and fluid restriction in hyponatremic patients. A realistic goal is to replenish vitamin K in hypercoagulable patients and to measure vitamin D levels (serum 25 hydroxycholecalciferol) and replenish it when needed. Most cirrhotic patients, even those with intermittent hepatic encephalopathy, can tolerate 80 g/day of protein.

Surgical Assessment

There remain few (if any) surgical contraindications to liver transplantation, depending on the experience of the surgical team. Any prior surgery in the right upper quadrant increases the risk of surgery and probable blood loss. Extensive thrombosis of the portal venous system, including the superior mesenteric vein, may preclude transplantation. Careful radiologic assessment is mandatory in these patients. Angiography remains the gold standard, but in many cases, magnetic resonance (MR) scanning with gadolinium angiography has replaced formal angiography, avoiding intravenous contrast in patients with marginal renal function.

Psychological Assessment

Psychological assessment is most important in patients with a history of illicit drug use or alcoholism. More than 80% of transplant programs in North America include an assessment by a psychiatrist or addiction specialist in the evaluation of patients with alcoholic liver disease. Assessment is directed to determine the likelihood that the candidate will remain abstinent from addictive substances both before the transplant and in his or her life thereafter. Although it remains controversial as an indicator of future abstinence, most liver transplant programs in North America and Europe either require or place a value on a period of abstinence in determining whether to place an alcoholic patient on the waiting list. Many programs will use a more nuanced approach that also assesses the patient's acceptance of alcoholism, their social support to remain abstinent, and their use of behavior modifying programs such Alcoholics Anonymous. The capacity of such assessments to accurately distinguish future drinkers from abstainers remains in doubt.

Assessment of the Candidate's Wishes

Liver transplant programs bear responsibility to inform and educate prospective recipients and their families of the risks and benefits of liver transplantation. It is important to provide the patient with the opportunity to withdraw from transplant assessment if he or she does not wish to proceed. Conversely, whenever the transplant program determines that the patient is not a suitable candidate, the program should facilitate the patient in receiving a second opinion regarding his or her suitability, if he or she should so wish.

PREDICTING THE OUTCOME OF LIVER TRANSPLANTATION

The outcome of liver transplantation is dependent on donor organ and recipient factors. Donor factors that reduce graft success include donor age and transplantation of a liver allograft from a female donor into a male recipient. It is widely held that the fat content of the donor liver influences early graft function, perhaps by facilitating the generation of reactive oxygen species.

As shown in Table 31–2, the cause of the underlying liver disease significantly affects the outcome after liver transplantation. The best outcomes are observed in patients with chronic cholestatic disorders and in chronic liver failure from cirrhosis of many causes. In contrast, the outcome is somewhat worse in patients transplanted for fulminant liver failure and is significantly worse in patients with malignant disease of the liver. Retransplantation carries a poorer outcome than does primary grafting, especially in patients undergoing retransplantation soon after the initial graft. The outcome of liver transplantation is influenced by the severity of illness of the recipient prior to surgery. Patient and graft survival is significantly impaired in recipients requiring intensive care unit management or in patients with multisystem failure before the transplant.

The Transplant Operation

The standard orthotopic liver transplant involves two related surgical procedures. The first procedure is the procurement of the liver graft from the heart-beating brain-dead donor and storage of the organ in cold preservation fluid for transport to the transplant center. The organ recovery procedure involves extensive coordination between multiple surgical teams in order to minimize the ischemia time of each organ procured. The duration of storage of the organ ex vivo is called the cold ischemia time. Cold ischemia times of less than 12 hours are ideal, after which the risk of early poor graft function or biliary damage increases. Younger donor livers tolerate longer ischemia times better than do older grafts.

The second procedure is the actual liver transplant. Many advances in surgical and anesthetic technique have been made in the relatively short history of liver transplantation, and the current procedure has little resemblance to the early operation of 20 years ago. The orthotopic liver transplant can be divided into three phases: (1) recipient hepatectomy, (2) the anhepatic phase, and (3) reperfusion. The first phase of the procedure is total hepatectomy of the recipient's native liver and is the most challenging and bloodiest part of the operation. The technical demands of the recipient hepatectomy are often determined by the severity of portal hypertension leading to formation of large, friable collateral vessels in the recipient's peritoneal cavity. The development of electrocautery dissection and the introduction of the argon beam coagulator have created a safe technique of controlled coagulation and dissection, minimizing blood loss. The presence of a surgical portacaval shunt, transjugular intrahepatic portosystemic shunt (TIPS), or previous surgical procedures in the right upper quadrant may increase the surgical complexity. Portal and systemic venovenous bypass is used by many centers. The goal of venovenous bypass is to decrease portal hypertension during the hepatectomy and anhepatic phase, thus controlling blood loss. The greatest benefit, however, may be the ability to warm the patient on bypass with a warming circuit, thus avoiding severe coagulopathy from hypothermia after reperfusion. In patients with hepatorenal syndrome and anuria, a bypass also allows for insertion of a filter within the circuit for ultrafiltration and removal of significant amounts of fluid during the bypass phase. The next phase is the anhepatic phase, during which time a large dose of corticosteroids are given. Patients without venovenous bypass have a marked decrease in venous return and may become hypotensive and require fluid or vasopressors. The new graft is sewn into the recipient during this time. There are five anastomoses involved: (1) the suprahepatic vena cava, (2) the infrahepatic vena cava, (3) the portal vein, (4) the hepatic artery, and finally (5) the biliary anastomosis, most commonly a choledochocholedochostomy. The third phase of the transplant begins after the portal vein anastomosis, at which time the liver is reperfused with blood. This is a critical part of the procedure and is characterized by varying degrees of what is called the reperfusion syndrome. This may be manifested as hypotension, bradycardia, arrhythmias, and rarely cardiac arrest, which is caused by a sudden influx of cold, hyperkalemic, acidotic blood into the heart. It is the tour de force of a transplant program to have experienced anesthesiologists to maintain the patient during this period of instability.

After reperfusion, careful hemostasis is obtained. The hepatic artery anastomosis is then completed, and the biliary choledochocholedochostomy is performed. In many centers, a percutaneous biliary drainage tube (T-tube) is placed across the biliary anastomosis. A choledochojejunostomy incorporating a Roux-en-Y loop is used in patients with an abnormal native common bile duct, such as in primary sclerosing cholangitis or biliary atresia, or in those patients with very small donor ducts.

Postoperative Care

The typical liver transplant recipient remains in the intensive care unit (ICU) for 24 to 48 hours on assisted ventilation for 24 hours or less. More extended stays in the ICU are dependent on the severity of illness prior to transplantation and may be dictated by developing multisystem organ failure. There are several signs within the first 12 hours that indicate whether the new liver is working well. Correction of acidosis, improvement in urine output, stable hemodynamics, quality bile output (if a T-tube is present), correction of coagulopathy without additional blood products, and improvement in mental status all verify a functioning graft.

Aminotransferases generally peak at 24 to 48 hours post transplant and decline gradually as the ischemia/reperfusion injury resolves. There is no characteristic pattern of liver tests that indicates the underlying cause of liver injury in the liver allograft. Reperfusion injury, acute cellular rejection, and recurrent viral hepatitis produce overlapping biochemical syndromes.

Graft Function

The relative risk of the different causes of graft dysfunction varies according to the interval from the transplant (Table 31–4). Failure of the allograft to function in the first 48 hours is called primary nonfunction. It is assumed to be related to donor organ characteristics or prolonged ischemia. It is important to exclude technical problems such as hemorrhage, occlusion of the vascular anastomoses, or dehiscence of the biliary anastomosis. The vascular integrity is assessed by Doppler sonography, MR angiography, or formal angiography. One advantage of the presence of a biliary drainage tube is the opportunity to image the biliary tract via a T-tube cholangiogram. Alternatively, endoscopic or percutaneous transhepatic cholangiography may be used. When a confident diagnosis of primary nonfunction is made, the patient should be relisted for transplantation. Primary nonfunction is akin to fulminant hepatic failure in an allograft recipient.

A common but less clearly defined problem is encountered when a graft recovers initially but fails to sustain the pattern of improvement, with resultant prolonged elevations of liver enzymes, prothrombin time, or serum bilirubin. This is sometimes called early poor graft function or delayed nonfunction. Once again, structural problems involving the vascular or biliary anastomoses must be excluded. Thereafter, it is often appropriate to perform a liver biopsy, especially to rule out acute cellular rejection as the cause of allograft dysfunction. Poor graft function may be multifactorial in origin and exacerbated by sepsis, total parenteral nutrition (TPN), hepatotoxic medications, and renal failure.

Table 31–4 Etiology of Graft Dysfunction After Transplantation

Time from Transplant	Diagnosis	Relative Importance
The first week	Primary nonfunction	*****
	Early poor function	*****
	Acute cellular rejection	***
	Biliary tract problems	***
	Hepatitis C/D/B	*
1 Week to 6 months	Acute cellular rejection	*****
	CMV hepatitis	**
	Hepatitis C/D/B	**
	Biliary tract problems	**
6 to 12 Months	Acute cellular rejection	***
	Hepatitis C/D/B	**
	Biliary tract problems	**
	Chronic ductopenic rejection	***

Adapted from McCaughan G: Immunologic complications: Rejection late after liver transplantation. In Neuberger J, Lucey MR (eds): Liver Transplantation: Practice and Management. London: BMJ Books, 1994.

As pointed out in the pretransplant section, patient and graft survival is compromised in patients who require care in the ICU or who have significant multisystemic failure immediately before the transplant. Sepsis in the early postoperative period often carries over from overt or covert infections in the pretransplant period. Invasive fungal infection is particularly ominous in the post-transplant recovery period and frequently portends death.

A particularly ominous development is failure to restore normal neurologic function in the first 24 to 48 hours. This may represent primary nonfunction of the new liver or (less likely) a new cerebral injury due to intracranial hemorrhage in a coagulopathic patient or the consequences of cerebral edema in a patient with fulminant hepatic failure. Cerebral injury caused by central pontine myelinolysis is recognized later after liver transplant and has been attributed to rapid restoration of serum sodium in the patient who is hyponatremic at the time of the transplant or secondary to cyclosporine or tacrolimus. Seizures in the first or second week after transplant may be caused by electrolyte disturbance or toxicity from cyclosporine or tacrolimus.

Occasionally, patients develop heart failure in the first 24 to 48 hours. This is probably because of underlying cardiomyopathy, which had been masked by the systemic hyporesistance of advanced liver failure. It may also be a manifestation of previously overlooked hemochromatosis. New-onset heart failure usually resolves with standard medical management.

The patient is maintained in hospital for 10 to 14 days and discharged home. Thereafter, the patient returns for frequent follow-up visits and serial measures of liver tests. As mentioned in the section on immunology, all patients receive immunosuppressive medications, initially in high doses and in gradually decreasing doses thereafter. Most patients also receive many other medications, including sulfamethoxazole-trimethoprim prophylaxis against *Pneumocystis carinii* pneumonia and prophylaxis against CMV in selected patients.

First 3 Months

Acute Cellular Rejection

After the initial 72 hours, consideration of acute cellular rejection as a cause of graft dysfunction increases. Approximately 50% of liver allograft recipients experience at least one episode of acute cellular rejection that necessitates adjustment of their immunosuppressive dosage. Eighty percent of acute cellular rejection episodes in liver allografts occur in the first 10 postoperative weeks. Acute cellular rejection manifests itself as a disturbance of liver tests, especially aminotransferases. It is sometimes accompanied by a systemic disturbance with fever and malaise, but usually the patient is unaware and the abnormality is recognised by screening blood tests only. The diagnosis should be confirmed by liver biopsy. Three features on biopsy are typical: a mixed, predominantly lymphocytic portal infiltrate, lymphocytic injury of the bile ducts ("ductitis"), and lymphocytic injury of the vascular endothelium ("endothelialitis"). The infiltrate often contains eosinophils. The hepatic lobule is spared. Determining whether the histologic features represent acute cellular rejection is often a matter of judgment.

Recurrent hepatitis C mimics acute cellular rejection, and the two can be difficult to tell apart. It is also difficult to decide whether to initiate further treatment in mild or patchy cases. The standard treatment response is a short course of high-dose corticosteroids. Clinical resolution of the elevated aminotransferases is the typical response of acute cellular rejection to bolus corticosteroids and is sometimes taken as confirmation of the diagnosis. This may be a facile interpretation, because high doses of steroids may cause the liver enzymes to decline in hepatitis C infection also. When liver enzymes don't resolve after a course of corticosteroids, the diagnosis of "steroid resistant rejection" may be made. Many patients undergo more than one liver biopsy in the course of an episode of acute cellular rejection. Steroid-resistant rejection is treated with more powerful immunosuppressive agents, including conversion from cyclosporine to tacrolimus, institution of therapy with monoclonal antibodies, or other immunosuppressive agents such as mycophenolate mofetil.

Other diagnoses that may account for graft dysfunction are listed in Table 31–4. Acute CMV infection affects liver allograft recipients in the first three postoperative months. Recipients of an allograft from CMV-positive donors are at greatest risk. Prophylaxis with IV ganciclovir is very effective, reducing both the frequency and severity of CMV in liver allograft recipients. It remains to be shown whether oral ganciclovir formulations will prove as effective.

New-onset cholestasis in the previously functioning graft suggests problems with the biliary tree. Bile duct leaks or strictures may result from occlusion of the hepatic artery. Hepatic artery thrombosis may also lead to the development of sterile hepatic abscesses. A rare but devastating problem is the formation of biliary casts from biliary sludge. Bile duct leaks may be treated by endoscopic stenting but frequently require operative intervention. Significant problems associated with hepatic artery thrombosis or biliary cast formation usually require retransplantation.

LONG-TERM MANAGEMENT

Restoration of Normal Life

The aim of liver transplantation is to restore the transplant recipient to healthy life. Few restrictions should be placed on patients after transplantation. Most liver transplant recipients report improvement in various measures of quality of life. Recipients of a successful transplant should return to work, school, and leisure activities when their stamina permits. Moderate use of alcohol is permitted, except in patients with a history of alcoholism. There should be no restrictions on returning to sexual activity. Most female patients who are capable of menstruation will initiate menstruation within 3 months of successful transplantation. Women should be advised to avoid pregnancy for at least 1 year after transplant, because it is during this time that immunosuppressant doses and the risk of acute cellular rejection are greatest. Pharmacologic contraceptives may be used, except by patients with previous Budd-Chiari syndrome, because of their propensity to thrombosis. Barrier contraceptives offer an alternative. Intrauterine contraceptive devices carry an unacceptable risk of infection. Successful pregnancy is possible after liver transplantation but should be considered a high-risk pregnancy and managed accordingly.

Health Maintenance

Annual health maintenance in adult recipients include cervical smears in all women, mammography in women who are 40 years of age or older, and PSA in all male recipients older than 45 years of age. All patients older than 45 years should be screened annually for colon cancer using guaiac cards. Patients with a prior history of primary sclerosing cholangitis and chronic ulcerative colitis and an intact colon should have an annual colonoscopy. Any evidence of mucosal dysplasia is an indication for a colectomy.

Live vaccines such as BCG, measles, mumps, rubella, varicella-zoster, yellow fever, oral thyphoid, and oral poliomyelitis are dangerous and should be avoided. On the other hand, inactivated vaccines, capsular antigens, and toxoids are safe. These include hepatitis A, hepatitis B, *Hemophilus influenzae,* pneumococcus, and influenza. All older recipients should receive influenza vaccination annually.

Disease Recurrence

Chronic Hepatitis C

Chronic hepatitis C infection is the most common indication for liver transplantation in the United States, accounting for approximately 1000 transplants per annum. All patients who are viremic at the time of transplantation retain the virus, with a variable effect on the transplanted liver. The impact of hepatitis C on the graft varies from little or no evidence of graft injury to a severe, often fatal cholestatic injury. Fluctuating increases in serum aminotransferase levels are the most common indicator of chronic hepatitis C in the transplanted liver. Survival outcome for liver transplant recipients infected by hepatitis C is unchanged compared with other recipients in the first 5 years. Five-year follow-up biopsies show that patients infected with hepatitis C may develop extensive fibrosis, and it is expected that recurrent hepatitis C will account for significant graft injury in the second 5-year follow-up period.

Hepatitis B Infection

Up to quite recently, chronic hepatitis B infection was considered to be a poor indication for liver transplantation. The frequency of recurrence of hepatitis B infection was high, and the outcome was worse than that for other indications. The most severe form of hepatitis B affecting liver grafts was entitled fibrosing cholestatic hepatitis and was characterized by distorted hepatocytes laden with massive amounts of hepatitis B surface antigen and core antigen. Fibrosing cholestatic hepatitis is frequently fatal. The administration of hyperimmune globulin (HBIg) during the operation and at regular intervals after transplantation has reduced the frequency and severity of recurrent hepatitis B infection, improved survival, and made fibrosing cholestatic hepatitis a rare phenomenon. The role of antiviral medications such as lamivudine or famciclovir in the prevention or treatment of recurrent hepatitis B infection in liver transplant recipients is unknown.

Malignancy

Pretransplant malignancies recur frequently after liver transplantation, accounting for the 35.4% 5-year survival for all malignant neoplasia as shown in Table 31–2. The grafted liver is the most common site for recurrence of hepatoma. Once recurrence has been identified, most transplant programs would minimize the oncogenic stimulus from immunosuppression by reducing the immunosuppressive protocol as much as possible. This is a delicate balance that carries the risk of acute cellular rejection. None of the possible antitumor regimens including systemic chemotherapy, chemoembolization, direct injection of alcohol, external beam radiation, or some combination of the above has been shown to be beneficial in the control of recurrent tumor after liver transplantation.

Medical Complications of Immunosuppressive Therapy

Much of the medical care of post-transplant patients is concerned with management of medical complications of immunosuppressive therapy. Many patients experience hypertension requiring antihypertensive chemotherapy. This is more severe in patients with a pretransplant history of hypertension. Cyclosporine and tacrolimus are the main causes of hypertension, but corticosteroids may also play a part in its genesis. Hypertension may complicate the use of a calcineurin inhibitor, even when trough blood levels are in the therapeutic range. When this happens, it is necessary to control hypertension pharmacologically, rather than reduce the immunosuppressive doses.

The calcineurin inhibitors are also the main causes of renal failure, which often accompanies hypertension, and is in part dose dependent. Advancing renal failure despite control of hypertension and drug trough levels in the desired range should prompt a change of immunosuppressive regimen, rather than sacrifice of the kidneys.

Insulin-dependent diabetes mellitus is related to use of corticosteroids. There is a suggestion, albeit unproven, that tacrolimus is more diabetogenic than cyclosporine. Weight gain is one of the most troubling metabolic complications of immunosuppression. It is unclear whether it is more likely with a particular combination of agents, although the appetite-stimulating effect of corticosteroids is one important factor. Gout is another significant metabolic complication of immunosuppressants. On the other hand, cyclosporine has more injurious effects on the integument than does tacrolimus, with patients experiencing hirsuitism, gum hypertrophy, and changes in facies. The latter phenomena may be sufficiently disabling to children and some women to warrant conversion to tacrolimus-based immunosuppression. Hyperlipidemia complicates the use of cyclosporine or corticosteroids. Hypercholesterolemia may require HMG CoA reductase inhibitors such as pravastatin. Indeed, there are suggestive data that pravastatin may reduce the incidence of chronic arteriopathic rejection in heart transplant recipients, although it is not known whether there is a similar benefit for liver transplant recipients.

Many patients are osteopenic on entry into the post liver transplant recovery period. Female sex, a history of cholestatic liver disease, and a prior history of corticosteroid use all contribute to bone loss in this population. Bone loss is further exacerbated in the first 6 to 12 months after transplant. Pathologic fractures or avascular necrosis of the femoral head are described, especially in the first year. Thereafter, bone density actually increases in concert with good allograft function. Corticosteroids are the main reason for worsening osteopenia after liver transplantation. Indeed, the desire to protect already thin bones is one of the principal stimuli to withdraw or reduce corticosteroids after transplantation.

Headache is the most common troublesome neurologic effect of immunosuppressive therapy. Headache is most severe in patients with a prior history of migraine. It is equally common with cyclosporine- and tacrolimus-based protocols. Tremor occurs with both cyclosporine and tacrolimus and is usually a clinical manifestation of toxic blood levels above the therapeutic range.

Post-transplant lymphoproliferative disorder (PTLD) is a particular problem in solid organ transplant recipients. It refers to a spectrum of proliferation of lymphoid cells infected by EBV. At its most benign, it is merely a lymphocytic infiltrate that resolves when immunosuppression is scaled down. At its most severe, it is an aggressive monoclonal non-Hodgkin's lymphoma. It may present as a mass in the liver or as a extrahepatic lymphoid mass in the brain, intestine, or other solid structure. PTLD may arise soon after transplant or may be delayed by months or even years of apparently successful graft survival. PTLD is more common in children and in patients who have received high doses of immunosuppression, especially anti-CD 3 monoclonal antibody. These high-risk patients should be screened routinely using EBV PCR. Many centers will treat an asymptomatic rising PCR by reducing immunosuppression and instituting antiviral therapy such as ganciclovir. PTLD is treated by reducing immunosuppression as much as possible, and in those cases resembling lymphoma, by chemotherapy. The outlook is dependent on the aggression of the tumor and the degree of resolution on reduction or withdrawal of immunosuppression.

SUGGESTED READINGS

Andreu M, Sola R, Sitges-Serra A, et al: Risk factors for spontaneous bacterial peritonitis in cirrhotic patients with ascites. Gastroenterology 104:1133–1138, 1993.

1997 Annual Report of the U.S. Scientific Registry for Transplant Recipients and the Organ Procurement and Transplantation Network—Transplant Data: 1988–1996. UNOS, Richmond, VA, and the Division of Transplantation, Office of Special Programs, Health Resources and Human Services Administration, U.S. Department of Health and Human Services, Rockville, MD.

Beresford T: Psychiatric assessment of alcoholic candidates for liver transplantation. In Lucey MR, Merion RM, Beresford TP (eds): Liver Transplantation and the Alcoholic Patient. Cambridge, UK: Cambridge University Press, 1994, pp 24–49.

Charlton MR, Seaberg EC, Wiesner RH, et al: Predictors of patient and graft survival following liver transplantation for hepatitis C. Hepatology; 28:823–830, 1998.

Everhart J, Beresford T: Liver transplantation for alcoholic liver disease: A survey of transplantation programs in the United States. Liver Transplantation Surg 3:220–226, 1997.

Fattovich G, Guistina G, Degos F, et al: Morbidity and mortality in compensated cirrhosis type C: A retrospective follow-up study of 384 patients. Gastroenterology 112:122–128, 1997.

Fisher LR, Henley KS, Lucey MR: Acute cellular rejection after liver transplantation: Variability, morbidity and mortality. Liver Transpl Surg 1:10–15, 1995.

Gane EJ, Portmann BC, Naoumov N, et al: Long-term outcome of hepatitis C infection after liver transplantation. N Engl J Med 334:815–820, 1996.

Gines A, Escorsell A, Gines P, et al: Incidence, predictive factors and prognosis of the hepatorenal syndrome in cirrhosis with ascites. Gastroenterology 105:229–236, 1993.

Gines P, Quintero E, Arroyo V, et al: Compensated cirrhosis: Natural history and prognostic factors. Hepatology 7:122–128, 1987.

Henley KS, Lucey MR, Appelman HD, et al: Biochemical and histopathological correlation in liver transplant: The first 180 days. Hepatology 16:688–693, 1992.

Kennedy I, Sells RA, Daar AS, et al: The case for 'presumed consent' in organ donation. Lancet 341:1650–1652, 1998.

Lucey MR, Brown KA, Everson GT, et al: Minimal criteria for placement of adults on the liver transplant waiting list: A report of a national conference organized by the American Society of Transplant Physicians and the American Association for the Study of Liver Diseases. Liver Transpl Surg 3:628–637, 1997.

Lucey MR, Carr K, Beresford TP, et al: Alcohol use after liver transplantation in alcoholics: A clinical cohort study. Hepatology 25:1223–1227, 1997.

Mazzaferro V, Regalia E, Doci R, et al: Liver transplantation for the treatment of small hepatocellular carcinomas in patients with cirrhosis. N Engl J Med 334:693–699, 1996.

McCaughan G: Immunologic complications: Rejection late after liver transplantation. In Neuberger J, Lucey MR (eds): Liver Transplantation: Practice and Management. London: BMJ Books, 1994.

Neuberger J, Tang H: Relapse after transplantation: European studies. Liver Transpl Surg 3:275–279, 1997.

Propst A, Propst T, Zangeri G, et al: Prognosis and life expectancy in chronic liver disease. Dig Dis Sci 40:463–472, 1995.

Samuel D, Muller R, Alexander G, et al: Liver transplantation in European patients with hepatitis B surface antigen. N Engl J Med 329:1842–1847, 1993.

32

Liver Transplantation: Long-Term Post-Transplant Management

Mary F. Hebert
Connie L. Davis
Ajit P. Limaye
Kris V. Kowdley
Robert L. Carithers, Jr.

L iver transplantation has become extremely successful over the past decade. Carefully selected patients have an 85% to 90% chance of surviving the first year and 75% to 80% likelihood of living 5 years or longer after transplantation. Because more than 4000 liver transplants are performed annually in the United States, the number of patients with successful liver transplants continues to grow. As a consequence, the demand for long-term management of these patients has steadily increased. Furthermore, many liver transplant recipients now receive most of their postoperative management from gastroenterologists, general internists, and family physicians in the community. The types of problems encountered in liver transplant recipients have shifted from early complications directly associated with the transplant toward long-term side effects of immunosuppressive therapy and a variety of general medical problems.

In this chapter, we have outlined the most common complications seen in liver transplant recipients while also emphasizing occasional (but serious) complications that must be dealt with quickly. We have concentrated heavily on the complications of immunosuppressive therapy and preventive medicine, because these have become the most important issues facing physicians who provide long-term care for liver transplant recipients.

OVERVIEW

Liver transplant recipients can develop a number of unique hepatobiliary complications. In addition, their original liver disease can recur. They also frequently develop complications related to immunosuppressive therapy, such as hypertension, glucose intolerance, electrolyte disturbances, and hyperlipidemias. A good working knowledge of these commonly encountered complications is important for optimum

long-term care of liver transplant recipients. Finally, because so much has been invested in these patients, it is important to develop a comprehensive long-term plan for early detection and prevention of potentially lethal infections and malignancies.

HEPATOBILIARY COMPLICATIONS

A small but significant subset of liver transplant recipients have long-term complications directly related to the transplant. The most common of these are cellular (acute) rejection and biliary tract complications. Less frequent but potentially more serious complications include ductopenic (chronic) rejection of the graft and delayed vascular complications such as hepatic artery or portal vein thrombosis.

Allograft Rejection

Two types of graft rejection occur after liver transplantation. Cellular rejection is an acute inflammatory rejection of the graft, which often becomes apparent within days to weeks after transplantation (Fig. 32–1). A second, less common form of rejection involves gradual disappearance of small bile ducts throughout the grafted liver. This ductopenic rejection can occur as early as a few weeks after transplantation but typically is not seen until months to years later.

Rejection of the transplanted liver can occur at any time. With the recent use of more powerful immunosuppressive agents, the first episode of cellular rejection is not often seen until after the patient has been discharged after the transplant operation. Rejection can also develop months to years after transplantation. Late rejection episodes are usually associated with depressed cyclosporine or tacrolimus levels

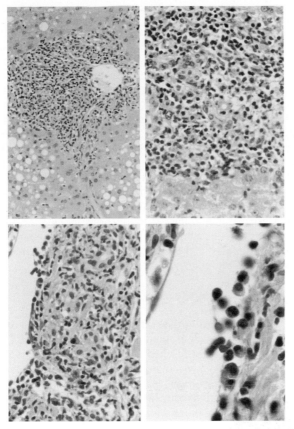

Figure 32–1
Classical histologic features of cellular rejection. (From Maddrey WC, Sorrell MF [eds]: Transplantation of the Liver, 2nd ed. E. Norwalk, CT: Appleton & Lange, 1995, p. 177. © Appleton & Lange, 1995.)

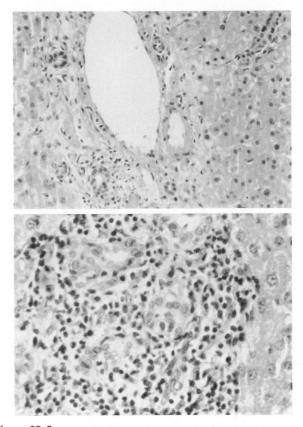

Figure 32–2
Liver biopsy before *(top)* and after *(bottom)* treatment of cellular rejection.

caused by patient noncompliance, poor absorption, or increased metabolism of these drugs.

Cellular Rejection

Cellular rejection typically presents with only mild nonspecific increases in aminotransferases (AST and ALT), γ-glutamyl transpeptidase (GGTP), alkaline phosphatase, and bilirubin values. Liver biopsy is essential for diagnosis. Characteristic histologic features of cellular rejection include lymphocytic invasion of the biliary epithelium and vascular endothelium (Fig. 32–1). Experienced pathologists have little difficulty recognizing cellular rejection; however, this is not a diagnosis that can be reliably rendered by pathologists who infrequently encounter liver transplant biopsies.

If the diagnosis can be established quickly, most patients respond to a short course of increased corticosteroid therapy with rapid biochemical and histologic resolution (Fig. 32–2). Most rejection episodes that fail to resolve with corticosteroid therapy respond to a 7- to 14-day course of monoclonal OKT3 antibody (muromonab-CD3) therapy or to other more aggressive immunosuppressive therapy. However, if not recognized promptly, cellular rejection can result in graft loss or progression to ductopenic rejection. Retransplantation then is often the only option. These concerns

underlie the need for continuous patient compliance and lifetime monitoring of liver function tests and immunosuppressive drug levels.

Ductopenic Rejection

Ductopenic rejection is characterized by slowly progressive cholestasis with marked elevation of GGTP, alkaline phosphatase, and bilirubin values. Serial liver biopsies show prominent cholestasis with gradual disappearance of small intralobular bile ducts and surprisingly little inflammatory infiltrate (Fig. 32–3). The pathogenesis of this condition is poorly understood, and treatment is generally ineffective. If the diagnosis can be established before patients are deeply jaundiced, tacrolimus therapy has successfully reversed the process in a few patients. However, progressive duct destruction usually continues, and most patients require retransplantation.

Biliary Tract Complications

Biliary tract complications are quite common after liver transplantation. Technical, anatomic, and vascular factors all contribute. The biliary tree is particularly susceptible to ischemic damage in patients who have undergone liver transplantation. Normally, approximately two thirds of the arterial blood supply to the common hepatic and upper common bile duct is derived from collateral vessels that originate in the duodenum. Only a third of the blood supply comes from the

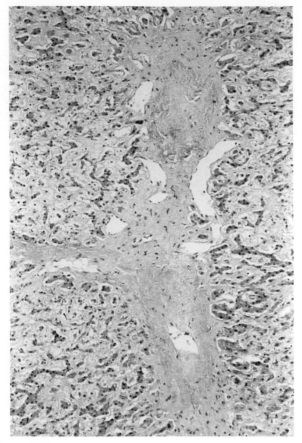

Figure 32–3
Ductopenic rejection. Note the absence of inflammatory infiltrate. (From Maddrey WC, Sorrell MF [eds]: Transplantation of the Liver, 2nd ed. E. Norwalk, CT: Appleton & Lange, 1995, p 178. © Appleton & Lange, 1995.)

right hepatic artery and intrahepatic collaterals. Because of this dual blood supply, ischemic biliary tract injury is quite uncommon in the nontransplant setting. However, because the common duct is transected at the time of procurement, almost all of the blood supply to the donor bile ducts comes from the right hepatic artery. As a consequence, perioperative hepatic artery thrombosis can interrupt the blood supply to the donor ducts and result in significant ischemic biliary disease. Furthermore, because of diminished collaterals, the bile ducts are susceptible to ischemic injury even in the absence of overt hepatic artery thrombosis.

Two types of biliary anastomosis are commonly utilized after liver transplantation: a duct-to-duct choledochocholedocostomy and a Roux-en-Y choledochojejunostomy. The latter anastomosis is usually performed in patients with underlying extrahepatic biliary tract disease, such as biliary atresia, primary sclerosing cholangitis, or secondary biliary cirrhosis. A major limitation of the choledochojejunostomy is poor access to the bile ducts, because endoscopic retrograde cholangiopancreatography (ERCP) usually cannot be performed in patients with a long Roux loop. These patients usually require percutaneous transhepatic cholangiography (PTC) for visualization of the biliary tree.

Frequency and Types of Biliary Tract Complications

In the early days of liver transplantation, biliary complications were reported in up to 50% of patients and were associated with mortality rates as high as 30%. Refinements in surgical technique, enhanced organ preservation, and improvements in nonoperative management of biliary complications all have contributed to a dramatic reduction in the severity of biliary complications after liver transplantation. Nevertheless, they remain the most frequently encountered postoperative complications related to the surgical operation.

The most common biliary tract complications are bile leaks and strictures. Bile leaks most frequently occur either at the T-tube entry site or at the biliary anastomosis. Bile duct strictures can be either anastomotic or nonanastomotic. Other less common biliary complications include the development of casts or stones, sphincter of Oddi dysfunction or papillary stenosis, and extrinsic compression from mass lesions.

Bile Leaks

Bile leaks can occur in the early postoperative period or can be delayed for weeks to months after transplantation. Early leaks often result from ischemia and frequently occur at the anastomosis (Fig. 32–4). In extreme cases, ischemic necrosis of the entire donor biliary system can result in the development of diffuse intrahepatic bilomas. Although these patients can be managed for months to years with percutaneous drainage, retransplantation is ultimately required. Leakage from the T-tube insertion site, which is also common, can often be treated by temporarily opening the T-tube to drainage. Pa-

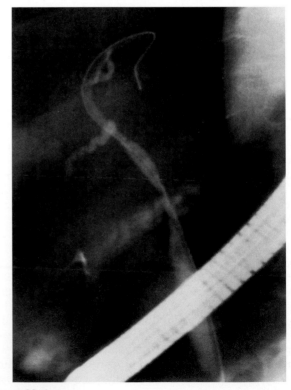

Figure 32–4
Anastomotic leak.

tients with reduced size grafts can have bile leakage from the raw surface of the liver, and patients with unrecognized accessory cystic duct remnants may also have problems with early postoperative bile leaks. These leaks can usually be treated conservatively either with T-tube drainage or percutaneous drainage. Patients with anastomotic or large-caliber leaks can be treated with endoscopic stent placement, which can be performed in the presence of a T-tube. Patients with a choledochojejunostomy or those who fail endoscopic therapy may benefit from surgical revision of the anastomosis. However, endoscopic approaches are preferred if the patient is clinically stable, because small leaks can be difficult to diagnose intraoperatively.

The most common cause of late bile leaks is removal of the T-tube, which is usually performed from 6 weeks to 4 months after transplantation. Patients typically develop severe abdominal pain and peritoneal signs within minutes to hours after removal of the T-tube. Although abdominal pain sometimes lasts only 3 to 4 hours, most patients have persistent pain and require parenteral narcotics. ERCP with stent placement across the leak is generally very effective in relieving symptoms and allowing the leak to close. Patients usually become free of pain several hours after the procedure and can often be discharged from the hospital shortly thereafter. Because of the high incidence of bile leaks associated with T-tube removal, some transplant centers now perform duct-to-duct anastomoses without a T-tube. This approach appears to be safe; however, additional follow-up is needed to determine whether late complications such as anastomotic strictures are increased.

Biliary Strictures

Biliary strictures are usually first detected 4 to 12 months after transplantation. Some patients are asymptomatic or have an insidious presentation with cholestatic liver enzymes or histologic features of extrahepatic obstruction noted on liver biopsy. Other patients present with frank cholangitis or nonspecific signs of infection, such as fever or myalgias. Patients with biliary tract strictures may also develop bacteremia after a liver biopsy, a complication that warrants an evaluation of the biliary tract. A high index of suspicion is necessary for diagnosis because biliary strictures after transplantation often do not result in duct dilatation on ultrasonography.

Strictures can be anastomotic or nonanastomotic. Because anastomotic narrowing is common after duct-to-duct reconstruction, it is important to determine whether the narrowing has clinical significance. Thorough knowledge of the patient's clinical history, pattern of biochemical abnormalities, and findings on liver biopsy must be taken into consideration to place cholangiographic findings in the appropriate clinical context. If symptomatic, these strictures can usually be managed successfully with ERCP using balloon dilatation or stent placement. In patients who cannot be managed with ERCP, revision of the bile duct anastomosis to a choledochojejunostomy is usually adequate. However, because anastomotic strictures may be due to biliary ischemia, it is also important to assess hepatic artery patency using ultrasound with Doppler flow studies. Patients who have strictures at a choledochojejunostomy anastomosis often have prominent symptoms and frequently have overt

evidence of cholangitis. Early intervention with percutaneous cholangiography and stent placement is frequently necessary to relieve symptoms and control the infection.

Strictures can also develop in other areas in the biliary tree after liver transplantation. Common locations include the bifurcation of the right and left hepatic ducts, as well as combinations of hilar and anastomotic strictures. Occasionally, diffuse strictures develop (Figs. 32–5 and 32–6). Potential causes of this phenomenon include late hepatic artery thrombosis, prolonged cold ischemia time, the use of ABO incompatible grafts, and recurrent primary sclerosing cholangitis. A variety of endoscopic and radiologic techniques can be used for dilatation and stent placement in these patients (Fig. 32–7). Using these techniques, complications of diffuse strictures can be controlled in many patients for years. However, retransplantation may ultimately be necessary.

Vascular Complications

Although vascular complications are relatively uncommon after liver transplantation, they can result in serious sequelae, such as diffuse strictures or necrosis of the biliary tree, recurrent bacteremia, catastrophic intra-abdominal hemorrhage, or recurrent variceal bleeding.

Hepatic Artery Thrombosis and Fistulas

Hepatic artery thrombosis is often a silent event that is discovered serendipitously on ultrasonography or because it is suspected as the underlying cause of bile leaks, biliary strictures, or recurrent bacteremia. Urgent reoperation and administration of streptokinase or other anticoagulants have occasionally been useful, although uncertainty about the timing of hepatic artery thrombosis frequently makes their use perfunctory. Many patients with delayed diagnoses require retransplantation because of irreversible injury to the

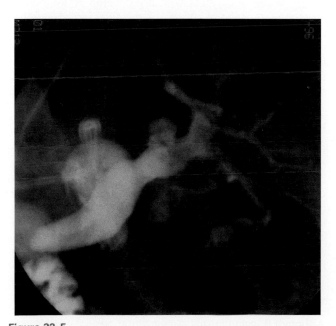

Figure 32–5
Diffuse strictures and leaks secondary to hepatic artery thrombosis.

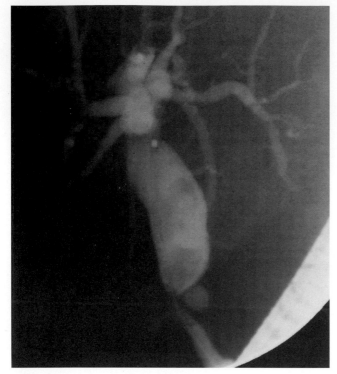

Figure 32–6
Anastomotic stricture with sludge.

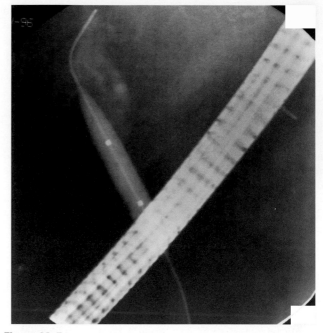

Figure 32–7
Balloon dilatation of stricture.

donor biliary tree; however, this is rarely an emergency procedure, because most patients can be managed for long periods with stent placement and percutaneous drainage of bilomas.

Pseudoaneurysms and hepatobiliary fistulas, infrequent but dreaded complications of liver transplantation, often present with catastrophic bleeding, hypovolemia, and shock. Pseudoaneurysms typically develop at the hepatic anastomosis. Rupture results in massive intra-abdominal bleeding or, if a hepatobiliary fistula has developed, can present as gastrointestinal bleeding from hemobilia. Although most patients are asymptomatic prior to rupture, one third have sentinel signs of abdominal pain or gastrointestinal bleeding.

Portal Vein Thrombosis

Portal vein thrombosis is usually discovered serendipitously on follow-up ultrasonography or because of recurrent variceal bleeding after transplantation. Portal vein repair and clot removal are usually impossible because of delayed discovery of the condition. Sclerotherapy, banding, splenectomy, and distal splenorenal shunts have all been used successfully to manage recurrent variceal bleeding in this setting. Retransplantation is required only if bleeding cannot be controlled or if progressive hepatic failure ensues.

Vena Caval Obstruction

Although it is an unusual complication, vena caval obstruction should be suspected whenever a patient develops persistent ascites or massive lower extremity edema after trans-

plantation. If ascites and edema are caused by vena caval occlusion, balloon dilatation can be used to successfully relieve the obstruction.

RECURRENT DISEASE

Recurrent disease has been a major impediment to long-term survival for patients with certain conditions. Significant recurrent disease has been encountered most frequently in patients transplanted for hepatobiliary malignancies and for cirrhosis secondary to chronic hepatitis B virus (HBV) or C virus (HCV) infections. Although theoretically possible, recurrent disease is uncommon in patients transplanted for autoimmune disorders, such as autoimmune hepatitis, primary biliary cirrhosis, and primary sclerosing cholangitis.

Malignancies

When transplantation is performed because of large unresectable hepatocellular cancers, recurrent tumor occurs in 90% of patients within 2 years of surgery. Although these patients often have excellent quality of life in the interim, tumor recurrence in the grafted liver usually heralds the onset of rapidly progressive disease followed by widespread metastases and early mortality. The prognosis for patients who undergo transplantation for unresectable cholangiocarcinoma is even more dismal.

In contrast, when an incidental tumor is found during the pretransplant evaluation or in the resected liver of a patient undergoing transplantation, the prognosis is much better. These patients rarely develop recurrent disease. In fact, some argue that transplantation, rather than hepatic resection, should be performed for small hepatocellular carcinomas.

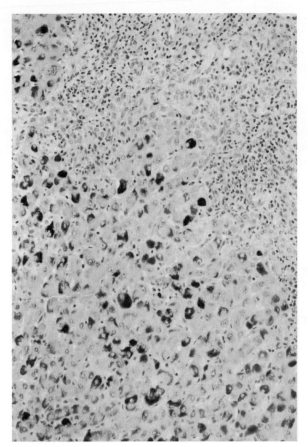

Figure 32–8
Recurrent hepatitis B.

Hepatitis B

Recurrent hepatitis B is also a major problem after liver transplantation. Patients at the highest risk for severe disease are those who are HBeAg-positive with circulating HBV DNA at the time of transplantation. Patients with fulminant hepatitis B and those also infected with hepatitis D virus are much less likely to develop severe recurrent infection.

Recurrent hepatitis B is usually heralded by the asymptomatic return of HBsAg followed by reappearance of HBV DNA and aminotransferase elevations. Although injury to the liver is mild in many patients, a few develop an unusual form of disease characterized by progressive hepatic fibrosis and profound cholestasis (fibrosing cholestatic hepatitis). Liver biopsy in these patients is remarkable for diffuse cellular swelling and fibrosis, accompanied by a relative lack of inflammatory infiltrate. Special stains reveal profound accumulation of HBV antigens within the liver (Fig. 32–8). Most patients with fibrosing cholestatic hepatitis die within the first 12 to 18 months after transplantation. In the past, the survival of patients transplanted for chronic hepatitis B was significantly lower than that for patients transplanted for other conditions.

The continuous use of high-dose hepatitis B immunoglobulin (HBIG) intraoperatively and postoperatively has dramatically altered the outcome of patients with hepatitis B after liver transplantation. However, this preparation, which must be given indefinitely, is extremely expensive. Lamivu-

dine, famciclovir, and other antiviral agents offer great promise that hepatitis B can be controlled effectively in the perioperative period with less expense than the continuous use of HBIG.

Hepatitis C

Recurrent hepatitis C is invariable in patients who are viremic before transplantation. However, despite high levels of circulating virus, only half of patients experience hepatocellular injury within the first year after transplantation. Injury to the liver is often mild, although some patients develop rapidly progressive disease with profound cholestasis and cirrhosis. A difficult issue in managing patients with recurrent hepatitis C is differentiating cellular rejection from recurrent hepatitis. Even the most experienced pathologists have difficulty making this distinction. As a result, patients with recurrent hepatitis C can be treated inappropriately with high-dose immunosuppression for suspected episodes of rejection, with a resultant increase in bacterial sepsis and mortality. If these misadventures can be minimized, the overall survival of patients with recurrent hepatitis C appears to be no different from patients transplanted for other conditions. However, the long-term outcome of these patients is uncertain.

IMMUNOSUPPRESSIVE THERAPY AND ASSOCIATED COMPLICATIONS

Several powerful immunosuppressive agents are now available for the management of liver transplant patients. Although these agents have greatly improved the overall outcome of transplantation, they have a number of side effects. In fact, the majority of long-term complications of liver transplantation are caused by the side effects of these medications. As a result, a good working knowledge of these drugs and their side effects is essential to the management of liver transplant recipients.

Major Immunosuppressive Agents

The immunosuppressive agents in common use today include cyclosporine, tacrolimus (FK-506), corticosteroids, azathioprine, and mycophenolate mofetil. Various combinations of these agents used for long-term immunosuppression include cyclosporine and prednisone; cyclosporine, prednisone, and azathioprine; tacrolimus alone or in combination with prednisone; and mycophenolate mofetil in combination with cyclosporine, tacrolimus, or prednisone. No particular regimen has been shown to be superior, and each is associated with significant side effects.

Cyclosporine

Cyclosporine, which has been in widespread use since 1980, is a lipophilic cyclic polypeptide that consists of 11 amino acids. The drug can be administered intravenously or orally. Oral bioavailability varies considerably from one patient to another but averages 30% in healthy volunteers. Absorption is often decreased in patients with vomiting or diarrhea. Because bile is necessary for the absorption of cyclosporine, either biliary diversion or cholestasis can result in decreased absorption and low cyclosporine levels.

Cyclosporine levels can be measured by a variety of techniques in either whole blood, serum, or plasma. Because each technique gives different results, it is important to measure levels in an individual patient using the same method. Most transplant programs aim to maintain trough levels between 150 and 350 ng/mL (using the whole blood HPLC assay) in the early postoperative period, with a goal of keeping long-term levels between 100 and 150 ng/mL.

The most common side effects of cyclosporine include nephrotoxicity, neurotoxicity, hypertension, hyperkalemia, hypomagnesemia, hirsutism, headaches, tremors, gingival hyperplasia, hyperlipidemia, and hyperuricemia.

Tacrolimus

Tacrolimus, a macrolide lactone, is more potent than cyclosporine; therefore, smaller doses and lower blood levels are required for equivalent immunosuppression. Like cyclosporine, the oral bioavailability is approximately 30% in healthy volunteers. However, in contrast to cyclosporine, bile is not necessary for absorption, and tacrolimus blood levels tend to increase when patients develop cholestasis. This may be partly due to an accumulation of metabolites that cross-react with the assay.

Tacrolimus levels can be measured in whole blood or plasma. Because tacrolimus is concentrated in red blood cells, whole blood levels are much higher than plasma levels. In general, whole blood assays for tacrolimus levels are more accurate and are preferred. Both an enzyme-linked immunosorbent assay (ELISA) and a microparticle enzyme immunoassay are available for determining tacrolimus levels. Most transplant centers aim to maintain trough whole blood levels between 5 and 15 ng/mL.

The common side effects of tacrolimus are similar to those seen with cyclosporine. Nephrotoxicity, headaches, tremors, hypertension, hyperkalemia, hypomagnesemia, hyperlipidemia, and hyperuricemia are common complications of both drugs. Tacrolimus appears to cause less gingival hyperplasia, hirsutism, and hypertension, but more glucose intolerance, gastrointestinal complaints, and hair loss than cyclosporine.

Corticosteroids

Long-term use of corticosteroids is associated with a number of side effects including hyperglycemia, hypertension, changes in body fat distribution, glaucoma, cataracts, osteoporosis, spinal compression fractures, and aseptic necrosis of the femoral head. In children, growth is impaired. Because of these many complications, many transplant programs have attempted to reduce the dose of corticosteroids by adding azathioprine or mycophenolate mofetil or by discontinuing corticosteroids altogether.

Azathioprine

Azathioprine is an antimetabolite that inhibits RNA and DNA synthesis and cell proliferation. Major side effects include bone marrow suppression with subsequent leukopenia, thrombocytopenia, and occasionally anemia. As a result, it is important to monitor blood counts regularly. The usual dose

of azathioprine is 1 to 2 mg/kg/day. The drug is metabolized to 6-mercaptopurine (6-MP) and various other metabolites.

Mycophenolate Mofetil

Mycophenolate mofetil is a prodrug that is rapidly converted to mycophenolic acid, a powerful inhibitor of de novo purine synthesis that limits both T and B cell proliferation. Major side effects include anorexia, nausea, abdominal discomfort, diarrhea, peptic ulcer disease, gastritis, anemia, leukopenia, and thrombocytopenia.

Drug Interactions of Clinical Importance

All of the major immunosuppressive agents have major drug interactions which, if not recognized, can result in serious toxicity and even fatality. As a result, a working knowledge of major drug interactions is particularly important when caring for liver transplant recipients.

Drug Interactions Involving Cyclosporine and Tacrolimus

Cyclosporine and tacrolimus undergo both hepatic and intestinal metabolism via cytochrome P-450 IIIA (CYP3A) to various metabolites. This enzyme can be profoundly inhibited or induced by a variety of pharmaceutical agents. Oral bioavailability of these drugs is also influenced by p-glycoprotein, which acts as a counter-transport pump that actively transports cyclosporine and tacrolimus back into the intestinal lumen.

Intestinal metabolism accounts for up to 50% of the overall metabolism of orally administered cyclosporine. The quantity of intestinal p-glycoprotein appears to be the key to explaining the variability of oral cyclosporine metabolism among patients. It appears that p-glycoprotein works to maximize exposure to intestinal enzymes, thus decreasing the importance of intestinal enzyme quantity. Induction of CYP3A and p-glycoprotein results in rapid metabolism, low bioavailability of cyclosporine and tacrolimus, and increased risk of rejection. In contrast, inhibition of CYP3A and p-glycoprotein can result in diminished metabolism and increased bioavailability of cyclosporine and tacrolimus with the potential for enhanced toxicity.

Cyclosporine Drug Interactions

Many agents have been shown to increase cyclosporine levels (Table 32–1). Antifungal agents, calcium channel blockers, and macrolide antibiotics are of the greatest clinical relevance, because these agents are frequently used in transplant recipients. The effect of orally administered en-

Table 32–1   Agents That Greatly Increase Cyclosporine Levels

Ketoconazole	Dramatic increase in levels within 24 hours
Erythromycin	Dramatic increase in levels within 1 week
Diltiazem	Moderate to dramatic increase in levels within 3 days
Verapamil	Moderate to dramatic increase in levels
Nicardipine	Moderate to dramatic increase in levels
Clarithromycin	Moderate to dramatic increase in levels

zyme inhibitors is even greater on intestinal enzymes than on hepatic enzymes, resulting in a marked increase in bioavailability of orally administered cyclosporine. Thus, for any given dose of cyclosporine, blood levels will be higher.

Among the antifungal agents, ketoconazole causes the greatest increase in cyclosporine levels, followed by itraconazole and fluconazole. Ketoconazole causes a significant decrease in cyclosporine clearance and an even greater effect on oral bioavailability.

The calcium channel blockers are variable in their effect on cyclosporine levels. Verapamil, diltiazem, and nicardipine all appear to lead to increased cyclosporine levels and potential toxicity. Alternative calcium channel blockers such as nifedipine and isradipine have gained favor in transplant patients because they do not have a major effect on cyclosporine levels.

Erythromycin also causes a dramatic increase in cyclosporine levels. Concomitant use of this drug results in a mild decrease in cyclosporine clearance but a marked increase in bioavailability of orally administered cyclosporine. This is consistent with erythromycin having a greater effect on p-glycoprotein and intestinal metabolism than on hepatic metabolism.

A number of agents also decrease cyclosporine levels, potentially leading to inadequate immunosuppression and increased risk of rejection (Table 32–2). Antiseizure and antituberculosis medications are particularly important. As an example, rifampin reduces cyclosporine levels through induction of hepatic metabolism, intestinal metabolism, and p-glycoprotein.

Tacrolimus Drug Interactions

Published information on tacrolimus drug interactions is limited. However, effects similar to those seen with cyclosporine are expected (Table 32–3). Low-dose ketoconazole (200 mg/day) therapy has little effect on hepatic metabolism of tacrolimus; however, it causes a significant increase in bioavailability through a clinically important effect on intestinal p-glycoprotein and intestinal metabolism. Rifampin is the only drug reported to date to decrease tacrolimus levels. However, it is anticipated that many agents that decrease cyclosporine levels will be shown to do the same for tacrolimus.

Drug Interactions Involving Azathioprine and Mycophenolate Mofetil

Azathioprine is metabolized to 6-mercaptopurine (6-MP), which is an active metabolite. 6-MP is further metabolized by xanthine oxidase into various inactive metabolites. Allopurinol, which exerts its effect on uric acid metabolism by

Table 32–2   Agents That Greatly Decrease Cyclosporine Levels

Phenobarbital	Dramatic decrease in levels within 1–2 weeks
Phenytoin	Dramatic decrease in levels within 1–2 weeks
Rifampin	Dramatic decrease in levels within 1 week
Carbamazepine	Moderate to dramatic decrease in levels

Table 32–3   Agents That Profoundly Affect Tacrolimus Levels

Ketoconazole	Dramatic increase in levels
Erythromycin	Dramatic increase in levels
Fluconazole	Mild increase in levels
Rifampin	Dramatic decrease in levels

inhibiting xanthine oxidase, also inhibits the metabolism of 6-MP. This interaction can result in severe bone marrow suppression with subsequent leukopenia, thrombocytopenia, and anemia. At least one patient has died of severe bone marrow suppression because of a physician's unawareness of this interaction. In addition, 1 in 300 patients have an inherited deficiency of thiopurine S-methyltransferase, one of the major enzymes responsible for inactivation of azathioprine and 6-MP, and can develop severe bone marrow suppression when normal doses of these drugs are prescribed.

Mycophenolate mofetil is metabolized to mycophenolic acid, which is further metabolized to mycophenolic acid glucuronide (MPAG). This compound appears to undergo significant enterohepatic recirculation. MPAG can also be eliminated via glomerular filtration and renal tubular secretion. Antacids and cholestyramine appear to decrease both the absorption and enterohepatic recirculation of MPAG. Potential interactions could also occur with other agents that alter renal secretion or interrupt enterohepatic recirculation.

COMMON MEDICAL PROBLEMS

Liver transplant recipients can experience a number of medical problems. Awareness of these potential problems and their management is essential to providing optimum long-term care for these patients.

Infections

Because of the need for lifetime immunosuppression, infections can be a major cause of morbidity and mortality after liver transplantation. The clinical signs and symptoms of infection can be greatly attenuated in patients on immunosuppression. Thus, a high level of clinical suspicion must be maintained when evaluating any clinical deterioration in a transplant recipient. Most serious opportunistic infections occur within the first 6 months after transplantation; thereafter, patients remain at risk for "typical" community-acquired infections (e.g., pneumonia, cellulitis, urinary tract infection).

The major risk for life-threatening infections is within the first few months after the transplant and is highest in patients with long, complicated hospitalizations. During this period fungal infections with *Aspergillus* and *Candida* can be lethal. Patients can also develop overwhelming pneumonia or sepsis from various bacterial infections. After the first postoperative month, the patients at greatest risk for serious infections are those who require excessively high levels of immunosuppression for recurrent episodes of rejection. Patients who can be maintained on minimal doses of immunosuppression have few infections, and those infections that do occur are often typical community acquired infections that respond well to standard antimicrobial therapy.

Prophylactic Regimens

The use of aggressive prophylactic regimens following liver transplantation has changed both the timing and frequency of many infections. Most patients receive ganciclovir prophylaxis immediately after transplantation if either they or the donor are seropositive for cytomegalovirus (CMV). If both the donor and recipient are CMV negative, patients typically receive acyclovir in the early postoperative period to prevent severe herpes simplex and varicella-zoster infections. In addition, most patients receive trimethoprim-sulfamethoxazole for 6 to 12 months after transplantation to prevent *Pneumocystis carinii* infections.

Viral Infections

Despite the aforementioned prophylactic measures, transplant recipients remain at risk for the development of systemic disease secondary to the reactivation of latent viral infections. This most commonly occurs after aggressive courses of immunosuppression for recurrent episodes of rejection.

Cytomegalovirus

CMV, which is the most important viral infection in liver transplant recipients, typically occurs 1 to 4 months after transplantation. CMV-negative recipients can develop a primary infection from the donor organ or from blood products administered before, during, or after the transplant. CMV-positive recipients can have either reactivation of latent infection or superinfection from CMV acquired in the perioperative period.

The typical manifestations of CMV infection include malaise, diffuse myalgias, fever, leukopenia, and thrombocytopenia. Patients often have modest elevations of aminotransferases, raising the possibility of allograft rejection. A liver biopsy can be very helpful to differentiate between these two conditions. CMV hepatitis is characterized by focal collections of inflammation within the hepatic parenchyma, often containing CMV inclusion bodies (Fig. 32–9). The diagnosis can be confirmed by detection of CMV viremia.

Other less common but more serious manifestations of CMV infection include gastrointestinal involvement, pneumonia, and chorioretinitis. If diagnosed in a timely fashion, CMV can usually be treated effectively with a 10- to 21-day course of intravenous ganciclovir.

Herpes Viruses

Herpes simplex virus (HSV) and varicella-zoster infections are common in transplant recipients. Herpes simplex reactivation can result in either painful oral ulcerations (HSV type 1) or as genital ulcerations (HSV type 2). Herpes zoster due to reactivation of varicella-zoster is also common in transplant recipients. Each of these infections responds well to treatment with intravenous or oral acyclovir.

Epstein-Barr Virus

Clinically apparent Epstein-Barr virus (EBV) infection is uncommon after liver transplantation. However, EBV infection acquired before or at the time of transplantation, is associated with the development of post-transplant lymphoproliferative disease (PTLD). The clinical presentation of PTLD is often that of a polyclonal or monoclonal lymphoma with a particular predisposition to the gastrointestinal tract. This syndrome is seen more commonly in patients who have received high-dose immunosuppression with cyclosporine, tacrolimus, or OKT3. Reduction of immunosuppression, immunotherapy with interferon, and chemotherapy have been successfully employed for treatment. The use of antiviral therapy is controversial.

Bacterial Infections

Bacterial infections are common during the immediate postoperative period. However, the risk of such infections rapidly diminishes over time unless the patient has biliary obstruction. In such patients, recurrent cholangitis can be a major management problem. It is important to specifically evaluate the hepatobiliary system in any liver transplant recipient with otherwise unexplained bacteremia. Uncommon, but potentially lethal, bacterial infections encountered in the transplant recipient include pneumococcal sepsis and *Listeria* meningitis. Pneumococcal sepsis is seen most commonly in splenectomized patients. This rapidly progressive disease is often lethal. The devastating nature of this infection underscores the need for regular immunization in transplant recipients. *Listeria* meningitis should be suspected in immunosuppressed patients who complain of new onset headaches, particularly in those who have a fever. The clinical course is often indolent. Typically, there is modest cere-

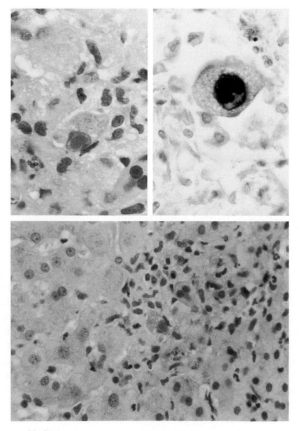

Figure 32–9
CMV hepatitis.

brospinal fluid (CSF) leukocytosis (<1000 cells/mm³), and a careful examination of Gram stains reveals gram-positive rods. Although many patients respond well to treatment with either penicillin or ampicillin, many experts now recommend the combination of one of these agents with gentamicin. Trimethoprim-sulfamethoxazole is an effective alternative in selected patients.

Fungal Infections

Aspergillus, Candida, and *Pneumocystis carinii* are the most common and serious fungal infections in liver transplant recipients. *Aspergillus* and *Candida* infections usually occur in the first or second post-transplant month in patients with severe, prolonged postoperative hospitalizations. The lung is the most common site of *Aspergillus* infection, and dissemination to the brain, skin, or bone can be seen. Prompt initiation of antifungal therapy with amphotericin B with or without adjunctive surgical débridement is the mainstay of management.

Other delayed fungal infections include cryptococcal meningitis and *Pneumocystis* pneumonia. Cryptococcal meningitis can have an indolent course with subtle clinical features. However, if untreated, the disease is ultimately fatal. Patients usually have a headache, but meningismus and focal neurologic findings are unusual. The CSF often contains elevated protein and depressed glucose levels with mild leukocytosis (100 to 500 cells/mm³). Direct visualization of organisms using India ink–stained preparations of CSF, detection of cryptococcal antigen, or culture confirms the diagnosis. The treatment of choice is amphotericin B with or without 5-fluorocytosine (5-FC).

Patients with *Pneumocystis* pneumonia typically present with the rapid development of fever, a nonproductive cough, and dyspnea. A chest x-ray typically reveals a diffuse, symmetric pattern of infiltrates that is often perihilar in distribution. Patients often have significant hypoxemia. A definitive diagnosis often requires a bronchoscopy to identify the organisms. Patients can usually be treated effectively with trimethoprim-sulfamethoxazole.

Renal Insufficiency

Renal impairment is common after liver transplantation. The most frequent causes include cyclosporine or tacrolimus treatment, use of other nephrotoxic medications, pretransplant renal ischemia caused by severe hepatic dysfunction, and intrinsic renal disease. The glomerular filtration rate declines from an average of 100 mL/min pretransplant to 60 mL/min posttransplant due to cyclosporine or tacrolimus use alone. Thereafter, renal function generally remains stable in most patients at least during the first 5 years after transplantation. On average, 25% to 40% of patients maintain serum creatinine values of 1.5 mg/dL or above, although serum creatinine is a poor marker of renal function in these patients. Renal histology ranges from no changes to interstitial fibrosis, tubular atrophy, and vascular sclerosis. Cyclosporine withdrawal improves renal function in patients who have renal dysfunction but good hepatic function 1 year after transplantation. Fish oil supplementation may improve the glomerular filtration rate and renal blood flow in cyclosporine-treated patients, but large-scale trials have not been performed and patient acceptance is low.

Renal ischemia after liver transplantation is greatly accentuated by treatment with nonsteroidal anti-inflammatory drugs (NSAIDs), especially if there is evidence of hepatic dysfunction. As a consequence, the use of NSAIDs should be avoided if at all possible. Although the degree of renal ischemic injury caused by hepatorenal syndrome (HRS) is difficult to quantitate, 7% of patients with HRS require dialysis within 4 years compared with only 2% of those without HRS before transplantation.

Several patients with end-stage liver disease also have intrinsic renal disease. Glomerular lesions include mesangial sclerosis with deposition of IgG and IgM, glomerulosclerosis without immunoglobulin deposition, and mesangial IgA deposition. Membranoproliferative glomerulonephritis and cryoglobulinemia can be seen in patients with chronic hepatitis C, and membranous glomerulopathy is seen in patients with hepatitis B infection. Clinical evidence of renal disease may be present before transplant or may be recognized only in the postoperative period.

Low-grade proteinuria after liver transplantation can be seen with cyclosporine or tacrolimus therapy or may be associated with intrinsic renal disease. HCV-infected patients often manifest significant proteinuria within 3 to 6 months of transplantation. The underlying renal lesion is usually membranoproliferative glomerulonephritis. The utility of treatment with interferon for HCV-related renal disease following liver transplantation is still unknown.

Electrolyte Disturbances

Electrolyte disturbances are quite common in liver transplant recipients. Most patients have sodium retention because of varying degrees of renal insufficiency and the use of cyclosporine or tacrolimus. However, hypernatremia and hyponatremia are uncommon once the patient has recovered from surgery. In contrast, hyperkalemia and hypomagnesemia can be persistent problems.

Hyperkalemia is a common consequence of both cyclosporine and tacrolimus therapy. Most patients have mild increases in potassium levels; however, patients occasionally develop severe hyperkalemia and require therapy to prevent cardiac arrhythmias. Because of the frequency of hyperkalemia, it is important to avoid the use of NSAIDs, salt substitutes, and potassium-sparing diuretics (e.g., spironolactone and amiloride). Angiotensin-converting enzyme inhibitors should also be used cautiously because of their propensity for hyperkalemia.

Hypertension

Hypertension, which is infrequently present before transplantation, occurs in 20% to 60% of patients after the operation. Normally, 24-hour blood pressure profiles are characterized by a diurnal increase and nocturnal decrease. In solid organ transplant recipients, the nocturnal drop in pressure may be lost. This is important because the loss of nocturnal fall in blood pressure has been correlated with an increased risk for cardiovascular complications. Hypertension requiring treatment appears to be less frequent in patients receiving tacrolimus compared with cyclosporine. However, the number of hypertensive patients is comparable in those receiving cyclosporine in capsular and microemulsion formulations.

The etiology of hypertension is multifactorial, including increases in extracellular volume, endothelin, cytosolic calcium, and thromboxane A_2 and decreases in magnesium, nitrous oxide, and prostacyclin. Cyclosporine effects on the renin-angiotensin system have been variable but, in general, cause systemic suppression but intrarenal stimulation of this system. Likewise, adrenergic mechanisms do not seem to play a role. Steroid use aggravates the hypertension by increasing extracellular volume. Although hypertension is thought to be initiated and maintained by the immunosuppressive medications, withdrawal of these agents after long-term treatment is not guaranteed to result in improved blood pressure control.

Post-transplant hypertension is generally associated with high systemic vascular resistance and, therefore, lends itself to initial treatment with calcium channel blockers such as nifedipine and isradipine. Careful monitoring of cyclosporine levels is required if verapamil, diltiazem, or nicardipine are used. β-Blockers are useful in patients who have increased cardiac output after calcium channel blocker therapy; however, their use can be associated with fatigue. Angiotensin-converting enzyme inhibitors are generally not effective first-line antihypertensive agents because of the suppressed systemic angiotensin system in these patients; however, there is evidence that they may reduce intrarenal cyclosporine toxicity. When they are used, care must be given to avoid hyperkalemia. Diuretics can be helpful supplements in the control of hypertension, but the risk for further renal dysfunction and hyperuricemia is increased. Potassium-sparing diuretics should not be used unless there is significant potassium wasting.

Neurologic Complications

Headaches, insomnia, tremors, peripheral neuropathies, and various vague neurologic complaints are common in liver transplant recipients. In some cases, these symptoms are the result of excessive levels of cyclosporine or tacrolimus and respond quickly to a reduction in the administered doses of these drugs. However, in many patients, symptoms are present or persist in the presence of optimum or even low levels of these drugs. Relief for these patients is much more difficult to achieve.

Headaches are a particularly distressing symptom for many liver transplant recipients. Patients with previous migraine headaches often have an increase in the severity and frequency of their headaches after liver transplantation. Other patients with no history of migraines may develop severe, unremitting headaches after transplantation. Amitriptyline and propranolol have been useful in some patients.

Each patient with new onset headaches after liver transplantation should have a complete neurologic evaluation or exclude other more serious causes of headaches; however, thereafter, repeated extensive and expensive evaluations should be avoided unless there has been a distinct change in symptoms.

Oral and Skin Manifestations

Liver transplant recipients can have a variety of disturbing oral and skin manifestations. Included among these manifestations are gingival hyperplasia induced by cyclosporine and nifedipine. Fortunately, gingival hyperplasia is not an infrequent side effect of tacrolimus, which can be substituted for cyclosporine in patients with this condition. Hirsutism is another distressing side effect of cyclosporine therapy that is not experienced by patients who take tacrolimus. Instead, these patients may experience hair loss.

Oral and genital herpes infections, herpes zoster, verrucae, and fungal infections of the nails are not uncommon in patients receiving long-term immunosuppression. The herpes infections respond well to acyclovir therapy. Fungal infections of the nails may be treated with systemic antifungal therapy in select high risk patients. Careful attention to drug interactions is necessary.

Transplant recipients are at high risk for the development of both basal and squamous cell carcinomas of the skin. Suspicious lesions should be biopsied, and patients should be counseled about the need to limit exposure to sunlight and the liberal use of sun blockers when they are outdoors.

Hyperuricemia and Gout

Although hyperuricemia is commonly seen after liver transplantation, clinical manifestations of gout are unusual. This is fortunate, because treatment for gout in transplant recipients can be quite difficult and is associated with a high risk of complications. The underlying cause of hyperuricemia appears to be multifactorial, but renal insufficiency and the use of cyclosporine and tacrolimus therapy appear to be the major contributors.

Considerable caution should be used in treating hyperuricemia and gout because of the high probability of side effects with commonly used drugs. Allopurinol can result in profound, life-threatening leukopenia in patients taking azathioprine. NSAIDs can result in rapid worsening of renal function in patients taking cyclosporine or tacrolimus, and these drugs should be used judiciously, if at all. Colchicine is probably the safest agent for treating gout in transplant recipients, although diarrhea can result in poor absorption of cyclosporine and tacrolimus.

Bone Disease

Osteoporosis with pathologic fractures can be a major cause of morbidity in patients with primary biliary cirrhosis, primary sclerosing cholangitis, and autoimmune hepatitis. Many of these patients have severe demineralization before transplantation because of their disease or the long-term use of corticosteroids. Immobilization after the transplant combined with high-dose corticosteroids often results in further bone loss as well as vertebral and other pathologic fractures. Early mobilization and minimization of corticosteroids are helpful in such patients. A number of other approaches to minimize bone loss are being explored. The biophosphonates (e.g. etidronate) have been shown to have promise in preliminary studies. Fortunately, many patients begin to develop increased bone mass 6 to 12 months after transplantation, and clinical problems caused by osteoporosis gradually disappear.

Diabetes Mellitus

Newly diagnosed diabetes occurs in 15% to 20% of liver transplant recipients. The agents thought to be responsible include corticosteroids, cyclosporine, and tacrolimus. Careful control of hyperglycemia is important. Oral hypoglycemic agents can be useful, but effective control often requires the use of insulin. Early reports to eliminate corticosteroid therapy in recipients with good graft function have shown favorable results in eliminating the need for insulin therapy in some patients.

Obesity

Obesity is an increasing and disturbing problem in the community of liver transplant recipients. Many patients with morbid obesity following liver transplantation were obese before surgery. After surgery, their pathologic eating habits are often exaggerated by corticosteroid therapy. Early and aggressive intervention by an experienced dietitian is the most beneficial approach to this difficult problem. Treatment with tacrolimus can be useful in some patients because of the anorexia that some patients experience when taking this drug.

Hyperlipidemias

Hyperlipidemia is common after solid organ transplantation. Potential causes include obesity, genetic predisposition, and immunosuppressive medications, especially cyclosporine, tacrolimus and corticosteroids. Hyperlipidemia appears to be most pronounced with sirolimus. Accelerated coronary artery disease has been well documented after cardiac and renal transplantation. Although increased risk of coronary disease has not been documented in liver transplant recipients, it is not clear whether this represents a different biology of disease or a shorter follow-up for most liver transplant recipients compared with cardiac and renal transplant recipients.

Given these uncertainties, it is not clear how aggressive to be in approaching the lipid disturbances that are seen after liver transplantation. Everyone would agree that dietary counseling and manipulation should be done; however, these efforts are rarely effective in patients with severe lipid disturbances. Some studies suggest that lipid levels are lower in patients who receive tacrolimus rather than cyclosporine therapy; however, other studies do not show a similar effect. Elimination of the use of corticosteroids may also be helpful, although this does not uniformly result in lower lipid levels.

Whether every patient should receive aggressive pharmacologic therapy for lipid disorders after liver transplantation remains to be established in terms of efficacy, safety, and cost-effectiveness. Each of the major classes of lipid-lowering agents has the potential for major side effects in transplant recipients. Bile acid resins may interfere with absorption of cyclosporine, tacrolimus, and other medications. Gemfibrozil and lovastatin are both associated with an increased risk of myositis and rhabdomyolysis when used in conjunction with cyclosporine. Nicotinic acid has various side effects, including severe hepatotoxicity. Of all the alternatives available, the best choices appear to be diet plus low-dose HMG-CoA reductase inhibitors such as pravastatin.

Post-Transplant Malignancies

Transplant recipients have a high risk for various malignancies, including squamous cell skin and lip cancers, cervical cancer, and lymphomas. Patients with primary sclerosing

Table 32–4 Screening Tests Recommended for Liver Transplant Recipients

Careful skin and oral examination	Annually, biopsy of suspicious lesions
Ophthalmologic examination	Annually for glaucoma and cataracts
Breast examination	Annually in women
Mammogram	Annually in women aged 40–59
Flexible sigmoidoscopy	Every 3–5 years beginning at age 50 or if fecal occult blood positive
Colonoscopy with multiple biopsies	Annually in patients with primary sclerosing cholangitis and ulcerative colitis
Papanicolaou smear	Annually for 3 years, then every 3 years in sexually active women of childbearing age
Blood pressure and body weight determinations	Annually
Creatinine clearance and 24-hour urine protein	Annually

cholangitis and long-standing ulcerative colitis appear to be at particularly high risk for colonic dysplasia and diffuse colon cancer. Regular, aggressive screening of these patients with colonoscopy and biopsies is essential to prevent the insidious development of colon cancer. If severe dysplasia is discovered on screening colonoscopy, a colectomy can be done safely within 10 to 12 weeks after the transplant.

PREVENTIVE MEDICINE

As patients survive longer after liver transplantation, routine screening procedures and regular immunizations have become increasingly important for their care. Outlined below are suggested guidelines for regular screening visits and immunizations for these patients.

Screening Procedures

Transplant recipients should receive all screening procedures recommended for their age and sex. Because of the

Table 32–5 Recommended Immunizations for Liver Transplant Recipients

Tetanus-diphtheria	All adults at 10-year intervals
Influenza	Annually in all transplant recipients
Pneumococcus*	Especially important in splenectomized patients
Hepatitis B*	If not received before transplantation
Hepatitis A	Anti-HAV–negative patients planning foreign travel and living in communities with prolonged hepatitis A outbreaks
Cholera, plague, inactivated typhoid	If indicated before foreign travel

*Should be administered before transplantation if possible.

Table 32–6 Immunizations Contraindicated in Transplant Recipients

Measles	Live virus vaccine
Rubella	Live virus vaccine
Yellow fever	Live virus vaccine
Oral polio	Live virus vaccine—neither patients nor children in household*
Typhoid Ty21a	Live virus vaccine

*Inactivated polio vaccine available for transplant recipients and children in household.

potentially increased risk of skin and oral cancers, a careful skin and oral examination and reinforcement of the need for sun blocks should be performed annually. Women should also have an annual Pap smear. Other recommendations are listed in Table 32–4.

Immunizations

Liver transplant recipients should receive routine pneumococcal, influenza, and tetanus immunizations (Table 32–5). However, live vaccines such as measles-mumps-rubella (MMR) and oral polio vaccine should not be given to transplant recipients (Table 32–6). Furthermore, children in the household of a transplant recipient should receive inactivated polio vaccine rather than live oral vaccine. Transplant recipients who are planning overseas travel should receive cholera, plague, hepatitis A, and inactivated typhoid vaccinations if indicated. However, they should avoid vaccination with live vaccines such as typhoid Ty21a and yellow fever vaccine.

SUMMARY

Liver transplantation has made a dramatic impact on the care of patients with end-stage liver disease and has offered many terminally ill patients the opportunity for long-term survival. The challenge that we now face is to maximize the quality and duration of this survival through careful and meticulous care of these patients after transplantation.

SUGGESTED READINGS

Anand AC, Hubscher SG, Gunson BK, et al: Timing, significance, and prognosis of late acute liver allograft rejection. Transplantation 60:1098–1103, 1995.

Araya V, Rakela J, Wright T: Hepatitis C after orthotopic liver transplantation. Gastroenterology 112:575–582, 1997.

Bennett WM, DeMattos A, Meyer MM, et al: Chronic cyclosporine nephropathy: The Achilles' heel of immunosuppressive therapy. Kidney Int 50:1089–1100, 1997.

Bismuth H, Chiche L, Adam R, et al: Liver resection versus transplantation for hepatocellular carcinoma in cirrhotic patients. Ann Surg 218:145–151, 1993.

Brentnall TA, Haggitt RC, Rabinovitch PS, et al: Risk and natural history of colonic neoplasia in patients with primary sclerosing cholangitis and ulcerative colitis. Gastroenterology 110:331–338, 1996.

Campana C, Regazzi MB, Buggia I, Molinaro M: Clinically significant drug interactions with cyclosporin: An update. Clin Pharmacokinet 30:141–179, 1996.

Davis CL, Gretch DR, Perkins JD, et al: Hepatitis C-associated glomerular disease in liver transplant recipients. Liver Transpl Surg 1:166–175, 1995.

Demetris AJ, Seaberg EC, Batts KP, et al: Reliability and predictive value of the National Institute of Diabetes and Digestive and Kidney Diseases Liver Transplantation Database nomenclature and grading system for cellular rejection of liver allografts. Hepatology 21:408–416, 1995.

Furlan V, Perello L, Jacquemin E, et al: Interactions between FK-506 and rifampicin or erythromycin in pediatric liver recipients. Transplantation 59:1217–1218, 1995.

Gane EJ, Portman BC, Naoumov NV, et al: Long-term outcome of hepatitis C infection after liver transplantation. N Engl J Med 334:815–820, 1996.

Greif F, Bronsther OL, Van Thiel DH, et al: The incidence, timing, and management of biliary tract complications after orthotopic liver transplantation. Ann Surg 219:40–45, 1994.

Grellier L, Mutimer D, Ahmed M, et al: Lamivudine prophylaxis: A new strategy for prevention of reinfection in liver transplantation for hepatitis B cirrhosis. Lancet 348:1212–1215, 1996.

Hibberd PL, Rubin RH: Clinical aspects of fungal infection in organ transplant recipients. Clin Infect Dis 19:S33–S40, 1994.

Kennedy DT, Hayney MS, Lake KD: Azathioprine and allopurinol: The price of an avoidable drug interaction. Ann Pharmacother 30:951–954, 1996.

Kobashigawa JA, Kasiske BL: Hyperlipidemia in solid organ transplantation. Transplantation 63:331–338, 1997.

Lake KD, Canafax DM: Important interactions of drugs with immunosuppressive agents used in transplant recipients. J Antimicrob Chemother 36:11–22, 1995.

Lampen A, Christians U, Guengerich FP, et al: Metabolism of the immunosuppressant tacrolimus in the small intestine: Cytochrome P-450, drug interactions, and interindividual variability. Drug Metab Dispos 23:1315–1324, 1995.

Lewis WD, Jenkins RL: Biliary strictures after liver transplantation. Surg Clin North Am 74:967–978, 1994.

Newell KA, Alonso EM, Whitington PF, et al: Posttransplant lymphoproliferative disease in pediatric liver transplantation: Interplay between primary Epstein-Barr virus infection and immunosuppression. Transplantation 62:370–375, 1996.

Porayko MK, Kondo M, Steers JL: Liver transplantation: Late complications of the biliary tract and their management. Semin Liver Dis 15:139–155, 1995.

Quagliarello VJ, Scheld WM: Treatment of bacterial meningitis. N Engl J Med 336:708–716, 1997.

Samuel D, Muller R, Alexander G, et al: Liver transplantation in European patients with the hepatitis B surface antigen. N Engl J Med 329:1842–1847, 1993.

Seifeldin R: Drug interactions in transplantation. Clin Ther 17:1043–1061, 1995.

Stegall MD, Everson GT, Schroter G, et al: Prednisone withdrawal late after adult liver transplantation reduces diabetes, hypertension, and hypercholesterolemia without causing graft loss. Hepatology 25:173–177, 1997.

Textor SC: De-novo hypertension after liver transplantation. Hypertension 22:257–267, 1993.

Venkataramanan R, Swaminathan A, Prasad T, et al: Clinical pharmacokinetics of tacrolimus. Clin Pharmacokinet 29:404–430, 1995.

Watkins PB: Drug metabolism by cytochrome P-450 in the liver and small bowel. Gastroenterol Clin North Am 21:511–526, 1992.

Wiesner RH: Advances in diagnosis, prevention, and management of hepatic allograft rejection. Clin Chem 40:2174–2185, 1994.

Wiesner RH, Ludwig J, van Hoek B, Krom RAF: Current concepts in cell-mediated hepatic allograft rejection leading to ductopenia and liver failure. Hepatology 14:721–729, 1991.

Yates CR, Krynetski EY, Loennechen T, et al: Molecular diagnosis of thiopurine S-methyltransferase deficiency: Genetic basis of azathioprine and mercaptopurine intolerance. Ann Intern Med 126:608–614, 1997.

33

Imaging of the Liver

Jeff L. Fidler
David D. Stark

Multiple techniques are currently available for imaging the liver. These individual modalities have unique advantages and limitations inherent to their design and physical properties of image acquisition. Over the past few years, dramatic improvements in technology have improved the quality of cross-sectional imaging in the abdomen and, specifically, the liver. Because of the rapidity in the advancement of technology, the potential clinical applications are yet to be fully understood and are undergoing extensive evaluation. Therefore, the clinician often faces a dilemma as to which modality to perform in the work-up of a given abnormality and which imaging algorithm is the most cost effective.

In this chapter, we discuss the imaging techniques available, their indications, advantages, and limitations. We also discuss the imaging features of several selected disease processes and the sensitivity and specificity of the different modalities, and we provide recommendations regarding the approach to imaging these patients.

IMAGING MODALITIES

The techniques currently available to image the liver include ultrasound, scintigraphy, computed tomography (CT), and magnetic resonance imaging (MRI). The choice of a particular technique is dictated by the clinical question. The objectives of imaging consist of detection, characterization, and staging or quantification of the disease process.

Ultrasound: Ultrasound acquires images of the body by transmitting sound waves through tissues and sampling the waves that return to the transducer. Tissues propagate these waves at different speeds based on their acoustic impedance and reflect the waves at different angles based on the angle of incidence of the sound wave to the individual tissue. This property allows specific localization and characterization of different tissues. Unfortunately, these properties are very complex and can cause numerous artifacts. Therefore, expertise is critical regarding performance and interpretation of these examinations in order to prevent misdiagnoses.

The unique advantages of ultrasound include the ability to perform the examination in real-time and the multiplanar capability. Improvements in transducer technology have led to the development of higher frequency transducers, which offer improved spatial resolution and are currently available for endoscopic or intraoperative use. This allows proximity to the region of interest and the formation of extremely high resolution images. When combined with Doppler techniques, information on blood flow direction and velocity can be obtained. This information can be displayed as numeric values with statistical analysis or as color representing velocity of blood flow superimposed on the anatomic gray scale images.

The main limitation of ultrasound relates to the restriction of sound wave penetration through certain tissues, such as bowel gas, bone, and fatty tissues that obscure visualization beneath them. This can lead to many blind spots in the abdomen; fortunately, however, this is not a major issue in imaging of the liver.

Its widespread availability, cost, and versatility make ultrasound a reasonable initial screening tool for most hepatobiliary disorders. Specifically, ultrasound is useful when evaluating the size of the liver and the parenchyma for diffuse infiltrative disorders that can alter the normal echotexture. Ultrasound is also useful for detection of certain mass lesions, dilatation of the bile ducts, and evaluation of vascular anatomy, patency, and hemodynamics.

Scintigraphy: Images of the liver are obtained by injecting intravenous radiopharmaceutical agents that are taken up by the liver parenchyma. These radiopharmaceutical agents are unstable and emit electromagnetic radiation (radioactive decay), which is detected by scintillation cameras. Images are usually acquired in a coronal projection (planar acquisition); however, specialized cameras allow individual slices to be reconstructed in various planes (single photon emission computed tomography [SPECT]).

The advantages of scintigraphic studies include the administration of physiologically targeted radiopharmaceutical agents. Many radiopharmaceutical agents are available for imaging the liver, and the choice of the agent depends on the suspected abnormality. For example, technetium sulfur colloid is taken by the reticuloendothelial system and produces a liver/spleen scan that can evaluate the size and configuration of the liver or detect focal mass lesions, which appear as photopenic or "cold" lesions within the parenchyma. Tagged red blood cells are blood pool agents that can be used to evaluate perfusion to specific lesions in the liver. Agents that are taken up by the hepatocytes and excreted into the biliary system can evaluate the function and excretion of the liver parenchyma and for obstruction of the biliary tract. Radioactive tagged monoclonal antibodies and 18-fluoro-2-deoxy-glucose (FDG) are currently undergoing evaluation to detect metastatic disease to the liver. The application of these targeted radiopharmaceutical agents allow relatively high sensitivity for detection of small concentrations of the radiopharmaceutical agents.

The major limitations to nuclear medicine studies include the lack of spatial resolution, which relates to several factors, including the use of radiopharmaceutical agents as the energy source, diffuse vascular distribution of the agent, sparse and disperse gamma emissions, scatter of the emitted energy, and low-resolution imaging devices. Efforts to improve spatial resolution using SPECT and positron emission tomography (PET) have not significantly changed the current approach to imaging of the liver.

With the recent advancements in CT, MRI, and ultrasound, scintigraphy is playing a decreasing role in the evaluation of the liver. However, there are certain scenarios where scintigraphy is utilized. These include lesion characterization, such as confirmation of hemangioma using tagged red blood cell scan and adjunctive imaging for the confirmation of focal nodular hyperplasia (FNH) using technetium sulfur colloid. Parenchymal perfusion, function, and excretion can be evaluated and may be useful in the evaluation of liver transplant patients. Evaluation for acute cholecystitis and biliary dyskinesia is commonly performed with technetium-labeled iminodiacetic acid scans.

Computed Tomography: CT images are acquired by rotating an ionizing radiation source around the patient and reconstructing images based on attenuation differences. Two basic acquisition techniques are currently available. Dynamic incremental scanning is performed by rotating the radiation source around the patient at a selected collimation (thickness) with acquisition of a single slice. Subsequently, the table is then advanced at a predetermined level (gap), and the next slice is obtained. Recent advances have improved the technology of the gantry or ring that orbits the patient. With the development of "slip-ring" technology, im-

ages can be obtained by continuous rotation of the radiation source and continual table advancement, thus producing a volume acquisition with a "screw-like" appearance. This technique is referred to as spiral or helical CT.

Attenuation differences between pathology and normal parenchyma on CT may be minimal unless there is evidence of bone destruction or formation of gas. Radiopharmaceutical agents have been extensively researched to improve lesion conspicuity. Iodinated contrast agents have been developed that have rapid excretion and negligible protein binding. When these agents are injected intravenously, they penetrate capillaries and have an extracellular distribution. The result is increased parenchymal contrast, allowing improved differentiation from pathology.

The liver is a unique organ in that it has a dual blood supply (portal and hepatic arterial). Various imaging protocols have been evaluated to exploit this pathophysiology and improve lesion conspicuity. Because approximately 80% of the liver perfusion is received from the portal venous system, and 20% is received from the hepatic arterial system, peak liver enhancement is seen during the portal venous phase (usually in the range of 60 to 90 seconds). Because of the rapidity of spiral CT, a complete examination of the liver can be obtained during the peak enhancement period. Also, new software is currently available that allows automatic acquisition to begin when peak enhancement occurs, thus reducing the number of suboptimal scans secondary to altered hemodynamics. Tumors and other pathologic conditions have usually altered perfusion and, therefore, appear as an area of low attenuation within the liver during the portal venous phase. However, because of biologic variations in hemodynamics, some lesions have similar attenuation to normal liver parenchyma. Becuase most tumors are supplied by the arterial system, there has been an emphasis on imaging the liver during the early phase when arterial flow predominates. This technique of scanning during the arterial and portal venous phase is referred to as "dual phase" imaging. By utilizing this technique, certain hypervascular tumors with increased flow may be demonstrated as areas of high attenuation on the early arterial phase. This technique has been shown to be useful in evaluating hepatocellular carcinoma and certain hypervascular metastases.

Because of the wide variation of tumor enhancement and the less than satisfactory result for individual lesion identification utilizing dynamic bolus techniques, other methods to administer contrast at angiography with selected cannulation of the hepatic artery (CT arteriography [CTA]) or by the superior mesenteric artery and splenic artery (CT arterial portography [CTAP]) are commonly performed. These techniques offer improved contrast and sensitivity in individual lesion detection; however, due to variations in the portal venous perfusion, they are plagued by many perfusion defects that can cause false-positive diagnoses of lesions.

The advantages of CT include the rapidity of acquisition and the ability to visualize the entire abdomen and pelvis. The technique is not operator-dependent; therefore, errors in acquisition of pertinent information are reduced. Extremely high-resolution images can be obtained as thin as 1 mm in thickness. With volume acquisition, images can be reconstructed at overlapping intervals and reformatted in various planes. With new software techniques, three-dimensional images can be produced allowing the clinician a new perspective of the spatial locations. Images obtained during the arterial phase of injection can be reconstructed, producing arteriographic images and potentially obviating the performance of invasive arteriography.

The principal limitations of CT are related to the acquisition of data in the transverse plane. When organs have borders with complex shapes, adjacent tissues can be included in the individual pixel. These tissues can lead to partial voluming artifacts, which can obscure tissue boundaries and mimic pathology. With the ability to reconstruct and reformat data with helical CT, this limitation may be reduced. Another major limitation includes the use of iodinated contrast, which is contraindicated in certain medical conditions or in individuals with contrast allergies. Altered portal venous hemodynamics can lead to suboptimal enhancement of the liver, decreasing the sensitivity of the examination.

The main role of CT is in the identification of liver masses, characterization of certain lesions such as hemangiomas, and staging of tumors. CT is also diagnostic in certain diffuse diseases, and CT angiography can be applied to vascular anatomy and patency.

Magnetic Resonance Imaging (MRI):   MRI is done by placing the patient in a uniform magnetic field and then applying and sampling repetitive radiofrequency waves. When the patient is placed inside the magnetic field, the hydrogen nuclei inside the body align themselves with the magnetic field. To create an image, a radiofrequency (RF) pulse must be applied. This RF pulse is generated from a coil and causes the nuclei to be rotated out of alignment. When the RF pulse is terminated, the nuclei attempt to realign with the magnetic field. During this process of "relaxation," a signal is produced in the coil. This signal is then processed and created into an image. Different tissues and pathology have various relaxation times. By varying the intervals of pulse application and time to listen to the signal (T_1 and T_2 weighting), these tissues and disorders can be differentiated.

MRI technology has dramatically improved over the last several years. Improvements in coil design have led to the development of smaller dedicated coils that can be used for specific body parts, improving spatial resolution, signal to noise, and smaller field of views, thus optimizing the examination. Improvements in the magnet have led to stronger, faster magnets with marked reduction in scan time, which now allows examination of the liver in a single breath hold. Improvements in software design have led to improved tissue contrast and lesion conspicuity. Three-dimensional images of the biliary tract (MR cholangiography [MRC]) can now be obtained rapidly without the injection of contrast media. With faster scans and newer software, noninvasive angiography by MRI (MRA) is becoming widely used. The ability to identify normal flow direction and velocity, patency, and anatomy is currently being utilized in the work-up of abdominal disease and gives valuable information regarding portal venous hemodynamics.

As with CT, various pharmaceutical agents have been evaluated to improve identification and characterization of lesions. The most widely used agents are the gadolinium chelates, which are extracellular agents. Other agents, such as iron oxide, which are taken up by the reticuloendothelial system, and hepatoselective agents, such as mangafodipir trisodium (MN-DPDP) and other gadolinium-based agents, are undergoing extensive research. Preliminary data suggest that these agents may be useful in improving the detection and characterization of lesions.

The advantages of MRI include the inherent tissue contrast without the use of intravenous contrast and the ability to change various parameters to optimize the examination for a specific clinical question. Images can be obtained in coronal, sagittal, axial, or oblique planes, and three-dimensional volume acquisitions can be performed that can then be reconstructed in various planes of view. Gadolinium-enhanced MRI can be performed in individuals who cannot undergo contrast-enhanced CT secondary to iodine allergy or impairment in renal function.

Although MRI is very robust, the technique does have several limitations. Current costs restrict its use to that of a problem-solving modality. Motion artifacts, which are most notable in the upper abdomen, are becoming less of a limitation with faster scanning techniques.

The physical geometry of the bore of the magnet restricts scanning larger patients and can lead to claustrophobia in others. Because of this limitation, vendors are now producing magnets with larger bores or an "open" design. This improved access to the patient also allows the performance of MRI-guided biopsies and surgical procedures. Finally, patients with contraindications, such as a pacemaker, aneurysm clip, or certain other ferromagnetic devices, are restricted from undergoing an MRI examination.

The main use of MRI is for lesion identification, characterization, and staging. MRI is the most sensitive noninvasive imaging study for lesion identification and is complimentary to CTAP in the preoperative evaluation of patients for hepatic resection. MRI is useful in the characterization and differentiation of hemangioma from metastases and evaluation of the liver for detection of lesions in the setting of fatty infiltration.

MRI can confirm fatty infiltration of the liver, diffuse infiltrative processes (including hemochromatosis), and use of MR techniques for evaluation of vascular anatomy and patency. The role of MRC is currently being investigated. Several studies have demonstrated its usefulness in detecting common bile duct stones and stenoses, and MRC may be able to replace direct cholangiography in selected cases.

IMAGING OF SELECTED DISEASES

Diffuse Disease of the Liver

Several diseases processes can cause diffuse infiltration of the liver parenchyma and may present with similar clinical signs and symptoms. The diagnosis is usually confirmed by liver biopsy; however, cross-sectional imaging may allow identification and characterization of these diseases and potentially prevent an invasive biopsy. In this section, we discuss the more commonly occurring diffuse diseases of the liver and their radiographic appearance.

Hepatic Steatosis: Hepatic steatosis has multiple etiologies and may present in a variety of radiographic patterns, including diffuse, nodular, geographic, or focal areas of infiltration. On sonography, these areas of fatty infiltration

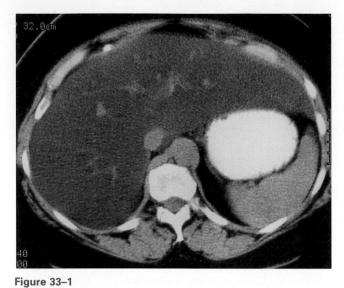

Figure 33–1
Hepatic steatosis. Unenhanced computed tomography scan demonstrates markedly lower attenuation of the liver relative to the spleen, which is consistent with fatty infiltration.

demonstrate increased echogenicity with decreased visualization of the intrahepatic vessels and reduced through transmission. However, this increased echogenicity is nonspecific and may be seen in hepatitis or fibrosis. On unenhanced CT scans, steatosis presents as areas of low attenuation. Criteria have been established to compare attenuation values of the liver in relation to the spleen. On unenhanced CT scans, liver attenuation less than the spleen is diagnostic (Fig. 33–1).

Occasionally, focal fatty infiltration can mimic a space-occupying mass. MRI is useful in the confirmation of hepatic steatosis in this setting. Fat demonstrates high signal intensity on T_1-weighted images; however, because of the relative sparse quantity deposited in the liver in relation to the rest of the body, the majority of hepatic steatosis will not demonstrate high signal and, therefore, is difficult to detect on conventional spin echo sequences. The most sensitive technique to demonstrate fatty infiltration is chemical shift imaging. Fat and water "rotate" at different rates in a magnetic field, and, by changing various parameters, images can be obtained when fat and water are either in phase (together) or out of phase (separated). Areas with small quantities of fat within an individual voxel will show a relative decrease in signal on the opposed phase images compared with the in-phase images. By comparing these two images, fatty infiltration can then be confirmed (Fig. 33–2). Other techniques, such as inversion recovery sequences, have also been utilized. MR spectroscopy (MRS) has been shown to be equivalent to CT in quantification of fat, and these two modalities may be used to serially follow a patient for regression or progression.

Cirrhosis: Cirrhosis is caused by irreversible hepatic fibrosis with destruction of the underlying hepatic architecture. The early radiographic changes of cirrhosis may consist only of fatty infiltration. However, as the disease progresses and the fibrosis increases, certain morphologic

changes appear. The liver becomes small with a nodular contour; there is atrophy of the right lobe and medial segment of the left lobe; and hypertrophy of the caudate and lateral segment of the left lobe occurs. These changes are well demonstrated on ultrasound, CT, and MRI (Fig. 33–3). By using parameters based on the ratio of individual lobe size, ultrasound has been shown to have a sensitivity and specificity of approximately 95% in the diagnosis of cirrhosis and CT, a sensitivity of 84%, and specificity of approximately 100%. However, in certain types of cirrhosis, the morphologic appearance of the liver may not significantly change, thus reducing the sensitivity of these parameters. MRI can provide additional findings with superior tissue contrast and can provide information regarding the severity of disease.

Hemodynamic alterations identified on Doppler ultrasound in cirrhosis include flattening of the normal pulsatility of the hepatic vein wave form, increased pulsatility of the portal vein wave form, and alterations in directional flow.

Regenerating nodules are common in cirrhosis. Because of the inherent improved tissue contrast, these nodules may be more conspicuous on MRI. Extensive work has been done in Japan in an attempt to differentiate the spectrum of benign regenerating nodules, dysplastic or precancerous nodules, and early hepatocellular carcinomas based on signal characteristics. However, there is an overlap, and nodules that are detected should be monitored closely for the development of hepatocellular carcinoma.

Iron Overload: Iron deposition in the liver can be secondary to several etiologies, including genetic hemochromatosis (GH), transfusional iron overload, and segmental areas of deposition in cases of altered intrahepatic portal perfusion. MRI is inherently sensitive to iron deposition, which decreases the T_2 and T_2 relaxation times and produces areas of low signal on T_2-weighted and gradient echo images (Fig. 33–4).

The possibilities of obtaining a noninvasive diagnosis of iron deposition have led to several studies evaluating MRI in the diagnosis of GH with sensitivities and specificities higher than 90%. However, because of variations in magnet strength and parameters in these studies, no standardized data are currently available, and reproducible quantification parameters are lacking. Therefore, the diagnosis is usually made by liver biopsy. MRI does allow the ability to monitor patients undergoing therapy by following serial signal intensities.

Other organs with increased iron will show a similar low signal, which helps to evaluate the overall distribution of iron deposition. This can help to distinguish hemochromatosis from other causes, such as transfusional iron overload.

Masses

Metastases: The liver is one of the most common organs affected by metastatic disease. Thus, the majority of research involving the liver has focused on the identification of metastases. Detection of small metastases has been challenging, because of variations in the biologic nature of various histologic tumor types and even differences between in-

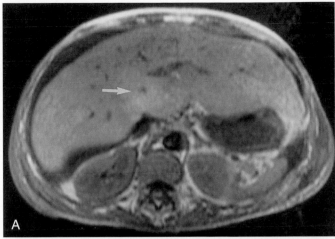

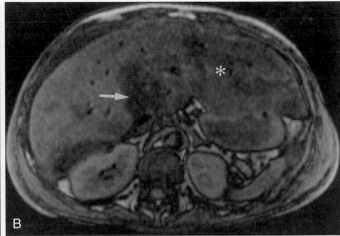

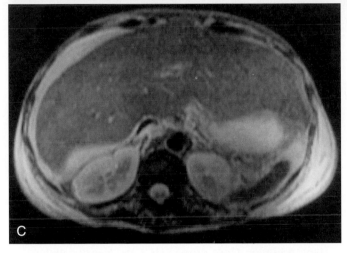

Figure 33–2
Hepatic steatosis. Demonstration of two areas of fatty infiltration of the liver on a magnetic resonance imaging scan. A T_1-weighted image *(A)* shows a focal area of higher intensity near the junction of the right and left lobes *(arrow)*. Chemical shift images *(B)* show a lower signal in density in this region and a more diffuse low signal in the left lobe *(asterisk)*. This relative drop in signal intensity on chemical shift imaging confirms the diagnosis of fat. This T_2-weighted image *(C)* shows no abnormal areas of increased signal in these areas, demonstrating further evidence of the benign etiology.

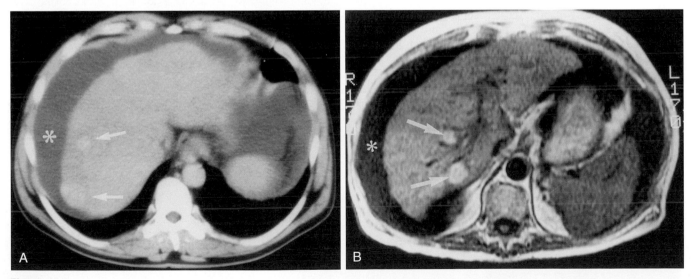

Figure 33–3
Cirrhosis. *A,* Computed tomography scan. *B,* A T_1-weighted image from a magnetic resonance imaging scan shows the classic morphologic appearance in cirrhosis, consisting of a small liver with a nodular contour and associated ascites *(asterisk)*. Note two regenerating nodules in the right lobe *(arrows)*. (From Fidler JL, Stark DD: Non-invasive techniques for the evaluation of liver diseases. In Wu GY [ed]: Liver diseases: Diagnosis and treatment. Totowa, New Jersey: Humana Press, 1998, pp 51–66.)

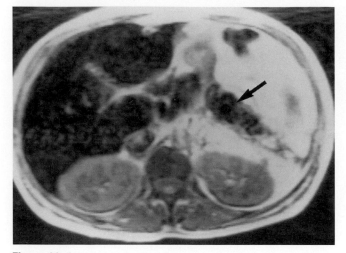

Figure 33–4
Hemochromatosis. T$_1$-weighted magnetic resonance image demonstrates marked low signal intensity in the liver and spleen. For comparison, the liver should be a similar intensity as the adjacent renal cortex.

dividual lesions within a single histologic type. Much of this variation relates to the vascularity of the tumor and the relative blood supply from the arterial or portal venous systems (Fig. 33–5). This physiology has led to the development and evaluation of different protocols, with imaging the liver in different times during hepatic enhancement, which was discussed previously.

The accuracy of the various imaging techniques is widely debated in the literature and institutionally biased. The major problem is the lack of a gold standard in comparing these modalities.

Because of the availability, cost, accepted sensitivity, and ability to screen the entire chest, abdomen, and pelvis, CT should be the initial study performed, even though it is not the most sensitive technique. Because most patients with metastases have multiple lesions, the accuracy of CT in distinguishing patients with metastases is higher than 80%. However, for detection of individual lesions, the sensitivity is much less.

MR is probably more sensitive than CT, however, results vary and are determined by coil selection, pulse sequence protocol, and the types of magnets utilized. At the present time, MRI should be utilized when there are confusing findings on CT, when there is a contraindication to contrasted CT, or in the setting of diffuse fatty infiltration, which can limit detection of a lesion on CT.

CTAP is the most sensitive technique, excluding intraoperative ultrasound. In patients who are considered to be surgical candidates, either CTAP or MRI (or a combination of the two studies) should be performed because of their improved lesion detection. MRI is complimentary to CTAP, thus allowing possible differentiation of perfusion anomalies from metastases with a combined sensitivity of approximately 97%.

The radiographic appearance of metastases varies and is often nonspecific. Certain features may suggest the presence of metastases, including the demonstration of calcification that is seen most often with mucinous carcinoma, such as metastatic colon cancer. Low-density areas may correlate with areas of necrosis. The morphologic pattern of contrast enhancement or signal patterns demonstrating heterogeneity or rings is a useful finding that distinguishes solid neoplasms from cysts or hemangiomas (Figs. 33–6 and 33–7).

Primary Liver Tumors

Hepatocellular Carcinoma (HCC): Hepatocellular carcinoma frequently occurs in association with chronic liver disease and cirrhosis (Fig. 33–8). Because of the presence of a background of chronic hepatitis, steatosis, and cirrhosis, detection is more difficult than with other primary tumors.

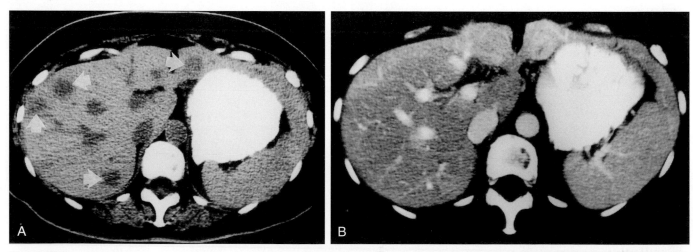

Figure 33–5
Metastases. Pre- *(A)* and post- *(B)* contrasted computed tomography images in a patient with breast cancer metastases *(arrows)*. Note the relative increased enhancement of these lesions, which are more conspicuous on the pre-contrast images. (From Fidler JL, Stark DD: Non-invasive techniques for the evaluation of liver diseases. In Wu GY [ed]: Liver diseases: Diagnosis and treatment. Totowa, New Jersey: Humana Press, 1998, pp 51–66.)

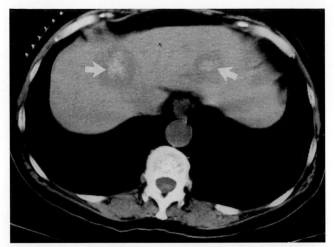

Figure 33–6
Metastases. Fine calcifications, which can be seen with metastases from mucinous adenocarcinomas *(arrows).*

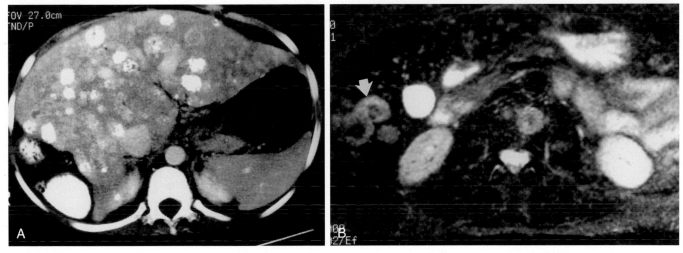

Figure 33–7
Metastases. *A,* A computed tomography demonstration of multiple calcified metastases. *B,* A T$_2$-weighted image from a magnetic resonance imaging scan demonstrates heterogeneous lesions in the right lobe of the liver with a ring of high signal intensity *(arrow).*

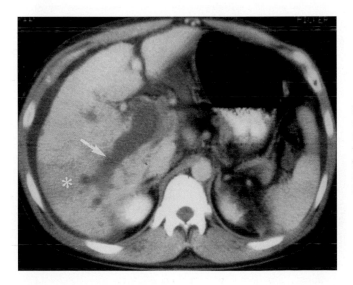

Figure 33–8
Hepatocellular carcinoma. A contrast computed tomography scan demonstrates a cirrhotic-appearing liver with an infiltrative hepatoma in the right lobe *(asterisk)* and associated portal vein thrombus *(arrow).* (From Fidler JL, Stark DD: Non-invasive techniques for the evaluation of liver diseases. In Wu GY [ed]: Liver diseases: Diagnosis and treatment. Totowa, New Jersey: Humana Press, 1998, pp 51–66.)

The evaluation for detection of hepatomas occurs in three major clinical settings: (1) screening patients with chronic liver disease, (2) preoperative evaluation for patients undergoing partial hepatectomy, and (3) detection of clinically significant hepatomas in patients undergoing liver transplant. A wide range of accuracy of the individual imaging techniques has been reported in the literature. For routine screening and follow-up of patients with chronic liver disease, a combination of ultrasound, CT, and α-fetoprotein levels have been shown to have a moderate sensitivity of approximately 84% in detecting small hepatomas; however, a significant number of individual nodules can be missed. Other studies have been shown to have fairly low sensitivity of CT in the identification of hepatomas. The addition of arterial phase images on CT and MR protocols has allowed detection of additional lesions that are not visible on the portal venous phase and conventional MR pulse sequences (Figs. 33–9 and 33–10). MRI may provide further information when differentiating HCC from regenerating nodules.

In patients who are being evaluated for partial hepatectomy, identification of individual lesions is critical; therefore, more sensitive and invasive techniques, such as conventional arteriography, lipoidal CT, and intraoperative ultrasound, are used, and the exact techniques are institutionally determined.

When screening patients who are undergoing liver transplant evaluation, we have found that ultrasound in combination with α-fetoprotein levels is an acceptable imaging algorithm. We reserve CT or MRI for confusing cases or for use with patients who have a high clinical suspicion of HCC, when ultrasound is not diagnostic.

Cavernous Hemangioma: Cavernous hemangiomas are exceedingly common and are present in 15% to 20% of the adult population. These lesions are commonly found on imaging techniques. When these lesions are detected in an in-

dividual with a malignancy, they can mimic metastases. Because of the frequency of this dilemma, several studies have been done to evaluate the sensitivity and specificity of CT, MRI, and tagged red blood cells when differentiating hemangiomas from metastases.

The imaging features reflect the histology and hemodynamics of the tumor, which is characterized by a cavernous collection of blood spaces. Blood flow is very slow and almost undetected, except for peripheral sites of entry. With intravenous contrast administration, hemangiomas demonstrate a classic pattern of peripheral nodular enhancement, centripetal filling, and uniform enhancement with retention of the blood pool product (Fig. 33–11).

Using the aforementioned criteria, CT has a sensitivity and specificity of 80% and almost 100%, respectively. The appearance of hemangioma on MRI is that of a well-defined lesion with a very strong signal (equivalent to fluid) on heavily T_2-weighted images (Fig. 33–12). Enhancement with gadolinium is similar to that seen on a CT scan. Using these criteria, the specificity is similar to tagged red blood cell scans and is higher than 95%. MRI, although more expensive than tagged red blood cell scans in the confirmation of hemangioma, does offer some advantages. MRI can detect smaller lesions that are slightly less than 1 cm, whereas tagged red blood cell scans using SPECT techniques can only detect lesions on the order of 1 to 1.5 cm. MRI offers improved visualization of lesions near larger vessels, which may be subtle on tagged red blood cell scans because of the blood pool activity within the vessel. MRI also allows identification of other unsuspected lesions that would be missed by performing tagged red blood cell scans.

Miscellaneous Tumors: The sensitivity of CT in detecting other primary tumors of the liver is quite high; however, many of the features are nonspecific and do not allow definitive characterization. Certain tumors may have features that can suggest the diagnosis. For example, hepatic adeno-

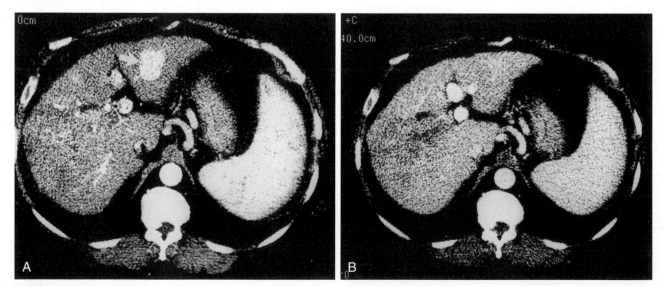

Figure 33–9
Hepatocellular carcinoma. Hepatocellular carcinoma in the left lobe of the liver is more conspicuous on the arterial phase computed tomography images *(A)* than the portal venous phase *(B)*.

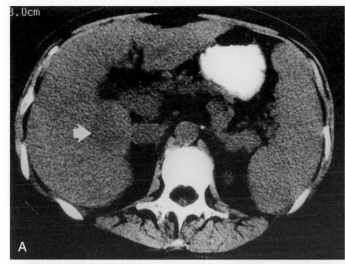

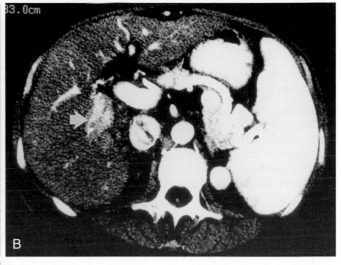

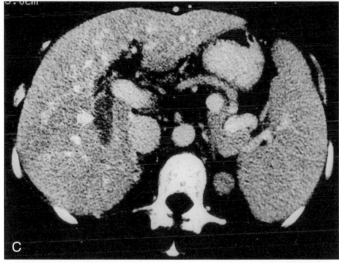

Figure 33–10
Hepatocellular carcinoma. Demonstration of hyper-enhancement on a "dual phase" computed tomography scan. *A,* Precontrast images show a hepatocellular carcinoma to be of relative lower attenuation *(arrow).* Note the marked hyperenhancement on the arterial phase *(B)* and the low attenuation on the conventional portal venous phase *(C).*

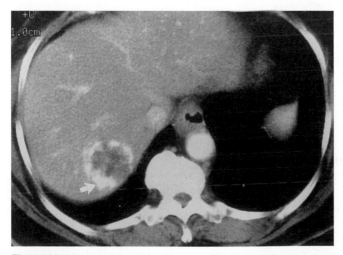

Figure 33–11
Hemangioma. Computed tomography demonstration of the classic early enhancement appearance showing nodular discontinuous peripheral enhancement *(arrow).*

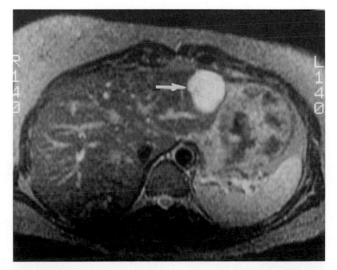

Figure 33–12
Hemangioma. Magnetic resonance imaging appearance of a hemangioma consists of a well-defined high signal intensity mass *(arrow).*

mas may contain areas of fat, necrosis, and hemorrhage. The presence of a central scar suggests the diagnosis of focal nodular hyperplasia (Fig. 33–13); however, can be seen with in fibrolamellar carcinoma and adenomas.

Vascular Abnormalities

Ultrasound can provide exquisitely sensitive information regarding the hemodynamics of the liver, such as vascular patency, velocity, and directional flow, and should be the initial study of choice when evaluating suspected vascular abnormalities. Ultrasound has a sensitivity of approximately 87% in the diagnosis of Budd-Chiari syndrome. Characteristic findings include the absence of the normal hepatic veins with areas of stenoses, webs, or thrombus. Abnormal Doppler wave forms may consist of absent or reversed flow in hepatic vein tributaries or the inferior vena cava (IVC), turbulent flow, or continuous flow. Ultrasound is 100% sensitive and 93% specific in the diagnosis of main portal vein thrombus and has been shown to be 97% sensitive in the diagnosis of significant arterial vascular disease in post-liver transplant patients.

MRI, with the ability to image flowing blood and determine the direction and velocity of flow, is generally complimentary to ultrasound in the evaluation of hepatic vessels. However, MR should be used in select cases in which ultrasound is nondiagnostic or confusing. Because of its expanded field of view, MRI shows associated collateral vessels throughout the abdomen.

With the rapid, high-resolution images obtained with helical CT, intravenous enhanced spiral CT scans can exquisitely demonstrate vascular anatomy and patency, especially of the arterial system (Figs. 33–14 and 33–15). Delayed images during portal venous phase can evaluate the venous structures, however, occasionally flow defects within these vessels can mimic thrombus.

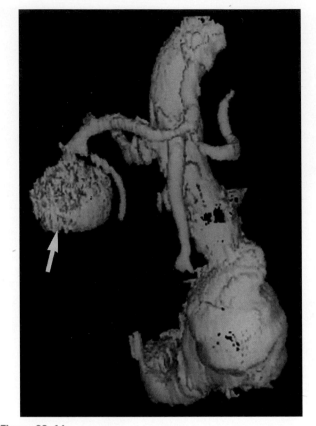

Figure 33–14
Computed tomography angiography. An anterior projection of a 3-D computed tomography angiogram demonstrates a large hepatic artery pseudoaneurysm *(arrow)*. Also note the large infrarenal abdominal aortic aneurysm.

Biliary Abnormalities

Gallstones: The primary modality that should be used to confirm the presence of cholelithiasis is ultrasound. Sonography has a sensitivity of greater than 95% in the diagnosis of cholelithiasis and can detect approximately 70% to 80% of choledocholithiasis. Gallstones within the distal part of the common bile duct are slightly more difficult to detect secondary to overlying bowel gas. On ultrasound, gallstones appear as echogenic structures with posterior acoustic shadowing. Because of the numerous possible pitfalls, meticulous technique and knowledge of these drawbacks are a necessity. To allow distention of the gallbladder and improve detection of gallstones, patients should be asked to fast for at least 4 to 6 hours before the examination.

When using a high-resolution technique, CT can detect a significant number of calcified or dense gallstones because of the contrast between the calcium and bile (Fig. 33–16). However, many gallstones demonstrate similar attenuation as bile, thus decreasing their rate of detection. Intravenous contrast agents that are excreted in the bile have been found to increase contrast between the stone and surrounding bile and improve detection; however, because of numerous side effects, these agents are not widely used in clinical practice.

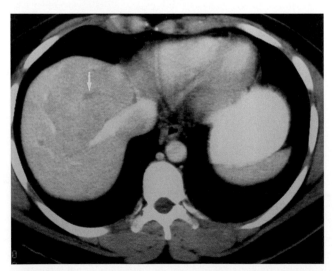

Figure 33–13
Focal nodular hyperplasia. An enhanced computed tomography scan demonstrates an isodense mass in the dome of the liver with a central star, which is characteristic of focal nodular hyperplasia.

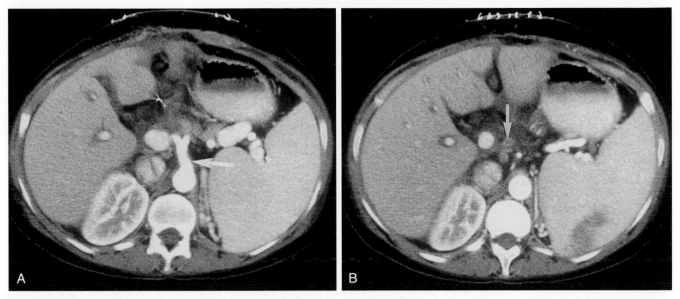

Figure 33–15
Hepatic artery thrombosis. The hepatic artery was unable to be identified by ultrasound in this patient who is status post liver transplant. Axial images from a computed tomography angiogram show the celiac axis *(A, arrow)* and a thrombus *(B)* within the proximal hepatic artery *(arrow).*

MRC has been shown to be useful in the diagnosis of gallstones with a sensitivity for detecting choledocholithiasis of 70% to 100% (Fig. 33–17).

Acute Cholecystitis: In patients with suspected acute cholecystis, sonography or hepatobiliary scintigraphy should be the initial imaging study performed. An advantage of ultrasound over scintigraphy is that ultrasound al-

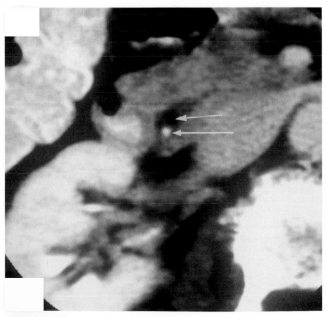

Figure 33–16
Choledocholithiasis. A computed tomography demonstration of choledocholithiasis with a calcified gallstone *(long arrow)* within the dependent portion of the distal common bile duct *(short arrow).*

lows a generalized screening of the right upper quadrant, which may detect other abnormalities that mimic acute cholecystitis. Findings of acute cholecystitis on ultrasound include the presence of gallstones with focal tenderness over the gallbladder (sonographic Murphy's sign), gallbladder distention, gallbladder wall thickening, air within the wall or lumen of the gallbladder, internal membranes, and pericholecystic fluid (Fig. 33–18). The most reliable sign is the presence of gallstones and the positive sonographic Murphy's sign with a positive predictive value of 92% and a negative predictive value of 95%.

In acute cholecystitis, hepatobiliary scintigraphy (technetium-labeled iminodiacetic acid scans) demonstrates lack of visualization of the gallbladder secondary to obstruction of the cystic duct. Hepatobiliary scintigraphy has a high sensitivity and specificity of more than 95%.

Occasionally, patients may have nonspecific clinical findings and are referred for CT examination. CT findings have been described and are similar to those found on ultrasound, including gallbladder wall thickening, pericholecystic stranding, gallbladder distention, pericholecystic fluid, subserosal edema, high attenuation bile, and sloughed membranes (Fig. 33–19). In one study, CT allowed detection of approximately 50% of cases of acute cholecystitis; however, the absence of findings does not exclude the diagnosis, and further imaging with ultrasound or scintigraphy should be performed.

Biliary Obstruction: Biliary obstruction can be secondary to many etiologies, including extrinsic or intrinsic masses, inflammation, and strictures. The evaluation of individuals with suspected biliary obstruction should begin with right upper quadrant sonography. Ultrasound allows detection of bile duct dilatation and can usually determine the site of obstruction in more than 90% of the cases and the cause in more than 70% of the cases. CT may provide use-

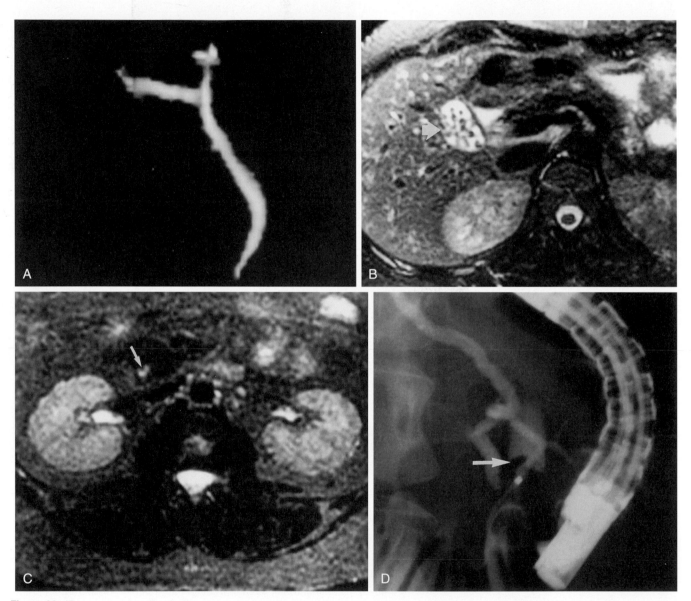

Figure 33–17

A, **Magnetic resonance cholangiography.** A normal-appearing magnetic resonance imaging (MRI) cholangiogram. *B,* **Cholelithiasis.** Note the appearance of gallstones on the MRI. The typical gallstone is a low signal intensity structure seen within the high-intensity bile, such as in the gallbladder *(arrow). C,* **Choledocholithiasis.** A tiny, 2- to 3-mm, low-signal intensity structure is seen on the axial images from a magnetic resonance cholangiogram in the distal common bile duct *(arrow).* This tiny gallstone was confirmed on subsequent endoscopic retrograde cholangiopancreatography *(D).*

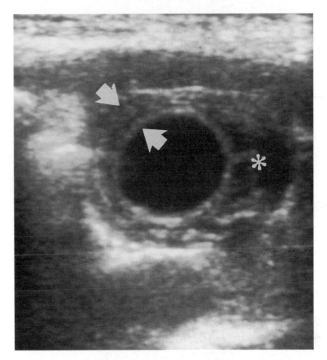

Figure 33–18
Acute cholecystitis. An ultrasound demonstrates a greatly thickened gallbladder wall *(arrows)* with intramural fluid *(asterisk)*. These findings combined with a positive "sonographic Murphy sign" are diagnostic of acute cholecystitis.

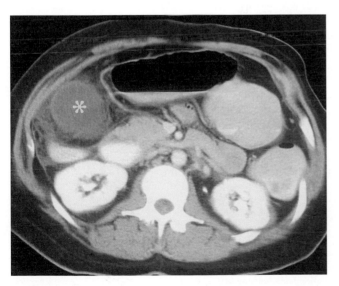

Figure 33–19
Acute cholecystitis. A computed tomography demonstration of acute cholecystitis shows the gallbladder *(asterisk)* to have an ill-defined wall. Note the surrounding high attenuation inflammatory changes in the pericholecystic fat. For comparison, the normal fat should be very dark as in the subcutaneous tissues.

ful information when the ultrasound is inconclusive or incompletely evaluates or stages the abnormality detected. MRC can provide a noninvasive technique to obtain cholangiographic images and the detection of bile duct strictures.

SUGGESTED READINGS

Baker ME, Silverman PM: Nodular focal fatty infiltration of the liver: CT appearance. AJR Am J Roentgenol 145:79–80, 1985.

Baron RL, Oliver JH III, Dodd GD III, et al: Hepatocellular carcinoma: Evaluation with biphasic, contrast-enhanced, helical CT. Radiology 199:505–511, 1996.

Bluemke DA, Soyer P, Fishman EK: Non-tumorous low-attenuation defects in the liver on helical CT during arterial portography: Frequency, location and appearance. AJR Am J Roentgenol 164:1141–1145, 1995.

Boland L, Gainani S, Libass S, et al: Diagnosis of Budd-Chiari syndrome by pulsed Doppler ultrasound. Gastroenterology 100:1324–1331, 1991.

Choi BI, Takayasu K, Han MC: Small hepatocellular carcinomas and associated nodular lesions of the liver: Pathology, pathogenesis and imaging findings. AJR Am J Roentgenol 160:1177–1187, 1993.

Dodd GD, Memel DS, Zajko AB, et al: Hepatic artery stenosis and thrombosis in transplant recipients: Doppler diagnosis with resistive index and systolic acceleration time. Radiology 192:657–661, 1994.

Fidler JF, Paulson EK, Layfield L: CT Evaluation of acute cholecystitis: Findings and usefulness in diagnosis. AJR Am J Roentgenol 166:1085–1088, 1996.

Gandon Y, Guyader D, Heautot JF, et al: Hemochromatosis: Diagnosis and quantification of liver iron with gradient-echo MR imaging. Radiology 193:533–538, 1994.

Gore RM: Diffuse liver disease. In Gore RM, Levine MS, Loufer I (eds): Textbook of Gastrointestinal Radiology. Philadelphia: WB Saunders, 1994, pp 1968–2017.

Guibaud L, Bret PM, Reinhold C, et al: Bile duct obstruction and choledocholithiasis: Diagnosis with MR cholangiography. Radiology 197:109–115, 1995.

Hahn PF, Stark DD, Saini S, et al: The differential diagnosis of ringed hepatic lesions in MR imaging. AJR Am J Roentgenol 154:287–290, 1990.

Jain KA, McGahan JP: Spectrum of CT and sonographic appearance of fatty infiltration of the liver. Clin Imaging 17:162–168, 1993.

Kane AG, Redwine MD, Cossi AF: Characterization of focal fatty change in the liver with a fat-enhanced inversion-recovery sequence. J Magn Reson Imaging 3:581–586, 1993.

Kobayashi K, Sugimoto T, Makino H, et al: Screening methods for early detection of hepatocellular carcinoma. Hepatology 5:1100–1105, 1985.

Lee JL, Saini S, Compton CC, Malt RA: MR demonstration of edema adjacent to a liver metastasis: Pathologic correlation. AJR Am J Roentgenol 157:499–501, 1991.

Longo R, Pollesello P, Ricci C, et al: Proton MR spectroscopy in quantitative in vivo determination of fat content in human liver steatosis. J Magn Reson Imaging 5:281–285, 1995.

Longo R, Ricci C, Masutti F, et al: Fatty infiltration of the liver: Quantification by localized magnetic resonance spectroscopy and comparison with computed tomography. Invest Radiol 28:297–302, 1993.

Matsui O, Kadoya M, Kameyama T, et al: Adenomatous hyperplastic nodules in the cirrhotic liver: Differentiation from hepatocellular carcinoma with MR imaging. Radiology 173:123–126, 1989.

McFarland EG, Mayo-Smith WW, Saini S, et al: Hepatic hemangiomas and malignant tumors: Improved differentiation with heavily T_2-weighted conventional spin-echo MR imaging. Radiology 193:43–47, 1994.

Miller WJ, Barn RL, Dodd GD III, Federle WP: Malignancies in patients with cirrhosis: CT sensitivity and specificity in 200 consecutive transplant patients. Radiology 193:645–650, 1994.

Murakami T, Kuroda C, Marukawa T, et al: Regenerating nodules in hepatic cirrhosis: MR findings with pathologic correlation. AJR Am J Roentgenol 155:1227–1231, 1990.

Muramatsu Y, Nawano S, Takayasu K, et al: Early hepatocellular carcinoma: MR imaging. Radiology 181:209–213, 1991.

Nelson BC, Chezmar JL, Bernardino ME: Comparison of angiography, CTA-portography, delayed CT and MRI for the pre-operative evaluation of hepatic tumors. Radiology 172:27–34, 1989.

Ohashi I, Hanafusa K, Yoshida T: Small hepatocellular carcinomas: Two-phase dynamic incremental CT in detection and evaluation. Radiology 189:851–855, 1993.

Oi H, Murakami T, Kim T, et al: Dynamic MR imaging and early phase helical CT for detecting small intrahepatic metastases of hepatocellular carcinoma. AJR Am J Roentgenol 166:369–374, 1996.

Okazaki N, Yoshida T, Yoshino M, Matue H: Screening of patients with chronic liver disease for hepatocellular carcinoma by ultrasonography. Clin Oncol 10:241–246, 1984.

Paulson EK, Baker ME, Hilleren DJ, et al: CT arterial portography: Causes of technical failure and variable liver enhancement. AJR Am J Roentgenol 159:745–749, 1992.

Quinn SF, Benjamin GG: Hepatic cavernous hemangiomas: Simple diagnostic sign with dynamic bolus CT. Radiology 182:545–548, 1992.

Ralls PW, Colletti PM, Lapin SA, et al: Real-time sonography in suspected acute cholecystitis: Prospective evaluation of primary and secondary signs. Radiology 1455:767–771, 1985.

Rizzi PM, Kane, PA, Ryder SD, et al: Accuracy of radiology in detection of hepatocellular carcinoma before liver transplant. Gastroenterology 107:1425–1429, 1994.

Semelka RC, Brown ED, Ascher SM, et al: Hepatic hemangiomas: A multi-institutional study of appearance on T_2-weighted and serial gadolinium-enhanced gradient-echo MR images. Radiology 192:401–406, 1994.

Siegelman ES, Mitchell DG, Outwater E, et al: Idiopathic hemochromatosis: MR imaging findings in cirrhotic and precirrhotic patients. Radiology 188:637–641, 1993.

Siegelman ES, Mitchell DG, Rubin R, et al: Parenchymal versus reticuloendothelial iron overload in the liver: Distinction with MR imaging. Radiology 179:361–366, 1991.

Small, WC, Mehard WB, Langmo LS, et al. Preoperative determination of the resectability of hepatic tumors: Efficacy of CT during arterial portography. AJR Am J Roentgenol 161:319–322, 1993.

Soto JA, Barish MA, Yucel EK, et al. Magnetic resonance cholangiography: Comparison with endoscopic retrograde cholangiopancreatography. Gastroenterology 110:589–597, 1996.

Soyer P, Lacheheb D, Levesque M: False-positive CT portography: Correlation with pathologic findings. AJR Am J Roentgenol 160:285–289, 1993.

Soyer P, Levesque M, Elias D, et al: Preoperative assessment of resectability of hepatic metastases from colonic carcinoma: CT portography versus sonography and dynamic CT. AJR Am J Roentgenol 159:741–744, 1992.

Takayasu K, Moriyama N, Muramatsu Y, et al: The diagnosis of small hepatocellular carcinomas: Efficacy of various imaging procedures in 100 patients. AJR Am J Roentgenol 155:49–54, 1990.

Takayasu K, Furukawa H, Wakao F, et al: CT diagnosis of early hepatocellular carcinoma: Sensitivity, findings, and CT pathologic correlation. AJR Am J Roentgenol 164:885–890, 1995.

Whitney WS, Herfkens RJ, Jeffrey RB, et al: Dynamic breath-hold multiplanar spoiled gradient-recalled MR imaging with gadolinium enhancement for differentiating hepatic hemangiomas from malignancies at 1.5 T. Radiology 189:863–870, 1993.

Winter TC III, Takayasu K, Muramatsu Y, et al: Early advanced hepatocellular carcinoma: Evaluation of CT and MR appearance with pathologic correlation. Radiology 192:379–387, 1994.

Yamashita Y, Mitsuzaki K, Yi T, et al: Small hepatocellular carcinoma in patients with chronic liver damage: Prospective comparison of detection with dynamic MR imaging and helical CT of the whole liver. Radiology 200:79–84, 1996.

34

Management of Bleeding Varices

Alex S. Befeler

Zahid A. Saeed

The genesis, anatomy, pathophysiology, and management of varices that have never bled, i.e., primary prophylaxis, are covered in Chapter 17. The present chapter covers the management of varices once they have bled. Of all the causes of gastrointestinal hemorrhage, variceal bleeding is associated with the highest mortality rate. There is 20% to 30% mortality associated with each episode of variceal bleeding, and approximately 70% of patients die within 1 year of the index bleeding episode without definitive intervention. Patients who survive the immediate threat of exsanguination continue to have a worse prognosis than do those who have not bled. They are at high risk for both early (in hospital) and late (after discharge from hospital) recurrent bleeding. The risk factors for early recurrent bleeding are age greater than 60 years, renal failure, hemoglobin less than 8 g/dL on admission, and overaggressive volume resuscitation. The risk factors for late recurrent bleeding are degree of hepatic failure, continued alcohol abuse, large variceal size, renal failure, and hepatocellular carcinoma. Despite potentially dangerous side effects of the available therapies and the fact that the therapies may not consistently prolong survival, the natural history of varices after they have bled dictates that measures be taken to either eliminate the varices or to lower the portal pressure.

DIAGNOSIS OF VARICEAL BLEEDING

When presented with a patient with upper gastrointestinal bleeding who is known to have varices or has evidence of cirrhosis, the clinician must assume that the source of bleeding is variceal and institute immediate empirical management. To allow further therapy on a rational basis, the diagnosis of variceal hemorrhage must be confirmed or excluded as soon as feasible by endoscopy, because up to 30% of upper gastro-

intestinal bleeding in cirrhotic patients is nonvariceal. The diagnosis of variceal bleeding is certain if one visualizes a varix with active bleeding (Fig. 34–1), a fibrin plug (Fig. 34–2) (known as the "white nipple sign"), or a fresh clot adherent to a varix. Bleeding stops spontaneously in more than 50% of patients; therefore, most endoscopies do not show active bleeding or a fibrin plug. Thus, in many patients, the diagnosis of variceal hemorrhage is presumptive; that is, based on the presence of varices with red signs (Fig. 34–3) and the absence of other plausible sources of bleeding.

GOALS OF THERAPY

The immediate goal is to control active bleeding. Because recurrent bleeding is frequent, the next goal of therapy is to prevent rebleeding. Some of the deaths associated with variceal bleeding may be attributed to the severity of liver disease that underlies the portal hypertension, and other deaths are a direct consequence of bleeding or its complications. Although deaths caused by liver disease are often inevitable, unless the patient undergoes a successful liver transplantation, deaths caused by bleeding can potentially be prevented. Thus, when evaluating the benefits of available therapies, factors to consider in the decision-making process include the ability of a particular therapy to control active bleeding, to prevent rebleeding, and to improve survival, all at the lowest cost in terms of morbidity inherent to the complications of each therapy.

AVAILABLE THERAPIES

The following section gives the possible options for the treatment of variceal bleeding. A discussion of the comparative efficacy of the various options appears in the next sec-

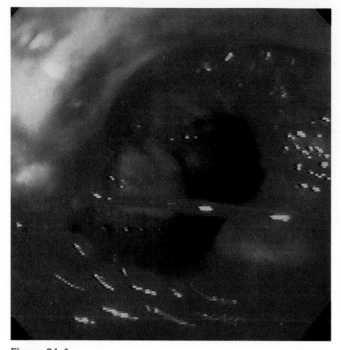

Figure 34–1
Endoscopic photograph of an actively bleeding esophageal varix. (Courtesy of Dr. Michael Blackstone.)

tion. The final section presents the authors' recommendations for a treatment algorithm.

Supportive Measures

The immediate therapy in a patient experiencing an upper gastrointestinal bleeding episode caused by varices is directed toward the correction of the patient's hypovolemia and of any associated coagulopathy. This is best accomplished in an intensive care unit, where moment-to-moment hemodynamic changes can be rapidly assessed and treated. The infusion of intravenous saline, packed red blood cells, platelets, and fresh frozen plasma is best achieved by the placement of two or more large-bore peripheral intravenous lines and frequently a central venous line (to monitor volume replacement). The resuscitation should be assessed by maintenance of a stable blood pressure, reduction in heart rate, good urine output, good peripheral perfusion, adequate central venous pressure if available, and a hematocrit between 25% and 30%. Care must be taken to avoid over-resuscitation, because it may increase portal pressure and precipitate recurrent variceal bleeding. Endotracheal intubation may be necessary to protect the airway in those patients at risk for aspiration because of altered mental status or repeated hematemesis. The altered mental status is often a result of excess nitrogen load delivered to the gut in the form of blood; therefore, the stomach should be aspirated of all blood via a nasogastric tube, and lactulose should be given to purge the bowel.

Tamponade

Balloon tamponade tubes were probably the first effective devices used to treat active variceal hemorrhage, but they produce many complications. They are currently used as a last resort when other therapy fails or as a temporizing measure to permit time for resuscitation before instituting definitive therapy. The Sengstaken-Blakemore tube and its latest modification, the Minnesota tube, are the tamponade devices that are most often used today (Fig. 34–4). They each have both gastric and esophageal balloons which, when inflated in the proper manner, provide compression to gastroesophageal varices between the balloon and the diaphragm. The Minnesota tube has the additional advantage of an esophageal suction port, which theoretically reduces the risk of aspiration. Compression of the varices leads to arrest of the bleeding. The tamponade tubes are ineffective for isolated gastric varices, because they are unable to apply adequate pressure to the proper location.

Before placing the tube into the patient, the balloons must be tested by inflating them with air and measuring their pressures at various volumes. The tube is inserted through the mouth in a usually previously intubated patient and into the stomach based on markings on the tube. Air is gradually insufflated, and pressures are monitored until the gastric balloon is filled. The tube is then withdrawn until resistance is produced. The end of the tube is then connected to a traction device or to a helmet on the patient to maintain the resistance. The gastric and esophageal ports are aspirated to assess if the bleeding has stopped. If there is continued bleeding, the esophageal balloon may be inflated to the lowest pressure which arrests the bleeding and is less than 45 mm Hg. The position should be checked with a radiograph after placement and after any adjustments. Pressures and tube markings should be checked periodically. The esophageal balloon, if used, should be deflated periodically to reduce the risk of esophageal necrosis. Given the high rate of serious complications, the tubes should only be placed by practitioners who are experienced in their use.

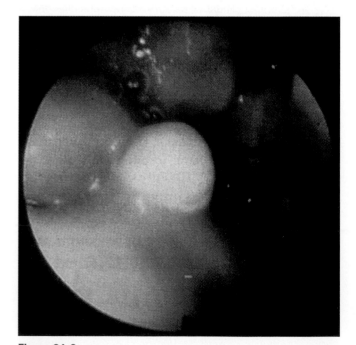

Figure 34–2
Endoscopic photograph of a fibrin plug known as the "white nipple sign."

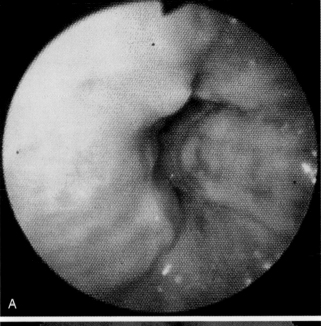

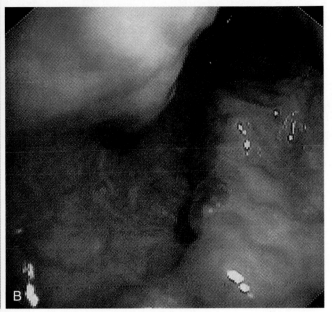

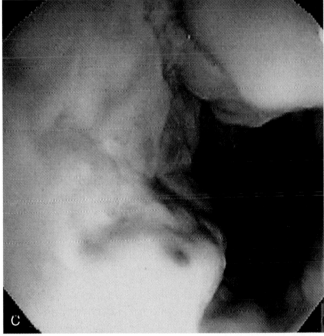

Figure 34–3
A, Endoscopic photograph of red wheal marks that appear as longitudinal red streaks on varices. *B,* Endoscopic photograph of a hematocystic spot that appears as a raised red spot or "blood blister" on varices and more red wheal marks. *C,* Endoscopic photograph of cherry red spots that appear as flat red spots on varices.

The tube should only be left in until resuscitation and definitive therapies are instituted and no longer than 24 hours. Complications occur in up to 35% of patients with approximately a 20% complication-related mortality. Complications include aspiration pneumonia, pressure necrosis of the stomach and esophagus, airway occlusion (due to migration), patient agitation, and chest pain.

Pharmacologic Therapies

In an actively bleeding patient with documented portal hypertension, pharmacologic therapy directed at decreasing portal pressure and thus the rate of bleeding from a variceal source is frequently used as volume resuscitation is in progress. This is done usually on the patient's admission to the hospital or in the emergency room because of its ease of availability compared with other therapies. Another advantage of pharmacologic therapy is that it is effective in nonvariceal bleeding and, therefore, may be comfortably instituted before a definitive endoscopic diagnosis. In addition, the initiation of pharmacologic therapy may increase the effectiveness of subsequent endoscopic therapy.

Chapter 17 by Sanyal describes the pathophysiology of variceal bleeding. Wall tension determines the risk of variceal rupture. Pharmacologic therapy decreases variceal blood flow through splanchnic arteriolar constriction. The decreased variceal blood flow produces lower portal pressure, measured clinically by hepatic venous pressure gradi-

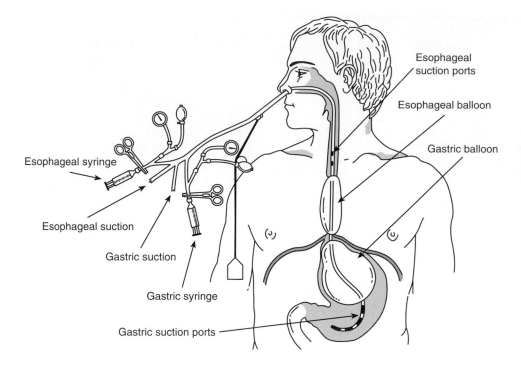

Figure 34–4
A Minnesota tube positioned correctly in a patient. It has esophageal and gastric balloons and suction ports. (Reproduced and modified from Levison SL: Insertion of Minnesota tube. In Drossman DA [ed]: Manual of Gastroenterologic Procedures, 2nd ed. New York: Raven Press, 1987, pp 21–29.)

ent (HVPG), and thus lowers wall tension. Several studies show that lowering HVPG to less than 12 mm Hg leads to a decreased risk of variceal hemorrhage. The most commonly used vasoconstrictor agents are vasopressin and somatostatin and their analogues. Nonselective β-blockers and nitrates also decrease portal pressure.

Vasopressin and Terlipressin

Vasopressin produces both splanchnic and systemic vasoconstriction. It is the effect on the splanchnic circulation that results in decreased portal blood flow and portal pressure, thus lowering variceal wall tension. The effect of vasopressin in reducing portal blood flow is dose dependent.

The starting dose for vasopressin is 0.2 to 0.4 units/min intravenously (IV). The dose is titrated up by 0.1 to 0.2 units/min every 30 to 60 minutes until bleeding stops or the maximum dose of 1 unit/min is reached.

There are numerous severe side effects of vasopressin. Cardiovascular effects include increased vascular resistance, decreased coronary blood flow, increased cardiac afterload, bradycardia, impaired cardiac contractility, and reduced cardiac output, which can all lead to severe arrhythmias and myocardial infarction. Severe noncardiac side effects associated with vasopressin include respiratory arrest, cerebral hemorrhage, stroke, bowel and limb ischemia, activation of fibrinolysis, and local tissue necrosis. The incidence of these complications, although dose dependent, occurs in approximately 25% of patients and has resulted in the decreased use of vasopressin as a single agent in the treatment of this disorder. Combination therapy with nitroglycerin decreases the side effects associated with vasopressin therapy alone. Several studies demonstrated that the simultaneous administration of vasopressin and nitroglycerin significantly decreases the cardiotoxic effects associated with vasopressin and may improve the control of var-

iceal hemorrhage possibly by a portal hypotensive effect. Nitroglycerin is effective whether administered transdermally, sublingually, or IV. The IV route is preferred because it allows accurate titration of the effective dose as volume resuscitation occurs. The dose of nitroglycerin is 10 to 400 µg/min IV titrated to maintain a systolic blood pressure greater than 90 to 100 mm Hg.

Terlipressin is a synthetic analogue of vasopressin and has the same mechanism of action. After absorption, it is slowly activated to the vasoactive form, which may decrease its cardiovascular side effects, although this is controversial. At present, terlipressin is unavailable in the United States.

Somatostatin and Octreotide

Somatostatin, a hypothalamic peptide, decreases portal pressure by causing selective splanchnic vasoconstriction. The mechanism is uncertain but probably involves direct vasoconstrictive effects and inhibition of glucagon, a vasodilatory peptide. Octreotide is a synthetic analogue of somatostatin with a prolonged biologic half-life that otherwise appears to behave in a similar manner. When given as an IV bolus, these medications produce rapid and more dramatic decreases in portal pressure over continuous infusion. Somatostatin and octreotide have about a 3% incidence of side effects, which include hyperglycemia, hypoglycemia (rarely), pancreatic exocrine insufficiency (rarely), and gastrointestinal upset.

The effective dose of somatostatin in controlling variceal hemorrhage is between 250 and 300 µg/hr. A 250- to 500-µg bolus of somatostatin decreases transmural variceal pressure within 30 to 90 seconds and is recommended when therapy is initiated or when rebleeding occurs. The more potent and longer acting analogue, octreotide acetate, controls variceal hemorrhage when infused at 25 to 75 µg/hr.

Before starting a continuous infusion of octreotide, a bolus of 50 μg is usually given to immediately decrease variceal pressure. If rebleeding occurs, a repeat bolus and increased dose of continuous octreotide should be tried.

Nonselective β-Blockers (Propranolol and Nadolol)

Nonselective β-blockers prevent variceal bleeding by decreasing portal pressure. The portal pressure is dependent on the portal inflow, which is determined by the mesenteric arteriolar resistance. Nonselective β-blockers block the β-adrenergic–mediated vasodilatation of the mesenteric arterioles and permit unopposed α-adrenergic vasoconstriction. This results in a decrease in portal flow, leading to a decrease in portal pressure below the threshold of 12 mm Hg, which is needed for variceal bleeding. Decreasing cardiac output may also play a role. Most trials use either propranolol or nadolol. Dosages are gradually titrated to achieve a 25% decrease in baseline heart rate or a heart rate between 50 and 60 beats/min while maintaining a blood pressure greater than 90/60 mm Hg. Using these goals, about half of the patients will fail to achieve sufficient lowering of their HVPG to prevent bleeding. Significant side effects include hypotension, exacerbation of bronchospasm, congestive heart failure, deterioration of mental function, and impotence. Approximately 20% of patients are unable to tolerate the medication. β-Blockers are usually not given during active variceal bleeding because of their hypotensive and bradycardic effects.

Nitrates

Nitrates lower portal pressure by a number of potential mechanisms. The primary effect is venodilatation that results in decreased cardiac output (through decreased venous return) and decreased postsinusoidal resistance, both of which lower portal pressure. At higher doses, arterial dilatation leads to hypotension and reflex splanchnic vasoconstriction. Pulmonary capillary bed nitrate-dependent baroreceptors also cause splanchnic vasoconstriction. Nitrates are only used in combination with either vasopressin or β-blockers. For use with β-blockers, generally the β-blockers are given until their goal doses are reached. Then isosorbide mononitrate is titrated up from 10 mg PO bid to 40 mg PO bid as tolerated by side effects and blood pressure. Typical side effects include lowered blood pressure, headaches, and possible tachyphylaxis.

Others

Other medications such as metoclopramide and domperidone are not well established for the treatment of active variceal hemorrhage and, therefore, cannot be recommended.

Endoscopic Therapies

Sclerotherapy

Endoscopic sclerotherapy was first reported in 1939. During sclerotherapy, a sclerosing solution is injected via a needle passed through the working channel of an endoscope either into a varix (intravariceal) or around a varix (paravariceal)

(Fig. 34–5). Typically, 1 to 2 mL of sclerosant is injected at each site beginning in the actively bleeding varix and then continuing into all varices from just proximal to the gastroesophageal junction to about 5 cm above using a total of 10 to 20 mL of sclerosant. Varices are eventually obliterated after multiple sclerotherapy sessions are performed at 1- to 2-week intervals. Initial hemostasis is thought to be a result of local edema mechanically compressing the bleeding varix. The sclerosing solution later induces a necroinflammatory response that leads to thrombosis of the vessel, fibrosis, and eventually obliteration of the varix. There are hypothetical advantages both for making injections intravariceally and paravariceally. By adding renograffin and methylene blue to the sclerosing solution, investigators demonstrated that despite the endoscopist's intent to perform intravariceal sclerotherapy, most often there was an inadvertent combination of intravariceal and paravariceal injections. Commonly used sclerosing agents include 5% sodium morrhuate, 5% ethanolamine oleate, 1% to 3% sodium tetradecyl sulfate, 1% polidocanol (not available in the United States), and different concentrations of ethanol. The results of studies directly comparing the efficacies and complication rates of commonly used sclerosing agents showed that no single agent is consistently better than another.

Sclerotherapy is associated with a high incidence of local and systemic complications. Common early minor complications include chest pain, fever, transient dysphagia, odynophagia, and pleural effusions. Esophageal ulcers are seen at previously sclerosed sites in 90% of the patients on the day after treatment, 70% at 1 week, 30% at 2 weeks, and 10% at 3 weeks. About 10% of these ulcers ultimately bleed. Prophylactic proton pump inhibitors probably limit this complication. Late esophageal strictures occur in approximately 10% of patients and can be managed with endoscopic dilatation. Rare but significant side effects include

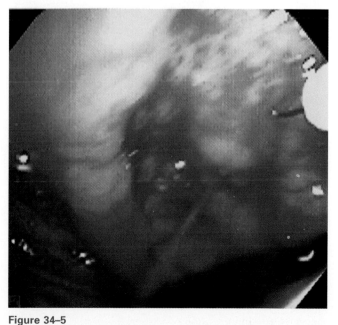

Figure 34–5
Endoscopic photograph of a bleeding esophageal varix undergoing intravariceal sclerotherapy.

aspiration pneumonia (up to 5% in unintubated emergency cases), adult respiratory distress syndrome, early and late esophageal perforation, mediastinitis, bacterial peritonitis, spinal cord paralysis, and pericarditis. There are other rare complications that are essentially "too numerous to count." About 10% of patients develop serious complications that are mainly pulmonary in nature, and 1% to 2% die as a direct result.

Rubber Band Ligation

Endoscopic rubber band ligation of varices was first proposed in the 1980s as an extension of experience with ligation of hemorrhoids. Ligation devices consist of a hollow cylindrical chamber that attaches to and extends the tip of an endoscope. The endoscopist places the chamber into contact with the tissue, then applies suction drawing tissue into the hollow chamber. A rubber band prestretched over the outer wall of the chamber is released by means of a triggering wire that passes through the working channel of the scope, thus ligating the portion of tissue within the chamber (Fig. 34–6). The first available ligation devices for varices were "single shot," requiring withdrawal of the endoscope for reloading after each ligation, thus necessitating placement of an overtube. Multiple ligation devices are now available that allow ligation of up to 10 sites without the need for removing the endoscope or placement of an overtube.

Ligation causes ischemic necrosis of ligated tissue. By 3 to 7 days, ischemic tissue sloughs off, leaving behind shallow ulcers. During this time, thrombosis occurs in the underlying vessel and an intense inflammatory reaction is accompanied by the formation of granulation tissue in the surrounding mucosa and submucosa. The ulcers heal in 2 to 3 weeks. These ulcers leave depressions that persist for 50 to 60 days. These changes correspond to re-epithelization and ultimately to fibrosis. Significant side effects (especially with multiple ligation devices) are rare and occur in less than 3% of patients. These side effects include dyphagia, transient chest pain, aspiration, and bleeding from esophageal ulcers. Strictures are a much rarer occurrence than with sclerotherapy.

Transjugular Intrahepatic Portosystemic Shunt

Transjugular intrahepatic portosystemic shunt (TIPS) became widely available and technically successful in the early 1990s with the advent of expandable metal stents. TIPS is a radiologically placed expandable metal stent that connects the hepatic and portal veins, thus decreasing portal hypertension without the mortality and morbidity associated with an open surgical procedure. Decreased portal hypertension leads to the cessation of variceal bleeding.

To create a TIPS, various modifications can be made to the following general technique. The portal vein and hepatic veins are assessed for patency with Doppler ultrasound. Some radiologists request a computed tomogram with IV contrast to assess the orientation of the portal and hepatic veins; others perform arterial portography and right hepatic venography at the time of the TIPS. Under conscious sedation or general anesthesia, the hepatic vein is catheterized via the internal jugular vein (Fig. 34–7). A needle is then passed into the liver parenchyma and gradually withdrawn with suction applied (sometimes with ultrasound guidance). A flash of blood indicates entrance into the portal venous system, which is confirmed with IV contrast. The tract is then dilated with a balloon over a guidewire, and an expandable metal stent is placed. The pressure gradient between the portal vein and the inferior vena cava is measured before and after the procedure. The stent diameter is expanded, or a parallel stent is placed to achieve a portocaval gradient less than 12 mm Hg. The procedure requires significant technical expertise and should be performed only in centers with experienced radiologists. Care must be taken not to place the stent into the inferior vena cava or the main portal vein, because this will make future orthotopic liver transplantation more difficult to accomplish.

Mortality from TIPS occurs in about 1% to 2% of patients, mainly from technical complications that result after puncture of the hepatic capsule or biliary tree, which lead to intraperitoneal bleeding or hemobilia, respectively. Other less common major complications include puncture of other organs adjacent to the liver, sepsis, heart failure, shunt migration, shunt thrombosis, hepatic infarction, and progressive liver failure. Many patients develop mild transient hemolysis. About 20% of patients develop new or worsened portosystemic encephalopathy, 80% of which will respond to lactulose. Possible risk factors for the development of encephalopathy include increased age, female gender, nonalcoholic etiology of liver disease, and hypoalbuminemia. TIPS leads to decreased hepatic blood flow, which results in varying decrements in hepatic function. Late complications consist mainly of stent dysfunction from tissue ingrowth, leading to recurrent portal hypertension, which occurred in 82% of patients in one study. Stent dysfunction can be corrected with angioplasty and placement of a new stent within

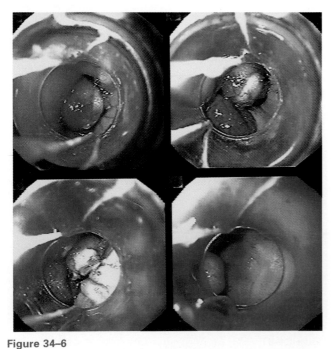

Figure 34–6
Endoscopic photograph of esophageal varices after rubber band ligation.

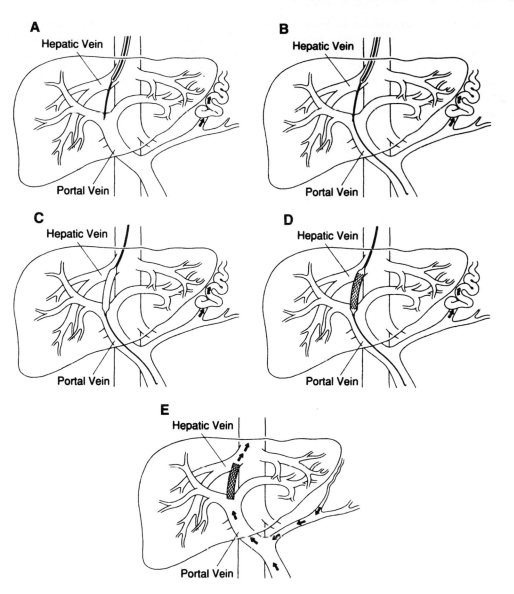

Figure 34–7
Transjugular intrahepatic portosystemic shunt (TIPS). *A,* A catheter is placed into the internal jugular vein through the vena cava and into the right hepatic vein. A needle is passed via the catheter through the liver parenchyma and into a branch of the portal vein. (The *arrow* indicates portal blood flow into the varices.) *B,* A guidewire is placed through the needle and into the portal vein. *C,* A balloon is passed over the guidewire and inflated to create a tract through the liver parenchyma. *D,* An expandable metal stent is placed via a delivery catheter across the tract, thus connecting the portal and systemic systems. *E,* The stent permits increased blood flow through the liver, thus causing decompression of the varices. (The *arrows* show a change in the direction of the blood flow.) (From Young HS: Gastrointestinal bleeding. Scientific American Medicine, Vol 1. Dale DC, Federman DD, Eds. Scientific American, Inc., New York, 1998, Sect 4, Subsect X, p 1. All rights reserved.)

the old stent or by placement of a parallel stent. Doppler ultrasonography is approximately 70% sensitive in detecting shunt dysfunction and should be done every 3 to 6 months. Any abnormalities in flow or diameter of shunt should be followed by hepatic venography and pressure measurements. Some radiologists recommend periodic hepatic venography every 6 months instead of ultrasonography, because 60% of patients eventually need revision of their TIPS. The National Digestive Disease Advisory Board Consensus conference proposed that TIPS should be performed to control active variceal bleeding that is unresponsive to endoscopic and pharmacologic therapy or recurrent variceal bleeding uncontrolled by two endoscopic procedures 24 hours apart. A properly placed TIPS does not alter early or late outcomes of orthotopic liver transplantation (OLT).

Angiographic Embolization

First described in 1974, transhepatic embolization of varices is rarely performed any more, because of the availability of more effective, less technically demanding, and less morbid measures. Angiographic embolization initially involved the cannulation of the portal vein via a method of percutaneous puncture of the liver. Catheters were then advanced into the short gastric and coronary veins with subsequent embolization utilizing gelfoam, chemical embolizing agents, or metal coils. Currently, embolization of varices is used as an occasional adjunct to TIPS, especially to eliminate gastric varices. Complications vary from 20% to 50% depending on the series and include pain, fever, portal vein thrombosis, pulmonary and systemic emboli, intra-abdominal hemorrhage, and death. Varices can re-form weeks to months after embolization and lead to recurrent bleeding.

Surgical Therapies

Surgical therapies for variceal bleeding are based on one of three pathophysiologic goals: (1) decompression of varices; (2) devascularization of varices; or (3) hepatic replacement.

Complete decompression of the portal system by creating end-to-side (portacaval) shunts or side-to-side (portacaval, mesocaval, mesorenal, or mesoatrial) or partial decompression by interposition H-graft shunts between portal venous and systemic venous circulations are highly effective at reducing the hepatic venous pressure gradient (HVPG) and thus variceal wall tension (Fig. 34–8). Additionally, side-to-side shunts permit drainage of the hepatic sinusoids through a patent portal vein that effectively treats ascites. Both kinds of shunts eliminate portal blood flow into the liver and result in progressive deterioration of hepatic function and increased risk of hepatic encephalopathy. Hepatic function is the major determinant of the long-term prognosis in cirrhotic patients. Partial decompression shunts and selective shunts attempt to preserve portal blood flow and thus eliminate the contribution of decreased portal blood flow to hepatic failure. Partial decompression shunts utilize a small diameter H-graft to create a connection between the mesenteric or portal vein and the inferior vena cava. The goal of partial decompression shunts is to lower

the HVPG below the 12 mm Hg threshold for variceal bleeding while maintaining blood flow to the liver (Fig. 34–9). Selective shunts attempt to maintain portal hypertension as seen by the liver and decompress the gastroesophageal variceal beds by dividing the portal circulation into two systems—one feeding the liver and the other the gastroesophageal varices. The distal splenorenal or "Warren" shunt and the coronary caval shunt are two techniques used to achieve this goal. The distal splenorenal shunt disconnects the splenic vein from the portal system and connects it to the renal vein, thus draining gastroesophageal varices through the splenic vein and into the systemic circulation (see Fig. 34–8D). The coronary caval shunt requires a splenectomy and an interposition graft between the left gastric vein and the inferior vena cava, thus draining gastroesophageal varices through the left gastric vein into the systemic circulation. Selective shunts can become complete shunts if all the

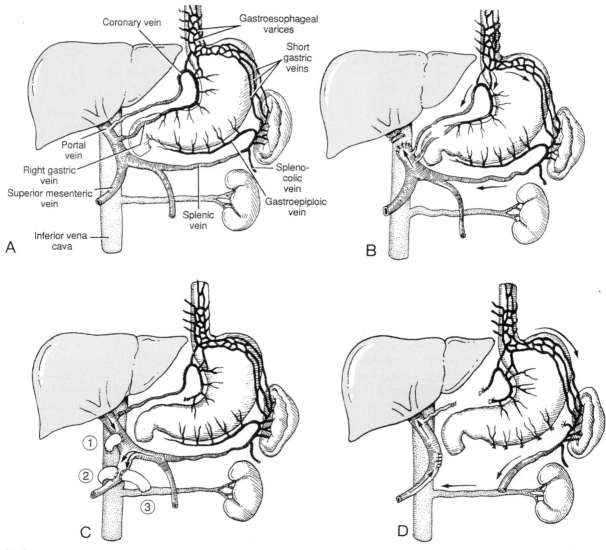

Figure 34–8

A, Normal portal venous anatomy. *B,* End-to-side portacaval shunt. *C,* Side-to-side interposition H-graft shunts. (1) Portacaval shunt, (2) mesocaval shunt, (3) mesovenal shunt. *D,* Distal splenovenal shunt. (From Young HS, Gregory PB: Bleeding varices. In Kaplowitz N [ed]: Liver and Biliary Diseases. Baltimore: Williams & Wilkins, 1996, p 572. Modified from Sabiston DC Jr [ed]: Textbook of Surgery, 13th ed. Philadelphia: WB Saunders, 1986, pp 1100–1103.)

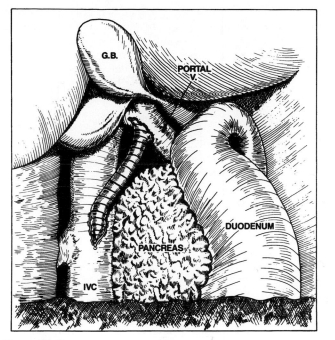

Figure 34–9
Small-diameter H-graft (partial decompressive shunt). (From Sarfeh IJ, Ryphius EB, Mason GR: A systematic appraisal of portacaval H-graft diameters: Clinical and hemodynamic parameters. Ann Surg 204:358, 1986.)

connections between the two portal systems are not divided at the initial surgery or if they re-form from growth of new varices. If the patient is a potential liver transplant candidate, the shunt should not involve the liver hilus, because this could make future OLT difficult or impossible.

Complications of shunts, in general, include recurrent bleeding, hepatic encephalopathy, surgical morbidity, surgical mortality, and worsening hepatic function. Overall, perioperative mortality for emergency shunt surgery is 50%. Mortality depends upon surgical experience, severity of blood loss before operation, and preoperative hepatic function. Elective shunts have a lower mortality. A discussion of the theoretical advantages of one surgical technique over another is beyond the scope of this chapter.

Various devascularization procedures are available from the simple to the very complex. They all employ direct disruption of blood flow into gastric and esophageal varices as their mechanism of action without altering blood flow into the liver. They include some or all of the following techniques: (1) esophageal transection and reanastomosis in order to disrupt esophageal variceal channels; (2) ablation of gastric and esophageal varices; or (3) splenectomy or ligation of the splenic vein. These procedures are popular in some centers in the Far East, but experience with them in the United States is very limited. All of the operative techniques are highly dependent on the skills and experience of the surgeon performing the procedure.

Hepatic replacement is the ultimate treatment for variceal bleeding because it corrects hepatic failure and returns portal pressure to the normal range, thus abolishing the risk of variceal bleeding. Refractory variceal bleeding is recognized as a primary indication for OLT by the United Net-

work for Organ Sharing (UNOS) in patients with underlying decompensated cirrhosis. It is also a clinical criterion that can be used to raise an otherwise equal patient to a higher status on the transplant list. Current expected 1- and 5-year survival rates of OLT are 80% to 85% and 65% to 75%, respectively. Chapter 31 discusses OLT in detail. The current shortage of donors limits OLT as a treatment for variceal bleeding.

EFFICACIES OF VARIOUS THERAPIES

Numerous randomized trials are published in complete and abstract form that address the problem of variceal bleeding. A complete review of each trial is beyond the scope of this chapter. What follows is a summary of the results with special emphasis on the development of recommendations for the treatment of variceal bleeding in the early 21st century.

Important measures of efficacy include the ability to control active bleeding, thus decreasing the frequency of rebleeding and prolonging survival without causing undue morbidity. Factors to bear in mind when interpreting reported results include: (1) Bleeding stops spontaneously in a significant proportion of patients; (2) There are various definitions for the terms "control of bleeding" and "rebleeding episode"; (3) There are different temporal relationships between bleeding and when the therapy was given; (4) There are different levels of severity of the underlying liver diseases and concurrent illnesses. Because these potential biases could affect the results, it is best to infer only from trials in which patients were prospectively randomized.

Control of Active Bleeding

Various approaches to the management of actively bleeding patients are currently in use in clinical practice including vasopressin, vasopressin plus nitroglycerin, terlipressin, somatostatin, octreotide, tamponade, sclerotherapy, variceal ligation, TIPS, embolization of varices, surgical shunts, and various combinations of the aforementioned treatments. The following section focuses on studies that evaluate treatments for patients with actively bleeding esophageal varices.

Pharmacologic Treatment and Tamponade

Several controlled trials studied the ability of vasopressin alone to stop active variceal bleeding, but they yielded conflicting results for bleeding control and none showed improved survival. Meta-analysis of four trials using IV vasopressin suggested efficacy but was strongly weighted by an early trial that only looked at 1-hour bleeding rates (Fig. 34–10). Intra-arterial vasopressin worked no better than IV vasopressin. The addition of nitroglycerin to vasopressin resulted in significant improvement in bleeding control and lower complication rates compared with vasopressin alone but had no effect on survival (see Fig. 34–10). Meta-analysis of four trials comparing terlipressin (glypressin) with and without nitrates to placebo showed significant improvement in bleeding control and mortality. When comparing terlipressin with vasopressin with and without nitroglycerin, two of five trials showed improved bleeding control, but this was not significant in meta-analysis and there was no improvement in mortality (see Fig. 34–10).

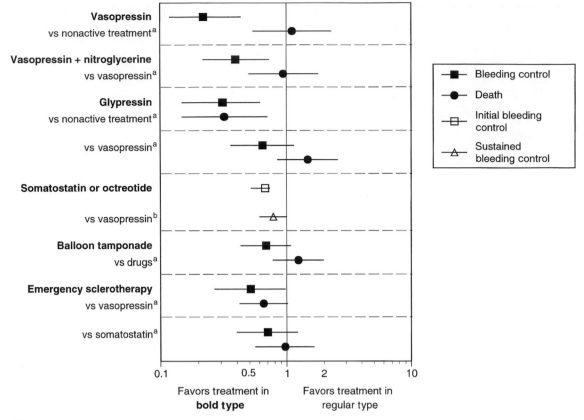

Figure 34–10
Meta-analyses comparing treatments for acute variceal bleeding.
[a]Pooled odds ratio on the log scale with 95% confidence intervals. (From D'Amico G, Pagliaro L, Bosch J: The treatment of portal hypertension: A meta-analytic review. Hepatology 22:332–354, 1995.)
[b]Relative risk on the log scale with 95% confidence intervals. (From Imperiale TF, Teran JC, McCullough AJ: A meta-analysis of somatostatin versus vasopressin in the management of acute esophageal variceal hemorrhage. Gastroenterology 109:1289–1294, 1995.)

Two controlled trials studied the ability of somatostatin to control variceal bleeding, one showing significant efficacy and both showing no effect on mortality. The study that showed no effect had a very high rate of spontaneous bleeding cessation (83%), probably due to defining a 4-hour bleeding-free period as bleeding cessation. This study also only gave somatostatin for 30 hours compared with 5 days in the other study. Meta-analysis of six trials comparing somatostatin or its analogue octreotide with vasopressin showed significantly improved initial and sustained bleeding control for somatostatin and significantly fewer side effects (see Fig. 34–10). Several trials showed no difference in efficacy between somatostatin or octreotide and terlipressin.

Tamponade balloons are up to 90% effective in initially arresting active bleeding due to gastroesophageal varices but achieve long-term hemostasis in only about 50% of patients. Meta-analysis of seven trials comparing balloon tamponade with medications (e.g., vasopressin, somatostatin, octreotide, or terlipressin) showed no significant differences in bleeding control or mortality (see Fig. 34–10). Tamponade balloons tend to have high rates of rebleeding once the balloons are deflated and are associated with frequent severe side effects as previously described.

Sclerotherapy

Six randomized studies comparing sclerotherapy with "conservative management," including supportive measures, balloon tamponade, or vasopressin with or without nitroglycerin, consistently showed that active bleeding was more frequently controlled (74% to 100%) with sclerotherapy versus conservative management (42% to 84%). Meta-analysis confirmed improved bleeding control with sclerotherapy compared with vasopressin (see Fig. 34–10). Balloon tamponade as an adjunct to sclerotherapy adds no improvement to bleeding control or survival. Meta-analysis of five trials comparing sclerotherapy versus balloon tamponade showed significantly improved bleeding control for the former. Meta-analysis of five trials comparing sclerotherapy versus somatostatin or octreotide therapy, showed no clear advantage of either treatment for bleeding control or survival (see Fig. 34–10). The addition of octreotide to sclerotherapy resulted in significant improvement in early bleeding control in four of five trials with one trial showing improved 5-day but not 15-day mortality. The best results tended to be in trials using continuous IV infusions of octreotide. The exact method by which periendoscopic octreotide therapy increases the effectiveness of endoscopic therapy is unclear. Octreotide may improve the clinical condition by making the patient more hemodynamically stable for endoscopy and providing a clearer endoscopic field of view, thus allowing for improved endoscopic visualization and administration of therapy. Continuation of this pharmacologic agent after endoscopic therapy for at least 5 days appears to prevent early rebleeding.

Ligation

The first reports of patients treated with band ligation showed that the efficacy was comparable with sclerotherapy with overall hemostasis rates ranging from 67% to 96%. In 1995, a meta-analysis of trials that compared ligation to sclerotherapy showed similar rates of control of active bleeding with less complications for ligation. The use of octreotide therapy before or at the time of endoscopic ligation significantly decreased the variceal rebleed rate and the need for balloon tamponade in several studies.

Transjugular Intrahepatic Portosystemic Shunt

TIPS is generally not used as first-line treatment for active variceal bleeding but as rescue therapy for patients who fail to respond to pharmacologic and endoscopic therapies. A large survey of centers using TIPS reported a 91% rate of success in controlling active variceal bleeding, most of which were refractory to other measures.

Surgery

Surgical options for the control of active variceal bleeding include surgical devascularization of gastroesophageal varices, portacaval shunts, and OLT. Comparisons of surgical techniques with medical or radiologic therapy are difficult to make because of the lack of high-quality randomized studies. A fair comparison may be impossible because early and late rebleeding and mortality are difficult to distinguish and compare. A randomized trial of staple transection of the esophagus and sclerotherapy showed no difference in early bleeding control or mortality, whereas another showed improved early bleeding control with surgery but no differences in short-term mortality. Emergency portacaval shunts result in almost 100% control of active bleeding at the expense of about a 30% to 50% perioperative mortality rate depending on the severity of the underlying liver disease. Generally, both early (3% to 19% versus 10% to 50%) and late rebleeding (0 to 19% versus 35% to 75%) were lower after shunt surgery than with sclerotherapy, but there was no difference in the mortality rate. Success of surgical intervention is highly dependent on a surgeon experienced with the chosen technique.

OLT is rarely used to treat active variceal bleeding given the shortage of donor organs and the availability of other alternatives. It is probably the most effective method to control bleeding and prolong survival for patients with severely decompensated cirrhosis.

Prevention of Rebleeding (Secondary Prophylaxis)

After the initial control of variceal bleeding there are several options to prevent recurrent bleeding from varices, including β-blockers with and without mononitrates, sclerotherapy, band ligation, TIPS, and surgery.

Pharmacotherapy

Meta-analysis of 12 trials comparing nonselective β blockers to supportive care showed significantly improved control of bleeding with rebleeding rates ranging from 21% to 76% versus 47% to 84% in the long term (Fig. 34–11). There is a nonsignificant trend toward improved survival favoring treatment with β-blockers. See the following sections for comparison of β-blockers to other treatments.

Sclerotherapy

Patients with variceal bleeding can have rebleeding both early and late. Sometimes it is difficult to arrive at conclusions about early versus late rebleeding, because definitions for early rebleeding are arbitrary and many studies do not state if the rebleeding occurred before or after varices were eradicated. Recurrence of varices occurs from 19% to 67% in various studies but does not always result in rebleeding. Studies were unable to show decreased rates of early bleeding for sclerotherapy compared with conservative therapy but did show consistently and usually significantly lower late bleeding rates, ranging from 8% to 58% (average of 28%) for sclerotherapy versus 28% to 80% (average of 49%) for conservative management. Meta-analysis of eight trials confirmed significantly reduced rebleeding and improved survival compared with conservative therapy (see Fig. 34–11).

Meta-analysis of nine trials comparing sclerotherapy to β-blockers showed significant reduction in rebleeding for sclerotherapy with no difference in mortality (see Fig. 34–11). The combination of trials is probably not valid because of heterogeneity among the trials; six trials showed decreased bleeding with sclerotherapy (two significantly), whereas three trials showed increased bleeding. Another meta-analysis evaluating nine trials (including eight from the aforementioned meta-analysis) comparing sclerotherapy with β-blockers showed no difference in episodes of upper gastrointestinal bleeding or mortality after sclerotherapy, but a significantly reduced variceal bleeding rate was noted. A single well-done randomized controlled trial comparing sclerotherapy with combination nadolol and isosorbide mononitrate therapy showed significant reduction in portal hypertensive-related bleeding and variceal bleeding for the medication group. Mortality differences were almost significant ($P = .07$). In the medication group of this study, patients with a greater than 20% decrease in HVPG had a significantly lower rebleeding rate. This study must be confirmed before a combination medical therapy can be accepted as being superior.

Meta-analysis of nine studies (published only in abstract) comparing sclerotherapy with combination sclerotherapy and β-receptor antagonists showed a significant reduction in all causes of upper gastrointestinal rebleeding rate for combination therapy by one of two statistical methods but no reduction in variceal rebleeding or mortality. Rebleeding tends to be less severe with combination therapy. This analysis suggests that combined treatment with sclero-

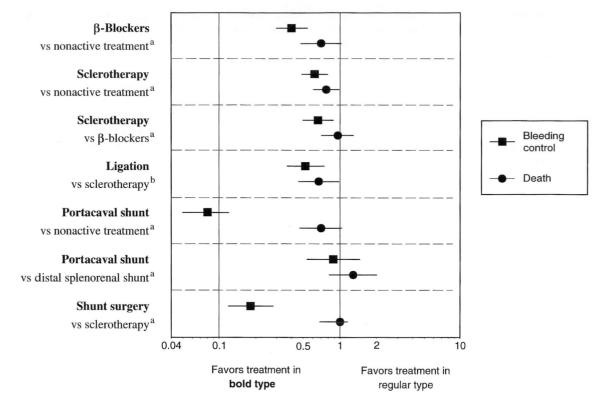

Figure 34–11

Meta-analyses comparing treatments for the prevention of rebleeding of varices.
[a]Pooled odds ratio on the log scale with 95% confidence intervals. (From D'Amico G, Pagliaro L, Bosch J: The treatment of portal hypertension: A meta-analytic review. Hepatology 22:332–354, 1995.)
[b]Common odds ratio on the log scale with 95% confidence intervals. (From Laine L, Cook D: Endoscopic ligation compared with sclerotherapy for treatment of esophageal variceal bleeding: A meta-analysis. Ann Intern Med 123:280–287, 1995.)

therapy and β-blockers may be more effective, especially in high-risk patients. See the following sections for comparisons of sclerotherapy to ligation, TIPS, or surgery.

Ligation

In 1995, a meta-analysis of seven trials comparing ligation with sclerotherapy showed significantly reduced rates of rebleeding, overall mortality, and mortality caused by rebleeding for ligation (see Fig. 34–11). Several more recent trials confirmed these results. Additionally, ligation requires fewer sessions to achieve variceal eradication and has fewer complications.

Interest in methods that might allow more rapid eradication of varices led to combining sclerotherapy and ligation at the same endoscopic session. Three of four trials evaluating combination therapy showed no difference in bleeding control or mortality with the addition of sclerotherapy to ligation. They did show either increased time to variceal eradication or increased time of endoscopy session or increased complication rates for combination therapy. Several trials showed significantly increased rates of variceal recurrence with ligation compared with sclerotherapy, but this finding has not translated into an increased risk of late rebleeding or mortality. One study showed lower rates of recurrent varices and recurrent bleeding but no difference in the mortality rate using ligation until varices were small

(grade 2) followed by low-dose sclerotherapy compared with ligation alone. This method of treatment must be confirmed with additional long-term studies to ascertain if clinically significant benefits can be achieved by reducing variceal recurrence rates. There are currently no studies that compare variceal ligation alone or in combination with other modalities versus pharmacotherapy. Because ligation is superior to sclerotherapy and sclerotherapy is generally superior to pharmacotherapy, it is safe to assume that ligation is superior to pharmacotherapy.

Transjugular Intrahepatic Portosystemic Shunt

TIPS is effective as a rescue therapy for patients who failed pharmacologic and endoscopic therapy. Because of its ability to prevent bleeding in refractory patients, there are currently 11 randomized controlled trials (including four abstracts) that compare TIPS to various medical and surgical treatments as secondary prophylaxis of variceal bleeding. Five of seven trials comparing TIPS to sclerotherapy with or without β-blockers showed significantly reduced rebleeding rates, and one showed improved survival with TIPS. One study showed improved survival with sclerotherapy, but 24% of active variceal bleeders were eliminated from the study because they could not be controlled initially with sclerotherapy and 15% of the sclerotherapy group eventually received TIPS due to recurrent bleeding. The trial showing improved survival with TIPS is only published in abstract form and had fewer patients followed for generally a shorter time than did the other trials. Four trials showed significantly increased rates of hepatic encephalopathy for TIPS. Overall, TIPS is generally more effective at preventing recurrent bleeding but has no effect on survival and produces more hepatic encephalopathy. There is one published trial and one abstract comparing TIPS to ligation, and both showed improved bleeding control for TIPS but no difference in survival. About 15% of patients in the endoscopically treated groups required TIPS for refractory recurrent bleeding. One trial comparing TIPS with combination of propranalol and isosorbide mononitrate showed improved bleeding control for TIPS but no difference in mortality. The current data show no clear survival advantage for TIPS as initial treatment for secondary prophylaxis over other therapies, when TIPS is used as rescue for failure to control recurrent bleeding with other therapies. It, therefore, becomes a choice for the clinician and the patient to choose their preferred intervention after considering the potential morbidities, increased rates of rebleeding versus encephalopathy, and perhaps decreased hepatic function.

Surgery

Successful surgical decompression of the portal circulation should completely prevent variceal rebleeding if the shunt remains patent. Meta-analysis of four studies comparing the portacaval shunt with conservative management showed significant reduction in rebleeding (9% to 20% versus 65% to 98%) and nearly significant reduction in mortality, but at the expense of significant increase in hepatic encephalopathy (0 to 4% versus 11% to 18%) (see Fig. 34–11). The reduction in mortality is probably clinically significant, because only one study showed worse survival with shunts and this trial may have had some bias at randomization. Meta-analysis of six trials comparing various portacaval shunts with distal splenorenal shunt shows no significant differences in rebleeding, survival, or encephalopathy (Fig. 34–11). A more recent trial was in agreement with the meta-analysis. A trial comparing the total portacaval shunt with the partial portacaval shunt using a small-diameter H-graft shows no difference in rebleeding or mortality but significantly decreased encephalopathy with the H-graft. Meta-analysis of seven trials (comparing shunt surgeries with sclerotherapy) shows significantly less rebleeding with surgery (3% to 23% versus 31% to 59%), but no differences in mortality and significantly increased encephalopathy (see Fig. 34–11). A randomized controlled trial of 70 patients comparing a small-diameter H-graft shunt with TIPS showed lower rates of "shunt failure" for H-graft shunts but no differences in mortality or encephalopathy. We await results of other trials comparing shunts with TIPS and ligation.

Early rebleeding (up to 6 weeks) was significantly lower (7% versus 42%) in patients who survived staple transection of the esophagus compared with sclerotherapy in a study of 101 patients; however, sclerotherapy was limited to a single session for the index bleed and subsequent treatments were not given. There is a recent case series of 10 patients who successfully underwent laparoscopic gastric devascularization with splenectomy for refractory esophageal varices.

OLT is highly successful at preventing recurrent bleeding and improving the survival of patients with decompensated cirrhosis, but organ availability limits this therapy.

Approach to Patient Care

When presented with a patient with suspected variceal bleeding, the first step is to stabilize the patient hemodynamically (Fig. 34–12). This is accomplished by the placement of adequate IV access and infusions of saline and blood products as described in the section on supportive care earlier. Treatment with either octreotide or somatostatin (given as a bolus followed by a continuous drip) should be started during the initial resuscitation process, because these drugs have minimal side effects and are effective in variceal and nonvariceal bleeding. Additionally, these drugs decrease both early variceal rebleeding rates and the need for balloon tamponade when combined with endoscopic therapy. This treatment should be continued for 5 days.

Early esophagogastroduodenoscopy (EGD) is essential to confirm the diagnosis and institute appropriate specific therapy, especially because up to 30% of cirrhotic patients will have a nonvariceal source of bleeding. If there are actively bleeding esophagogastric varices, a multiple ligator device should be used to treat the bleeding vessel followed by treatment of other varices present. If there is failure to achieve hemostasis, an attempt should be made at sclerotherapy during the same endoscopic session. If this attempt fails, treatment should include a repeat bolus with somatostatin or octreotide and placement of a Minnesota tube to stabilize the patient hemodynamically (Fig. 34–13). This time period should be used to evaluate the patient for a TIPS or surgery. The choice depends on the experience level of the interventional radiologist and the surgeon. If both persons are experienced, then a patient with Child-Pugh class A cirrhosis should have a surgical shunt. The choice of shunt procedure depends on the surgeon's preference and whether the patient will be a future candidate for OLT. Portacaval shunts lead to increased morbidity with liver transplantation and should be avoided if OLT is a consideration. Either distal splenorenal or H-graft mesocaval shunts are probably better overall for most patients, but they are more technically demanding. These patients should then be followed closely for evidence of early hepatic decompensation and referred for OLT at that time. Esophageal staple gun transection is another alternative, but there is very little experience with this procedure in the United States. TIPS is a viable alternative if experienced surgeons are not available or if the patient is too unstable for surgery. If the patient is in Child-Pugh class B or C, then TIPS is a good bridge to future transplantation, because it is less invasive and less likely to interfere with OLT.

If the endoscopic therapy controls the bleeding, the patient should have repeated variceal ligation every 2 to 3 weeks until the varices are eradicated. The patient should have repeat endoscopy every 3 months for the first year and every 6 months thereafter to assess for and treat recurrent varices. The addition of a β-blocker, possibly combined with isosorbide mononitrate treatment, should theoretically reduce the risk of rebleeding. This is suggested by a meta-analysis that showed decreased overall gastrointestinal bleeding with the addition of β-blockers to sclerotherapy.

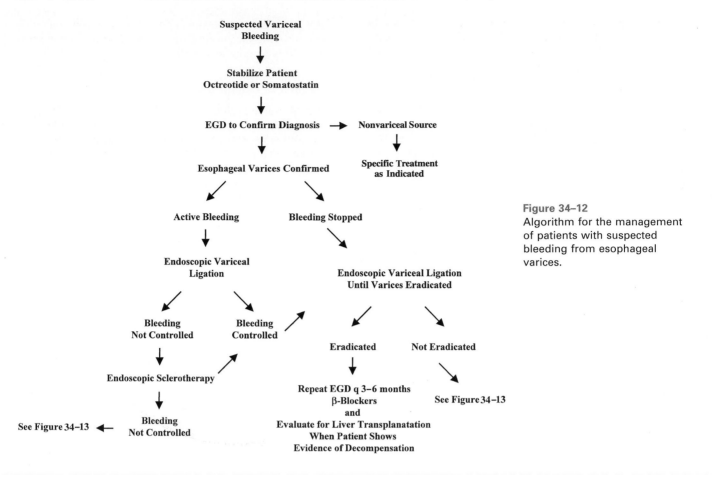

Figure 34–12
Algorithm for the management of patients with suspected bleeding from esophageal varices.

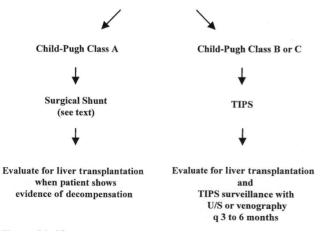

Figure 34–13
Algorithm for the management of patients with uncontrolled variceal bleeding.

Furthermore, this treatment scheme addresses two distinct mechanisms of variceal bleeding that may improve the expected 30% long-term rebleeding rate. We anticipate future trials to address this issue and would consider use of these medications in high-risk patients. The patient should be evaluated for liver transplantation when he or she demonstrates any evidence of hepatic decompensation, if he or she is otherwise an appropriate candidate.

Gastric Varices

Gastric varices can form as a result of cirrhosis, noncirrhotic portal hypertension, splenic vein thrombosis, and after endoscopic treatment of esophageal varices. Hemorrhage from gastric varices is usually more severe and has an even worse prognosis than does hemorrhage from esophageal varices. Endoscopy may underestimate the prevalence of gastric varices. Gastric varices were found in 57% of 230 patients studied by portal vein catheterization, but there is no way to be certain if all of the gastric varices that were found were clinically significant. The incidence of gastric variceal bleeding is not clearly known and has ranged from 2% to 60% in various series.

There are many small series that address gastric variceal bleeding, but they are hard to interpret because they fail to classify the different types of varices. Some more recent series use the Baveno consensus conference classification of gastric varices as described in Chapter 17. The importance of classifying gastric varices is shown by a large prospective series of 568 patients. Gastroesophageal varices type 1 (GOV1) are esophageal varices that extend onto the lesser curve of the stomach (Fig. 34–14). Approximately 60% disappeared after obliteration of the esophageal varices by sclerotherapy in the large series, but of the remaining varices 28% bleed. GOV1 responded to sclerotherapy both for active bleeding and for eradication of varices. Gastroesophageal varices type 2 (GOV2) are esophageal varices that extend onto the fundus (see Fig. 34–14). They only partially responded to sclerotherapy of the esophageal varices in both the acute bleeding and eradication phases and bleed 55% of the time. Isolated gastric varices type 1 (IGV1) are fundal varices that do not reach the cardia (see Fig. 34–14). They bled 78% of the time and did not respond reliably to sclerotherapy. Isolated gastric varices 2 (IGV2) can be anywhere in the stomach except the proximal lesser curve and fundus (see Fig. 34–14). They bled in less than 10% of cases; however, when they did bleed, it was often severe. Endoscopic features associated with increased risk of bleeding of gastric fundal varices (GOV2 and IGV1) included large size, red color spots, and a higher Child class.

Several small series report successful treatment of gastric varices with large volumes (average of 6.8 mL, up to 30 mL per varix) of standard sclerosing agents. Initial bleeding control ranged from 26% to 83%, with rebleeding from 25% to 53%, and mortality from 24% to 67%. When the type of gastric varices were given, all outcomes were worse for IGV1 versus GOV1 and GOV2. Injection of isobutyl-2-cyanoacrylate (bucrylate) or N-butyl-2-cyanoacrylate (histoacryl), tissue glues that polymerize on contact with blood to form a firm adherent clot, were successful for initial control of bleeding and prevention of rebleeding in several small series. Initial hemostasis was achieved in from 88% to 100% of patients; rebleeding rates ranged from 4% to 53% and overall mortality ranged from 8% to 38%. As with standard sclerotherapy, patients with GOV1 and GOV2 did better than did those with IGV1. Injection of tissue glue is associated with the same complications as standard sclerotherapy and may have increased risk for cerebral embolization. There are no randomized studies comparing tissue glue with standard sclerotherapy for control of bleeding gastric varices. One trial (published as an abstract), which involves 25 patients, compares tissue glue with sclerotherapy using ethanol for secondary prophylaxis of IGV1 and IGV2. Tissue glue worked significantly better in obliterating varices (79% vs 35%) and preventing rebleeding (79% vs 36%) with no differences in need for surgery or mortality. Tissue glue is not currently available in the United States. One series of 11 patients using thrombin injected via a sclerotherapy needle into nine IGV1 and two GOV1 showed 100% initial hemostasis, with a 9% rebleeding rate and 0% mortality. Thrombin has the advantage of causing no local ulcerations. Two small series with short follow-up using ligation via detachable snares showed 100% initial bleeding control and no rebleeding. There are case reports of successful band ligation for gastric varices. One series (published as an abstract) comparing patients who received TIPS for refractory bleeding from esophageal or gastric varices showed no differences in initial bleeding control (>95%), rebleeding rates (<15%), and mortality (<42%). Others series suggest that TIPS may be less effective for gastric varices compared with esophageal varices. Several series show successful bleeding control for various types of gastric varices with acceptable mortality (<33%) using gastric devascularization with and without splenectomy.

Overall, most studies on gastric varices are difficult to compare, because they do not carefully define the severity of underlying cirrhosis and the location of the gastric varices. These are probably the two most important determinants of outcome. There is insufficient literature to make strong recommendations of one treatment modality over another. Tissue adhesives probably work better than standard sclerotherapy and ligation, although they are unavailable for use in the United States. Currently, most centers use TIPS or surgical procedures to treat significant bleeding from gastric varices.

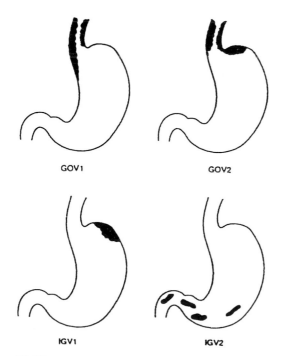

Figure 34–14
Classification of gastric varices based on the Baveno consensus conference. (From Sarin SK, Lahoti D, Saxena SP, et al: Prevalence, classification and natural history of gastric varices: A long-term follow-up study in 568 portal hypertension patients. Hepatology 16:1343–1349, 1992.)

SUGGESTED READINGS

Bernard B, Lebrec D, Mathurin P, et al: Propranolol and sclerotherapy in the prevention of gastrointestinal rebleeding in patients with cirrhosis: A meta-analysis. J Hepatol 26:312–324, 1997.
Besson I, Ingrand P, Person B, et al: Sclerotherapy with or without octreotide for acute variceal bleeding. N Engl J Med 333:555–560, 1995.
Burroughs AK, Hamilton G, Phillips A, et al: A comparison of sclerotherapy with staple transection of the esophagus for the emergency control of bleeding from esophageal varices. N Engl J Med 321:857–862, 1989.
Cipolletta L, Bianco MA, Rotondano G, et al: Emergency endoscopic ligation of actively bleeding gastric varices with a detachable snare. Gastrointest Endosc 47:400–403, 1998.

D'Amico G, Pagliaro L, Bosch J: The treatment of portal hypertension: A meta-analytic review. Hepatology 22:332–354, 1995.

Freedman AM, Sanyal AJ, Tisnado J, et al: Complications of transjugular intrahepatic portosystemic shunt: A comprehensive review. Radiographics 3:1185–1210, 1993.

Grace ND: Diagnosis and treatment of gastrointestinal bleeding secondary to portal hypertension. Am J Gastroenterol 92:1081–1091, 1997.

Grace ND, Groszmann RJ, Garcia-Tsao G, et al: Portal hypertension and variceal bleeding: An AASLD single topic symposium. Hepatology 28:868–880, 1998.

Hartigan PM, Gebhard RL, Gregory PB: Sclerotherapy for actively bleeding esophageal varices in male alcoholics with cirrhosis. Veterans Affairs Cooperative Variceal Sclerotherapy Group. Gastrointest Endosc 46:1–7, 1997.

Henderson JM: Surgical measures in prevention of recurrent variceal bleeding. Gastrointest Endosc Clin North Am 2:151–166, 1992.

Hsieh JS, Huang CJ, Huang TJ: Management of isolated gastric varices by devascularization and proximal gastrectomy in cirrhotic patients. HPB Surg 7:201–209, 1994.

Imperiale TF, Teran JC, McCullough AJ: A meta-analysis of somatostatin versus vasopressin in the management of acute esophageal variceal hemorrhage. Gastroenterology 109:1289–1294, 1995.

Kim T, Shijo H, Kokawa H, et al: Risk factors for hemorrhage from gastric fundal varices. Hepatology 25:307–312, 1997.

Laine L, Cook D: Endoscopic ligation compared with sclerotherapy for treatment of esophageal variceal bleeding: A meta-analysis. Ann Intern Med 123:280–287, 1995.

Lo GH, Lai KH, Cheng JS, et al: The additive effect of sclerotherapy to patients receiving repeated endoscopic variceal ligation: A prospective, randomized trial. Hepatology 28:391–395, 1998.

Orloff MJ, Orloff MS, Orloff SL, et al: Three decades of experience with emergency portacaval shunt for acutely bleeding esophageal varices in 400 unselected patients with cirrhosis of the liver. J Am Coll Surg 180:257–272, 1995.

Ramond M-J, Valla D, Mosnier J-F, et al: Successful endoscopic obturation of gastric varices with butyl cyanoacrylate. Hepatology 10:488–493, 1989.

Rosemurgy AS, Goode SE, Zwiebel BR, et al: A prospective trial of transjugular intrahepatic portasystemic stent shunts versus small-diameter prosthetic H-graft portacaval shunts in the treatment of bleeding varices. Ann Surg 224:378–386, 1996.

Saeed, ZA: Endoscopic therapy of bleeding esophageal varices: Ligation is still the best. Gastroenterology 110:635–638, 1996.

Saeed ZA, Stiegmann GV, Ramirez FC, et al: Endoscopic variceal ligation is superior to combined ligation and sclerotherapy for esophageal varices: A multicenter prospective randomized trial. Hepatology 25:71–74, 1997.

Sarin SK: Diagnostic issues: Portal hypertensive gastropathy and gastric varices. In DeFranchis R (ed): Portal hypertension II. Proceedings of the second Baveno International consensus workshop on definitions, methodology and therapeutic strategies. Oxford: Blackwell Science, 1996, pp 30–55.

Sarin SK: Long-term follow-up of gastric variceal sclerotherapy: An eleven-year experience. Gastrointest Endosc 46:8–14, 1997.

Sarin SK, Lahoti D, Saxena SP, et al: Prevalence, classification and natural history of gastric varices: A long-term follow-up study in 568 portal hypertension patients. Hepatology 16:1343–1349, 1992.

Technology Assessment Committee of the ASGE: Transvenous intrahepatic portosystemic shunt (TIPS). Gastrointest Endosc 47:584–587, 1998.

Thomas PG, D'Cruz AJ: Distal splenorenal shunting for bleeding gastric varices. Br J Surg 81:241–244, 1994.

Villanueva C, Balanzo J, Novella MT, et al: Nadolol plus isosorbide mononitrate compared with sclerotherapy for the prevention of variceal rebleeding. N Engl J Med 334:1624–1629, 1996.

Zoller WG, Gross M: Beta-blockers for prophylaxis of bleeding from esophageal varices in cirrhotic portal hypertension: Review of the literature (Review). Eur J Med Res 1:407–416, 1996.

35

Endoscopy in the Management of Biliary Tract Disorders

Klaus Mergener
John Baillie

Endoscopic retrograde cholangiopancreatography (ERCP) is a major tool in the investigation and treatment of biliary tract disease. ERCP rapidly evolved from a purely diagnostic technique into a therapeutic one with the development of endoscopic sphincterotomy (independently reported by Kawai and Classen) in 1974. The development of large-channel therapeutic duodenoscopes allowed endoscopists to place endoprostheses of 10 French gauge or larger in the biliary tree starting around 1980. Since then, diagnostic and therapeutic ERCP has greatly evolved to allow us to treat a wide spectrum of biliary and pancreatic disorders. Such sophistication demands well trained and experienced endoscopists to ensure that these procedures are applied appropriately and with the least morbidity. As gauged by the complication rate, ERCP is the most dangerous procedure routinely performed by endoscopists. There has been considerable debate regarding the appropriate training in hepatobiliary and pancreatic disorders and the use of ERCP. It is clear that previous guidelines for ERCP training based solely on the number of procedures were inadequate. The professional background of the individual performing endoscopy, whether he or she is a gastroenterologist, surgeon, or radiologist, is less important than the quality of the training that he or she receives.

Although ERCP remains the "gold standard" for investigating the biliary tree and pancreatic ductal system, it is just one of several imaging modalities available. These modalities range from the relatively noninvasive type, such as transabdominal ultrasound, computed tomography (CT), and magnetic resonance cholangiopancreatography (MRCP), to percutaneous transhepatic cholangiography (PTC), which is the most invasive procedure. An evolving imaging technique that is of particular interest to the endoscopist is endoscopic ultrasound (EUS). This technique has significant applica-

tions in hepatobiliary and pancreatic disorders, although it is fair to say that to date it has been used more widely to study the pancreas than to elucidate biliary tract disease. The choice of imaging techniques depends on the clinical situation, the availability of equipment, and the interest and expertise of the radiologists involved. In this chapter, we review the principal indications for ERCP in disorders of the biliary tract. When appropriate, we will outline management algorithms and, in particular, adjunctive radiologic procedures.

GENERAL INDICATIONS

The gastrointestinal (GI) endoscopist is often required to perform ERCP to evaluate abnormal liver function tests, frank jaundice, and biliary-type pain (Table 35-1). As with many liver problems, a good history and physical examination plus basic laboratory tests can often provide a reliable diagnosis. It is particularly important to distinguish parenchymal liver disease from cholestasis caused by mechanical biliary obstruction or a canalicular level biochemical defect. Cross-sectional imaging such as transabdominal ultrasound or CT scanning can provide useful information about the presence or absence of intra- and extrahepatic bile duct dilatation. Abnormal masses within the liver, such as tumors and cysts, are also well seen with these imaging techniques. However, they are less sensitive for stones within the biliary tree and may not detect infiltrating processes, in which the contrast between the pathologic tissue and the liver parenchyma is poor. MRCP, once thought to be of little value as an imaging technique in the GI tract, is helping to elucidate many hepatic abnormalities. T_2-weighted images, which cause water density liquids to appear brightly on images, are particularly useful for investigating fluid-filled cavities as

Table 35–1   Diagnostic Indications for Endoscopic Retrograde Cholangiopancreatography

Biliary

Choledocholithiasis
Biliary strictures
Malignancy of the biliary tree (cholangiocarcinoma)
   Collection of bile for cytology and brushings
   Biopsy of the bile duct
Pre- and postsurgical evaluation of the biliary tree (selected cases)
Detection of congenital abnormalities (e.g., choledochal cysts)
Detection of gallbladder and cystic duct pathology
Evaluation of space-occupying lesions in the liver (e.g., abscesses, cysts)
Evaluation of unexplained liver function test abnormalities
Manometry of the sphincter of Oddi

Pancreatic

Evaluation of acute, relapsing, and chronic pancreatitis
Evaluation of complications of pancreatitis
   Pseudocysts
   Strictures
   Stones
   Fistulas
Evaluation of pancreas divisum
Pancreatic malignancy
   Brushings and biopsy of the pancreatic duct
   Collection of pancreatic juice for cytology
   Stenting of malignant strictures
Pre- and postsurgical evaluation of the pancreas (selected cases)
Assessment of pancreatic ascites

well as particularly vascular structures, such as hemangiomas. A targeted biopsy under CT guidance provides tissue for cytology and histology to allow diagnosis of hepatic, biliary, and pancreatic masses as well as enlarged lymph nodes adjacent to these organs. ERCP is often used when there is diagnostic doubt, such as when biliary stones and strictures are suspected but cannot be confirmed by other imaging modalities. ERCP also offers the additional benefit of therapeutic intervention in selected cases (Table 35–2).

Endoscopists with skill and experience in ERCP rarely

Table 35–2   Biliary Tract Indications for Therapeutic Endoscopic Retrograde Cholangiopancreatography

Choledocholithiasis (including mechanical and contact lithotripsy)
Extraction of cystic duct and (rarely) gallbladder stones
Dilatation and stenting of benign and malignant bile duct strictures
Stenting of obstructing ampullary tumors
Biliary decompression in sphincter of Oddi dysfunction/ papillary stenosis (sphincterotomy)
Removal of intrabiliary foreign bodies (e.g., flukes, worms)
Treatment of biliary leaks

fail to access the bile duct. However, there are situations in which this may be technically difficult or impossible. For example, after rearrangement of the gastric anatomy (e.g., Billroth II gastrectomy), normal access to the duodenal papilla may be lost. Also, strictures or masses affecting the duodenum may render ERCP problematic. When ERCP fails or is technically impossible, direct access to the bile ducts is possible by the transhepatic percutaneous route. PTC may be technically difficult when the bile ducts are not dilated, but in experienced hands it is a very valuable technique. The vogue in the 1980s for so-called combined or "rendezvous" procedures, whereby vascular radiologists and endoscopists "meet" with guidewires and snares in the duodenum to effect diagnostic and therapeutic procedures, has declined with the recognition that such procedures are often associated with significant morbidity. Modern interventional radiologists rarely, if ever, need endoscopists to assist them with their biliary stenting procedures. However, as radiologists have yet to perfect a safe and effective way to perform sphincterotomy by the percutaneous route, endoscopists are still sometimes invited to participate in combined procedures for this specific indication (Fig. 35–1A, B).

PATIENT PREPARATION

Informed consent—preferably in writing—should be obtained before all endoscopic procedures. The discussion must be particularly detailed in the case of ERCP, given its complexity and the risk of potentially life-threatening complications such as pancreatitis, bleeding, and perforation. There is a great deal of variation in the quoted morbidity and mortality rate of ERCP. Many of these data are based on old surveys and require updating in the light of improved technology and skill levels. However, the morbidity of ERCP is generally quoted to be in the range of 3% to 10% with mortality rates ranging from 0.1% to 1%. One prospective study of complications of biliary sphincterotomy at the time of ERCP found an overall complication rate of 9.8% with a procedure-related mortality of 0.4%. Particular risk factors for complications included suspected dysfunction of the sphincter of Oddi, the presence of cirrhosis, and performance of a "precut" sphincterotomy. As patients are almost always sedated for ERCP, particular attention has to be paid to prior or existing medical problems that may affect the type of sedation given. A few patients who have exhibited intolerance of conscious sedation require general anesthesia. In addition, most children tolerate ERCP better with a general anesthetic of short duration than they do when intravenous sedatives are given.

Antibiotic Coverage

There are no data to support the routine use of prophylactic antibiotics in patients undergoing ERCP. Although the data supporting antibiotic therapy for prophylaxis against cholangitis in patients with known biliary obstruction, suspected choledocholithiasis, biliary leaks, and so forth are scant, most endoscopists give antibiotics in this case. We use a combination of ampicillin and gentamicin (substituting vancomycin for ampicillin in patients who are allergic to penicillin); alternatively, a broad-spectrum cephalosporin is sufficient in most cases. Clearly, great care must be taken when

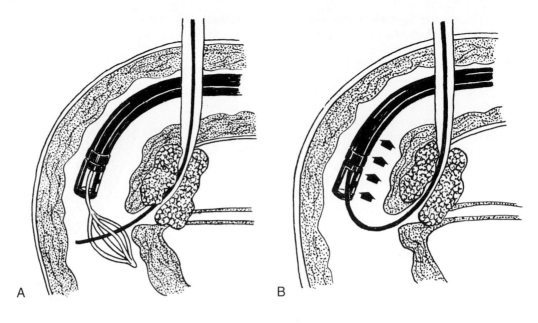

Figure 35–1
Combined ("rendez vous") procedure. *A,* A guidewire, which was advanced percutaneously through the bile duct, is grasped by an endoscopic basket under direct vision. *B,* The guidewire is withdrawn through the duodenoscope to provide easy access for endoscopic catheters. (*A* and *B,* From Baillie J: Gastrointestinal Endoscopy: Beyond the Basics. Boston, MA: Butterworth-Heinemann Press, 1997.)

administering gentamicin to patients with renal insufficiency. In this setting, a lower than normal dose is appropriate, and drug levels must be monitored carefully. If a complication such as contained or free perforation of the biliary tree is suspected following ERCP, antibiotic coverage should be broadened to include an agent active against anaerobic organisms (e.g., metronidazole). No benefit can be gained from adding antibiotics to contrast media used during ERCP. The effect of antibiotics depend on their tissue concentration; simply injecting antibiotics into the biliary tree has no useful effect against organisms that may cause cholangitis. Although most endoscopists use parenteral antibiotics, data suggest that oral ciprofloxacin may be equally effective. We recommend collection of bile for culture and sensitivity determination in cases where sepsis is suspected or known to be present (e.g., from positive results on blood cultures).

Contrast Allergy

It has been the practice of endoscopists for many years to administer antihistamines and corticosteroids as prophylaxis against contrast allergy in patients undergoing ERCP. This is a controversial subject; there are scant data supporting this practice. Although the routine use of low osmolality, nonionic contrast media has been advocated, there are insufficient data to support this. These contrast agents are expensive and, therefore, should be reserved for patients with a known history of major allergic reactions to iodinated contrast. Even then, it is not clear that severe contrast reactions can be prevented by this approach. Many endoscopy units adopt a practice similar to their radiology colleagues of giving corticosteroids (e.g., prednisone) in three or five divided doses over the preceding 24 to 36 hours.

Coagulopathy

Prior to ERCP, a detailed history of bleeding disorder should be obtained, and routine coagulation indices (e.g., pro-

thrombin time, partial thromboplastin time) should be measured. This is particularly important when endoscopic sphincterotomy is anticipated. Most endoscopists accept 2 to 3 seconds prolongation of the prothrombin time, but beyond this time remedial action is required if a sphincterotomy is to be performed. We ask our patients to discontinue the use of aspirin and nonsteroidal anti-inflammatory drugs for 1 week before ERCP if these agents are not absolutely essential. For patients who are taking aspirin as antistroke prophylaxis, we usually let them continue their therapy because the risk of a thrombotic cerebrovascular incident probably outweighs that of postsphincterotomy hemorrhage. When an urgent ERCP has to be performed in the setting of major coagulopathy, establishing biliary drainage by nasobiliary drain or stent insertion without sphincterotomy is often sufficient to relieve the acute problem. A good example of this is when a patient with common bile duct stones (choledocholithiasis) has cholangitis, leading to systemic sepsis with disseminated intravascular coagulation. The simple act of placing a stent to allow the obstructed bile duct to drain will quickly improve matters. Once coagulation has returned to normal, either spontaneously or after administration of clotting factors, a further ERCP can be done to remove the stent followed by sphincterotomy and stone extraction. Patients with known disorders of specific clotting factors (e.g., hemophilia, Christmas disease) or platelets (e.g., thrombocytopenia) should be managed jointly with a hematologist or expert in coagulation disorders.

ERCP—The Procedure

ERCP is an endoscopic procedure performed with the aid of fluoroscopy, which can either be done using a fixed x-ray/fluoroscopy table or a mobile fluoroscopy system. After the patient is sedated with intravenous agents (usually a benzodiazepine with or without a narcotic such as meperidine), and sometimes the administration of topical lidocaine to the posterior pharynx, the duodenoscope is advanced through the esophagus and stomach to the descending duodenum. This may be performed with the patient in the prone position or starting in the semiprone position and then rotated flat (Fig. 35–2). Once the duodenoscope tip is in position adjacent to the duodenal papilla, it is shortened in a straightening maneuver. Considerable experience is required to use a duodenoscope effectively. Duodenoscopes have an instrument channel through which guidewires, catheters, and various accessories (e.g., stone baskets and balloons) can be advanced. At the tip of the duodenoscope there is a small metal elevator, or "bridge," that allows the endoscopist to vary the angle at which equipment exits from the instrument channel. The elevator has an important role in the successful cannulation of bile duct and pancreatic duct orifices, because access to these is highly dependent on appropriate orientation of the cannula. For diagnostic and simple therapeutic procedures, the so-called diagnostic duodenoscopes (with instrument channels in the range of 2.8 mm diameter) are adequate. For stenting with endoprostheses larger than 7 French gauge, therapeutic duodenoscopes are required; these have larger instrument channels with an internal diameter up to and beyond 4.2 mm. For a limited number of specialized indications, such as contact lithotripsy of stones and direct access to hilar tumors, very small endoscopes (miniscopes or so-called "baby" scopes) can be advanced through the instrument channel of a therapeutic duodenoscope into the bile duct. This so-called "mother and baby" scope approach requires two operators and a prior sphincterotomy to afford biliary access. The use of miniscopes is limited to tertiary referral centers whose volume of unusual cases can justify the expense of purchasing and maintaining these delicate instruments.

Difficult Anatomy

In experienced hands, cannulation of the bile duct and pancreatic duct can be achieved in most cases. An expert endoscopist usually has a biliary cannulation success rate higher than 90%. However, the endoscopic approach to the biliary tree and pancreatic ductal system can be rendered difficult or impossible by surgical rearrangement of the gastric and upper small bowel anatomy. For example, after Billroth II gastrectomy, diagnostic and therapeutic ERCP are usually still possible, but a different and more difficult technique is required. The afferent limb of the gastroenterostomy must be identified and instrumented, and the duodenal papilla must be approached from "below" (Fig. 35–3). A

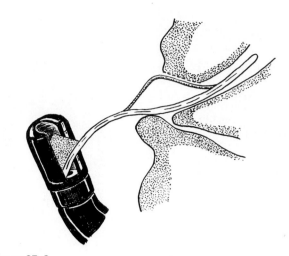

Figure 35–3
Biliary cannulation in a patient following a Billroth-II gastrectomy requires a special technique. Cannulation is assisted by use of a Billroth-II papillotome.

Roux-en-Y gastrojejunostomy increases the level of difficulty; perhaps only one in five ERCPs can be successfully completed in this setting. Therefore, the decision whether or not to perform ERCP in the case of these patients must be individualized. Periampullary diverticula are not uncommon, especially in elderly patients, and these may make cannulation more difficult to accomplish. However, with skilled technique, most diverticula do not present insurmountable difficulties. A choledochoduodenostomy, which is the simplest form of surgical biliary bypass, was used extensively in the past as part of the treatment for common bile duct stones. The usual site for the surgical anastomosis between the bile duct and the intestine is the posterior duodenal bulb, where the orifice is usually easily identified and cannulated. If the choledochoduodenostomy orifice is sufficiently large, spillage of contrast back into the duodenum presents a problem. This can be overcome by cannulating the orifice with a balloon catheter and inflating the balloon to occlude the opening. Cholangiography can then be done in the standard fashion.

Complications of ERCP

In the past, the morbidity of ERCP was commonly reported to be approximately 10% with a 1% mortality. Clearly, in the light of improving technical skills and better equipment, these figures have improved. The data from Freeman and associates suggest a complication rate of 9.8%, with a procedure-related mortality of 0.4% in patients undergoing sphincterotomy. The incidence of complications depends on many factors, ranging from the indication for the procedure, whether it is diagnostic or therapeutic, what interventions were performed (e.g., sphincterotomy, biliary manometry), the skill level of the endoscopist, and so forth. Although it is difficult to prove, complications may have some direct relationship to the skill and experience of the endoscopist. In the past, it has been difficult to compare studies reporting complications because of lack of uniform definitions.

Currently, the most commonly used definitions of ERCP

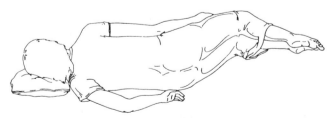

Figure 35–2
A patient positioned for endoscopic retrograde cholangiopancreatography starting in the semi-prone position. Note the position of the left arm behind the back to facilitate fluoroscopy and rolling the patient fully prone.

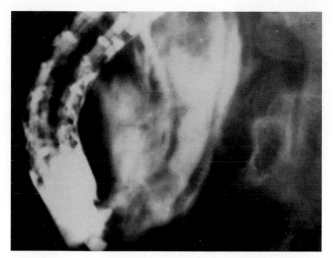

Figure 35–4
Complication of endoscopic retrograde pancreatography. This x-ray taken after endoscopic sphincterotomy shows contrast in the retroduodenal space and air outlining the distal common bile duct. This is a retroperitoneal perforation complicating sphincterotomy.

complications are those promulgated by Cotton. Pancreatitis remains the the most common complication of diagnostic and therapeutic ERCP and can be fatal in some cases. Vigorous efforts to identify effective prophylaxis against pancreatitis (e.g., using glucagon, octreotide, and corticosteroids) have largely been disappointing. One prospective double-blind, multicenter European trial employing intravenous infusion of gabexate (not yet available in the United States) had encouraging results. A retrospective study of post-ERCP pancreatitis suggested that secretin might be effective in reducing the incidence of this complication. A prospective study is being conducted to evaluate this hypothesis. Initial trials of the platelet activating factor (PAF) inhibitor, lexipafant, suggested benefit if this agent was administered within 24 to 36 hours of the onset of pancreatitis. Unfortunately, a subsequent European trial showed no benefit, and the manufacturer has discontinued funding for clinical evaluation of this drug. Other complications of ERCP include bleeding following endoscopic sphincterotomy, retroduodenal perforation (Fig. 35–4), and sepsis. The latter is a problem when therapeutic endoscopy fails to establish unobstructed biliary drainage. For this reason, all endoscopists attempting to undertake ERCP must be able to effect simple biliary drainage by placing a nasobiliary drain or stent or by performing endoscopic sphincterotomy. A comprehensive review of ERCP complications is beyond the scope of this chapter, and the interested reader is referred to several recent reviews.

NORMAL CHOLANGIOGRAM

Injection of radiographic contrast medium into the biliary tree through the main duodenal papilla (Fig. 35–5) provides excellent anatomic detail. In most cases, the following structures can be identified: the common bile duct, the common hepatic duct, the cystic duct leading to the gallbladder, the bifurcation (hilum), the right and left main intrahepatic

ducts and the secondary and tertiary ducts leading from these. Because of the patient's position, the left intrahepatic ducts are usually filled preferentially, and good visualization of the right system may require repositioning. Endoscopists must be aware of the variability in biliary anatomy, including high and low takeoff of the cystic duct from the extrahepatic biliary tree. The upper limit of normal diameter for the common bile duct (measured by convention in the midduct) is 6 to 8 mm. Most accept a small increase in diameter after cholecystectomy (with an upper limit of 10 mm). It is not uncommon for elderly patients to have gross dilatation of the bile duct without clear pathology. However, in younger patients, a common bile duct exceeding 10 mm in diameter is considered pathologic. Release of bile into the duodenum is not continuous but regulated by the activity of the sphincter of Oddi, a ring of smooth muscle at the level of the ampulla. Sphincter of Oddi dysfunction may be associated with a syndrome of recurrent biliary pain with or without abnormal liver tests or dilatation of the bile duct. In most individuals, the common bile duct is joined by the main pancreatic duct at the level of the ampulla, where they share a final common channel into the duodenum. In patients with pancreas divisum, however, the main pancreatic (dorsal) duct empties through the minor duodenal papilla.

CHOLELITHIASIS AND CHOLEDOCHOLITHIASIS

Overview

The management of stones in the biliary tree has been one of the most successful applications of therapeutic ERCP. Approximately 20 million Americans have gallstones and around 2 million cholecystectomies are performed annually. Symptoms relating to gallstones are a common cause of

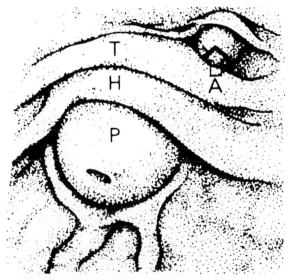

Figure 35–5
The anatomic landmarks of the major and minor duodenal papillae are required knowledge for endoscopic retrograde cholangiopancreatography. P, Main duodenal papilla; H, Hooding fold; T, Transverse fold; A, Accessory (minor) papilla.

hospital admission with estimated direct health care costs exceeding $2 billion yearly. There are two basic types of gallstones: cholesterol stones and pigment stones (the latter are divided into brown stones and black stones). Cholesterol gallstones account for 75% to 80% of the gallstones in the United States. They are found most commonly in middle-aged women, overweight individuals, and patients with ileal disease or after small bowel resection. Pigment stones consist principally of calcium bilirubinate, phosphate, and carbonate salts. They are associated with chronic bacterial or parasitic infections (brown stones) or chronic hemolytic disorders (black pigment stones). Gallstones usually form within the gallbladder. Most individuals with gallstones are asymptomatic. However, acute cholecystitis can develop when a stone lodges in the neck of the gallbladder (Hartmann's pouch) or in the cystic duct. Patients who have had a prior episode of biliary colic have a 60% to 70% chance of developing recurrent gallstone-related problems. Removal of the gallbladder (usually by the laparoscopic approach) is now recommended for this group of patients.

Most common bile duct stones form within the gallbladder and migrate into the bile duct. However, de novo formation of stones within the biliary tree can occur both before and after cholecystectomy (Fig. 35–6). Patients with periampullary diverticula are at increased risk of developing bile duct stones. A unique variant of choledocholithiasis is oriental cholangiohepatitis.

Although this is rare in the United States, chronic infestation of the bile duct with parasites such as *Clonorchis sinensis* and *Fasciola hepatica* is very common in certain parts of the world, including Southeast Asia. The presence of ova and dead worms in the biliary tree promotes the formation of stones. Indeed, these may be found within the stones when they are sectioned and examined microscopically. Stones in the intrahepatic ducts are difficult to access endoscopically and sometimes also radiologically. In patients with recurrent cholangitis related to intrahepatic stone disease, surgical resection may be necessary.

Common problems associated with bile duct stones are acute or intermittent biliary obstruction causing pain, infection (cholangitis), obstructive jaundice, and biliary pancreatitis. The management of common bile duct stones is dictated by the clinical setting. ERCP with stone extraction is possible in many cases; elective ERCP is usually the treatment of choice for documented common bile duct stones. Acute cholangitis complicating gallstone pancreatitis represents a medical emergency and is an indication for urgent ERCP for biliary decompression. Routine ERCP prior to laparoscopic cholecystectomy cannot be recommended; it is not cost-effective and the risk of complications outweighs the benefits. However, for selected patients, particularly those who have had complicated gallstone pancreatitis, ERCP can be performed to clear the bile duct before surgery, allowing the surgeon a single procedure.

Stone Extraction

Sphincterotomy

Endoscopic sphincterotomy revolutionized the management of common bile duct stones. Before its introduction, common duct stones had to be removed surgically by an "open" procedure that carried a considerable morbidity. The endoscopic approach to common bile duct stones is successful in at least 90% of cases in expert hands, and morbidity and mortality rates compare favorably with the surgical approach. In the same expert hands, endoscopic sphincterotomy can be performed with a mortality rate of less than 0.5% and a procedure-related morbidity rate of less than 10%. Endoscopic sphincterotomy is the most invasive procedure routinely performed by GI endoscopists. A sphincterotome is a modified cannula with an exposed wire at the distal end through which an electric current is transmitted. The sphincterotome is inserted into the bile duct, and short bursts of current are applied to incise the SO as well as the roof of the intraduodenal segment of the bile duct. Various less controlled techniques (grouped under the term "pre-cut papillotomy") have been developed to access the biliary tree in difficult cases (Fig. 35–7A–D). Pre-cut techniques carry a significant morbidity and should only be used by experts for therapeutic access. In Freeman's study, 9.8% of patients undergoing endoscopic sphincterotomy had a complication, including pancreatitis (5.4%), bleeding (2%), cholangitis (1%), and perforation (<0.5%). The incidence of late complications of biliary sphincterotomy in studies with extended follow-up for more than 5 to 10 years ranges between 10% and 24%; these complications include stenosis of the sphincterotomy site, recurrent bile duct stones, and cholangitis. This rate of complications compares favorably with the results of surgical exploration and drainage of the

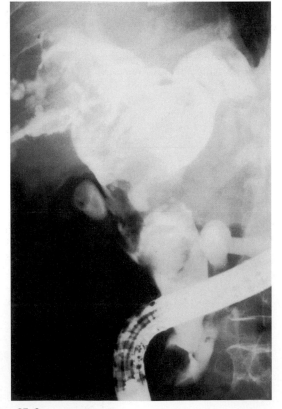

Figure 35–6
Massive choledocholithiasis involving both the intrahepatic and extrahepatic biliary tree, seen at ERCP. A right percutaneous biliary catheter is also present.

Figure 35–7
Precut papillotomy. *A,* Needle knife papillotome is poised, ready to incise the roof of the papillary structure in order to release an impacted stone. The *dotted line* indicates the preferred (safest) axis of cut. *B,* Some operators prefer to make an incision upward, or cephalad. *C,* Some operators prefer to make the incision downward, toward the papillary orifice. This approach cuts down on to the stone, which may be somewhat safer than a "blind" cephalad incision. *D,* After the initial incision using the needle knife, the papillotomy is extended using a standard sphincterotome seated in the bile duct.

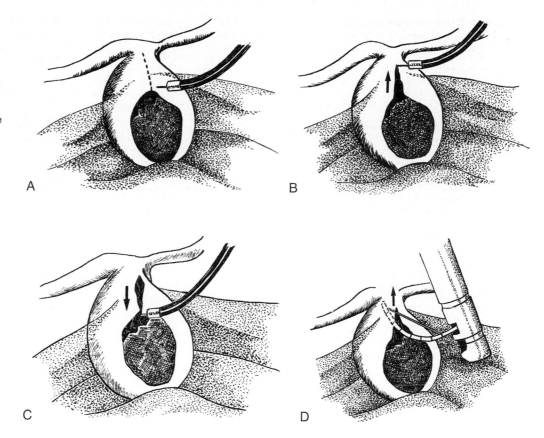

common bile duct. Most of the late complications of ERCP can be managed by additional endoscopic therapy.

Stone Extraction After Sphincterotomy

After successful endoscopic sphincterotomy, removal of common bile duct stones can be achieved in 80% to 95% of patients. Although small stones may pass spontaneously after sphincterotomy, it is unwise to rely on this. Various endoscopic balloons and basket catheters are available to retrieve stones. Forceful traction against resistance should be avoided because this risks traumatic extension of the sphincterotomy. Occasionally, a stone is trapped in a basket in the bile duct such that it cannot be removed or disengaged. In the past, this was a very serious problem because the patient might have to undergo surgery to have the impacted stone and basket removed. Fortunately, over-the-catheter lithotripsy devices can overcome this problem. A commonly used system has a cranking device that pulls the wires of the basket against and into a metal oversleeve. Either the stone or the basket breaks, resolving the problem.

Stone Extraction Through the Intact Papilla

Although sphincterotomy is frequently used to enlarge the opening to the CBD for stone extraction, it has been demonstrated that small stones can be recovered safely through the intact duodenal papilla using balloon or basket catheters. This avoids the immediate and late complications for sphincterotomy, which are particularly likely in the presence of a nondilated bile duct. It is desirable to preserve the bili-

ary sphincter, especially in young patients. The first reported series of patients was from Duke University; a few (mild) complications were encountered, and all of the relatively small stones (<8 mm in diameter) were removed. Mac-Mathuna and associates subsequently reported the use of balloon dilatation to allow large stones (up to and exceeding 20 mm in diameter) to be removed from the common bile duct without sphincterotomy. Surprisingly few complications were seen, but this approach is yet to be widely adopted. MacMathuna and colleagues published work comparing the pathologic effects of sphincterotomy with those of balloon dilatation of the papilla. Using an animal model, they showed that the effects on the local tissue of stretching the biliary sphincter with a balloon were transient and reversible, whereas permanent changes result from sphincterotomy. Stone extraction without sphincterotomy—especially when performed for large stones—can cause significant edema of the papilla and make it difficult to remove all of the stones and debris. When the papilla is already swollen, as in gallstone pancreatitis with an obstructing calculus, sphincterotomy may be necessary to improve biliary drainage, thus balloon dilatation is not always the ideal approach. Data from a U.S. multicenter trial has greatly reduced enthusiasm for so-called balloon sphincteroplasty (BS). When compared with standard endoscopic sphincterotomy, BS had a three-fold higher risk of procedure-related pancreatitis. In this study, all of the severe cases of pancreatitis were seen following BS, and two of these patients died. When large stones are present, mechanical or contact lithotripsy are usually necessary to fragment the stone to facilitate its extraction. Currently, those endoscopists who use the balloon dilatation technique as an alternative to sphincterotomy usually reserve it for easily accessible small stones (<5 to 8 mm in diameter) in young patients in whom it is particularly desirable to avoid sphincter ablation.

Attempts to relax the biliary sphincter with pharmacologic agents have been disappointing despite encouraging early reports that short-acting nitrates allowed the sphincter to relax and facilitated cannulation. The success of botulinum toxin in selected cases of achalasia led investigators to inject the duodenal papilla with this agent in the hope of relaxing the sphincter. Unfortunately, the results were mixed, most likely because it is difficult to accurately target the sphincter mechanism for injection at ERCP. Work on pharmacologic modulation of the duodenal papilla continues, with particular interest in the role of nitrous oxide (NO), which appears to be involved in the regulation of SO contraction.

Difficult Bile Duct Stones

Common bile duct stones that exceed 15 mm in diameter present difficulties for retrieval, because they will not easily pass through a standard sphincterotomy site. Smaller stones can also present difficulties when they are situated proximal to a bile duct stricture or in a tortuous, dilated bile duct (where they may be difficult to capture in a basket). Finally, intrahepatic bile duct stones are notoriously difficult to remove because of their inaccessibility. In some cases, percutaneous procedures or even surgical intervention may be required to deal with difficult biliary calculi. Various techniques are available to facilitate the removal of bile duct stones. These include mechanical lithotripsy, contact lithotripsy (electrohydraulic laser), extracorporeal shock wave lithotripsy, and chemical dissolution. By using one or more of these techniques, almost all biliary calculi can be removed.

Mechanical Lithotripsy

Mechanical lithotriptors consist of a reinforced basket with a mechanical cranking device. After the stone is captured within the wires of the basket, the proximal end of the cable is attached to a crank. This is slowly tightened to close the basket around the stone and break it by mechanical force. Modern mechanical lithotriptors are highly effective with success rates being documented from 75% to 100%. Such is the reliability of mechanical lithotriptors that contact and other forms of lithotripsy are infrequently used now.

Electrohydraulic Lithotripsy

Electrohydraulic lithotripsy has been employed for many years by urologists, who use it to fragment stones in the urinary bladder, renal pelvis, and ureters. This technology has been adapted for endoscopic use by miniaturizing the devices so that they can fit through an instrument channel. They can also be used through percutaneous tracks into the liver, through a mature T-tube tract, or retrogradely into the bile duct through a choledochoscope. In electrohydraulic lithotripsy, rapid conversion of a liquid into its gaseous form results in sudden volume expansion, creating a forceful shock wave that fractures the gallstone. As it is possible to

damage the bile duct wall by misplaced application of energy, this technique is usually done under direct vision using a choledochoscope. This miniaturized endoscope is introduced through the instrument channel of a duodenoscope into the bile duct. The lithotripsy probe is then advanced through a tiny channel in the choledochoscope and its tip directed against the stone. Once suitably small fragments have been created (this can be a rapid process), conventional stone retrieval techniques (e.g., basket, balloon) are used to complete the stone removal. Overall, electrohydraulic lithotripsy is safe and effective; success rates are reported to be approximately 80%. However, equipment costs and the need for a second, well-trained endoscopist to handle the choledochoscope limits the availability of this technique to a few specialist centers.

Laser Lithotripsy

Laser energy can be used to fragment bile duct stones in a mechanism similar to that of electrohydraulic lithotripsy (i.e., the creation of a short wave from a burst of energy at the stone surface). The standard laser used by endoscopists, the neodymium: yttrium-aluminum-garnet (Nd:YAG) laser, is unsuitable for this purpose, however. A laser that emits its energy in discrete pulses—such as a tunable dye laser—is ideal. Typically, a frequency of around 10 Hz (10 pulses/sec) is used. The laser fiber is advanced through the instrument channel of the choledochoscope, and its tip brought into direct contact with the stone to be treated. To reduce the risk of collateral damage to the bile duct wall, so-called "smart lasers" have been developed and tested. The laser has a built-in automatic stone detection system that prevents it firing at anything except a stone. This minimizes the risk of bile duct injury and obviates the need for choledochoscopy. The laser fiber can also be advanced through a modified balloon catheter, and the lithotripsy process can be monitored under fluoroscopy. Laser lithotripsy of bile duct stones can be very effective. However, it is a very expensive technology; the equipment is delicate and costly to maintain; and the procedure is time-consuming and requires several operators. For all of these reasons, its use is limited to a few specialist centers.

Extracorporeal Shock Wave Lithotripsy (ESWL)

ESWL of common bile duct stones represents yet another adaptation of a procedure developed by urologists. ESWL was pioneered in Europe for the treatment of gallbladder stones. However, it is also a useful management option for treating difficult common bile duct stones, especially when contact methods for stone fragmentation are unavailable or have been unsuccessful. ESWL procedures for bile duct stones are usually carried out under fluoroscopy, with contrast being injected into the bile duct through a nasobiliary drain (Fig. 35–8) or percutaneous catheter. Some ESWL devices use ultrasound rather than fluoroscopy to detect their targets. Ultrasound imaging of common bile duct stones is less reliable than fluoroscopy of ducts containing contrast. If a sphincterotomy has already been performed, air in the biliary tree can also add to the difficulty of performing ultrasound examination. Although ESWL is no longer in widespread use for the treatment of gallbladder stones (having

profound sedation and other systemic effects (e.g., hemolysis). For this reason, MTBE is not used in the biliary tree. A search continues for an agent that will reliably disaggregate mixed bile duct stones, but none has been identified to date.

Stents for Stones

When endoscopic techniques fail to completely clear the bile duct of stones, good biliary drainage must be established before finishing the procedure. An endoscopic prosthesis (stent) or nasobiliary drain should be placed in the bile duct to prevent biliary obstruction and its sequel, cholangitis (Fig. 35–9). Thereafter, the patient may be brought back for a further procedure when local edema or bleeding has settled or referred to an expert in another center. Ursodeoxycholic acid may be a useful adjunctive treatment. Alternatives are percutaneous procedures or surgery in patients who are fit enough to have this done. However, many elderly, frail patients are poor candidates even for repeat endoscopy, and this has prompted the use of stents for long-term management of retained bile duct stones. On the whole, this is a successful strategy, although a recent large prospective study from Amsterdam suggests that prolonged stenting has risks (mainly recurrent cholangitis). Because almost all stents occlude if left in the bile duct long enough, stenting for bile duct stones should be regarded as a temporizing maneuver until a more permanent solution is found for the patient's problem.

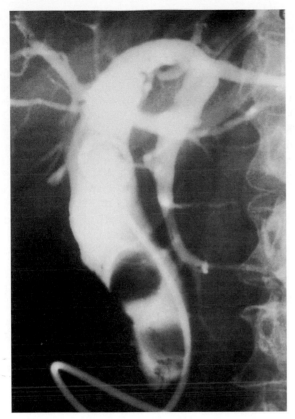

Figure 35–8
Cholangiogram showing retained bile duct stones (two lucencies in the distal duct). A nasobiliary drain has been placed to ensure biliary drainage and to facilitate cholangiography for extracorporeal shockwave lithotripsy (ESWL).

been superseded by laparoscopic cholecystectomy), most centers where ESWL is available for urologic use can "borrow" time on the lithotripter to treat difficult bile duct stones.

Chemical Dissolution Agents

Dissolving bile duct stones by infusing chemical agents through a nasobiliary drain or percutaneous catheter is an attractive concept, but in practice the results have been disappointing. The earliest dissolution agent used was mono-octanoin, a fatty acid derivative, which was infused over a 5- to 8-day period. The dissolution rates for pure cholesterol stones were in the range of 40% to 60%, but the treatment often had to be discontinued because of the patient's intolerance of the agent (e.g., nausea, abdominal cramps, diarrhea) or the nasobiliary tube. This technique is not suitable for mixed stones, which comprise a significant proportion of common bile duct stones. When methyl *tert*-butyl ether (MTBE) was being evaluated for treating cholesterol stones in the gallbladder, there was interest in modifying this approach to deal with common bile duct stones. Unfortunately, it proved impossible to reliably contain this volatile and potentially toxic agent within the bile duct. MTBE leaking from the bile duct into the duodenum can cause a severe duodenitis, and if enough of the ether is absorbed, it causes

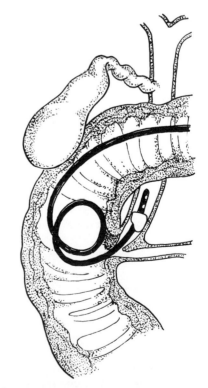

Figure 35–9
Schematic showing nasobiliary drain with the tip in the bile duct beyond a stone; this preserves biliary drainage and prevents cholangitis following endoscopic retrograde cholangiopancreatography with incomplete or failed stone extraction.

ERCP IN RELATION TO LAPAROSCOPIC CHOLECYSTECTOMY

Laparoscopic cholecystectomy (LC) has now been widely adopted as the treatment of choice for symptomatic cholelithiasis. This has had an impact on the practice of biliary endoscopy in numerous ways. When LC was first introduced, endoscopists saw many patients with iatrogenic bile duct injuries as well as cystic duct leaks. This early rush of complications reflected the learning curve for surgeons performing this laparoscopic procedure. Although LC-related biliary problems have greatly diminished with increasing experience, endoscopists still see them occasionally.

Common Bile Duct Stones

It has been important to develop an algorithm for the management of suspected or proven bile duct stones in patients undergoing LC (Fig. 35–10). There are ample data in the surgical literature to allow stratification of patients with cholelithiasis into low- (<5%), medium-, and high- (>20%) risk for common bile duct stones (choledocholithiasis). The risk factors for choledocholithiasis include cholestatic liver function tests, jaundice, dilated bile duct on ultrasound with or without stones seen, and cholangitis. Interestingly, recent pancreatitis is not a reliable risk factor, because small stones causing gallstone pancreatitis usually pass spontaneously (i.e., they are usually gone by the time a radiologic study is done to look for them). Many surgeons request ERCP before LC to assess the bile duct for stones and, if necessary remove, them. This strategy allows the surgeon to plan a single procedure. Thus, if the endoscopist fails to cannulate the bile duct or remove stones that have been visualized, the surgeon can perform an intraoperative cholangiogram (IOC) or, when appropriate, convert a laparoscopic to an open procedure to remove bile duct stones. In our opinion, routine pre-LC ERCP cannot be justified. The yield of bile duct stones is low in the absence of the aforementioned risk factors, and ERCP exposes patients to the risk of complications, which for some patients greatly exceed those of laparoscopic surgery. Because every surgeon who performs laparoscopic cholecystectomy should have

the training and skills to perform IOC, ERCP to outline the biliary anatomy is an unjustifiable use of this procedure. As evidenced by existing studies, patients who have gallstone pancreatitis with biliary obstruction (jaundice, cholangitis) may benefit from early ERCP to decompress the biliary tree. In this small group of patients, pre-LC ERCP is justified. Also, in patients in whom there is some genuine doubt about the likely success of ERCP (e.g., in those who have had prior Billroth II gastrectomy), a preoperative study may be justified to plan the subsequent management. The preferred management of suspected choledocholithiasis is for the patient to proceed direct to LC with IOC being performed. Those patients who have stones demonstrated by IOC can have ERCP for bile duct clearance before they go home, usually the day after surgery. Clearly, the current use of ERCP in relation to LC is greatly influenced by the skill of the individual endoscopist and by the willingness and ability of the surgeon to perform IOC.

Bile Duct Leaks

Bile leaks most commonly follow gallbladder surgery but can result from ductal disruption associated with blunt or sharp trauma or iatrogenic injury (e.g., liver biopsy). A patient who develops abdominal pain and low-grade fever soon after LC requires investigation for a possible bile leak or other complication of the procedure. Noninvasive, cross-sectional abdominal imaging with ultrasound scanning or CT may detect a localized collection of bile (biloma) or sometimes bile lying free in the peritoneum. Any significant collection of bile requires percutaneous or surgical drainage. Although a radioisotope biliary excretion study (e.g., hepato-iminodiacetic acid [HIDA] scan) may provide evidence of a bile leak, cholangiography is required to define the exact site. ERCP is the preferred approach in most centers. PTC is reserved for patients in whom endoscopic access has been unsuccessful or who have leaked from sequestered parts of the liver (i.e., that are not in communication with the main ductal system). Most bile duct leaks after LC result from slipped clips or other closure devices that have been applied to the cystic duct stump (Fig. 35–11). Injuries to the common bile duct, common hepatic duct, or more proximal bile ducts from cautery or misplaced clips can result in leakage as well as early and delayed biliary strictures. High bile duct injuries such as those involving the hilum and intrahepatic ducts can result in parts of the liver being sequestered; that is, their ductal drainage systems no longer communicate with the rest of the biliary tree. Depending on the site and nature of the injury, there may be an associated leak that cannot be demonstrated by retrograde cholangiography. When a patient clearly has a bile duct leak, as evidenced by persistent biloma, and ERCP fails to demonstrate a site of extravasation, this particular problem should be considered. As the area involved is usually decompressed by the leak, there are no dilated ducts to be seen on cross-sectional imaging. Therefore, a percutaneous cholangiogram must be performed. Because PTC is technically difficult when the bile ducts are not dilated, the services of a skilled vascular radiologist are necessary.

When a cystic duct leak is identified at ERCP, placement of a stent across the duodenal papilla is usually adequate therapy (Fig. 35–12). Routine performance of a sphincter-

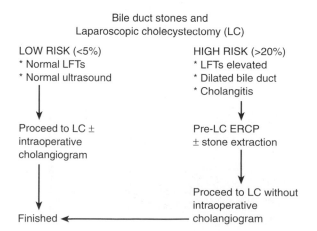

Figure 35–10
Algorithm for management of suspected bile duct stones in relation to a laparoscopic cholecystectomy.

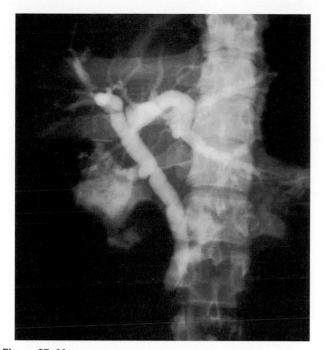

Figure 35–11
Cystic duct stump leak following a laparoscopic cholecystectomy. The "cloud" of contrast emerging from the cystic duct stump is a leak into the subhepatic space.

otomy for cystic duct leaks is unjustifiable, because it exposes the patient to additional risks and is unnecessary. Sphincterotomy should be reserved for patients who have mechanical obstruction at the level of the papilla, such as those with an obstructing stone or true papillary stenosis. It is probably unnecessary to insert a stent that is long enough to bridge the origin of the cystic duct. The simple act of bridging the papilla and providing a low-pressure route for bile to exit seems adequate. There are no data to indicate that a large stent is any better than a small one, but we tend to put in the largest stent that comfortably fits across the papilla (usually a 10 French gauge). Bile duct leaks usually close within days of this treatment, and we routinely ask patients to return in 2 to 4 weeks' time to have the stent removed. Biliary stents should not be left in place for longer than 3 months because of the risk of occlusion with subsequent cholangitis. In a few patients, stenting does not result in resolution of the leak. If a 7 French stent has been placed, the size of the stent may be increased to a 10 French stent in the hope that a larger caliber stent will provide better flow. Alternatively, some endoscopists perform a sphincterotomy at this point.

Persistent leaks are an indication for PTC to assess the presence of an unsuspected accessory duct that was not apparent on the initial examination. There is great variation in the anatomy of the bile ducts, and some patients with leaks have had injuries or transection of accessory bile ducts, the best known being the accessory duct of Luschka. Finally, patients who have very persistent leaks require surgery to deal with these. Sometimes, the leak site is so large that it will not close spontaneously. We have seen this in the setting of avulsed cystic duct stumps and more proximal extrahepatic bile duct injuries. Before surgery to deal with these

problems, percutaneous cholangiography and drain placement are usually necessary.

The published results of endoscopic management of biliary leaks suggest that this is a largely successful and cost-effective management strategy. Drastic injuries to the bile duct, which end in complete transection, result in leaks that cannot be resolved using endoscopic or percutaneous biliary drainage. These injuries require early surgery for repair, which usually requires a biliary diversion. Bile leaks are also seen after liver transplantation. The leak may occur at the bile duct anastomosis or result from persistence of the choledochocutaneous fistula formed by the T-tube. These leaks usually respond to endoscopic therapy, although experience shows that stents or drains must be left in place much longer than in nonimmunosuppressed patients to guarantee healing. Anastomotic breakdown (which is usually an ischemic process) requires surgery. Figure 35–13*A* and *B* outline management algorithms for bile duct leaks depending on whether or not the leak is demonstrated by ERCP.

Benign Bile Duct Strictures

Causes of benign bile duct strictures are listed in Table 35–3. Iatrogenic injury at the time of open or laparoscopic gallbladder surgery is probably the most common cause of benign biliary strictures (Fig. 35–14). Postsurgical strictures are not uncommon after orthotopic liver transplantation, particularly at the site of anastomosis of the bile ducts (Fig. 35–15). Complete transection of a bile duct by a surgical clip or suture is a catastrophic injury that declares itself

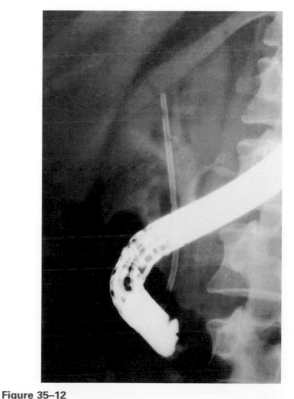

Figure 35–12
A 7 French gauge polyethylene biliary stent has been placed in the bile duct with its distal tip in the duodenum to manage a cystic duct stump leak after laparoscopic cholecystectomy.

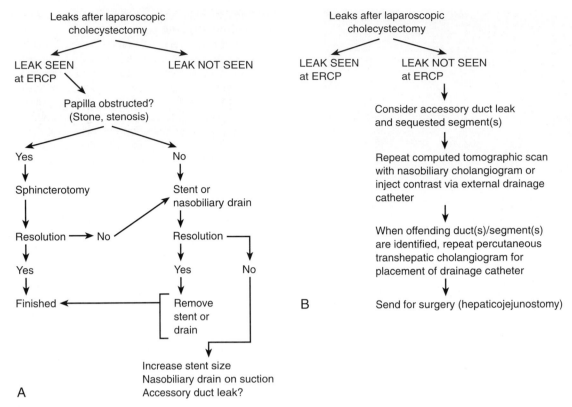

Figure 35–13
Management of bile leaks after laparoscopic cholecystectomy. *A,* Management algorithm when leaks can be seen at endoscopic retrograde cholangiopancreatography (ERCP). *B,* Management algorithm when leaks are not seen at ERCP.

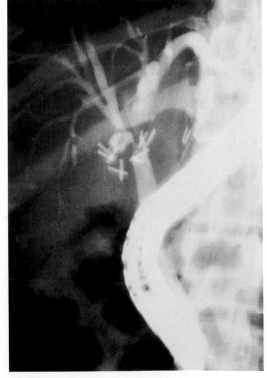

Figure 35–14
Iatrogenic biliary stricture at the liver hilum following a laparoscopic cholecystectomy. The injury is in the vicinity of multiple surgical clips.

quickly (Fig. 35–16) within days, the patient exhibits signs and symptoms of biliary obstruction, including jaundice and itching. Lesser degrees of ductal injury (short of transection) may result in early or late strictures. Many of these injuries result from trauma to local vasculature, causing an ischemic injury. Ischemic strictures may present from days to years after the initial insult. Other causes of bile duct strictures such as external compression due to chronic pancreatitis, pseudocysts, or stones in the gallbladder neck or cystic duct (i.e., Mirizzi's syndrome, Fig. 35–17) need to be considered.

The first step in evaluating a benign biliary stricture is to ascertain that this stricture is truly benign. If there is any doubt about the nature of a newly diagnosed stricture, tissue sampling should be performed using brush cytology, fine needle aspiration (FNA), or biopsy. Doubt about the nature

Table 35–3   Causes of Benign Bile Duct Strictures

Congenital (including biliary atresia)
Acquired
  Trauma—nonoperative or operative (including ischemia)
  Sclerosing cholangitis (primary and secondary)
  Liver transplantation
  Chronic pancreatitis
  Pancreatic pseudocysts
  Mirizzi's syndrome
  Vascular indentation
  Congenital hepatic cysts

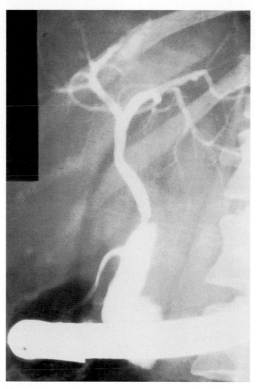

Figure 35–15
Anastomotic bile duct stricture (seen at the junction of the donor and recipient bile ducts) after an orthotopic liver transplantation. This cholangiogram also shows a leak caused by the persistence of the T-tube track, a problem that is not common in these chronically immunosuppressed patients. (From Baillie J: Gastrointestinal Endoscopy: Beyond the Basics. Boston, MA: Butterworth-Heinemann, 1997.)

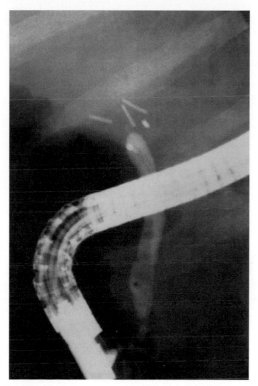

Figure 35–16
Complete transection of the extrahepatic bile duct, an iatrogenic injury resulting from laparoscopic cholecystectomy.

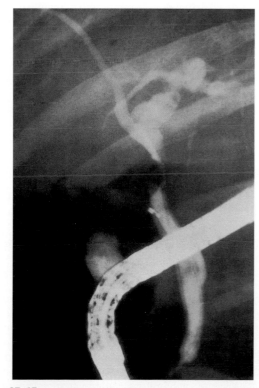
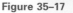

Figure 35–17
Mirizzi's syndrome. The smooth, extrinsic compression of the common hepatic duct mimics malignancy, but in this case it is due to the presence of a stone lodged in the cystic duct or the neck of the gallbladder.

of a stricture arises when there has been no clear history of trauma (operative or otherwise) or predisposing factor, such as inflammatory bowel disease with associated sclerosing cholangitis. Most benign postoperative biliary strictures are ischemic. These strictures almost always progress, although spontaneous resolution has occasionally been reported. These unusual recoveries may result from resolution of edema rather than from reversal of fibrosis. The early recognition of biliary strictures is crucial to avoid long-term complications, including cholangitis, secondary biliary cirrhosis, and portal hypertension. If the stricture is in the extrahepatic bile duct or at the bifurcation (hilum) (see Fig. 35–14), it is justifiable to attempt endoscopic or percutaneous radiologic dilatation with or without stenting. Strictures (especially those that are multiple) involving the smaller intrahepatic bile ducts are not amenable to these interventions. Once accessible strictures have been dilated using either balloon catheters or graduated (step) dilators, endoprostheses (stents) are often inserted to maintain their patency. These stents are left in place for 3 to 6 months; then they are removed. A biliary stricture that persists after two or even three dilatations and stent placements is unlikely to resolve spontaneously. Patients with such resistant strictures should be advised to undergo surgical diversion in order to avoid the longer-term risks of biliary obstruction and sepsis. Patients who suffer injuries to the bile duct at the time of lapa-

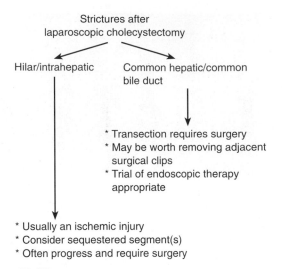

Figure 35–18
Algorithm for management of biliary strictures following laparoscopic cholecystectomy.

roscopic cholecystectomy seldom do well from attempts from primary repair. Those patients who fail endoscopic therapy (a significant proportion) often proceed to have surgical biliary diversion, typically hepaticojejunostomy. Given the significant medicolegal implications of iatrogenic injury to the bile ducts, it is very important that treatment be tailored to the individual's needs (Fig. 35–18). Although it may be in the best interest of a frail, elderly patient to have a prolonged trial of endoscopic therapy, younger patients may be served better by early reconstructive surgery. Patients who have persistent benign strictures without obvious cause should be monitored closely for the development of malignancy. This is particularly the case in patients with known or suspected primary sclerosing cholangitis (PSC), which is associated with an increased risk for cholangiocarcinoma. These tumors are often difficult to diagnose, because they may grow along the bile duct without a significant mass visible on cross-sectional imaging, such as CT.

PRIMARY SCLEROSING CHOLANGITIS

PSC is a chronic cholestatic disorder characterized by diffuse inflammatory fibrosis of the intra- and extrahepatic bile ducts. Although the pathogenesis of PSC remains unclear, it is one of several conditions commonly associated with inflammatory bowel disease, especially ulcerative colitis (Table 35–4).

The cholangiographic appearances of PSC are almost (but not quite) unique; ERCP has increased the number of patients being diagnosed with PSC at an asymptomatic stage. Thinning of the intrahepatic bile ducts with multifocal strictures and areas of dilatation are characteristic in PSC (Fig. 35–19). In the extrahepatic bile duct, PSC may be manifest as a solitary stricture (Fig. 35–20), which may be dominant in terms of symptoms and biochemical abnormalities. ERCP helps to determine the severity and extent of intra- and extrahepatic involvement in PSC. As the disease progresses, patients may develop worsening cholestasis and

intermittent cholangitis. In the absence of effective medical therapy, perhaps a third of patients with PSC eventually require liver transplantation. PSC is a good indication for liver transplantation, because the operative morbidity and mortality are low with excellent survival. The intrahepatic strictures of PSC are generally diffuse and multifocal and, therefore, rarely amenable to endoscopic therapy. If a dominant extrahepatic stricture is the cause of recurrent cholangitis, endoscopic therapy with stricture dilatation and stenting should be considered, because it is likely to reduce the risk of cholestasis and infective complications.

For the endoscopist considering ERCP as a way to diagnose and treat PSC, the following questions are appropriate. First, what is the indication for the procedure? Although ERCP is indicated to make the initial diagnosis (often in the setting of unexplained liver function test abnormalities or pruritus), it is not acceptable to follow the progress of uncomplicated PSC with serial ERCPs at regular intervals. Therapeutic indications for ERCP include stricture dilatation and stenting (after cytologic brushing) as well as stone removal. These therapeutic interventions may symptomatically improve the patient, but there is no evidence that they reverse the underlying pathologic process. Patients with progressive liver disease in PSC who are destined for liver transplantation can be kept well by endoscopic or interventional radiology procedures until they are ready to receive a new liver. The next consideration for the endoscopist regarding the patient with PSC is whether or not the intended intervention may make the surgeon's job more difficult, either for biliary bypass or for liver transplantation. For this reason, most endoscopists believe that expandable metal mesh stents should not be put in the bile duct in benign disease. Before any endoscopic intervention in PSC, it is most important to provide antibiotic prophylaxis against gram-negative sepsis.

The next important question for endoscopists performing ERCP on patients with PSC is to determine if a new stricture is malignant. There is a strong association between

Table 35–4   Classification of Sclerosing Cholangitis

Primary

Unknown cause/associated with other diseases (e.g., ulcerative colitis)

Secondary

Known or suspected causes
   Surgical trauma
   Bile duct stones
   Cholangiocarcinoma
   Toxic chemicals (e.g., formaldehyde)
   Ischemia
   Intrahepatic arterial floxuridine (and derivatives)
   Liver transplant rejection
   Histiocytosis X
   AIDS (*Cryptosporidium* infection)

Adapted from Lu SC, Kaplowitz N: Diseases of the biliary tree. In Yamada T, et al (eds): Textbook of Gastroenterology. Philadelphia: JB Lippincott, 1991.

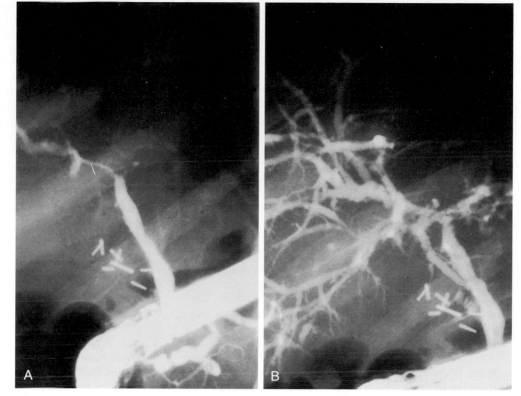

Figure 35–19
Sclerosing cholangitis (endoscopic retrograde cholangiopancreatography). *A,* Unaided retrograde cholangiography in a patient with primary sclerosing cholangitis (PSC) fails to reveal much of the intrahepatic biliary tree. *B,* Occlusion cholangiography—where contrast is injected under pressure beyond a balloon catheter (not visible) inflated in the extrahepatic bile duct—reveals the characteristic strictures and small duct irregularity of PSC.

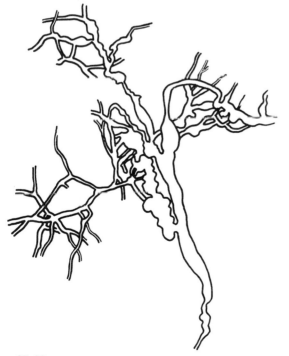

Figure 35–20
Primary sclerosing cholangitis (PSC). Tracing from an actual cholangiogram demonstrating intrahepatic disease plus a solitary extrahepatic stricture; only the latter is amenable to endoscopic therapy. (From Baillie J: Gastrointestinal Endoscopy: Beyond the Basics. Boston, MA: Butterworth-Heinemann, 1997.)

sclerosing cholangitis and the development of cholangiocarcinoma (risk of 7% to 9%). Often these tumors cannot be visualized on CT scanning (at least in their early stages), thus endoscopic brushing and other tissue sampling methods are important. Overall, the sensitivity of endoscopic brush cytology is in the range of 40% to 60%. The yield of malignant diagnoses can be increased by adjunctive techniques such as flow cytometry, ploidy studies, determination of K-*ras*-oncogene status, and so forth. Direct biopsy of accessible biliary tumors and core biopsies or aspiration specimens are also excellent tools for diagnosing malignancy. CA 19-9, a serologic marker for some malignancies, is helpful in the diagnosis of cholangiocarcinoma, although it lacks specificity. It has been said that dilatation of bile ducts above (proximal to) an extrahepatic biliary stricture is highly suggestive of the development of malignancy. There is some truth to this observation. Because sclerosing cholangitis is a chronic fibrosing condition, it is difficult for the bile ducts to dilate until there is significant pressure generated by obstruction. Certainly, in our experience, new bile duct dilatation is often a clue to malignancy. In patients who have progressive cholestasis and liver injury associated with extensive PSC, liver transplantation may be the definitive therapy. In such patients, endoscopic maneuvers such as dilatation and stenting of strictures are temporizing. In other patients whose PSC is not associated with chronic liver disease but who have problems with recurrent cholangitis, biliary bypass surgery remains an option. In view of the potential for patients with PSC to need some form of biliary surgery (up to and including transplantation), it is very important that endoscopic or percutaneous procedures do not make the surgeon's job more difficult. As previously stated, we believe that it is inappropriate to use currently available-expandable metal mesh stents for benign strictures in PSC, because these stents can prejudice the patient's future options for surgical intervention. It is not impossible to perform biliary surgery with an expandable metal mesh stent in place, but it certainly makes such operations technically demanding. This is a good example of why patients with PSC should be managed by a multidisciplinary team, including the gastroenterologist/endoscopist, hepatologist, and transplant surgeon.

SPHINCTER OF ODDI DYSFUNCTION

The flow of bile into the duodenum is not continuous but regulated by the sphincter of Oddi, a ring of smooth muscle fibers that encircle the distal common bile duct at the level of the ampulla. The physiology of the sphincter of Oddi is complex and incompletely understood but probably involves a combination of neural, paracrine, and endocrine inputs. We know that when the gallbladder contracts, the sphincter of Oddi relaxes to allow a bolus of bile to be expelled into the duodenum to aid digestion. Manometric measurement of the sphincter of Oddi can be performed during ERCP, using a specialized manometry catheter. The resting pressure of the sphincter of Oddi is 5 to 15 mm Hg. Phasic contractions occur 3 to 7 times per minute, which raise the pressure to 30 to 150 mm Hg. Sphincter of Oddi dysfunction is a relatively uncommon disorder but should be suspected in patients with episodic biliary-type pain after cholecystectomy. The Geenen-Hogan classification of sphincter of Oddi dysfunction is based on the presence or absence of typical pain, abnormal elevation of liver enzymes (aminotransferases), dilatation of the common bile duct, and delayed drainage of contrast from the biliary tree after ERCP (Table 35–5). Sphincter of Oddi dysfunction is recognized manometrically by high resting sphincter pressure (>40 mm Hg), sustained elevation in pressures during contraction, and abnormal responses to cholecystokinin (CCK) or a fatty meal. Dysfunction of the sphincter of Oddi comprises two separate entities, papillary stenosis (a structural abnormality) and sphincter of Oddi dyskinesia (a motor or motility disorder). These entities are difficult to diagnose and manage. Although perhaps 70% of patients with type I Geenen-Hogan sphincter of Oddi dysfunction get symptomatic improvement from endoscopic sphincterotomy, this falls to less than 20% in type III. Endoscopists with an interest in ERCP see patients with a wide variety of chronic pain syndromes, most of which are not caused by sphincter of Oddi dysfunction and which therefore do not benefit from endoscopic sphincterotomy. The risk of pancreatitis following ERCP, sphincter of Oddi manometry, and endoscopic sphincterotomy in Freeman's study was quite high (21.7%). Careful selection of patients for ERCP, manometry, and sphincterotomy is very important and rewards attention to stratification using radiologic, biochemical, and symptom criteria.

Papillary stenosis is a structural abnormality that describes fibrosis and subsequent narrowing of the sphincteric portion of the distal common bile duct. The pathophysiologic events that result in papillary stenosis are poorly understood. It may result from repeated trauma from passage of small biliary calculi. Papillitis, an inflammatory condition of the duodenal papilla, occurs mainly in immunosuppressed patients and is sometimes associated with viral infection (e.g., cytomegalovirus [CMV], human immunodeficiency virus [HIV]). Patients with papillary stenosis may have classic symptoms of biliary obstruction with constant or intermittent biliary-type pain. They also have abnormal liver tests and radiologic (e.g., ultrasound) evidence of biliary dilatation. The symptoms usually persist and sometimes worsen after cholecystectomy, which removes a distensible reservoir (gallbladder) and exacerbates the effects of impaired bile flow. This is one form of the postcholecystectomy syndrome. When one reviews the history of patients presenting with papillary stenosis, these patients have often undergone cholecystectomy for presumed gallstones. However, when examined by a pathologist, the gallbladder may appear normal. The fibrotic nature of the disorder makes endoscopic cannulation of the bile duct technically difficult in some cases. When the endoscopic approach fails, percutaneous access (alone or for a combined procedure) is an option. A few patients may require a formal surgical procedure, namely sphincteroplasty. Endoscopic sphincterotomy for papillary stenosis carries an increased risk of complications such as pancreatitis, bleeding, and perforation. However, when undertaken successfully, sphincterotomy often provides permanent relief of the patient's symptoms. Endoscopic stenting or balloon dilatation rarely improves matters and carries a high risk of causing pancreatitis in this particular patient population. These procedures cannot be recommended in papillary stenosis. In their classic paper in 1989, Geenen and Hogan suggested that sphincter stenosis and dysmotility should be considered together as part of an sphincter of Oddi dysfunction syndrome (see Table 35–5).

Table 35–5 Modified Geenen-Hogan Classification of Sphincter of Oddi Dysfunction (Excludes Delayed Drainage)

Geenen-Hogan Class	Pain	Abnormal LFTs on 2 or More Occasions	Dilated Common Bile Duct ≥12 mm in Diameter
I	Yes	Yes	Yes
II	Yes	Yes	No
	Yes	No	Yes
III	Yes	No	No

LFT, Liver function tests.

Patients in group I present with typical biliary pain, elevated liver test results documented on two occasions or more with a dilated bile duct (>12 mm in diameter) or delayed drainage of contrast (>45 minutes from the common bile duct) during ERCP. Using sphincter of Oddi manometry, motor dysfunction has been recorded in approximately 70% of these patients. In this group, stenosis of the sphincter appears to dominate. Endoscopic sphincterotomy in patients in group I almost always abolishes symptoms. For this reason, manometry is considered unnecessary, and the endoscopist can proceed directly to sphincterotomy.

Patients in group II have a biliary type of pain but only one of the two other criteria listed for group I. Sphincter of Oddi dysfunction occurs in approximately 50% of patients in group II; manometry can be helpful in this group. In a randomized, double-blind, prospective study of patients in group II, those with manometric abnormalities were significantly more likely to benefit from sphincterotomy than were patients with normal manometry.

Patients in group III present clinically with a pain syndrome only. The pain may be caused by sphincter of Oddi dysfunction but more often is functional or the result of some other, nonbiliary disorder (chest wall pain syndromes and esophageal pain are common). In patients in group III, sphincter of Oddi manometry is abnormal in less than 20% of cases. Even in this subgroup, only 50% improve after sphincterotomy. Given the greater risk of sphincterotomy in patients with sphincter of Oddi dysfunction compared with sphincterotomy for stone disease, biliary manometry and sphincterotomy in patients in group III should only be undertaken after careful clinical evaluation and detailed explanation of the risks and benefits.

Referral for evaluation of possible "biliary pain" represents a significant percentage of patients seen in dedicated biliary clinics. Often, these patients have already undergone extensive clinical, radiologic, and laboratory testing without a diagnosis being made. Unfortunately, chronic abdominal pain, which may involve the right upper quadrant, may arise from a large number of sources including the chest wall and pleura, esophagus, stomach and duodenum, colon, and kidneys. ERCP must be used judiciously, because the risk-benefit equation may be weighted against the patient if a diagnosis of biliary or pancreatic pathology is unlikely. The uncritical use of ERCP to investigate patients with dubious evidence of biliary or pancreatic problems results in unnecessary misery for patients who develop complications and is a fertile source of medical malpractice litigation in the United States. As biliary manometry is only available in specialist centers, patients with suspected sphincter of Oddi dysfunction should be referred to such centers for evaluation. Further research is needed to develop better strategies to stratify these patients for management and to assess the outcome and cost-effectiveness of treatment in these difficult to manage patients.

MALIGNANT BILE DUCT STRICTURES

Malignancies Affecting the Biliary Tree

Malignancies resulting in bile duct strictures can be divided into primary and secondary (Table 35–6) types: primary ma-

Table 35–6   Malignant Tumors of the Biliary Tree

Primary

Cholangiocarcinoma
Hepatocellular carcinoma
Gallbladder carcinoma

Secondary

Pancreatic tumors, including adenocarcinoma and lymphoma
Metastatic malignancy (e.g., colon, breast, bronchus)

lignancies are those arising from biliary epithelium or closely adjacent tissues and include cholangiocarcinoma, hepatocellular carcinoma, and gallbladder cancer. Secondary malignancies cause biliary strictures by extrinsic compression of the bile ducts; they include pancreatic tumors (e.g., adenocarcinoma, lymphoma) and metastatic malignancy (e.g., colon, breast, bronchus).

Because the management and prognosis of each of these types of malignancy is unique, a vigorous effort must be made to identify the tissue of origin. A few tumors that cause biliary strictures are amenable to surgical resection, but it is important to identify these cases because removal of the tumor may be the patient's only hope for cure or prolonged survival. Staging of such tumors may include CT scanning with or without portography (imaging of the portal vein) and hepatic arteriography. Vascular encasement or invasion (i.e., of the hepatic artery, superior mesenteric artery, or portal vein) are usually contraindications to attempting curative resection. Whereas curative surgery may be impossible, surgery for biliary and sometimes gastric bypass provides useful palliation in carefully selected cases. In patients with distal malignant bile duct strictures (ampullary cancer is a good example), laparoscopic biliary and gastric bypass may be an option, reducing the morbidity of the surgery and getting patients home as quickly as possible. The gallbladder should not be used for biliary bypass (i.e., cholecystenterostomy) unless the tumor and cystic duct orifice are at least 2 cm apart. Endoscopic and percutaneous stenting procedures remain the mainstay of palliation for malignant biliary obstruction.

Diagnostic Options

Clinical Considerations

In older patients, an unexplained bile duct stricture should be considered malignant until proved otherwise. Multiple biliary strictures are usually limited to sclerosing cholangitis, both primary and secondary (including AIDS cholangiopathy). New onset of jaundice, a dramatically worsening stricture, gross biliary dilatation upstream from the stricture, and systemic signs and symptoms (e.g., pain, itching, weight loss) must be considered suspicious for the development of cholangiocarcinoma. This is usually a disease of the sixth and seventh decade, although young patients with inflammatory bowel disease and sclerosing cholangitis may develop malignancy. Approximately 10% of patients with cholangiocarcinoma have ulcerative colitis or Crohn's disease. Patients with tumors arising above the bifurcation may not become jaundiced but usually have elevation in serum alkaline phosphatase and aminotransferases. Cross-sectional imaging (CT being the best) in such cases usually reveals segmental or lobar duct dilatation. These cases are worth identifying, because unilateral drainage of the biliary tree will afford symptomatic relief from pain and itching in most cases. The following sections discuss ancillary diagnostic tools used to identify bile duct cancer. Because 95% of bile duct cancers are adenocarcinomas, the focus is primarily on the diagnosis of these tumors.

Imaging Techniques (Other Than ERCP)

Many radiologic techniques are available to study the biliary tree, including transabdominal ultrasonography, CT, magnetic resonance imaging (MRI), arteriography and, most recently, EUS, and positron emission tomography (PET). Transabdominal ultrasound examination has a high sensitivity for detecting the level of biliary obstruction, and for detecting bile duct stones. Unfortunately, it is very operator dependent.

A lesion causing biliary obstruction at the level of the pancreatic head may be difficult to identify by ultrasound because of overlying bowel gas. Ultrasound benefits from being portable and relatively inexpensive. Doppler ultrasound has the additional benefit of demonstrating vascular flow. CT, which is considerably more complex and expensive, requires the administration of oral and intravenous contrast media, with small but not negligible contrast reaction risk. CT shows the structures adjacent to the biliary tree (including lymph nodes) very well, thus it is usually the imaging modality that suggests the underlying diagnosis. Spiral CT, delayed-phase imaging, CT portography, and CT arteriography can provide useful information about biliary tumors in selected cases (Fig. 35–21). Small cholangiocarcinomas can be difficult to visualize because of the lack of

contrast with adjacent tissues. Only about 30% of patients with cholangiocarcinoma have space-occupying lesions that are visible on standard CT scans. Hilar cholangiocarcinomas tend to be hyperdense mass lesions with irregular margins, which can often be demonstrated by delayed-phase CT scanning. This is because of differences in contrast retention between the tumor itself and surrounding fibrotic or sclerotic tissue. Under CT or ultrasound guidance, FNA biopsy of a mass at the level of bile duct obstruction often yields the diagnosis of malignancy.

MRI of the biliary tree has become a useful tool, because rapid scanning, respiratory compensation, and fat suppression techniques have greatly enhanced its resolution. One study from England showed that MRI was equivalent to ERCP in demonstrating the level of biliary obstruction. Heavily T_2-weighted resonance images make bile "light up" (because of its water content), accurately revealing the course of the entire biliary tree. MRI is proving to be useful in the pancreas also, showing parenchymal and ductal abnormalities that may not be accessible at ERCP. At some point, MRCP seems likely to replace much of diagnostic ERCP: MRI scans do not require the patient to be sedated or to receive intraductal contrast, nor do they cause pancreatitis. PET has shown promise in diagnosing biliary and pancreatic malignancy. In this technique, a sugar radiolabeled with a positron (antiparticle of the electron) emitting isotope (usually ^{18}F) is selectively retained by tumor cells, creating a "hot spot" when the tumor site is scanned for positron emissions. Although it has shown promise in early studies, PET scanning for biliary and pancreatic tumors remains a research tool. Arteriography is used mainly for tumor staging; determination of vascular involvement is the principal role for this test. EUS has been used to stage bile duct cancers. The sensitivity of EUS for estimating the depth of tumor invasion is approximately 85%. Miniature EUS probes designed for direct examination of the bile ducts via percutaneous tracts or the transpapillary route have proved potentially valuable but remain research tools.

Tissue Sampling

The definitive diagnosis of malignancy depends on tissue sampling. Techniques available to obtain tissue for diagnosis include exfoliative cytology, endoscopic forceps biopsy, endoscopic FNA, and radiologic FNA.

Exfoliative Cytology: Duodenal aspirates in patients with biliary and pancreatic cancer may contain malignant cells. However, this simple technique is limited by a 5% to 10% false-positive rate. Direct sampling of bile at ERCP has a disappointingly low sensitivity (6% to 26%) for detecting cancer. Prior dilatation of the stricture may increase the yield. Overall, the diagnostic yield of exfoliative cytology alone is low.

Brush Cytology: Using an endoscopic brush would be expected to increase the yield of malignant cells for biliary tumors (Fig. 35–22). Foutch reviewed the world literature and reported an overall sensitivity of 59%, with higher sensitivity in cholangiocarcinoma than in pancreatic cancer. Repeated brushing may increase the cytologic yield. Lee and colleagues evaluated endoscopic bile duct brush cytol-

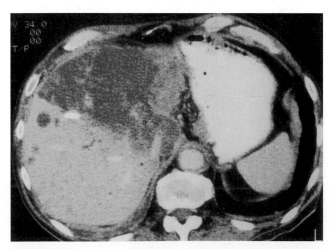

Figure 35–21
Contrast-enhanced computed tomography (CT) scan showing a large mass lesion involving part of the right lobe of the liver and most of the left (darker area of the liver scan). There are no significantly dilated bile ducts so that this patient's jaundice would not benefit from endoscopic or percutaneous biliary drainage.

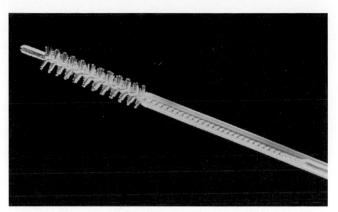

Figure 35–22
Cytology brush of the type used for biliary and pancreatic brush cytology.

ogy, stratifying samples into benign, low-grade, and high-grade dysplasia. Overall, the finding of dysplasia had a 37% sensitivity and 100% specificity for bile duct cancer.

The combination of brush cytology, FNA, and forceps biopsy has a greater sensitivity (~80%) than any single modality alone.

Fine Needle Aspiration (FNA) and Forceps Biopsy: Howell and associates reported a 61% sensitivity (16 of 26 patients) for endoscopic FNA of malignant biliary strictures. Kubota found a sensitivity of 81% for transpapillary stricture biopsy in 43 patients with pancreatic and biliary malignancy (Fig. 35–23). Kubota and Nimura have reported high diagnostic yields (>85%) for cholangiocarcinoma using forceps biopsy by the percutaneous route. Percutaneous FNA under radiologic guidance has very variable results but an acceptably low complication rate. Schechter and associates have described a percutaneous biliary "shave" technique using an atherectomy catheter through an existing biliary drainage tract; their sensitivity was 70% (15 of 19 patients). Sherman and coworkers performed "triple sampling" on 127 patients with the Geenen cytology brush, the Howell aspiration needle (two thrusts), and endobiliary forceps biopsy (3 to 4 bites). Overall, sensitivity was 71% with all three techniques; the authors recommend routinely using two of these sampling methods.

Molecular Markers for Biliary Malignancy: "Ploidy" refers to the DNA content of cells. The association between aneuploidy and malignant transformation makes evaluation of the ploidy status of biopsy samples potentially useful. Two techniques that can evaluate DNA content of cells are flow cytometry and absorptive cytometry; the latter requires a much smaller tissue sample and appears to be superior for diagnosing malignancy. Because of variable results from clinical studies, flow cytometry has yet to gain widespread acceptance as a tool for investigating biliary malignancy. Patients with aneuploidy appear to have a shortened survival when compared with those with diploid DNA content. Mutations in the k-*ras*-oncogene have been reported in 75% to 100% of pancreatic cancers. Tada and associates noted a high incidence of *ras* gene mutation in bile duct cancers. The mutation occurs at the codon 12 position. The role of

this mutation in the genesis of cholangiocarcinoma is unclear. Other mutations that have been described in pancreatic and biliary cancers include the p53 mutation and loss of integrity of chromosomes 5 and 17. The future role of studies of gene mutations is uncertain; more data are needed.

Staging of Bile Duct Tumors

The tumor, node, and metastasis (TNM) classification is being used increasingly to categorize cholangiocarcinoma into four stages: Stage I is limited to the mucosa; stage II has periductal invasion but without nodal disease or metastases; stage III has regional lymph node involvement; and stage IV involves adjacent structures or distant metastases. Malignancies of the bile duct are also classified according to their location. Upper one third tumors involve the common hepatic duct and confluence; middle one third tumors involve the common bile duct between the cystic duct and the upper border of the duodenum; and lower one third tumors arise from the common bile duct between the upper border of the duodenum to the papilla of Vater. The management of bile duct tumors depends greatly on their site of origin and pathology. Tumors involving the middle and upper thirds of the biliary tree are often nodular, whereas lower third tumors tend to be more papillary. For endoscopists, the Bismuth classification of hilar tumors is useful (Fig. 35–24): Type I tumors are located within the common hepatic duct; type II tumors involve the right and left main intrahepatic ducts; and type III tumors involve the secondary intrahepatic ducts (IIIA for the right ones, IIIB for the left ones). A more advanced stage, in which both the right and left sec-

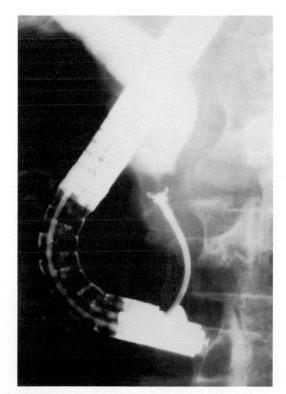

Figure 35–23
Malleable forceps being used at endoscopic retrograde cholangiopancreatography to biopsy a low bile duct tumor.

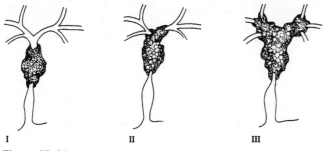

Figure 35–24
Bismuth classification of hilar bile duct tumors. (From Baillie J: Gastrointestinal Endoscopy: Beyond The Basics. Boston, MA: Butterworth-Heinemann, 1997.)

ondary bile ducts are involved, may be called stage IV. The following findings on imaging studies commonly indicate lack of resectability: (1) bilateral intrahepatic bile duct spread or multifocal disease; (2) involvement of the main trunk of the portal vein; (3) involvement of both branches of the portal vein or bilateral involvement of the hepatic artery and portal vein; and (4) vascular involvement on one side of the liver with extensive bile duct involvement on the other.

Biliary Stenting

Endoscopic stenting is now a well-established form of palliative treatment for malignant biliary obstruction (Fig. 35–25A, B). Hilar strictures are much more difficult to bridge than more distal strictures, which result in a higher rate of postprocedure cholangitis. Two prospective, randomized trials have compared plastic and metal endoprostheses for distal biliary obstruction by tumors. Overall survival was the same; however, the median time to stent occlusion was longer for metal stents (33% after 273 days) than for plastic ones (54% after 123 days). A second study showed occlusion rates of 22% for metal stents and 43% for plastic stents-

(during the lifetime of the patients). Patients stented for hilar obstruction suffer from recurrent jaundice and cholangitis more frequently than do those with other sites of obstruction. An advantage of the percutaneous approach in hilar malignancy is the ability to place two stents simultaneously through the right and left biliary systems. This can be done endoscopically but is a technical tour de force. Bilateral placement of metal mesh stents has become popular for hilar tumors. These stents have a tendency to occlude due to tumor ingrowth and fibrogranulomatous reaction (Fig. 35–26). The choice of palliation used for patients with unresectable cholangiocarcinoma depends on the overall condition of the patient and the predicted survival time. The 30-day mortality for endoscopic or percutaneous stenting is 14% to 25% with a mean survival of 3 to 6 months. Comparison of surgical and endoscopic palliation of distal common bile duct strictures reveals comparable survival and quality of life.

AMPULLARY (PAPILLARY) TUMORS

Malignant tumors of the duodenal papilla have more favorable resectability rates and prognosis than do pancreatic cancers. When treated by standard pancreaticoduodenectomy (Whipple procedure), the 5-year survival is approximately 35%. Local resection offers useful palliation but poorer long-term outlook. High-risk patients or those with unresectable lesions can be palliated by surgical bypass of the bile duct or duodenum or by endoscopic stenting. Ampullary tumors tend to be seen in patients older than 50 years of age; there is an association with familial adenomatous polyposis and Gardner's syndrome. Ampullary tumors usually present with jaundice, which may fluctuate. This is more common than weight loss, which in turn is more common than anemia.

EUS has a useful role in the diagnosis and staging of ampullary tumors. Endoscopic biopsies of an ampullary carcinoma are diagnostic in 45% to 85% of cases. The yield can be increased by taking biopsies after biliary sphincterotomy.

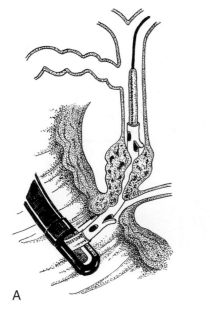
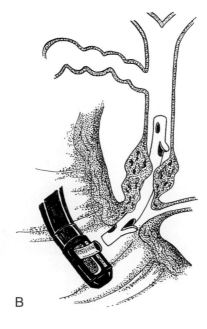

Figure 35–25
Endoscopic stenting of a biliary tumor. *A,* Using a triple-layer system (guidewire, inner catheter and stent), a No. 10 French gauge polyethylene ("Amsterdam") stent is positioned across a low bile duct stricture. *B,* After the inner catheter and guidewire are removed, the stent is left in position across the stricture with the distal end draining into the descending duodenum. (From Baillie J: Gastrointestinal Endoscopy: Beyond the Basics. Boston, MA: Butterworth-Heinemann, 1997.)

A   B

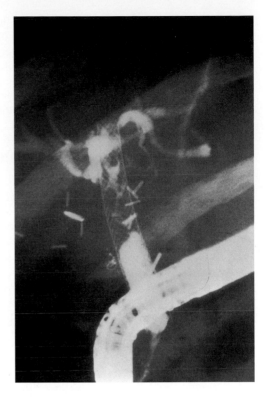

Figure 35–26
Occlusion of a metal mesh biliary stent by tumor ingrowth. This metal mesh stent (Wallstent™, Schneider, Minneapolis, MN) was placed across a common hepatic duct stricture due to cholangiocarcinoma. Within 3 months, the patient returned jaundiced, and ERCP reveals that the stent has occluded due to ingrowth of tumor through the interstices of the mesh.

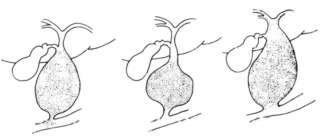

A   TYPE IA   TYPE IB   TYPE IC

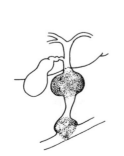

B   TYPE II   TYPE III

Figure 35–27
Todani classification of congenital biliary cysts. *A,* Type IA: Localized extrahepatic; type IB: Sequential dilatation; and type IC: Diffuse or cylindrical dilatation. *B,* Type II: Extrahepatic diverticulum, type III: Choledochocele. *C,* Type IVa: Multiple intrahepatic and extrahepatic cysts; Type IVb: Multiple extrahepatic cysts only. *D,* Type V: Solitary intrahepatic cyst.

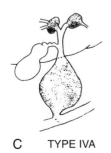

C   TYPE IVA   TYPE IVB

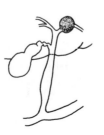

D   TYPE V

Some benign ampullary tumors are amenable to endoscopic snare excision. Early studies of endoscopic palliation of ampullary tumors favored papillotomy; however, endoscopic stenting without prior papillotomy affords relief from biliary obstruction in more than 90% of cases. Ampullary masses are not always tumors: Choledochoceles and duodenal duplication cysts are examples of ampullary pseudotumors.

MISCELLANEOUS: CONGENITAL BILE DUCT CYSTS AND CAROLI'S DISEASE

ERCP endoscopists may encounter congenital cystic dilatations of the biliary tree called choledochal cysts. The Todani classification is the most commonly employed (Fig. 35–27). Type III choledochal cysts, or choledochoceles, are dilatations of the common bile duct with the muscular portion of the duodenal wall. These may bulge into the lumen of the duodenum as a round, smooth defect associated with the ampulla of Vater. Choledochal cysts are frequently associated with anomalous pancreaticobiliary ductal union and an increased risk of bile duct malignancy. They occur in 1:100,000 to 1:150,000 live births and are most common in Asian populations. Most present before adulthood; the so-called classical triad of signs and symptoms is abdominal pain, jaundice, and a palpable abdominal mass. Choledochoceles are particularly likely to cause recurrent pancreatitis. The differential diagnosis of a choledochal cyst includes a duodenal duplication cyst, mesenteric cyst, pancreatic pseudocyst, gallbladder mucocele, and so forth. Cross-sectional imaging, such as ultrasound and CT scanning, is helpful in making a diagnosis, as are radionuclide scans (e.g., HIDA) and, of course, cholangiography (ERCP and PTC). The incidence of carcinoma in choledochal cysts is 3% to 20%. The risk increases with age. The outlook when cancer arises in a choledochal cyst is grim, with a 5% 2-year survival.

Caroli's disease is a congenital polycystic segmental dilatation of the biliary tree that is confined to the intrahepatic ducts in the absence of cirrhosis or portal hypertension. Most cases occur in association with congenital hepatic fibrosis, which is a familial disorder with autosomal recessive inheritance. Caroli's disease may be a premalignant condition.

SUGGESTED READINGS

Adam A, Benjamin IS: The staging of cholangiocarcinoma. Clin Radiol 46:299–303, 1992.

Aliperti G: Complications related to diagnostic and therapeutic endoscopic retrograde cholangiopancreatography. Gastrointest Endosc Clin North Am 6:379–407, 1996.

Allen MJ, Bovody TJ, Bugliosi TF, et al: Cholelitholysis using methyl tertiary butyl ether. Gastroenterology 88:122–125, 1985.

Almoguera C, Shibata D, Forrester K, et al: Most human carcinomas of the exocrine pancreas contain mutant c-k-ras genes. Cell 53:549–554, 1988.

Alveyn CG: Antimicrobial prophylaxis during biliary endoscopic procedures. J Antimicrob Chemother 31 Suppl B:101–105, 1993.

Andersen JR, Sorenson SM, Kruse A, et al: Randomized trial of endoscopic endoprosthesis versus operative bypass in malignant obstructive jaundice. Gut 30:1132–1135, 1989.

Ashburn HJ, Rossi RL, Munson JL: Local resection of ampullary tumors: Is there a place for it? Arch Surg 128:515–520, 1993.

Baillie J: Complications of endoscopy. Endoscopy 26:185–203, 1994.

Baillie J: Treatment of acute biliary pancreatitis (Editorial). N Engl J Med 336:286–287, 1907.

Bergman JJGHM, Rauws EAJ, Tijssen JGP, et al: Biliary endoprostheses in elderly patients with endoscopically irretrievable common bile duct stones: Report on 117 patients. Gastrointest Endosc 42:195–201, 1995.

Bergman JJGHM, Van der Mey S, Rauws EAJ, et al: Long-term follow-up after endoscopic sphincterotomy for bile duct stones in patients younger than 60 years of age. Gastrointest Endosc 44:643–649, 1996.

Bernstein J: What is Caroli's disease? Gastroenterology 68:417–418, 1975.

Binmoeller KF, Boaventure S, Ramsperger K, Soehendra N: Endoscopic snare excision of being adenomas of the papilla of Vater. Gastrointest Endosc 39:127–131, 1993.

Bismuth H, Corlette MB: Intrahepatic cholangioenteric anastomosis in carcinoma of the hilus of the liver. Surg Gynecol Obstet 140:170–176, 1975.

Bismuth H, Nakache R, Diamond T: Management strategies in resection for hilar cholangiocarcinoma. Ann Surg 215:31–38, 1992.

Bloustein PA: Association of carcinoma with congenital cystic conditions of the liver and bile ducts. Am J Gastroenterol 67:40–46, 1977.

Botoman VA, Kozarek RA, Nowell LA, et al: Long-term outcome after ES in patients with biliary colic and suspected sphincter of Oddi dysfunction. Gastrointest Endosc 40:165–170, 1994.

Bouregois N, Dunham F, Verhest A, et al: Endoscopic biopsies of the papilla of Vater at the time of endoscopic sphincterotomy: Difficulties in interpretation. Gastrointest Endosc 30:163–166, 1984.

Brink JA, Borello JA: MR imaging of the biliary system. Magn Reson Imaging Clin North Am 3:143–160, 1995.

Broe PJ, Cameron JL: The management of proximal biliary tract tumors. Adv Surg 15:47–62, 1981.

Broome U, Olsson R, Loof L, et al: Natural history and prognostic factors in 305 Swedish patients with primary sclerosing cholangitis. Gut 38:610–615, 1996.

Burt RW, Berenson MW, Lee RG, et al: Upper gastrointestinal polyps in Gardner's syndrome. Gastroenterology 86:295–301, 1984.

Carmona RH, Crass RA, Lim RC Jr, Trunkey DD: Oriental cholangitis. Am J Surg 148:117–124, 1984.

Cavallini G, Tittobello A, Frulloni L, et al: Gabexate for the prevention of pancreatic damage related to endoscopic retrograde cholangiopancreatography. N Engl J Med 335:919–923, 1996.

Chang L, French S, Kierro M, Lo SK: A prospective study comparing endobiliary biopsy, brush and aspiration cytology during ERCP in diagnosing biliary obstructive lesions (Abstract). Am J Gastroenterol 87:1282A, 1992.

Chaudhuri PK, Chaudhuri B, Schuler JJ, Nyhus LM: Carcinoma associated with congenital cystic dilation of the bile ducts. Arch Surg 117:1349–1351, 1982.

Chen LY, Goldberg HI. Sclerosing cholangitis: Broad spectrum of radiographic features. Gastrointest Radiol 9:39–47, 1984.

Classen M, Demling L: Endoskopische Sphinkterotomie der Papilla Vateri und Steinextraktion aus dem Ductus choledochus. Dtsch Med Wochenschr 99:496–497, 1974.

Collen MJ, Hanan MR, Maher JA, Stubrin SE: Modification of endoscopic retrograde cholangiopancreatography (ERCP) septic complications by the addition of an antibiotic to the contrast media: Randomized controlled investigation. Am J Gastroenterol 74:493–496, 1980.

Cotton PB: Endoscopic methods for the relief of malignant obstructive jaundice. World J Surg 8:854–861, 1989.

Cotton PB: Management of malignant bile duct obstruction. J Gastroenterol Hepatol 1:63–77, 1990.

Cotton PB: Pre-cut papillotomy—a risky technique for experts only (Editorial). Gastrointest Endosc 35:578–579, 1989.

Cotton PB, Forbes A, Leung JWC, Dineen L: Endoscopic stenting for long-term treatment of large bile duct stones: 2- to 5-year follow-up. Gastrointest Endosc 33:411–412, 1987.

Cotton PB, Kozarek RA, Schapiro RH, et al: Endoscopic laser lithotripsy of large bile duct stones. Gastroenterology 99:1128–1133, 1990.

Cotton PB, Lehman G, Vennes J, et al: Endoscopic sphincterotomy complications and their management: An attempt at consensus. Gastrointest Endosc 37:383–393, 1991.

Dancygier H, Classen M: Preoperative staging of a distal common bile duct tumor by endoscopic ultrasound. Gastrointest Endosc 95:219–222, 1988.

Davids PHP, Groen AK, Rauws EAJ, et al: Randomized trial of self-expanding metal stents vs polyethylene stents for distal malignant biliary obstruction. Lancet 430:1488–1492, 1992.

Davids PHP, Rauws EAJ, Coene PPLO, et al: Endoscopic stenting for post-operative biliary strictures. Gastrointest Endosc 38:12–18, 1992.

Dayton MT, Longmire WP, Tompkins RK: Caroli's disease: A premalignant condition? Am J Surg 145:41–48, 1983.

Dias LM, Silva R, Viana HL, et al: Biliary fascioliasis: Diagnosis, treatment and follow-up by ERCP. Gastrointest Endosc 43:616–620, 1996.

Diehl AK: Epidemiology and natural history of gallstone disease. Gastroenterol Clin North Am 20:1–19, 1991.

Dimagno EP, Regan PT, Clain JE, et al: Human endoscopic ultrasonography. Gastroenterology 83:824–829, 1982.

Ding SF, Delhanty JDA, Bowles L, et al: Loss of constitutional heterozygosity on chromosomes 5 and 17 in cholangiocarcinoma. Br J Cancer 67:1007–1010, 1993.

Fan S-T, Lai ECS, Mok FPT, et al: Early treatment of acute biliary pancreatitis by endoscopic papillotomy. N Engl J Med 328:228–232, 1993.

Fan ZM, Yamashida Y, Harada M, et al: Intrahepatic cholangiocarcinoma: Spin-echo and contrast-enhanced dynamic MR imaging. AJR Am J Roentgenol 161:313–317, 1993.

Farley DR, Weaver MS, Nagorney DM: "Natural history" of unresected cholangiocarcinoma: Patient outcome after noncurative intervention. Mayo Clin Proc 70:425–429, 1995.

Farouk M, Niotis M, Branum GD, et al: Indications for and the technique of local resection of tumors of the papilla of Vater. Arch Surg 126:650–652, 1991.

Flanigan DP: Biliary carcinoma associated with biliary cysts. Cancer 40:880–883, 1977.

Foutch PG: Diagnosis of cancer by cytologic methods performed during ERCP. Gastrointest Endosc 40:249–252, 1994.

Foutch PG, Harlan J, Sanowski RA: Endoscopic placement of biliary stents for treatment of high risk geriatric patients with common duct stones. Am J Gastroenterol 84:527–529, 1989.

Freeman ML, Nelson DB, Sherman S, et al: Complications of endoscopic biliary sphincterotomy. N Engl J Med 335:909–918, 1996.

Funch-Jensen P, Kruse A, Rauensback J: Endoscopic sphincter of Oddi manometry in healthy volunteers. Scand J Gastroenterol 87:759–762, 1987.

Geenen JE, Hogan WJ, Dodds WJ, et al: The efficacy of endoscopic sphincterotomy after cholecystectomy in patients with sphincter of Oddi dysfunction. N Engl J Med 320:82–87, 1989.

Gibson RN, Young E, Hadjis N, et al: Percutaneous transhepatic endoprostheses for hilar cholangiocarcinoma. Am J Surg 156:363–367, 1988.

Gilbert DA, DiMarino AJ Jr, Jensen DM, et al: Status evaluation: Biliary stents. American Society for Gastrointestinal Endoscopy: Technology Assessment Committee. Gastrointest Endosc 38:750–752, 1992.

Gress F, Chen YK, Sherman S, et al: Experience with a catheter-based ultrasound probe in the bile duct and pancreas. Endoscopy 27:178–184, 1995.

Hausegger KA, Kleinert R, Lammer J, et al: Malignant biliary obstruction: Histologic findings after treatment with self-expandable stents. Radiology 185:461–464, 1992.

Hayes DH, Bolton JS, Willis GW, et al: Carcinoma of the ampulla of Vater. Ann Surg 206:572–577, 1987.

Hintze RE, Adler A, Veltzke W: Outcome of mechanical lithotripsy of bile duct stones in an unselected series of 704 patients. Hepatogastroenterology 43:473–476, 1996.

Hixson LJ, Fennerty MB, Jaffee PE, et al: Peroral cholangioscopy with intracorporeal electrohydraulic lithotripsy for choledocholithiasis. Am J Gastroenterol 87:296–299, 1992.

Hogan WJ: Position paper: Sphincter of Oddi manometry. Gastrointest Endosc 45:342–348, 1997.

Hogan WJ, Geenen JE: Biliary dyskinesia. Endoscopy 1:179–183, 1988.

Howell DA, Beveridge RP, Bosco JJ, Jones M: Endoscopic needle aspiration biopsy at ERCP in the diagnosis of biliary strictures. Gastrointest Endosc 38:531–535, 1992.

Hurwitz M, Sawicki M, Samara G, Passaro E: Diagnostic and prognostic molecular markers in cancer. Am J Surg 164:299–306, 1992.

Ishizaki Y, Wakayama T, Okada Y, Kobayashi T: Magnetic resonance cholangiography for evaluation of obstructive jaundice. Am J Gastroenterol 88:2072–2077, 1993.

Jarvinen H, Nyberg M, Peltokallio P: Upper gastrointestinal tract polyps in familial adenomatosis coli. Gut 24:333–339, 1983.

Johansen K, Paun M: Duplex ultrasonography of the portal vein. Surg Clin North Am 70:181–190, 1990.

Johanson JF, Geenen JE, Hogan WJ, et al: Endoscopic therapy of a duodenal duplication cyst. Gastrointest Endosc 38:60–64, 1992.

Johnson GK, Geenen JE, Bedford RA, et al: A comparison of nonionic versus ionic contrast media: Results of a prospective, multicenter study. Midwest Pancreaticobiliary Study Group. Gastrointest Endosc 42:312–316, 1995.

Johnson SK, Geenen JE, Venu RP, et al: Treatment of non-extractable common bile duct stones with combination ursodeoxycholic acid plus endoprosthesis. Gastrointest Endosc 39:528–531, 1993.

Jordon D, Harpaz N, Thung SN: Caroli's disease and adult polycystic kidney disease: A rarely recognized association. Lancet 9:30–35, 1989.

Jowell PS, Baillie J, Branch MS, et al: Quantitative assessment of procedural competence: A prospective study of training in retrograde cholangiopancreatography. Ann Intern Med 125:983–989, 1996.

Kagawa Y, Kashihara S, Kuramoto S, Maetani S: Carcinoma arising in a congenitally dilated biliary tract: Report of a case and review of the literature. Gastroenterology 74:1286–1294, 1978.

Kato T, Fukatsu H, Ito K, et al: Fluorodeoxyglucose position emission tomography in pancreatic cancer: An unsolved problem. Eur J Nucl Med 22:32–39, 1995.

Kawai K, Akasaka Y, Murakami K, et al: Endoscopic sphincterotomy of the ampulla of Vater. Gastrointest Endosc 20:148–151, 1974.

Kelly TR, Wagoner DS: Gallstone pancreatitis: A prospective randomized trial of the timing of surgery. Surgery 104:600–605, 1988.

Kersting-Sommerhoff B, Helmberger H, Bautz W: Radiologic diagnosis and staging of gallbladder and bile duct tumors. Endoscopy 25:86–91, 1993.

Knyrim K, Wagner HJ, Pausch J, et al: A prospective, randomized, controlled trial of metal stents for malignant obstruction of the common bile duct. Endoscopy 25:207–212, 1993.

Kozarek RA: Laparoscopic cholecystectomy: What to do with the common duct (Editorial). Gastrointest Endosc 39:99–101, 1993.

Kozarek RA, Ball TJ, Patterson DJ, et al: Endoscopic treatment of biliary injury in the era of laparoscopic cholecystectomy. Gastrointest Endosc 40:10–16, 1994.

Kubota Y, Seki T, Yamaguchi T, et al: Bilateral internal drainage of biliary hilar malignancy via a single percutaneous track: Role of percutaneous transhepatic cholangioscopy. Endoscopy 24:194–198, 1992.

Kubota Y, Takaoka M, Tani K, et al: Endoscopic transpapillary biopsy for diagnosis of patients with pancreaticobiliary ductal strictures. Am J Gastroenterol 88:1700–1704, 1993.

Kurzawinski T, Deery A, Davidson BR: Diagnostic value of cytology for biliary stricture. Br J Surg 80:414–421, 1993.

Lai ECS, Tompkins RK, Roslyn JJ, Mann LL: Proximal bile duct cancer. Ann Surg 205:111–118, 1987.

Lee JG, Layfield L, Kerns BJ, et al: What you see is not what you get: The utility of image analysis in exfoliated bile duct cells for diagnosis of cancer (Abstract). Gastrointest Endosc 40:403, 1994.

Lee JG, Leung JW, Baillie J, et al: Benign, dysplastic or malignant—making sense of endoscopic bile duct brush cytology: Results in 149 consecutive patients. Am J Gastroenterol 90:722–726, 1995.

Lee JG, Schutz SM, England RE, et al: Endoscopic therapy of sclerosing cholangitis. Hepatology 21:661–667, 1995.

Lee SP, Kuver R: Gallstones. In Yamada T (ed): Textbook of Gastroenterology, 2nd ed. Philadelphia, JB Lippincott, 1995, pp 2187–2212.

Lee Y-M, Kaplan MM: Primary sclerosing cholangitis. N Engl J Med 332:924–933, 1995.

Leese T, Neoptolemos JP, Carr-Locke DL: Successes, failures, early complications and their management following endoscopic sphincterotomy: Results in 394 consecutive patients from a single center. Br J Surg 72:215–219, 1985.

Leung JWC, Chung SSC: Electrohydraulic lithotripsy with peroral choledochoscopy. BMJ 299:595–598, 1989.

Leung JWC, Sung JY, Chung SC, Metreweli C: Hepatic clonorchiasis—a study by endoscopic retrograde cholangiopancreatography. Gastrointest Endosc 35:226–231, 1989.

Looser C, Stain SC, Baer HU, et al: Staging of hilar cholangiocarcinoma by ultrasound and duplex sonography: A comparison of angiography and operative findings. Br J Radiol 65:871–877, 1992.

Lund J: Surgical indication in cholelithiasis: Prophylactic cholecystectomy elucidated on the basis of long-term follow-up on 526 non-operated cases. Ann Surg 151:153–162, 1960.

MacMathuna P, Siegenberg D, Gibbons D, et al: The acute and long-term effect of balloon sphincteroplasty on papillary structure: An animal study. Gastrointest Endosc 44:650–655, 1996.

MacMathuna P, White P, Clarke E, et al: Endoscopic sphincteroplasty: A novel and safe alternative to papillotomy in the management of bile duct stones. Gut 35:127–129, 1994.

Margulis SJ, Honig CL, Soave R, et al: Biliary tract obstruction in the acquired immunodeficiency syndrome. Ann Intern Med 105:207–210, 1986.

May GR, Cotton PB, Edmunds SE, Chong W: Removal of stones from the bile duct at ERCP without sphincterotomy. Gastrointest Endosc 39:749–754, 1993.

McGuire DE, Venu RP, Brown RD, et al: Brush cytology for pancreatic carcinoma: An analysis of factors influencing results. Gastrointest Endosc 44:300–304, 1996.

McLean GK, Burke DR: Role of endoprostheses in the management of malignant biliary obstruction. Radiology 170:961–967, 1989.

Mehal WZ, Culshaw KD, Tillotson GS, Chapman RW: Antibiotic prophylaxis for ERCP: A randomized clinical trial comparing ciprofloxacin and cefuroxime in 200 patients at high risk of cholangitis. Eur J Gastroenterol Hepatol 7:841–845, 1995.

Mergener K, Freed K, Keogan M, et al: ERCP after Roux-en-Y gastrojejunostomy rarely succeeds: Could MRCP be the answer? Gastrointest Endosc 45:abstract 140, 1997.

Michelassi F, Erroi F, Dawson PJ, et al: Experience with 647 consecutive tumors of the duodenum, ampulla, head of pancreas and distal common bile duct. Ann Surg 210:544–556, 1989.

Mohandas KM, Swaroop VS, Gullar SU, et al: Diagnosis of malignant obstructive jaundice by bile cytology: Results improved by dilating the bile duct strictures. Gastrointest Endosc 40:150–154, 1994.

Monson JRT, Donohue JH, McEntee GP, et al: Radical resection for carcinoma of the ampulla of Vater. Arch Surg 126:353–357, 1991.

Moody FG: Lithotripsy in the treatment of biliary stones. Am J Surg 165:479–482, 1993.

Mukai H, Nakajima M, Yasuda K, et al: Evaluation of endoscopic ultrasonography in the pre-operative staging of carcinoma of the ampulla of Vater and common bile duct. Gastrointest Endosc 38:676–683, 1992.

Mundorf J, Jowell PS, Branch MS, et al: Reduced incidence of post-ERCP pancreatitis in non-pancreas divisum patients who receive intravenous secretin during ERCP. Am J Gastroenterol 90:1611A, 1995.

Neoptolemos JP, Carr-Locke DL, London NJ, et al: Controlled trial of urgent endoscopic retrograde cholangiopancreatography and endoscopic sphincterotomy versus conservative treatment for acute pancreatitis due to gallstones. Lancet 2:979–983, 1988.

Neoptolemos JP, Hall C, O'Connor HJ, et al: Methyl-*tert*-butyl-ether for treating bile duct stones: The British experience. Br J Surg 77:32–35, 1990.

Neoptolemos JP, Talbot IC, Carr-Locke DL, et al: Treatment and outcome in 52 consecutive cases of ampullary carcinoma. Br J Surg 74:957–961, 1987.

Neuhaus H, Hoffmann W, Gottlieb K, Classen M: Endoscopic lithotripsy of bile duct stones using a new laser with automatic stone recognition. Gastrointest Endosc 40:708–715, 1994.

Nichols JC, Gores GJ, LaRusso NF, et al: Diagnostic role of serum CA 19-9 for cholangiocarcinoma in patients with primary sclerosing cholangitis. Mayo Clin Proc 68:874–879, 1993.

Nimura Y, Shionoya S, Hayakawa N, et al: Value of percutaneous transhepatic cholangioscopy. Surg Endosc 2:213–219, 1988.

Orenstein SR, Whittington PF: Choledochal cyst resulting in congenital cirrhosis. Am J Dis Child 136:1025–1027, 1982.

Osnes M, Rosseland AR, Aabakken L: Endoscopic retrograde cholangiography and endoscopic papillotomy in patients with a previous Billroth II resection. Gut 27:1193–1198, 1986.

Ostroff JW, Shapiro HA: Complications of endoscopic sphincterotomy. In Jacobsen IM (ed): ERCP: Diagnostic and Therapeutic Applications. New York: Elsevier Science, 1989, pp 61–73.

Ostrow JD: The etiology of pigmented gallstones. Hepatology 4:215s–222s, 1984.

Palmer KR, Hofmann AF: Intraductal monooctanoin for the direct dissolution of bile duct stones: Experience in 343 patients. Gut 27:196–202, 1986.

Pasricha PJ, Miskovsky EP, Kalloo AN: Intrasphincteric injection of botulinum toxin for suspected sphincter of Oddi dysfunction. Gut 35:1319–1321, 1994.

Pauletzki JG, Sharkey KA, Davison JS, et al: Involvement of L-arginine-nitric oxide pathways in neural relaxation of the sphincter of Oddi. Eur J Pharmacol 232:263–270, 1993.

Phinney PR, Austin GE, Kadell BM: Cholangiocarcinoma arising in Caroli's disease. Arch Pathol Lab Med 105:194–197, 1981.

Pitt HA, Thompson HH, Tompkins RK, Longmire WP: Primary sclerosing cholangitis: Results of an aggressive surgical approach. Ann Surg 196:259–268, 1982.

Polydorou AA, Cairns SR, Dowsett JF, et al: Palliation of proximal malignant biliary obstruction by endoscopic endoprosthesis insertion. Gut 32:685–689, 1991.

Prat F, Tennenbaum R, Ponsot P, et al: Endoscopic sphincterotomy in patients with liver cirrhosis. Gastrointest Endosc 43(2 pt 1):127–131, 1996.

Rabinovitz M, Zajko AR, Hassenein T, et al: Diagnostic value of brush cytology in the diagnosis of bile duct carcinoma: A study of 65 patients with bile duct strictures. Hepatology 12:747–752, 1990.

Ranzi T, Castagnone D, Velio P, et al: Gastric and duodenal polyps in familial polyposis coli. Gut 22:363–367, 1981.

Rosen CB, Nagarney RM: Cholangiocarcinoma complicating sclerosing cholangitis. Semin Liver Dis 11:26–30, 1991.

Rossi RL, Silverman ML, Braasch JW, et al: Carcinomas arising in cystic conditions of the bile ducts: A clinical and pathological study. Ann Surg 205:377–384, 1987.

Rustgi AK, Schapiro RH: Biliary stents for common bile duct stones. Gastrointest Endosc Clin North Am 1:79–91, 1991.

Ryan ME: Cytologic brushing of ductal lesions during ERCP. Gastrointest Endosc 37:139–142, 1991.

Ryan ME, Baldarf MC: Comparison of flow cytometry for DNA content and brush cytology for detection of malignancy in pancreaticobiliary strictures. Gastrointest Endosc 40:133–139, 1994.

Santucci L, Natalini G, Sarpi L, et al: Selective ERCP and pre-operative bile duct stone removal in patients scheduled for laparoscopic cholecystectomy: A prospective study. Am J Gastroenterol 91:1326–1330, 1996.

Sarris GE, Tsang D: Choledochocele: Case report, literature review and a proposed classification. Surgery 105:408–414, 1989.

Sauerbruch T, Stern M: Fragmentation of bile duct stones by extracorporeal shock waves: A new approach to biliary calculi after failure of routine endoscopic measures. Gastroenterology 96:146–152, 1989.

Schechter MS, Doemeny JM, Johnson JQ: Biliary ductal shave biopsy with use of the Simpson atherectomy catheter. J Vasc Interv Radiol 4:819–824, 1993.

Schneiderman D, Cello J, Laing F: Papillary stenosis and sclerosing cholangitis in the acquired immunodeficiency syndrome. Ann Intern Med 106:546–549, 1987.

Shaw MJ, Mackie RD, Moore JP, et al: Results of a multicenter trial using a mechanical lithotripter for the treatment of large bile duct stones. Am J Gastroenterol 88:730–733, 1993.

Sheng R, Sammon JK, Zajko AB, Campbell WC: Bile leak after hepatic transplantation: Cholangiographic features, prevalence and clinical outcome. Radiology 192:413–416, 1994.

Shepherd HA, Royle G, Ross APR, et al: Endoscopic biliary endoprostheses in the palliation of malignant obstruction of the distal common bile duct: A randomized trial. Br J Surg 75:1166–1168, 1988.

Sherman S, Esher EJ, Pezzi JS, et al: Yield of ERCP tissue sampling of biliary strictures by brush, forceps and needle aspiration methods (Abstract). Gastrointest Endosc 41:478, 1995.

Sherman S, Lehman G, Silverman W: Efficacy of endoscopic sphincterotomy and surgical sphincteroplasty for patients with sphincter of Oddi dysfunction. Gastrointest Endosc 37:71A, 1991.

Siegel JH, Ben-Zvi JS, Pullano WE: Mechanical lithotripsy of common duct stones. Gastrointest Endosc 36:351–356, 1990.

Siegenberg D, MacMathuna P, Soto JA, et al: The accuracy of magnetic resonance cholangiopancreatography (MRCP) approaches that for biliary tract imaging (Abstract). Gastrointest Endosc 41:313, 1995.

Sivak MV: Endoscopic management of bile duct stones. Am J Surg 158:228–238, 1989.

Sons HU, Bochard F: Carcinoma of the extrahepatic bile ducts: A postmortem case study of 65 cases and review of the literature. J Surg Oncol 34:6–12, 1987.

Staritz M, Poralla T, Dormeyer HH, Meyer zum Bueschenfelde KH: Endoscopic removal of common bile duct stones through the intact papilla after medical sphincter dilation. Gastroenterology 88:1807–1811, 1995.

Stoker J, Lameris JS, van Blamkenstein M: Percutaneous metallic self-expandable endoprostheses in malignant hilar biliary obstruction. Gastrointest Endosc 39:43–49, 1993.

Tada M, Omata M, Ohto M: High incidence of ras gene mutation in intrahepatic cholangiocarcinoma. Cancer 69:1115–1118, 1992.

Takayasu K. Ikeya S, Mukai K, et al: CT of hilar cholangiocarcinoma: Late contrast enhancement in 6 patients. AJR Am J Roentgenol 154:1203–1206, 1990.

Tani K, Kubota Y, Yamaguchi T, et al: MR imaging of peripheral cholangiocarcinoma. J Comput Assist Tomogr 15:975–978, 1991.

Tarnasky PR, England RE, Lail LM, et al: Cystic duct patency in malignant obstructive jaundice: An ERCP-based study relevant to the role of laparoscopic cholecystenterostomy. Ann Surg 221:265–271, 1995.

Tarnasky PR, Cunningham JT, Hawes RH, et al: Pitfalls of bile duct stone removal after balloon sphincter dilation. Am J Gastroenterol 91:822, 1996.

Terada T, Shimuzu K, Izumi R, Nakanuma Y: P-53 expression in formalin-fixed, paraffin embedded archival specimens of intrahepatic cholangiocarcinoma: Retrieval of p53 antigenicity by microwave oven heating of tissue sections. Mod Pathol 7:249–252, 1994.

Tio TL, Cheng J, Wijers OB, et al: Endoscopic TNM staging of extrahepatic bile duct cancer. Comparison with pathological staging. Gastroenterology 100:1351–1361, 1991.

Tio TL, Tytgat GN: Endoscopic ultrasonography of bile duct malignancy and the progressive assessment of local resectability. Scand J Gastroenterol 21:151–157, 1986.

Todani T, Watanabe Y, Narusue M, et al: Congenital bile duct cysts: Classification, operative procedures, and review of thirty seven cases including cancer arising from choledochal cyst. Am J Surg 134:263–269, 1977.

Tritapepe R, Di Padova C, Pazzoli M, et al: The treatment of retained biliary stones with monooctanoin: Report of 16 patients. Am J Gastroenterol 79:710–717, 1984.

Turner WW, Cramer CR: Recurrent oriental cholangiohepatitis. Surgery 93:397–401, 1983.

Vallera RA, Baillie J: Complications of endoscopy. Endoscopy 28:187–204, 1996.

Van Laethem J-L, Vertongen P, Deviere J, et al: Detection of c-K-ras gene codon mutations from pancreatic duct brushings in the diagnosis of pancreatic tumors. Gut 36:781–787, 1995.

Vauthey JN, Blumgart LH: Recent advances in the management of cholangiocarcinomas. Semin Liver Dis 14:109–114, 1994.

Wagner HJ, Knyrim K, Vakil N, et al: Plastic endoprostheses versus metal stents in the palliative treatment of malignant hilar biliary obstruction: A prospective and randomized trial. Endoscopy 25:213–218, 1993.

Waxman I: Characteristics of a malignant bile duct obstruction by intraductal ultrasonography. Am J Gastroenterol 90:1073–1075, 1995.

Wiersma MJ, Lehman GA, Sherman S, et al: Endoscopic brush cytology, fine needle aspiration and forceps biopsy in the evaluation of malignant biliary strictures. Gastrointest Endosc 39:336A, 1993.

Williams JA, Cubilla A, McLean BJ, Fortner JG: Twenty two year experience with periampullary carcinoma at Memorial Sloan Kettering Cancer Center. Am J Surg 138:662–665, 1979.

Williamson BW, Blumgart LH, McKellar NJ: Management of tumors of the liver: Combined use of arteriography and venography in the assessment of resectability especially in hilar tumors. Am J Surg 139:210–215, 1980.

Yamaguchi K, Enjoji M: Adenoma of the ampulla of Vater: Putative precancerous lesion. Gut 32:1558–1561, 1991.

Yamaguchi K, Enjoji M, Kitamura K: Endoscopic biopsy has limited accuracy in the diagnosis of ampullary tumors. Gastrointest Endosc 36:588–592, 1990.

Yamagushi M: Congenital choledochal cyst: Analysis of 1,433 patients in the Japanese literature. Am J Surg 140:653–657, 1980.

Yamashita Y, Takahashi M, Kanazawa S, et al: Parenchymal changes of the liver in cholangiocarcinoma: CT evaluation. Gastrointest Radiol 17:161–166, 1992.

Index